CLINICAL COMPETENCIES

Skills from Beginning through Advanced

LORRAINE FLEMING-McPHILLIPS, MS, MT, CMA (AAMA)

Quinebaug Valley Community College (retired)

Danielson, CT

Pearson

Boston   Columbus   Indianapolis   New York   San Francisco   Upper Saddle River   Amsterdam   Cape Town   Dubai
London   Madrid   Milan   Munich   Paris   Montreal   Toronto   Delhi   Mexico City   Sao Paulo   Sydney
Hong Kong   Seoul   Singapore   Taipei   Tokyo

Library of Congress Cataloging-in-Publication Data

Fleming-McPhillips, Lorraine.
  Clinical competencies: skills from beginning through advanced/Lorraine Fleming-McPhillips.
    p.; cm.
  Includes index.
  ISBN-13: 978-0-13-512973-9
  ISBN-10: 0-13-512973-7
  1. Medical assistants.   I. Title.
  [DNLM: 1. Allied Health Personnel.   2. Clinical Competence.   W 21.5 F598c 2011]
  R728.8.F54 2011
  610.73'7—dc22

2009053895

Publisher: Julie Levin Alexander
Publisher's Assistant: Regina Bruno
Editor-in-Chief: Mark Cohen
Executive Editor: Joan Gill
Development Editor: Bronwen Glowacki
Editorial Assistant: Mary Ellen Ruitenberg
Director of Marketing: Dave Gesell
Senior Marketing Manager: Harper Coles
Marketing Specialist: Michael Sirinides
Marketing Assistant: Judy Noh
Managing Production Editor: Patrick Walsh
Production Liaison: Julie Boddorf
Production Editor: Kelly Ricci

Manufacturing Manager: Ilene Sanford
Manufacturing Buyer: Pat Brown
Art Director: Kristine Carney
Interior Designer: Candace Rowley
Cover Designer: Candace Rowley
Director, Image Resource Center: Melinda Reo
Manager, Rights and Permissions: Zina Arabia
Manager, Visual Research: Beth Brenzel
Manager, Cover Visual Research and Permissions: Nancy Seise
Composition: Aptara®, Inc.
Full-Service Project Manager: Niraj Bhatt, Aptara®, Inc.
Printing and Binding: Courier Kendallville
Cover Printer: Lehigh-Phoenix Color

10 9 8 7 6 5 4 3 2 1

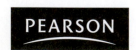

www.pearsonhighered.com

ISBN 13: 978-0-13-512973-9
ISBN 10:   0-13-512973-7

Brief Contents

CHAPTER 1
Introduction to Clinical Competencies   1

CHAPTER 2
Infection Control   8

CHAPTER 3
Vital Signs and Mensuration   20

CHAPTER 4
Assisting with Physical Examination   42

CHAPTER 5
Assisting with Medical Specialties   60

CHAPTER 6
Assisting with Pediatrics   99

CHAPTER 7
Assisting with Therapeutic Modalities and Rehabilitation   115

CHAPTER 8
Assisting with Minor Surgery   145

CHAPTER 9
Assisting with Medical Emergencies   169

CHAPTER 10
Clinical Laboratory Testing   197

CHAPTER 11
Urinalysis   209

CHAPTER 12
Microbiology   226

CHAPTER 13
Phlebotomy   236

CHAPTER 14
Hematology   256

CHAPTER 15
Serology/Immunology   275

CHAPTER 16
Blood Chemistry   287

CHAPTER 17
Diagnostic Imaging   301

CHAPTER 18
Pharmacology   309

CHAPTER 19
Intravenous Therapy   343

CHAPTER 20
Nutrition and Patient Education   365

CHAPTER 21
Cardiology and Pulmonology   379

Appendices   A-1

Glossary   G-1

Index   I-1

Dedication

I would like to dedicate this book to my husband, Norman, who made this book possible through his patience, understanding, and willingness to take over many of my household responsibilities. I also would like to mention my children, Mark, Holly, Amy, and Carrie, and my stepchildren, Norman, Eileen, and Brian, who cheered me on and offered praise and encouragement. Lastly I would like to thank Joan Gill for her confidence and faith in me and my writing abilities and Bronwen Glowacki for her help and ready responses to my many questions and requests.

LORRAINE (LORRIE) FLEMING-McPHILLIPS

Preface

During my many years teaching medical assisting students in career and college programs, I never discovered a text that had a complete compilation of all the skills needed to instruct these valuable multiskilled professionals. Moreover, health care delivery has undergone many changes, particularly in the classification of those providing care. Today we have patient care technicians, nursing assistants, medical assistants, and many others involved in health care delivery in hospitals, ambulatory care centers, offices, nursing homes, clinics, and schools. All these individuals require training and evaluation of skills.

Many texts provide basic skills or include material in ancillary competency books that are packaged with the main text. This makes rapid location of competencies difficult. I knew a stand-alone text including all the basic entry-level skills as well as advanced skills would be a valuable asset to all who participate in health care delivery today, and that is what this text accomplishes.

Clinical Competencies, 1st edition, can be utilized for a quick review of a skill not performed routinely, as a training manual for new employees, as a lab manual for students checking one another's competency performance, as an instructor's skill-evaluation text, and as a procedure manual for offices, clinics, hospitals, and ambulatory care centers.

The more than 250 competencies presented in this text are clustered into chapters as in most comprehensive texts. For example, Chapter 3: Vital Signs and Mensuration contains individual procedures for measuring oral, rectal, axillary, and aural temperatures using a variety of appropriate instruments. Each procedure offers a brief narrative explanation, a cross-reference to CAAHEP and ABHES competencies, a list of required equipment and supplies, and step-by-step explanations illustrated with clarifying black-and-white and color photos and diagrams. A performance checklist and performance evaluation sheet for each procedure are included on MyHealthProfessionsKit. The Appendices includes valuable information such as abbreviations, metric measurements, laboratory reference values, emergency procedures, lists of easily confused drug names, and abbreviations that cause errors.

The text adheres to the required skills designated by the CAAHEP Standards and Guidelines for Medical Assisting Educational Programs and the ABHES national curricula. It is my hope that all who use *Clinical Competencies,* 1st edition, will find it a valuable asset in their health care career.

LORRAINE (LORRIE) FLEMING-McPHILLIPS

Reviewers List

The invaluable editorial advice and direction provided by the following educators and health care professionals is deeply appreciated:

Sue Boulden, BSN, CMA (AAMA)
Medical Assisting Program Chair
Mount Hood Community College
Gresham, OR

Cindi Brassington, MS, CMA (AAMA)
Professor of Allied Health
Quinebaug Valley Community College
Danielson, CT

Adrienne L. Carter, MEd, RMA
Teacher
Riverside Community College
Moreno Valley, CA

Patricia Celani, CMA (AAMA)
Medical Instructor
Kaplan Career Institute
Pittsburgh, PA

Lisa Davis Drennan, RN
Instructor
Draughons Junior College
Bowling Green, KY

Donna Firn, CMA (AAMA)
Clinical Assistant
Delaware County Community College
Media, PA

Cindy L. Garman, CMA (AAMA), AASAM
Medical Program Director
Akron Institute
Akron, OH

Cheri Goretti, MA, MT (ASCP), CMA (AAMA)
Director of Medical Assisting Program
Quinebaug Valley Community College
Danielson, CT

Susan Horn, AAS, CMA (AAMA)
Medical Program Coordinator
Harrison College
Lafayette, IN

Dolly Horton, CMA (AAMA), MEd
Medical Assisting Coordinator
Mayland Community College
Spruce Pine, NC

Ann E. Kunze, BA, CMA (AAMA)
Program Director
Medical Careers Institute
Newport News, VA

Deborah H. McCloskey, MT (AMT), MT (HEW), CLS (NCA), PhD (abd)
Adjunct Professor, Laboratory Manager
Community College of Allegheny County
Pittsburgh, PA

Claudette Mitchell, MBA, LPN
MA Instructor & Research Nurse Coordinator
Bauder College & Moorehouse School of Medicine
Newnan, GA

Adrian Rios, EMT, CPT-1, RMA, NCMA, MA
Medical Assistant Program Director
Newbridge College
Santa Ana, CA

Lynn Slack, CMA (AAMA)
Medical Programs Director
Kaplan Career Institute
Pittsburgh, PA

Lavada L. Spangler, CMA (AAMA)
Instructor
ATI Career Training Center
North Richland Hills, TX

Sherry Stanfield, RN, BSN, MS
Assistant Program Director, Medical Assisting
Miller-Motte Technical College
North Charleston, SC

Donna Lee Stevenson, LPN, BA
Allied Health Department Chair
Remington College
Largo, FL

Tiffany Stewart, CPC, CCS, CMBS, AAS
Externship Evaluator
Delta Technical College
Horn Lake, MS

Deborah Sulkowski, CMA (AAMA)
Medical Department Chair
Pittsburgh Technical Institute
Oakdale, PA

Judith D. Symons
Medical Assistant Instructor
McCann School of Business
Pottsville, PA

Jacquelyn Taylor, NCRMA
MA Instructor
Sanford Brown Institute
Dallas, TX

About the Author

LORRAINE FLEMING-McPHILLIPS MS, MT (ASCP), CMA (AAMA)

Lorraine (known as Lorrie to family and friends) graduated with High Honors from the University of Connecticut with a Bachelor of Arts in Medical Technology. She earned her registration from the American Society of Clinical Pathologists upon graduation from the university and maintains that registration to present. Lorrie worked at a number of hospitals and private clinical laboratories as a general medical technologist for 11 years before beginning teaching medical assisting. She taught for 11 years specializing in medical assisting and phlebotomy education. In 1992 Lorrie continued her education and graduated in 1995 from the University of Connecticut with a Master of Science in Allied Health focusing on education and research. During her final year in the masters program she was selected as a member of Phi Kappa Phi National Honor Society.

As Lorrie was furthering her education she was chosen to establish a Medical Assisting Program at Quinebaug Valley Community College in Connecticut. During her 7 years at the college Lorrie developed the medical assisting program, which earned accreditation through the AAMA. As program chair she created other allied health programs, namely phlebotomy, health information management, coding specialist, and an Allied Health Certificate program. As Tech Prep Advisor, Lorrie established links with 7 area high schools to facilitate students' entry into allied health programs. Lorrie taught all of the core courses, clinical and administrative. She served on numerous committees and also developed a Medical Assisting Program and curricula for another college.

Lorrie has been a member of AAMA since 1992 and has maintained active certification since then. She served the organization on local and state levels in Connecticut including state president. After moving to Florida she became a member of the state and local AAMA. Currently Lorrie serves as a member of the Advisory Board for the Medical Assisting Program at Indian River State College, Fort Pierce, Florida.

Lorrie is married and has four children, three stepchildren and 17 grandchildren. She resides in Florida and spends summers in Connecticut at a small summer cottage with her husband Norman.

Acknowledgments

Cover Photo Credits

Daniel Naylor/iStockphoto; Harmonic Photo/iStockphoto; Adam Gault/OJO Images/Getty Images; Maria Gerasimenko/iStockphoto; Voronin76/Shutterstock; Elzbieta Sekowska/iStockphoto; Toby Maudsley/Iconica/Getty Images; Shannon Long/iStockphoto; iStockphoto

Interior Photo Credits

Al Dodge/Pearson Education/PH College, 74, 340; Brian Warling/Pearson Education/PH College, 68; Carl Leet/Pearson Education/PH College, 356; Elena Dorfman, 352; George Draper/Pearson Education/PH College, 175, 337, 342, 352, 360, 361, 362, 390; Jenny Thomas/Jenny Thomas Photography, 390; Jim Varney/Photo Researchers, Inc., 232; Michal Heron/Michal Heron Photography, 174, 179; Michal Heron/Pearson Education/PH College, 3, 141, 175, 237, 246, 250, 304, 340, 389, 392; Nathan Eldridge/Pearson Education/PH College, 173, 330, 332, 358; Network Graphics/Pearson Education/PH College, 328; Raymond B. Otero/Visuals Unlimited, 233; Richard Logan/Pearson Education/PH College, 184; Ron May/Pearson Education/PH College, 186, 293, 357; Shirlee Snyder, 330; VU/Southern Illinois/Visuals Unlimited, 62; Nonin Medical, Inc., 38; Audrey Berman, 180; Baxter Healthcare Corporation, 357; Becton Dickinson and Company, 244; Pearson Education/PH College, 31, 304, 327, 352; McKenzie Shirley B, 246, 263; Becton Dickinson Vacutainer Systems, 246; U.S. Department of Agriculture, 263; Pearson Education PH Chet, 390; Letitia Anne Peplau, 355

Contents

The Skills xviii

The Special Features xix

CHAPTER 1

Introduction to Clinical Competencies 1

HIPAA and the Patient's Bill of Rights 2

Professionalism 3

Documentation 3

Telephone Techniques 4

Procedure 1-1: Answering and Screening Telephone Calls 5

Procedure 1-2: Calling Pharmacy for Prescriptions 6

Procedure 1-3: Handling Emergency Calls 7

CHAPTER 2

Infection Control 8

Standard Precautions 9

Transmission-Based Precautions 11

Infection Control Procedures 11

Procedure 2-1: Disposing of Infectious Waste 12

Procedure 2-2: Performing Aseptic Hand Washing 12

Procedure 2-3: Performing Waterless-Based Hand Sanitizing 13

Procedure 2-4: Applying and Removing Nonsterile Gloves 14

Procedure 2-5: Sanitizing Instruments 15

Procedure 2-6: Wrapping Instruments for Autoclaving 15

Procedure 2-7: Sterilizing Instruments in Autoclave 16

Procedure 2-8: Chemically Sterilizing Instruments 17

Procedure 2-9: Performing Transmission-Based Precautions: Isolation Techniques 18

CHAPTER 3

Vital Signs and Mensuration 20

Temperature 21

Procedure 3-1: Measuring Oral Temperature with a Glass Nonmercury Thermometer 22

Procedure 3-2: Measuring Rectal Temperature Using Glass Nonmercury Thermometer 23

Procedure 3-3: Cleaning and Storing Glass Nonmercury Thermometer 24

Procedure 3-4: Measuring Oral Temperature Using Electronic or Digital Thermometer 25

Procedure 3-5: Measuring Rectal Temperature Using Electronic or Digital Thermometer 26

Procedure 3-6: Measuring Temperature Using Aural (Tympanic Membrane) Thermometer 26

Procedure 3-7: Measuring Dermal Temperature Using Disposable Thermometer 27

Procedure 3-8: Measuring Axillary Temperature 28

Procedure 3-9: Measuring Temperature with Temporal Artery Thermometer 28

Pulse 29

Procedure 3-10: Measuring Radial Pulse 30

Procedure 3-11: Measuring Apical Pulse 31

Respiration 32

Procedure 3-12: Measuring Apical–Radial Pulse (Two Person) 32

Procedure 3-13: Measuring Respirations 33

Blood Pressure 34

Procedure 3-14: Measuring Systolic Blood Pressure Using Palpatory Method 35

Procedure 3-15: Measuring Systolic/Diastolic Blood Pressure Using a Sphygmomanometer 36

Pain 37

Oxygen Saturation Measurement 38

Procedure 3-16: Measuring Oxygen Saturation Using a Pulse Oximeter 38

Anthropometry 39

Procedure 3-17: Measuring Adult Height and Weight 39

Procedure 3-18: Calculating Adult Body Mass Index 40

Procedure 3-19: Determining Fat Fold Measurement in Adults 40

CHAPTER 4

Assisting with Physical Examination 42

Positioning and Methods of Examination 43

Cleaning the Examination Room 43

Interviewing Patient for Physical Examination 43

Procedure 4-1: Cleaning the Examination Room 46

Procedure 4-2: Interviewing New Patient to Obtain Medical History to Prepare for Physical Examination 47

Procedure 4-3: Documenting a Chief Complaint During a Patient Interview 48

Assisting with Complete Physical Examination 49

Procedure 4-4: Positioning Patient in Supine Position 50

Procedure 4-5: Positioning Patient in Fowler's Position 50

Procedure 4-6: Positioning Patient in Dorsal Recumbent Position 51

Procedure 4-7: Positioning Patient in Lithotomy Position 52

Procedure 4-8: Positioning Patient in Prone Position 53

Procedure 4-9: Positioning Patient in Sims' Position 53

Procedure 4-10: Positioning Patient in Knee–Chest Position 54

Procedure 4-11: Assisting with Complete Physical Examination 55

Performing Scoliosis Examination 56

Caring for Vomiting Patient 56

Procedure 4-12: Performing Scoliosis Screening 57

Procedure 4-13: Assisting Vomiting Patient 57

Communicating Effectively with Elderly and Culturally Diverse Patients 58

Procedure 4-14: Communicating with Patients from Other Cultures 58

Procedure 4-15: Communicating Effectively with the Elderly 59

CHAPTER 5
Assisting with Medical Specialties 60

Allergy 61

Performing Scratch Testing 61

Procedure 5-1: Performing Scratch Testing 62

Procedure 5-2: Performing Patch Testing 63

Patch Testing 64

Intradermal Allergy Testing 64

Radioallergosorbent (RAST) Testing 64

Desensitizing Allergy Injection Treatment 64

Dermatology 64

Assisting with Skin Biopsy 65

Taking a Wound Culture 65

Procedure 5-3: Taking a Wound Culture 65

Gastroenterology 66

Procedure 5-4: Administering Disposable Enema 66

Assisting with Sigmoidoscopy 67

Assisting with Colonoscopy 67

Procedure 5-5: Assisting with Sigmoidoscopy Examination 68

Collecting Stool Specimen 69

Procedure 5-6: Assisting with Colonoscopy 69

Procedure 5-7: Instructing Patient in Collecting Stool Specimens 70

Testing for Occult Blood 70

Procedure 5-8: Testing for Occult Blood 70

Neurology 71

Procedure 5-9: Performing a Pupil Check 71

Assisting Physician with Neurological Examination 72

Assisting with Lumbar Puncture 72

Procedure 5-10: Assisting with Neurologic Screening Examination 72

Obstetrics and Gynecology 73

ADVANCED Procedure 5-11: Assisting with Lumbar Puncture 74

Breast Examination 75

Procedure 5-12: Instructing a Patient on Breast Self-Examination 75

Pelvic Examination and Pap Test 76

Procedure 5-13: Assisting with Pelvic Examination and Pap Test 76

Obtaining Specimens for Sexually Transmitted Diseases 77

Amplified DNA Probe Test for Chlamydia and Gonorrhea 77

Assisting with Prenatal Examinations 78

Procedure 5-14: Preparing Wet Mount/Wet Prep and KOH Slides 79

Procedure 5-15: Obtaining Material for Amplified DNA Probe Test for Chlamydia and Gonorrhea 79

Assisting with Postpartum Visit 80

Procedure 5-16: Assisting with Routine Prenatal Visit 81

Assisting with Colposcopy and Cervical Biopsy 81

Procedure 5-17: Assisting with Postpartum Examination 82

Procedure 5-18: Assisting with Colposcopy and Cervical Biopsy 82

Urinary Catheterization on a Female 83

Team Approach to the Male Reproductive System 83

Instructing Male Patient on Testicular Self-Examination 84

Procedure 5-19: Performing Urinary Catheterization on a Female 84

Procedure 5-20: Instructing Male Patient on Testicular Self-Examination 85

Urinary Catheterization on a Male 86

Ophthalmology 86

Screening for Visual Acuity with Snellen Eye Chart 86

Procedure 5-21: Performing Urinary Catheterization on a Male 87

Screening for Near-Vision Acuity 88

Screening for Color-Vision Acuity 88

Procedure 5-22: Screening Distance Visual Acuity with Snellen Chart 88

Procedure 5-23: Screening for Near-Vision Acuity 89

Irrigation of the Eye 89

Instilling Eye Medications 89

Assisting Vision-Impaired Patient 89

Procedure 5-24: Screening for Color-Vision Acuity 90

Procedure 5-25: Irrigating the Eye 90

Procedure 5-26: Instilling Eye Medications 91

Eye Patch Dressing 92

Otorhinolaryngology 92

Procedure 5-27: Applying Eye Patch Dressing 92

Assisting with Audiometry 93

Irrigating the Ear 93

Instilling Ear Medication 93

Procedure 5-28: Assisting with Audiometry 94

Procedure 5-29: Irrigating the Ear 94

Nose and Throat 95

Procedure 5-30: Instilling Ear Medication 95

Procedure 5-31: Instilling Nasal Medication 96

Assisting with Treatment for Epistaxis 97

Throat Culture 97

Procedure 5-32: Assisting with Treatment of Epistaxis 97

Procedure 5-33: Obtaining a Throat Culture 98

CHAPTER 6

Assisting with Pediatrics 99

Apgar Scoring 100

Patient Safety 100

Wrapping the Infant 100

Pediatric Vital Signs 101

Procedure 6-1: Wrapping an Infant or Small Child 101

Height, Weight 102

Procedure 6-2: Measuring Pediatric Vital Signs 103

Head and Chest Circumference 104

Procedure 6-3: Measuring the Weight and Length of Infants 105

Procedure 6-4: Measuring Infant Head Circumference 106

Growth and Development 106

Procedure 6-5: Measuring Circumference of Child's Chest 106

Immunizations 107

Procedure 6-6: Calculating Growth Percentiles 107

Sick-Child Visits 112

Procedure 6-7: Documenting and Maintaining Patient Immunization Record 113

Procedure 6-8: Applying Pediatric Urine Collection Device 113

CHAPTER 7

Assisting with Therapeutic Modalities and Rehabilitation 115

Range of Motion 116

Heat Therapies 116

Procedure 7-1: Performing and Instructing Range-of-Motion Exercises 116

Applying Hot Soaks 120

Procedure 7-2: Applying a Hot Compress 121

Applying Heating Pad or Aquathermic Pad 121

Procedure 7-3: Performing a Hot Soak Procedure 122

Cold Therapies 122

Procedure 7-4: Applying a Heating Pad 123

Ultrasound Therapy 123

Procedure 7-5: Applying a Cold Compress 124

Procedure 7-6: Applying an Ice Bag 124

Procedure 7-7: Applying a Cold Chemical Pack 125

ADVANCED Procedure 7-8: Administering an Ultrasound Treatment 126

Adaptive Equipment and Devices 127

Canes 127

Crutches 128

Procedure 7-9: Instructing a Patient to Use a Cane Correctly 128

Body Mechanics and Patient Transfer 130

Procedure 7-10: Measuring a Patient for Axillary Crutches 131

Procedure 7-11: Instructing a Patient to Use Crutches Correctly 132

Procedure 7-12: Instruct a Patient on Correct Use of Walker 133

Transferring Patients 134

Procedure 7-13: Performing Patient Wheelchair Transfer to Chair or Examination Table 135

Procedure 7-14: Transferring Patient from Examination Table or Bed to Wheelchair 136

Procedure 7-15: Ambulating Patient with One Assistant 137

Procedure 7-16: Assisting the Falling Patient 138

Cast Care 138

Procedure 7-17: Assisting with Cast Application 140

Procedure 7-18: Assisting with Cast Removal 140

Applying Immobilizing Devices 141

Procedure 7-19: Applying an Arm Sling 141

Procedure 7-20: Applying a Spiral Bandage 142

Procedure 7-21: Applying a Figure-Eight Bandage 143

Procedure 7-22: Applying Cervical Collar 144

CHAPTER 8

Assisting with Minor Surgery 145

Surgical Asepsis, Surgical Instruments, and Supplies 146

Procedure 8-1: Performing Surgical Hand Scrub/Sterile Scrub 148

Sterile Gloves 149

Procedure 8-2: Donning and Removing Sterile Gloves 149

Sterile Packets 151

Procedure 8-3: Opening a Sterile Packet 151

Procedure 8-4: Dropping a Sterile Item onto a Sterile Field 152

Procedure 8-5: Transferring Sterile Items with Sterile Transfer Forceps 152

Procedure 8-6: Pouring from a Sterile Container onto a Sterile Field 153

Assisting with Minor Surgery 154

Procedure 8-7: Assisting with Minor Surgery 154

Preparation of Patient's Skin 155

Procedure 8-8: Preparing a Patient's Skin for Minor Surgery 155

Cleansing Minor Wounds 156

Assisting with Sutures 157

Procedure 8-9: Cleaning a Minor Wound 157

Procedure 8-10: Assisting with Suturing 158

Dressing Change and Removing Sutures and Staples 159

Procedure 8-11: Changing a Sterile Dressing 159

Procedure 8-12: Removing Sutures and Staples 160

Procedure 8-13: Applying and Removing Sterile Adhesive Skin Closures 162

Wound Irrigation and Packing 162

Procedure 8-14: Irrigating a Wound 163

Procedure 8-15: Packing a Wound 164

Other Procedures 164

Biopsy Procedures 164

Procedure 8-16: Assisting with Excision of a Sebaceous Cyst 165

Procedure 8-17: Assisting with Aspiration of Joint Fluid 165

Procedure 8-18: Assisting with a Hemorrhoid Thrombectomy 166

Procedure 8-19: Preparing a Patient for Laser Surgery 167

Cryosurgery 168

CHAPTER 9

Assisting with Medical Emergencies 169

Emergency Action Planning 170

Emergency Equipment 170

Primary Assessment 171

Secondary Assessment 172

Recovery Position 173

Procedure 9-1: Placing a Victim in Recovery Position 173

Blocked Airway, Rescue Breathing, Maintaining Circulation 174

Procedure 9-2: Administering Abdominal Thrusts (Heimlich Maneuver) for a Conscious Adult 175

Procedure 9-3: Performing Abdominal Thrusts for a Conscious Child 176

Procedure 9-4: Performing Back Blows and Chest Thrusts for a Conscious Choking Infant 176

Procedure 9-5: Performing Back Blows and Chest Thrusts for an Unconscious Infant 177

Procedure 9-6: Administering Abdominal Thrusts (Heimlich Maneuver) for an Unresponsive Adult or Child 178

Procedure 9-7: Performing Rescue Breathing for an Adult 180

Procedure 9-8: Performing Rescue Breathing for a Child 180

Procedure 9-9: Performing Rescue Breathing for an Infant 181

Procedure 9-10: Performing CPR for an Adult 182

Procedure 9-11: Performing CPR for a Child 184

Procedure 9-12: Performing CPR for an Infant 184

Procedure 9-13: Using an Automated External Defibrillator (AED) 185

Procedure 9-14: Maintaining the Emergency/Crash Cart 186

Other Types of Medical Emergencies 187

Syncope 187

Assisting a Patient During an Asthma Attack 187

Procedure 9-15: Caring for a Fainting Patient 187

Anaphylaxis 188

Procedure 9-16: Assisting a Patient During an Asthma Attack 188

Procedure 9-17: Assisting with an Anaphylactic Emergency 188

Severe Bleeding 189

Burn Emergencies 189

Procedure 9-18: Controlling Severe Bleeding 190

Seizures 190

Poisoning 191

Procedure 9-19: Assisting with Burn Emergencies 192

Procedure 9-20: Assisting a Patient During a Seizure 192

Heat and Cold Emergencies 193

Bandages and Splints 194

Procedure 9-21: Applying a Tubular Gauze Bandage 194

Procedure 9-22: Applying an Arm Splint 195

Emergency Preparedness 195

Fire 195

Floods 196

Hurricanes 196

Terrorist Attack 196

Nuclear Blast 196

CHAPTER 10

Clinical Laboratory Testing 197

Clinical Laboratories 198

Clinical Laboratory Departments 199

Quality Control 200

Proficiency Testing 200

Laboratory Safety 200

Laboratory Requisitions 200

Chain of Custody 202

Patient Preparation and Specimen Handling 202

Patients' Test Results 202

Laboratory Testing Cycle and Time 202

Procedure 10-1: Completing a Laboratory Requisition and Preparing Specimen for Transport to Outside Laboratory 203

Procedure 10-2: Monitoring and Following Up on Patient Test Results 204

Procedure 10-3: Recording Quality Control Values on QC Control Record and Identifying Out-of-Control Values 205

Laboratory Equipment 206

Microscope 206

Centrifuge 206

Procedure 10-4: Using and Cleaning a Microscope 207

Incubator 208

Refrigerator and Freezer 208

Chemistry Analyzer 208

Automated Cell Counter 208

Urine Analyzer 208

CHAPTER 11

Urinalysis 209

Collecting a Urine Specimen 210

Random Urine Sample 210

First Voided Morning Specimen 210

Timed Urine Specimen 211

Procedure 11-1: Instructing a Patient How to Collect a 24-Hour Urine Specimen 211

2-Hour Postprandial Specimen 212

Clean-Catch Midstream Specimen 212

Procedure 11-2: Instructing a Male Patient How to Collect a Clean-Catch Midstream Urine Specimen 212

Procedure 11-3: Instructing a Female Patient How to Collect a Clean-Catch Midstream Urine Specimen 213

Urine Specimen for a Drug Screen 214

Procedure 11-4: Collecting a Urine Specimen for Drug Screening 214

Routine Urinalysis 215

Physical Characteristics 215

Appearance 215

Color 215

Odor 215

Quantity (Volume) 216

Specific Gravity 216

Procedure 11-5: Evaluating the Color, Clarity, and Volume of Urine 216

Procedure 11-6: Measuring Specific Gravity of Urine with Refractometer 217

Chemical Characteristics 218

Performing a Complete Urinalysis 218

Procedure 11-7: Testing Urine with Chemical Reagent Strips 219

Procedure 11-8: Performing a Complete Urinalysis 220

Confirmation of Chemical Reagent Stick Testing 221

Procedure 11-9: Performing Clinitest Tablet Test for Glucose and Other Reducing Substances in Urine 221

Procedure 11-10: Testing for Ketones in Urine Using Acetest (Nitroprusside Reaction) 222

Procedure 11-11: Testing for Protein in Urine Using Sulfosalicylic Acid (SSA) 223

Procedure 11-12: Testing Urine Using Ictotest (Diazo Tablet) for Bilirubin 223

Urine Pregnancy Testing 224

Procedure 11-13: Performing a Urine Pregnancy Test Using the Enzyme Immunoassay Method 225

CHAPTER 12

Microbiology 226

Naming Microorganisms 227

Specimen Collection 227

Preparing a Direct Smear 228

Procedure 12-1: Preparing a Direct Smear 228

Staining a Direct Smear 229

Procedure 12-2: Performing a Gram Stain 229

Culture and Sensitivity Testing 230

Procedure 12-3: Streaking a Blood Agar Plate for Colony Isolation   232

Rapid Strep Testing   233

Urine Cultures   233

Procedure 12-4: Performing a Urine Culture for Colony Count   233

Collecting Specimens for Ova and Parasites   234

Procedure 12-5: Obtaining a Stool Specimen for Ova and Parasites   234

Collecting Pinworm Specimens   235

Testing for Influenza   235

Procedure 12-6: Obtaining and Examining a Specimen for Pinworms   235

CHAPTER 13

Phlebotomy   236

Basic Procedural Steps   237

Basic Blood Drawing Equipment   237

Skin Puncture   237

Skin Puncture Devices   238

Procedure 13-1: Performing a Skin Puncture for an Adult or Child   239

Heelstick Procedure   240

Procedure 13-2: Performing a Heelstick for an Infant   241

Venipuncture Equipment   241

Procedure 13-3: Collecting a Heelstick Blood Specimen for PKU Screening   242

Procedure 13-4: Obtaining a Skin Puncture Specimen in a Microtainer Unit   243

Order of Draw   244

Needles, Holders, and Syringes   244

Butterfly/Winged Infusion Sets   246

Tourniquets   246

Patient Identification and Laboratory Test Orders   246

Procedure 13-5: Identifying the Patient Correctly Prior to a Phlebotomy Procedure   247

Venipuncture Sites   247

Procedure 13-6: Performing a Venipuncture Using the Evacuated Tube Collection Method   248

Procedure 13-7: Performing a Venipuncture Using the Syringe Method   249

Procedure 13-8: Performing a Butterfly/Winged Infusion Blood Draw from a Patient's Hand   251

Phlebotomy Problems   252

Syncope   252

Hematomas   252

Failure to Obtain Blood   252

Specimen Problems   253

Special Collection Procedures   253

Arterial Blood Gases   253

Capillary Blood Gases   253

Blood Cultures   253

Procedure 13-9: Collecting a Specimen for Blood Culture   253

Bleeding Times   254

Procedure 13-10: Performing a Bleeding Time Test with a Surgicutt Device   255

CHAPTER 14

Hematology   256

Blood Components   257

Microhematocrit   257

Procedure 14-1: Performing a Manual Microhematocrit   258

Procedure 14-2: Performing a Hematocrit Using HemataSTAT II Instrument   259

Hemoglobin   260

White and Red Blood Cell Counts   260

Procedure 14-3: Performing a Hemoglobin Determination Using HemoCue Method   261

White Blood Cell Count   262

Unopette   262

Procedure 14-4: Preparing a Dilution of Whole Blood Using a WBC Unopette System   263

Procedure 14-5: Performing a CBC Using QBC STAR Centrifugal Hematology   264

Peripheral Blood Smears   267

Procedure 14-6: Preparing a Peripheral Blood Smear   267

Procedure 14-7 Staining a Peripheral Blood Smear   269

ADVANCED Procedure 14-8: Performing a Differential Blood Smear Examination   269

Red Blood Cell Indices   271

Erythrocyte Sedimentation Rate (ESR)   271

Procedure 14-9: Performing an Erythrocyte Sedimentation Rate Using the Wintrobe Method   272

Procedure 14-10: Performing an Erythrocyte Sedimentation Rate Using the Westergren Method   273

Coagulation Studies   273

Coagulation Testing   274

CHAPTER 15

Serology/Immunology   275

Serology Tests   276

Quality Control   276

CLIA Waived Serology Tests   277

Mononucleosis Tests   277

Procedure 15-1: Performing a Test for Infectious Mononucleosis Using the BioStar Acceava Mono II Test   278

Strep Tests   279

Procedure 15-2: Performing BioStar Acceava Strep A Test   280

Testing for *Helicobacter pylori*   281

Procedure 15-3: Performing a QuickVue Test for *Helicobacter pylori*   281

Other Serology Tests   282

Blood Antigens   282

ADVANCED Procedure 15-4: Performing Agglutination Slide Testing for ABO Blood Grouping   284

ADVANCED Procedure 15-5: Performing Rh Typing by Slide Method   285

CHAPTER 16

Blood Chemistry   287

Blood Glucose   288

Blood Glucose Testing   289

Postprandial Blood Glucose Test   289

Glucose Tolerance Tests   289

Glycosylated Hemoglobin (HgbA1c)   290

CLIA Waived Glucose Tests   290

Procedure 16-1: Calibrating a Blood Glucose Meter (One Touch Ultra)   291

Procedure 16-2: Performing a Blood Glucose Test Using One Touch Ultra Device   291

Procedure 16-3: Performing Quality Control for Blood Glucose Testing Using SureStep Flexx Glucose Monitor   293

Procedure 16-4: Monitoring Blood Glucose with a SureStep Flexx Monitor   294

Procedure 16-5: Performing a Glycosylated Hemoglobin Test Using a Bayer DCA 2000+ Analyzer   294

Lipid Testing   296

Cholesterol   297

Procedure 16-6: Performing a Cholesterol Test Using a ProAct Testing Device   298

Procedure 16-7: Performing Lipid Profile and Glucose Testing Using a Cholestech LDX Analyzer   298

Other Chemistry Tests   300

CHAPTER 17

Diagnostic Imaging   301

Patient Positions   302

Procedure 17-1: Performing a General X-ray Examination   304

Contrast Studies   305

Sequencing Multiple Radiographic Procedures   306

Maintaining Radiographic Records   306

Procedure 17-2: Sequencing Multiple Radiographic/Diagnostic Imaging Examinations   307

Other Diagnostic Imaging Procedures   307

Procedure 17-3: Maintaining and Loaning Radiographic Records   308

CHAPTER 18

Pharmacology   309

Drug Safety   310

Drug References   310

Drug Classifications   310

Drug Prescriptions   311

Medication Measurement and Conversion   314

Calculating Dosages   315

Legal Implications   315

Monitoring Medications   316

Pharmacodynamics   316

Routes of Administration of Drugs   316

Adverse Reactions to Drugs   317

Administering Medications Safely   318

Procedure 18-1: Preparing for Medication Administration   320

Oral Medications   321

Procedure 18-2: Following Administration of Medication Protocol   320

Procedure 18-3: Preparing Oral Medications   321

Procedure 18-4: Preparing a Prescription for the Physician's Signature   322

Procedure 18-5: Administering Oral Medication to Adults   323

Other Routes of Administration   324

Procedure 18-6: Administering Oral Medication to a Child   324

Topical Medications   325

Suppositories   325

Procedure 18-7: Applying Topical Medication   325

Procedure 18-8: Applying Transdermal Medication   326

Procedure 18-9: Administering Rectal Suppositories   327

Procedure 18-10: Administering a Vaginal Suppository   328

Parenteral Medications   329

Parenteral Medication Equipment   329

Procedure 18-11: Reconstituting Powdered Medication   331

Procedure 18-12: Withdrawing Medication from a Vial   331

Procedure 18-13: Withdrawing Medication from an Ampule   332

Procedure 18-14: Preparing for Injection by Combining Medications in One Syringe Using Two Different Vials   333

Procedure 18-15: Preparing Two Medications in Two Syringes and Combining into One Syringe 334

Procedure 18-16: Setting up a Prefilled Disposable Medication Cartridge Syringe 334

Administering Parenteral Medication 335

Administering Intradermal Injections 335

Administering Subcutaneous Injections 335

Procedure 18-17: Administering an Intradermal Injection 336

Administering Intramuscular Injections 337

Procedure 18-18: Administering a Subcutaneous Injection 338

Administering Z-Track Injections 339

Procedure 18-19: Administering an Intramuscular Injection 340

Procedure 18-20: Administering a Z-Track Injection 341

CHAPTER 19

Intravenous Therapy 343

Legal Regulations 344

Intravenous Therapy for Fluid and Electrolyte Balance 344

Other Uses of Intravenous Therapy 345

Intravenous Delivery Methods 345

Central Vascular Access Devices 346

Peripheral Vascular Access Devices 346

Intravenous Containers and Administration Sets 346

Venous Access Devices 349

Puncturing the Vein 349

Securing the Venous Access Device 350

Preparing the IV Infusion 351

ADVANCED Procedure 19-1: Preparing an IV Infusion 351

ADVANCED Procedure 19-2: Preparing the Venipuncture Site for IV 353

ADVANCED Procedure 19-3: Starting an IV with a Winged Needle 354

ADVANCED Procedure 19-4: Inserting an Over-the-Needle Catheter 355

Adjusting the Flow Rate of an Infusion 356

ADVANCED Procedure 19-5: Adding Extension Tubing to an IV Set 358

ADVANCED Procedure 19-6: Monitoring an Intravenous Infusion 358

ADVANCED Procedure 19-7: Changing the IV Solution 359

Converting IV to Saline Lock 359

ADVANCED Procedure 19-8: Converting an IV to an Intermittent Infusion Lock 360

ADVANCED Procedure 19-9: Administering Medication to an IV Line by Injection "Push" 360

ADVANCED Procedure 19-10: Administering Medication Using a Secondary ("Piggyback") Bag 361

ADVANCED Procedure 19-11: Administering Medication Using a Peripheral Saline Lock 362

ADVANCED Procedure 19-12: Discontinuing an IV 363

CHAPTER 20

Nutrition and Patient Education 365

Essential Nutrients for Health 366

Carbohydrates 368

Proteins 369

Fats 369

Vitamins 369

Minerals 369

Fiber 369

Water 369

Calories 370

Food Pyramid Guidelines 370

Reading a Food Label 371

Dietary Guidelines 372

Dietary Modifications 373

Patient Education 374

Effective Teaching Plans 375

Procedure 20-1: Teaching a Patient to Read a Food Label 375

Procedure 20-2: Developing a Teaching Plan to Encourage an Increase in Daily Fiber 376

Wellness and Prevention 377

Procedure 20-3: Teaching Wellness and Disease Prevention to a Patient 377

CHAPTER 21

Cardiology and Pulmonology 379

Cardiology 380

Performing a 12-Lead Electrocardiogram 380

Applying a Holter Monitor 382

Procedure 21-1: Performing a 12-Lead Single-Channel or Multichannel Electrocardiogram 383

Exercise Tolerance Stress Testing 384

Procedure 21-2: Applying a Holter Monitor 385

Procedure 21-3: Assisting with Treadmill Stress Testing 386

Pulmonology 386

Spirometry Testing 386

Performing Spirometry Testing 387

Procedure 21-4: Performing Spirometry Testing 387

Peak Flow Measurement 388

Procedure 21-5: Teaching Peak Flow Measurement 388

Pulmonary Inhalation Treatments 389

Metered-Dose Inhalers 389

Procedure 21-6: Instructing a Patient to Use a Metered-Dose Inhaler (MDI)   390

Procedure 21-7: Administering a Nebulized Breathing Treatment   391

Administering Oxygen by Nasal Cannula   392

Procedure 21-8: Administering Oxygen by Nasal Cannula or Face Mask   392

Collecting a Sputum Specimen   393

Procedure 21-9: Collecting a Sputum Specimen   393

Appendices

A   Common Medical Abbreviations   A-1

B   JCAHO's Official "Do Not Use" List   A-3

C   ISMP's List of Error-Prone Abbreviations, Symbols, and Dose Designations   A-4

D   Normal Blood Values/Disease Conditions Evaluated for Abnormal Values   A-8

E   Celsius/Fahrenheit Temperature Conversions   A-13

F   Medical Terminology Word Parts   A-14

Glossary   G-1

Index   I-1

This text was designed to be a reference of procedures—from beginning through advanced.

Each skill is **MAPPED** to its corresponding **ABHES** and **CAAHEP** standard.

Procedures begin with the, **OBJECTIVE, STANDARD**, and **EQUIPMENT AND SUPPLIES** to focus you on the purpose and needs of the skill.

The **STEPS** guide you through the skill in an easy-to-follow, how-to format.

NOTES highlight important information or reminders.

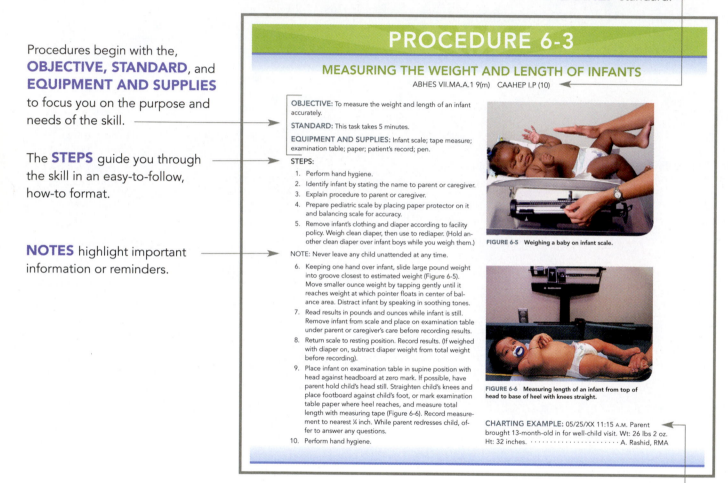

PROCEDURE 6-3

MEASURING THE WEIGHT AND LENGTH OF INFANTS
ABHES VII.MA.A.1 9(m)   CAAHEP I.P (10)

OBJECTIVE: To measure the weight and length of an infant accurately.

STANDARD: This task takes 5 minutes.

EQUIPMENT AND SUPPLIES: Infant scale; tape measure; examination table; paper; patient's record; pen.

STEPS:

1. Perform hand hygiene.
2. Identify infant by stating the name to parent or caregiver.
3. Explain procedure to parent or caregiver.
4. Prepare pediatric scale by placing paper protector on it and balancing scale for accuracy.
5. Remove infant's clothing and diaper according to facility policy. Weigh clean diaper, then use to rediaper. (Hold another clean diaper over infant boys while you weigh them.)

NOTE: Never leave any child unattended at any time.

6. Keeping one hand over infant, slide large pound weight into groove closest to estimated weight (Figure 6-5). Move smaller ounce weight by tapping gently until it reaches weight at which pointer floats in center of balance area. Distract infant by speaking in soothing tones.
7. Read results in pounds and ounces while infant is still. Remove infant from scale and place on examination table under parent or caregiver's care before recording results.
8. Return scale to resting position. Record results. (If weighed with diaper on, subtract diaper weight from total weight before recording).
9. Place infant on examination table in supine position with head against headboard at zero mark. If possible, have parent hold child's head still. Straighten child's knees and place footboard against child's foot, or mark examination table paper where heel reaches, and measure total length with measuring tape (Figure 6-6). Record measurement to nearest ¼ inch. While parent redresses child, offer to answer any questions.
10. Perform hand hygiene.

FIGURE 6-5 Weighing a baby on infant scale.

FIGURE 6-6 Measuring length of an infant from top of head to base of heel with knees straight.

CHARTING EXAMPLE: 05/25/XX 11:15 A.M. Parent brought 13-month-old in for well-child visit. Wt: 26 lbs 2 oz. Ht: 32 inches. · A. Rashid, RMA

You are shown how to document the procedure in the **CHARTING EXAMPLE**.

ADVANCED procedures are easy to spot!

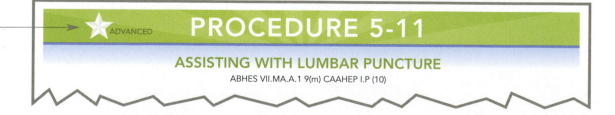

★ ADVANCED

PROCEDURE 5-11

ASSISTING WITH LUMBAR PUNCTURE
ABHES VII.MA.A.1 9(m) CAAHEP I.P (10)

The Special Features

Tables and boxes highlight important information throughout the text and within the procedures.

WHY? Why and when would you measure rectal temperature rather than oral or aural? Rectal temperature is measured for an unconscious patient, one who is nauseous, a small child, or a patient who has had oral surgery. Glass nonmercury thermometers are not used rectally for the most part because of the availability of other thermometers that are easier to use, require less time, and are less dangerous.

WHY? expands the rationale behind a procedure or step.

TABLE 3-1 Average Body Temperature Ranges at Various Body Locations

Type	Site	Range
Oral	Mouth	97.6°–99.6°F 36.5°–37°C
Rectal	Rectum	98.6°–100.6°F 37°–38.1°C
Axillary	Armpit	96.6°–98.6°F 35.9°–37°C
Tympanic Membrane	Ear	98.6°F 37°C
Temporal Artery	Forehead	98.6°–100.6°F 37°–38.1°C

TABLES present key topics in an at-a-glance format.

HIPAA Alert! In some facilities patients are weighed in a hallway or other less-than-private place. Be sure that any measurements are not observed by other patients.

HIPAA ALERT! Draws attention to possible privacy problems and their solutions.

Safety Alert! Remind patients not to lie on a heat source because it may cause burns to tissues in the area.

SAFETY ALERT! Warns of possible safety hazards.

Legal Alert! Only licensed personnel may give test results to a patient unless assistive personnel are specifically instructed to do so by the physician.

LEGAL ALERT! Focuses on possible legal implications of an action.

BOX 5-2 Guidelines for Assisting with Tissue Biopsy

- Observe strict surgical asepsis throughout the procedure.
- Assemble all supplies needed for procedure.
- Prepare patient by explaining procedure, including possibility of some discomfort.
- Follow office protocol for preparing skin site, and document.
- Assist physician as needed, observing standard precautions and using PPE.
- Immediately and thoroughly label any specimen removed.
- Clean procedure area and properly dispose of all waste materials.
- Document thoroughly in patient's record, including where specimen sent and patient education regarding care of biopsy site.
- Perform hand hygiene.

BOXES provide additional tips or guidelines.

1 Introduction to Clinical Competencies

PROCEDURES

Procedure 1-1 Answering and Screening Telephone Calls

Procedure 1-2 Calling Pharmacy for Prescriptions

Procedure 1-3 Handling Emergency Calls

TERMS TO LEARN

empathy

discretion

integrity

The rapidly changing health care environment has resulted in health care providers relying more heavily on assistive personnel than ever before. Multiskilled health care workers, such as medical assistants, perform valuable clinical and administrative skills in a variety of facilities. Job demands require assistive personnel to perform competently an astonishing number of skills. Although this text focuses on clinical competency skills, basic through advanced, first a brief review of the indispensable skills of communication, professionalism, and documentation is essential.

A key component to reliable health care is communication. The foundation of every patient interaction is some form of communication, whether written, verbal, or nonverbal. Medical records are read by a host of medical personnel, and therefore documentation of each and every interaction is essential. To function as a team, each member of the team must have the most up-to-date, accurate information about the patient.

Today's patients are consumers and demand more of a partnership with their physician and other health care team members than ever before. In addition, they are more informed consumers as a result of the abundance of information available through the Internet and other forms of media. Patients frequently ask questions, request information, and do not want to be kept waiting for appointments and test results.

Patient-centered care should be the main focus of all health care providers. Every occasion of contact the provider has with the patient should be handled in a manner that considers the patient's health, emotional well-being and right to privacy. Each caregiver must consider the cultural differences that patients present during each contact. In the United States baby boomers are reaching retirement age, and as a result the general population is older and living longer than ever before. An aging population presents challenges to caregivers. Many elderly patients live alone, may not eat a nutritionally sound diet, and may be slowing down physically and mentally. They may require extra time to fill out a form or may require assistance with dressing or paying a bill. Patience and kindness with each individual strengthens the bonds between staff and patient.

Medical assistants and other assistive personnel are often the first contacts patients have in a medical facility. The first impression one makes is a reflection of the facility and medical care in general. Every patient should be treated with respect and dignity at all times. A smile and pleasant manner and tone of voice help to create a positive experience. Each interaction is important whether face to face or over the phone.

HIPAA and the Patient's Bill of Rights

The Health Insurance Portability and Accountability Act (HIPAA) was enacted by the U.S. Congress in 1996. Title I of HIPAA protects health insurance coverage for workers and their families when they change or lose their jobs. Title II of HIPAA defines offenses relating to health care and sets civil and criminal penalties for these offenses. Title II creates several programs to control fraud and abuse within the health care system. Other provisions, known as the Administrative Simplification (AS) provisions, require the U.S. Department of Health and Human Services (HHS) to draft rules aimed at increasing the efficiency of the health care system. HHS creates standards for the use and dissemination of health care information, establishes national standards for electronic health care transactions, and specifies national identifiers for providers, health insurance plans, and employers. The HHS issued the Privacy Rule to put into practice the requirements of the HIPAA. The main goal of the Privacy Rule is to ensure that individuals' health information is protected while allowing the flow of health information necessary to provide quality health care and to protect public health. The Privacy Rule took effect in 2003 and regulates the use and disclosure of information by "covered entities" (health insurers, medical providers, employer-sponsored health plans, and health care clearinghouses) that perform certain transactions. The Privacy Rule establishes regulations for the use and disclosure of Protected Health Information (PHI) and gives individuals the right to confidentiality with respect to their health care data and the right to correct inaccuracies in any PHI. Further information can be found on the HHS website (www.hhs.gov/ocr/hipaa).

As a result of these directives, health care institutions and all individuals delivering care must protect individually identifiable health information in any form, whether electronic, paper, or oral, from incidental release to unauthorized entities. PHI refers to all individually identifiable health information, including demographic data, physical or mental status, health care provider names, and name of person who is financially responsible for payment.

Health care institutions must adhere to HIPAA and the Privacy Rule or risk fines and possible lawsuits. Workshops to educate staff on HIPAA compliance are important tools to safeguard patient privacy. Each patient must sign a release of information document on the first visit; otherwise the information cannot be released to other providers or to insurance companies for reimbursement.

No patient information may be shared with other entities without prior written authorization from the patient. Thus computer screen information, faxes, e-mails, and any other document containing private information must be designated as private and be shielded from the view of unauthorized individuals.

The right to privacy is an inherent patient right. The American Hospital Association developed a Patient's Bill of Rights, which describes the patient–physician relationship. Patient's rights include, among others, the following:

- The right to respectful considerate care
- The right to information about care, diagnosis, and prognosis
- The right to decide about treatment or refuse treatment
- The right to every consideration of privacy, and confidentiality of records and other health information
- The right to expect reasonable care and be informed about the policies of the health care facility with respect to billing and insurance

Professionalism

The relationship between health care provider and patient demands that health care providers exhibit professional characteristics. Qualities or characteristics of professionalism include **empathy**, **discretion**, confidentiality, and **integrity**. Integrity connotes that the caregiver is dependable, honest, dedicated to high principles, thorough, and punctual. An empathetic caregiver is sensitive to another's feelings and can imagine himself or herself in another's place. Discretion means that the caregiver is tactful in communicating with patients and co-workers.

All patient contacts, written and verbal, must be treated as confidential. Medical records, family issues, and any other matters pertinent to the health of the patient are confidential. The caregiver is morally and legally required to protect the patient's right to privacy.

Professionalism also requires the caregiver to be neatly dressed, exhibit good personal hygiene, speak in modulated tones, and refrain from chewing gum and wearing strong perfume or excessive jewelry.

Documentation

Documentation is one of the most important tasks performed in the medical environment (see Figure 1-1). Since the advent of managed care, medical records have been open to the many health care entities, courts of law, and insurance companies. Adherence to documentation guidelines is vital to ensure accurate information and avoid legal complications. The following are the basics of documentation:

- **The correct chart.** Be certain you have the chart for the correct patient, including correct spelling, date of

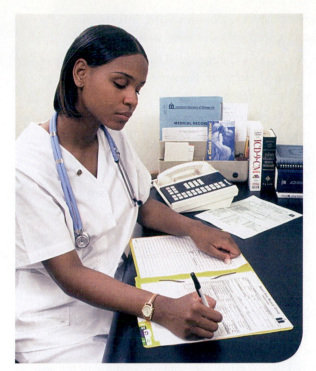

FIGURE 1-1 Clear and accurate documentation is the best defense against potential liability.

birth, and Social Security number. The patient's name should appear on each page.

- **Document accurately and objectively.** Record factual information only. Avoid judgments, speculations, opinions and assumptions.
- **Document every patient encounter.** Record all procedures, office visits, telephone calls, actions taken, appointment-related information, and evidence of noncompliance.
- **Document completely.** Record all facts. Listen carefully. Record specifics, including date and time of onset of symptoms and location of the problem. Rate all pain on a scale of 1 to 10.
- **Document date and time.** Record the date and time at each entry.
- **Black ink.** Use only black ink. Write legibly or print.
- **Use correct spelling.** Look up medical and nonmedical words whenever you are unsure.
- **Standard abbreviations.** Use only standard abbreviations. Look them up if you are unsure.
- **Circle positive and negative symbols.** Doing so makes the information more noticeable.
- **Document every line.** Do not skip lines. This prevents alteration of entries.
- **Sign.** Sign every entry with your first initial, last name, and credential(s).

- **Never postpone documenting information.** Postponing documentation may cause you to forget details.
- **Never make a diagnosis.** Diagnosis is the task of the licensed caregiver. Report only facts and symptoms using the patient's own words.
- **Never document for someone else or ask someone to document for you.** Legal problems may result.
- **Do not use correction fluid or scribble over an error.** Draw a single through a mistake. Initial it, then add the date, time, and correct information.
- **Sign and draw a line after each entry.**

Telephone Techniques

The telephone is the backbone of most medical facilities. It is a key communication pathway between the medical staff and patients. Telephone systems have changed dramatically in recent years. More automated systems are used and are the first contact patients have with the medical facility. Automated menu systems are sometimes difficult for patients to navigate, especially if they are feeling poorly. Regardless of the type of telephone system a facility uses, a menu selection near the beginning of the message should allow patients to speak with a receptionist.

First impressions made through phone systems are critically important to the delivery of health care (Figure 1-2). Answer the telephone with a pleasant businesslike voice, use good pronunciation, and articulate clearly. Impatience can be detected during a phone conversation, especially when the speaker is being bombarded with other demands for attention.

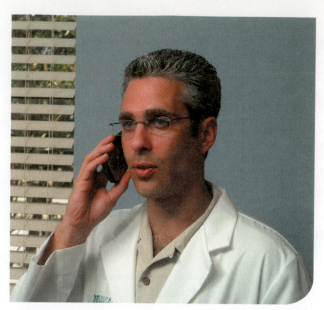

FIGURE 1-3 Many physicians use cell phones to stay in touch with their office.

Take accurate messages, including the caller's name; date, time, and reason for the call; and a callback number.

Telephone screening is the process used to determine the order in which patients' calls should be taken. Doctors and nurses make assessments daily in their treatment of patients on the phone and in person (Figure 1-3). Evaluation of patient phone calls in the medical office is different. Patients may be calling for an appointment, during which the physician will make an assessment and perhaps a diagnosis. Medical assistants and other assistive personnel are not licensed or trained to diagnose or assess, but they must use telephone screening techniques. Careful questioning of patients over the phone permits personnel to assess symptoms based on protocols established by the physician in charge. Assistive personnel may follow only physician-approved protocols when screening calls.

HIPAA Alert! All telephone conversations with patients should be conducted in an area that provides privacy so they cannot be overheard by other patients or unauthorized personnel.

Table 1-1 Telephone Screening Guidelines provides examples of calls that may be handled by medical assistants and calls that should be referred to the physician or other designated licensed personnel.

Telephone triage manuals are available commercially and may assist physicians in establishing protocols for their

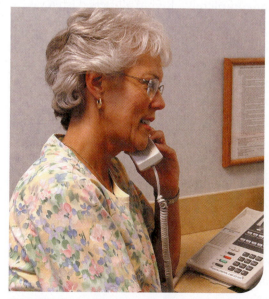

FIGURE 1-2 A pleasant smile can go a long way, even over telephone lines.

TABLE 1-1 Telephone Screening Guidelines

Calls Handled by Medical Assistants

Scheduling appointments and tests

Billing inquiries

Diagnostic test and laboratory test results from facilities

General information, office hours, directions

Referrals to other physicians

Insurance companies requesting information

Calls to Be Referred or Approved

Patient requesting tests results

Call from other doctors

Sales representatives

Medication requests or refills

Patients with medical questions

Patients who want to speak to doctor

Emergency calls

BOX 1-1 Information to Request from Patient

- Date and time of call
- Patient's name
- Caller's name if different from patient
- Telephone number
- Patient's physician
- General complaint
- History of present illness (what, where, when)
- Self-treatment
- Medications and over-the-counter medications
- Drug allergies
- Instructions to patient based on office protocol

specialty. Certain patients warrant emergency action, and a clear path of action must be available for all who answer telephones. Box 1-1 lists information to request from a patient during a telephone encounter.

In addition to screening telephone calls and taking messages, health care employees may need to place outgoing calls, such as calls to pharmacies for prescriptions or refills, requests for test results, requests for information from third parties, and calls to schedule test procedures and surgeries (see Figure 1-4). Accuracy and professionalism are important in all these interactions. Also see Procedure 1-1: Answering and Screening Telephone Calls.

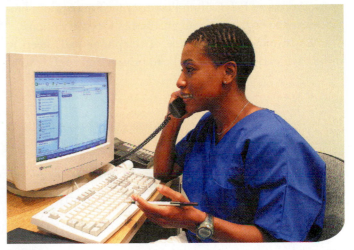

FIGURE 1-4 The medical assistant spends many hours on the telephone assisting patients.

PROCEDURE 1-1

ANSWERING AND SCREENING TELEPHONE CALLS

ABHES VII.MA.A.1 8(ee); VII.MA.A.1 9(o)   CAAHEP IV.P (7)

OBJECTIVE: To answer calls professionally gathering necessary information, documenting correctly, and following up on request of caller.

STANDARD: The time this task takes will vary with caller.

EQUIPMENT AND SUPPLIES: Telephone; message pad; pen; paper; telephone call protocol guide; appointment book; physician referral sheet.

STEPS:

1. Answer phone promptly using professional voice and designated message. (*Note:* Phone should not ring more than three times. If you need to put caller on hold, ask permission first. This gives caller a chance to identify the situation as an emergency.)

2. Ask caller's name, address, and phone number at once in case connection is disrupted.

3. Determine if call is an emergency. If emergency, follow designated protocol. Record information on a notepad. (See Box 1-1.)

4. Repeat information back to caller after recording on message pad.

5. Process the call to designated personnel (appointment scheduling, billing, physician callback, emergencies, physician to physician).

6. Ask caller if he or she has other questions.

7. Courteously say good-bye. Do not hang up until patient has hung up. Document information immediately; include any further actions to be taken. Deliver message to appropriate person or staff slot.

CHARTING EXAMPLE: 03/01/XX 9:05 A.M. Pt. called c/o "sinus infection" ×2 days "thick green nasal drainage"; no fever. Taking OTC sinus tab "no relief." Scheduled Pt. for 1:00 P.M. today per telephone screening protocol. ··········
······························· H. Campo, CMA (AAMA)

One frequent patient request involves obtaining prescriptions. Procedure 1-2: Calling Pharmacy for Prescriptions provides steps to be taken to call pharmacies for prescriptions.

When handling any type of telephone call, keep in mind each patient has the right to privacy and confidentiality and to be treated with respect. The procedure for handling emergency calls is documented in Procedure 1-3: Handling Emergency Calls.

PROCEDURE 1-2

CALLING PHARMACY FOR PRESCRIPTIONS

ABHES VII.MA.A.1 8(ee)   CAAHEP IV.P (7)

OBJECTIVE: To call in a patient prescription accurately and courteously.

STANDARD: This task takes about 5 minutes if pharmacy not overly busy.

EQUIPMENT AND SUPPLIES: Notepad; pen; paper; telephone; patient chart; prescription.

STEPS:

1. Accurately and courteously obtain necessary patient information during incoming call.

2. Document patient's chart with information and physician's prescription order. (If verbal order, read prescription information back to physician.)

3. For refill request, give physician patient's chart with phone message about refill on top.

4. If refill approved, call pharmacy. Ask to speak to pharmacy staff; for accuracy, have staff repeat prescription back to you.

5. Document chart with time and date of call and name of pharmacy staff person.

6. Notify patient by phone that prescription has been ordered. Provide instructions as needed and designated by physician. Ask patient to write down instructions.

7. Document patient phone call.

CHARTING EXAMPLE: 02/28/XX 10:20 A.M. Called in Rx to CVS Pharmacy 3924 Federal Hwy. Jupiter FL 561-781-9909. Spoke c̄ pharmacist M. Lopez: Levoxyl 0.50 mg, # 30 Sig 1 Tab tid ×30 days per written order of Dr. Worth. ············
······························· C. Blardo, CMA (AAMA)

HANDLING EMERGENCY CALLS

ABHES VII.MA.A.1 8(ee); VII.MA.A.1 9(e)   CAAHEP IV.P (7); XI.A (1)

OBJECTIVE: To determine the emergency status of a call and follow designated protocol correctly.

STANDARD: The time this task requires depends on nature of call.

EQUIPMENT AND SUPPLIES: Telephone; emergency call protocol; pen; notepad; telephone message forms; phone numbers of area emergency rooms; poison control centers; ambulance services.

STEPS:

1. Answer the phone within three rings using appropriate telephone techniques.
2. If call is a potential emergency, remain calm and obtain the following information:
   - Caller's name
   - Relationship to patient
   - Patient's name, age, address, telephone number
3. Read information back to caller for accuracy.
4. Obtain a description from patient of symptoms, accident, or both.
5. Ask about treatment given thus far.
6. Read back details of medical problem.
7. Refer to emergency protocol list and act accordingly.
8. Refer call to physician or other licensed personnel immediately.
9. If licensed personnel unavailable, instruct caller to go to hospital, call poison control, or call 911 for ambulance.
10. If caller is unable to follow directions, place on hold and call 911; return to caller and stay on line until help arrives.
11. When emergency is over, document fully in patient's chart.

CHARTING EXAMPLE: 03/02/XX 8:50 A.M. Pt. called c/o chest and left arm pain. N&V, SOB; Called EMS. Stayed on line until EMS arrived. Notified Dr. McGann of Pt. emergency · · · ·
· L. Schwartz, RMA

2 Infection Control

PROCEDURES

Procedure 2-1 Disposing of Infectious Waste

Procedure 2-2 Performing Aseptic Hand Washing

Procedure 2-3 Performing Waterless-Based Hand Sanitizing

Procedure 2-4 Applying and Removing Nonsterile Gloves

Procedure 2-5 Sanitizing Instruments

Procedure 2-6 Wrapping Instruments for Autoclaving

Procedure 2-7 Sterilizing Instruments in Autoclave

Procedure 2-8 Chemically Sterilizing Instruments

Procedure 2-9 Performing Transmission-Based Precautions: Isolation Techniques

TERMS TO LEARN

nosocomial

Universal Precautions

Standard Precautions

transmission-based precautions

droplet precautions

contact precautions

BOX 2-1 Standard Precautions: Equipment/Situations

Hand Hygiene	Hands must be washed or waterless sanitizing agents used before and after gloves are removed. Hands must be washed or waterless sanitizing agent used immediately if contaminated with blood or body fluids and between patient contacts.
Gloves	Must be worn when in contact with blood and all body fluids, secretions, and excretions (except sweat), regardless of whether blood is visible or not. Must be worn when in contact with mucous membranes, nonintact skin, and contaminated articles.
Gown	Must be worn during procedures or situations in which there may be exposure to blood, body fluids, mucous membranes, or draining wounds.
Mask/Eyewear	Must be worn by coughing patient and by health care providers during procedures that are likely to generate droplets of blood or body fluids (splashes or sprays).
Multiple-Use Equipment	Common multiple-use equipment such as blood pressure cuffs or stethoscopes must be cleaned and disinfected after use or when they become soiled with bodily fluids or blood. Single-use items are discarded.
Needles and Sharps	Must be discarded into a puncture-proof container. Needles should not be recapped or broken.

Microorganisms are found everywhere in our environment. Some are nonpathogenic, and others are disease producing or pathogenic. One of the main goals of health care employees is to limit the exposure of patients and themselves to pathogens. Healthy individuals may have some resistance to disease, but those who are suffering from illness are more susceptible to new infections.

Guidelines have been developed by several government agencies to protect patients and health care workers from exposure to pathogens. In 1970 the Centers for Disease Control (CDC) published a manual of isolation techniques for hospitals. This was updated in 1975. The term **Universal Precautions** refers to routine infection control precautions developed in 1985 to prevent the transmission of hepatitis B virus, human immunodeficiency virus (HIV), and other bloodborne pathogens. In 1996 the CDC developed and published new guidelines for isolation precautions in hospitals, and these were called **Standard Precautions**. The Standard Precautions combine major features of Universal Precautions and body substance isolation precautions into one set of recommendations.

CDC precautions are enforced by the U.S. Occupational Safety and Health Administration (OSHA). These OSHA standards are law and must be followed by all health care agencies in which employees could be "reasonably anticipated" to come into contact with potentially infectious materials such as blood, saliva, and tissues. Each facility must have a program in place to determine exposure probability, methods of compliance (safety measures in place),

and postexposure evaluation. Employers are responsible for having available sharps containers, sinks with running water, personal protective equipment (PPE) and biohazard waste containers. Standard Precautions equipment and examples of situations in which they must be used are found in Box 2-1.

The CDC issued isolation guidelines that emphasized a two-tier approach to controlling infection. The first tier of prevention is the CDC's Standard Precautions (Figure 2-1). These steps are utilized with all individuals seeking medical care regardless of their diagnosis. Standard Precautions seek to prevent transmission of disease through body fluids and require health care providers to treat all body fluids as if they are infected with pathogens. Hand sanitizing is one of the best means of reducing the spread of microorganisms in a health care facility and at home. The second tier of CDC guidelines focuses on infected patients or those suspected of being infected. These guidelines require precautions known as transmission-based precautions (discussed later in this chapter).

Standard Precautions

Standard Precautions apply to all body fluids, blood, nonintact skin, and mucous membranes. Body fluids include the following:

- Blood
- Body fluids with visible blood

STANDARD PRECAUTIONS
FOR INFECTION CONTROL

Assume that every person is potentially infected or colonized with an organism that could be transmitted in the healthcare setting.

Hand Hygiene

Avoid unnecessary touching of surfaces in close proximity to the patient.

When hands are visibly dirty, contaminated with proteinaceous material, or visibly soiled with blood or body fluids, wash hands with soap and water.

If hands are not visibly soiled, or after removing visible material with soap and water, decontaminate hands with an alcohol-based hand rub. Alternatively, hands may be washed with an antimicrobial soap and water.

Perform hand hygiene:
Before having direct contact with patients.
After contact with blood, body fluids or excretions, mucous membranes, nonintact skin, or wound dressings.
After contact with a patient's intact skin (e.g., when taking a pulse or blood pressure or lifting a patient).
If hands will be moving from a contaminated body site to a clean body site during patient care.
After contact with inanimate objects (including medical equipment) in the immediate vicinity of the patient.
After removing gloves.

Personal protective equipment (PPE)

Wear PPE when the nature of the anticipated patient interaction indicates that contact with blood or body fluids may occur.

Before leaving the patient's room or cubicle, remove and discard PPE.

Gloves

Wear gloves when contact with blood or other potentially infectious materials, mucous membranes, nonintact skin, or potentially contaminated intact skin (e.g., of a patient incontinent of stool or urine) could occur.

Remove gloves after contact with a patient and/or the surrounding environment using proper technique to prevent hand contamination. Do not wear the same pair of gloves for the care of more than one patient.

Change gloves during patient care if the hands will move from a contaminated body site (e.g., perineal area) to a clean body site (e.g., face).

Gowns

Wear a gown to protect skin and prevent soiling or contamination of clothing during procedures and patient-care activities when contact with blood, body fluids, secretions, or excretions is anticipated.

Wear a gown for direct patient contact if the patient has uncontained secretions or excretions.

Remove gown and perform hand hygiene before leaving patient's environment.

Mouth, nose, eye protection

Use PPE to protect the mucous membranes of the eyes, nose and mouth during procedures and patient-care activities that are likely to generate splashes or sprays of blood, body fluids, secretions and excretions.

During aerosol-generating procedures wear one of the following: a face shield that fully covers the front and sides of the face, a mask with attached shield, or a mask and goggles.

Respiratory Hygiene/Cough Etiquette

Educate healthcare personnel to contain respiratory secretions to prevent droplet and fomite transmission of respiratory pathogens, especially during seasonal outbreaks of viral respiratory tract infections.

Offer masks to coughing patients and other symptomatic persons (e.g., persons who accompany ill patients) upon entry into the facility.

Patient-Care equipment and instruments/devices

Wear PPE (e.g., gloves, gown), according to the level of anticipated contamination, when handling patient-care equipment and instruments/devices that are visibly soiled or may have been in contact with blood or body fluids.

Care of the environment

Include multi-use electronic equipment in policies and procedures for preventing contamination and for cleaning and disinfection, especially those items that are used by patients, those used during delivery of patient care, and mobile devices that are moved in and out of patient rooms frequently (e.g., daily).

Textiles and laundry

Handle used textiles and fabrics with minimum agitation to avoid contamination of air, surfaces and persons.

SPR7 · ©2007 Brevis Corporation · www.brevis.com

FIGURE 2-1 Standard Precautions for infection control.
Source: Printed with permission of Brevis Corporation, www.brevis.com.

- Tissue specimens
- Semen
- Vaginal secretions
- Amniotic fluid
- Cerebrospinal fluid
- Pleural fluid
- Pericardial fluid
- Interstitial fluid

Standard Precautions require proper hand hygiene and the use of PPE, such as the following:

- Gloves
- Cap
- Boots
- Mask
- Gown
- Eye protection

PPE provides barrier protection from body fluids. Hand hygiene recommendations include not wearing artificial fingernails or extenders when having direct contact with high-risk patients, such as those in intensive care or operating rooms. Natural fingernails should be kept ¼ inch or shorter in length.

Transmission-Based Precautions

Transmission-based precautions fall into three categories: airborne precautions, droplet precautions, and contact precautions. Airborne precautions often involve patient isolation in a private room if hospitalized and require use of mask and gown by all health care personnel who come in contact with the patient. By using transmission-based precautions, the risk of transmitting diseases such as tuberculosis and chickenpox is, hopefully, reduced. Hand washing and gloves are required as well.

Droplet precautions are used around patients suspected of being infected with organisms spread by droplets during sneezing, coughing, and talking. Some examples are such diseases as *Haemophilus influenzae* Type b, meningitis, pneumonia, pertussis, and streptococcal pneumonia. A mask should be worn if the caregiver is within 3 feet of the patient. Gown and gloves are worn when there is a chance of coming into contact with the blood or body fluids of suspected patents.

Contact precautions are used when infections are difficult to treat and microorganism transmission among patients and health care providers would be easy. Conditions such as intestinal infections, hepatitis, wounds, respiratory infections, herpes, scabies, and pediculosis are treated while using contact precautions. These precautions include isolating patients and wearing gown and gloves. If in contact with body fluids, mask and eyewear also should be worn. Health care providers should be aware that some diseases are transmitted by several routes, and all relevant precautions should be taken.

Some patients may be latex sensitive. Before touching a patient, he or she should be asked if they have a history of latex sensitivity. High-risk patients such as those with congenital defects and indwelling catheters must always be assessed for latex sensitivity. Patients with allergies to bananas, chestnuts, kiwis, and avocados may have cross-sensitivity to latex, so it is prudent to ask about those allergies as well. Symptoms to latex sensitivity include contact dermatitis, swelling, itching, and rhinitis and in some cases may include anaphylaxis. Latex-free gloves, syringes, IV tubing, and solution bags should be available to meet patients' needs.

Infection Control Procedures

An estimated two million infections are acquired during hospital stays annually according to the CDC. An infection acquired in the hospital is known as a **nosocomial** infection. Only a small number of states require hospitals to report incidences of nosocomial infections. The number-one way to reduce these types of infections is proper and timely hand washing.

Safety Alert! Nosocomial infections cause close to 100,000 deaths per year and billions of dollars in health care costs.

Procedures 2-1 through 2-9 delineate the steps for hand washing, disposing of infectious waste, applying and removing nonsterile gloves, sanitizing instruments, wrapping instruments for autoclaving, sterilizing instruments in an autoclave, performing chemical sterilization, and performing transmission-based precautions.

PROCEDURE 2-1

DISPOSING OF INFECTIOUS WASTE

ABHES VII.MA.A.1 10(c)   CAAHEP III.P (3)

OBJECTIVE: The student will dispose of infectious waste substances without causing contamination.

STANDARD: This task should take 2–3 minutes.

EQUIPMENT AND SUPPLIES: Infectious waste and infectious waste container with lid marked appropriately with universal biohazard symbol and label; red disposable plastic liners.

STEPS:

1. Check to ensure infectious waste container is lined with red disposable bag.
2. Discard infectious waste into the infectious waste container.
3. Before disposing of liquid waste, be sure it is contained in a closeable device prior to placing in infectious waste container.
4. Do not put contaminated glass into infectious waste container. (Place large glass items into puncture-proof container, and small glass items go into sharps container.)
5. When full, remove red trash bag and secure opening to protect trash-handling personnel and others from contamination.
6. Make sure red bags are not overstuffed to prevent rupture, spills, and leaks.
7. Do not mix noninfectious trash in same bin or container with infectious bags.
8. Store closed full red bags in designated area away from general patient area without blocking hallways, entrances, or other public areas.

PROCEDURE 2-2

PERFORMING ASEPTIC HAND WASHING

ABHES VII.MA.A.1 9(b)   CAAHEP III.P (4)

OBJECTIVE: To perform aseptic hand washing correctly to reduce spread of pathogens.

STANDARD: This task should take 2–3 minutes.

EQUIPMENT AND SUPPLIES: Soap in soap dispenser; nail cleaner; warm running water; paper towels; waste container.

STEPS:

1. Remove all rings, watches, and bracelets.
2. Stand close to sink without touching it.
3. Turn on faucet and adjust temperature of water. Avoid hot water to decrease risk of dermatitis.
4. Wet hands in running water, apply soap and work into lather by moving over palms and between fingers for at least 15 seconds, and work soap under fingernails and scrub wrists (Figure 2-2A).
5. Use nail cleaner during first hand washing of day, and clean under nails on each hand.
6. Rinse hands and wrists while keeping hands pointed downward with hands below elbows. Do not touch inside of sink.
7. Rewash if hands are heavily soiled.

8. Gently dry hands with paper towel with fingers and hands pointed upward, then discard paper towel when finished.

9. Use a dry paper towel to turn off faucet. Discard towel when finished (Figure 2-2B). Repeat procedures if hands touch sink at any time.

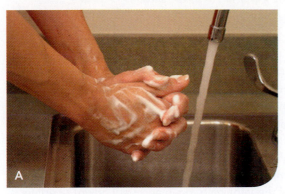
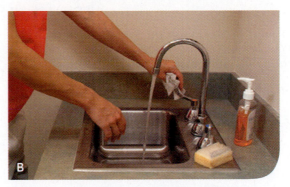

FIGURE 2-2 (A) Hold hands and wrists below elbows when washing hands; (B) use paper towel to turn off faucet.

PROCEDURE 2-3

PERFORMING WATERLESS-BASED HAND SANITIZING

ABHES VII.MA.A.1 9(i)   CAAHEP III.P (2)

OBJECTIVE: Sanitize hands using a waterless-based hand-washing substance to prevent spreading pathogens.

> **WHY?** Germicidal wipes, effective at killing 99.9% of harmful bacteria, are available and are approved by the EPA.

STANDARD: Task should take 1–2 minutes.

EQUIPMENT AND SUPPLIES: Waterless-based hand-cleaning substance containing 60% to 95% ethanol or isopropanol (foam, lotion, or gel).

STEPS:

1. Inspect hands for obvious signs of contamination or waste debris.

NOTE: If hands are visibly dirty they must be washed with soap and water.

2. Remove rings.

3. Apply waterless-based rub to the palm of one hand following manufacturer's guidelines for amount.

4. Spread evenly and rub vigorously over all surfaces of hands and fingers continuing to ½ inch above wrists.

5. Rub hands together until they are dry, about 30 seconds.

NOTE: OSHA recommends washing hands with soap and water after three applications of gel.

6. Allow hands and forearms to dry thoroughly before donning sterile gloves.

APPLYING AND REMOVING NONSTERILE GLOVES

ABHES VII.MA.A.1 9(i)   CAAHEP III.P (3)

OBJECTIVE: To apply nonsterile gloves and remove them appropriately to prevent the spread of pathogens.

STANDARD: This task should take 1–2 minutes.

EQUIPMENT AND SUPPLIES: Gloves; biohazard waste container.

STEPS:

1. Perform hand hygiene.
2. Choose appropriate size gloves for your hands (Figure 2-3A). Hold glove at the wrist opening and insert fingers, then pull glove up to wrist. Apply second glove in same manner, checking for holes and other flaws (Figure 2-3B). If any flaws are found, discard and obtain new gloves.
3. To remove gloves, grasp the glove covering your non-dominant hand at the palm and pull away (Figure 2-3C).
4. Pull glove off and hold it in the palm of the gloved dominant hand (Figure 2-3D).
5. While holding the soiled glove in your gloved hand, slide the index finger of the ungloved hand below the cuff of the remaining glove and peel down, inverting over the first glove. (Both gloves will be in a ball and inside out).
6. Dispose of gloves in biohazard waste container.
7. Perform hand hygiene.

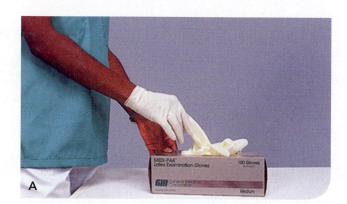

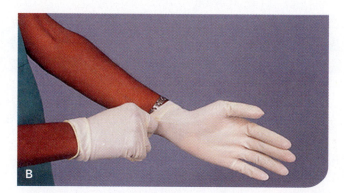

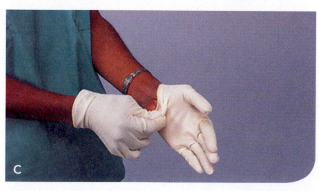

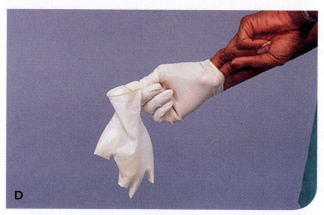

FIGURE 2-3 (A) Clean gloves need to be easily accessible for health care workers; (B) pick up gloves at wrist edge and slip fingers into openings; (C) remove gloves by pulling off without touching hand with soiled gloves; (D) place rolled-up glove in palm of second hand, and then remove glove.

PROCEDURE 2-5

SANITIZING INSTRUMENTS

ABHES VII.MA.A.1 9(o)4   CAAHEP III.P (6)

OBJECTIVE: To sanitize instruments, leaving no visible evidence of contamination.

STANDARD: This task should be completed in 10 minutes.

EQUIPMENT AND SUPPLIES: Disposable gloves; lab safety glasses; laboratory apron (fluid resistant); utility gloves (rubber); nylon scrub brush; towel; sink; running water; container to hold all instruments; low-sudsing (low pH) detergent or germicidal agent.

NOTE: All instruments should be rinsed under warm running water immediately after use to remove gross signs of contamination (blood, tissue, or body fluids). They should be submerged in water with low pH detergent until ready to be sanitized.

STEPS:

1. Apply nonsterile gloves, then rubber gloves and face protection.
2. Rinse all instruments in a large container filled with water and low-sudsing detergent.
3. Rinse instruments in clear water, separating delicate sharp instruments from general instruments.
4. Scrub each instrument under running water with brush and low-sudsing detergent.
5. Open all instruments, and scrub all hinged and serrated edges.
6. Rinse instruments thoroughly under hot water.
7. Roll instruments in towel, and dry them, checking the condition of each for defects and soil.
8. Dry instruments further with disposable paper towels.
9. Prepare for disinfection or sterilization.
10. Remove gloves and perform hand hygiene.

PROCEDURE 2-6

WRAPPING INSTRUMENTS FOR AUTOCLAVING

ABHES VII.MA.A.1 9(h)   CAAHEP III.P (5)

OBJECTIVE: To wrap sanitized instruments for autoclaving.

STANDARD: This procedure should take about 10 minutes.

EQUIPMENT AND SUPPLIES: Autoclave wrapping material or sterilization pouch; sterilization indicator strips; autoclave tape.

NOTE: Sterilization pouch may be used for individual instruments.

STEPS:

1. Perform hand hygiene.
2. Assemble instruments and supplies.
3. Place items in center of enough wrapping material to cover the entire article.
4. Place items in center, with open hinges and sharp items enclosed in a piece of gauze to prevent puncture of material.
5. Place indicator strip in center of packet.
6. Fold bottom point of wrapping material up and over instruments. Fold back a small flap for use when packet is unwrapped (Figure 2-4A).
7. Fold right side over until it covers items, and fold a small flap back as before (Figure 2-4B).
8. Fold left side over in same manner, including a small flap.
9. Fold bottom of package up until you have reached the top point (Figure 2-4C). Secure with a piece of autoclave tape (Figure 2-4D).

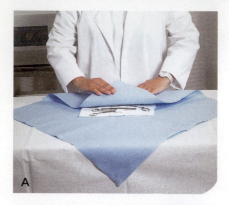 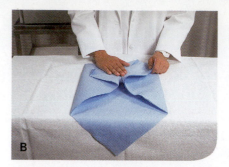

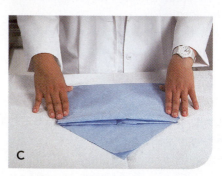 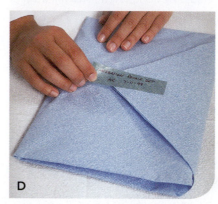

FIGURE 2-4 (A) Fold bottom point of wrap up over instruments. Fold small portion of point back over to use as a flap when unwrapping; (B) fold left side of wrap over instruments, and fold a small portion back for a flap; (C) fold up bottom of package, and continue until reaching top; (D) secure package with autoclave tape, then label with date, item name, and your initials.

10. Be sure the packet is folded snugly.
11. Label package with name of items, your initials, and the date.

NOTE: A variety of autoclave bags or pouches are available in different sizes. Some come in continuous rolls, and pieces can be cut off to fit the article, then ends are taped. Whatever type is used, label the bag with the name of the item, then date and initial it before inserting the instrument. Then add indicator strip and seal bag.

PROCEDURE 2-7

STERILIZING INSTRUMENTS IN AUTOCLAVE

ABHES VII.MA.A.1 9(o)4   CAAHEP III.P (5); III.P (6)

OBJECTIVE: To sterilize instruments in autoclave to prevent spread of pathogens.

STANDARD: This task takes approximately 1 hour.

EQUIPMENT AND SUPPLIES: Autoclave; instruments sanitized and wrapped for autoclaving; distilled water; autoclave directions.

STEPS:

1. Check level of water in the autoclave reservoir. Add distilled water as needed to the fill line.

2. Load autoclave. Load trays and packs on their sides. Place containers with lids on their sides with lids off or ajar. Load mixed loads with hard objects on bottom racks

and softer items on top racks. Keep large packs 2 to 4 inches apart and smaller packets 1 to 2 inches apart.

3. Read manufacturer's instructions and follow exactly. Most autoclaves follow protocols similar to the following:

   a. Turn control knob to "Fill" and observe carefully with door open until water reaches the chamber fill line.

   b. Turn knob to autoclave position. This shuts off the water.

   c. Close and lock the door.

   d. When pressure reaches 15 to 17 pounds and temperature reaches 250°F to 270°F, set timer for required time. Typical timing would be 30 minutes for wrapped trays and packages and 15 minutes for unwrapped items. Always check manufacturer's suggested times and facility protocol.

4. When timing is complete, turn control knob to " Vent."

5. When pressure reaches zero, open door about 1 inch and allow items in autoclave to dry completely before removing (about 30 to 45 minutes).

NOTE: Wet items and packages are considered contaminated and will have to be rewrapped and reautoclaved.

6. Turn autoclave knob to "Off."

7. Remove wrapped items and check autoclave tape on outside for color change. Store in dry closed cabinet for use. Always use sterile transfer forceps to remove unwrapped items, and place items on sterile field or in sterile storage area.

8. Record date, time, and types of items autoclaved in log and initial.

NOTE: Autoclaves, like any equipment, must be properly maintained and serviced according to manufacturer's directions. A maintenance log must be kept.

PROCEDURE 2-8

CHEMICALLY STERILIZING INSTRUMENTS

ABHES VII.MA.A.1 9(o)4   CAAHEP III.P (6)

OBJECTIVE: To chemically sterilize heat-sensitive instruments to prevent the spread of pathogens.

STANDARD: This task should take approximately 20 minutes.

EQUIPMENT AND SUPPLIES: Chemical disinfectant; goggles; disposable gloves; utility (rubber) gloves; sink glass, or stainless steel container with cover; sterile towels; sterile transfer forceps; sterile basin; sanitized articles.

NOTE: Before anything can be chemically sterilized, it must be sanitized properly as described in Procedure 2-5. Always read manufacturer's directions on the original chemical agent container.

STEPS:

1. Sanitize instrument appropriately.
2. Select type of chemical needed for instrument to be sterilized.
3. Read directions on the original germicidal agent label.

NOTE: If opening germicide for the first time write date on container and follow directions to prepare chemical agent.

4. Place chemical agent in appropriate container (large enough to submerge the instrument completely).
5. Cover tightly and record time, date, and your initials.
6. Do not open container during the sterilization process.
7. When sterilization timing is complete, remove instrument from container using sterile gloves or transfer forceps and rinse thoroughly with sterile water over a sterile basin. Hold instruments over basin a few moments to drain excess sterile water.
8. Dry instrument thoroughly with sterile towel and place on sterile field for use.

NOTE: Using a plastic-lined sterile drape prevents instrument from becoming wet, which could cause contamination.

9. Change chemical agent every 7 to 14 days or as recommended by manufacturer.
10. Perform hand hygiene after removing gloves.

PROCEDURE 2-9

PERFORMING TRANSMISSION-BASED PRECAUTION: ISOLATION TECHNIQUES

ABHES VII.MA.A.1 9(i)   CAAHEP III.P (3)

OBJECTIVE: To provide barrier protection for caregivers to prevent the spread of infectious diseases.

STANDARD: This task takes 5 minutes.

EQUIPMENT AND SUPPLIES: Disposable gowns; masks; caps; nonsterile gloves; sterile gloves; sink and running water; paper towels.

STEPS:

1. Review orders and agency protocols regarding isolation procedures.

NOTE: Office-based personnel may not use transmission-based precautions often, but they should be familiar with the necessary equipment and how to use it.

2. Assemble appropriate and necessary PPE.
3. Remove lab coat and jewelry.
4. Perform hand hygiene (Procedure 2-2).
5. Don appropriate disposable apparel.
   - Apply cap to cover hair and ears completely.
   - Apply gown over outer garments as follows: Hold gown in front of body. Place arms through sleeves. Pull sleeves on, covering wrists. Tie securely at neck and waist.
   - Apply mask by placing top of mask over bridge of nose and pinch metal strip to secure snug fit on nose,

tying if needed (Figures 2-5A, 2-5B, 2-5C, and 2-5D). Don protective eyewear.
   - Don nonsterile gloves, and pull up over gown cuffs to cover wrists completely.
   - Perform patient tasks as needed, and exit isolation area.

6. Remove barrier protections in the following order:
   - Untie waist of gown.
   - Remove gloves (Procedure 2-4).
   - Wash hands (Procedure 2-2).
   - Untie neck of gown. Remove gown by pulling down from shoulders, turning gown inside out and pulling out arms from sleeves.

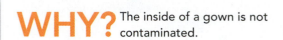

WHY? The inside of a gown is not contaminated.

   - Holding the gown away from you with contaminated area on inside, fold and place in biohazard waste container.
   - Remove protective eyewear.
   - Remove mask and discard.

7. Perform hand hygiene.

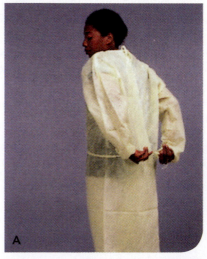 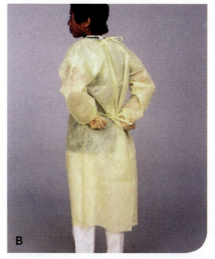

FIGURE 2-5   Technique for donning and removing a nonsterile gown. (A) Tie the neck piece of gown and overlap flaps; (B) tie the gown securely at the waist. Put on gloves, and pull cuffs over gown at wrists.

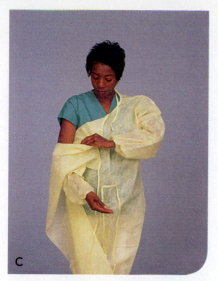

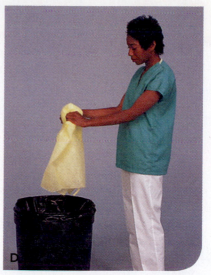

FIGURE 2-5 (Continued) (C) to take off gown, remove and dispose of gloves properly, then untie neck and waist, grasp shoulders, and turn gown inside out as it is removed; (D) fold up gown and discard. Do not reuse a gown. Wash hands.

3 Vital Signs and Mensuration

PROCEDURES

Procedure 3-1 Measuring Oral Temperature with Glass Nonmercury Thermometer

Procedure 3-2 Measuring Rectal Temperature Using Glass Nonmercury Thermometer

Procedure 3-3 Cleaning and Storing Glass Nonmercury Thermometer

Procedure 3-4 Measuring Oral Temperature Using Electronic or Digital Thermometer

Procedure 3-5 Measuring Rectal Temperature Using Electronic or Digital Thermometer

Procedure 3-6 Measuring Temperature Using Aural (Tympanic Membrane) Thermometer

Procedure 3-7 Measuring Dermal Temperature Using Disposable Thermometer

Procedure 3-8 Measuring Axillary Temperature

Procedure 3-9 Measuring Temperature with Temporal Artery Thermometer

Procedure 3-10 Measuring Radial Pulse

Procedure 3-11 Measuring Apical Pulse

Procedure 3-12 Measuring Apical–Radial Pulse (two person)

Procedure 3-13 Measuring Respirations

Procedure 3-14 Measuring Systolic Pressure Using Palpatory Method

Procedure 3-15 Measuring Systolic/Diastolic Blood Pressure Using Sphygmomanometer

Procedure 3-16 Measuring Oxygen Saturation Using a Pulse Oximeter

Procedure 3-17 Measuring Adult Height and Weight

Procedure 3-18 Calculating Adult Body Mass Index

Procedure 3-19 Determining Fat Fold Measurement in Adults

TERMS TO LEARN

homeostasis

frenulum linguae

pulse deficit

pulse pressure

anthropometry

One of the first interactions the medical staff has with patients occurs when measuring vitals signs and performing body measurements. Vital signs, also known as cardinal signs, are basic indicators of processes in the body that sustain life. Vital signs include temperature (T), pulse (P), respiration (R), blood pressure (BP), and pain. These signs reflect the general health of the patient. Vital signs are measured each time a patient is seen in most health care settings. Height and weight measurements also are usually performed with each office visit. All these measurements provide a baseline of data for future patient encounters. Care must be taken that all are performed accurately and documented correctly. Treatment effectiveness and patient compliance are assessed based on vital signs data and height and weight measurements.

Vital signs vary with time of day, patient's response (level of anxiety), eating and drinking immediately before being seen, mood, environmental temperature, and presence of disease. Weight and height may vary, depending on whether or not the patient is wearing shoes. Calculation of body mass index (BMI) is based on accurate measurement of height and weight and employment of a formula to obtain the result. BMI is particularly important in tracking patients with eating disorders.

Temperature

Temperature is regulated by producing and releasing heat from the body to maintain **homeostasis** or a balanced state. Several sites in the body may be used to obtain body temperature:

- Mouth (O)
- Ear (Tym)
- Rectum (R)
- Axilla (A)
- Temporal artery (TA)

Because the normal ranges vary slightly at different sites, when documenting body temperature it is important to indicate which site was used. Table 3-1 lists average body temperature ranges at various sites. Temporal artery (TA) measurement is a new noninvasive procedure involving a thermometer that measures the temperature over the temporal artery. Studies have shown that TA thermometer measurements are more accurate than measurements made with tympanic and rectal thermometers. TA thermometers may be used on adults as well as children. One brand of temporal artery thermometer is being used in some hospitals as it is more cost effective and accurate than ear thermometers and takes 0.1 second to respond.

TABLE 3-1 Average Body Temperature Ranges at Various Body Locations

Type	Site	Range
Oral	Mouth	97.6°–99.6°F 36.5°–37°C
Rectal	Rectum	98.6°–100.6°F 37°–38.1°C
Axillary	Armpit	96.6°–98.6°F 35.9°–37°C
Tympanic Membrane	Ear	98.6°F 37°C
Temporal Artery	Forehead	98.6°–100.6°F 37°–38.1°C

Arterial temperature is close to rectal temperature, about 1 degree higher than oral temperature and 2 degrees higher than axillary temperature. Temporal artery readings are not affected by factors such as smoking, drinking, and coughing that may interfere with oral measurement.

When measuring TA temperature assess the side of the head that is exposed, not the side covered by hair or resting on a pillow. The latter may cause a higher reading because heat is not allowed to dissipate. Slide the thermometer in a fairly straight line across the forehead midway between the eyebrows and the hairline. (Do not slide it down the side of the face.) At this point the temporal artery is less than 2 mm below the surface of the skin. The temporal artery thermometer is quick, accurate, noninvasive, and easy to use.

Several other types of thermometers are available for measuring body temperature. Nonmercury glass thermometers have replaced the mercury-filled thermometers in most institutions due to the toxicity of mercury. These may be used orally, rectally, or in the axillary area. They contain gallium or alcohol; however, because of the danger of breakage, nonmercury glass thermometers are not as extensively used as electronic, digital, or chemical thermometers.

Electronic thermometers are widely used in hospitals because they are accurate, sanitary, user friendly, and quick to provide results. Inexpensive digital thermometers are available for home use. Parents should be encouraged to switch to digital thermometers and make arrangements to dispose of glass mercury units. Tympanic thermometers can detect heat waves within the ear canal and calculate body temperature from the data. Disposable thermometers are available in a variety of forms. Chemical disposable thermometers use liquid dots, heat-sensitive bars, or patches applied to the forehead that change color to indicate body temperature. Certain types of chemical disposable thermometers may be used orally as well; some are single use, and others may be reused several times. Special heat-sensitive wearable thermometers may be applied to a patient's forehead for up to 2 days. The temperature is read by color change of the dots. Both tympanic and chemical disposable thermometers are easy to use on children.

Oral and rectal thermometers must be cleaned and stored separately. Axillary thermometers may be stored with oral ones. Cleaning and storage depend on the policy of the facility. Disposable covers or probes are used with digital, electronic, and tympanic thermometers. The units are cleaned according to the manufacturer's directions.

Procedures 3-1 through 3-9 list steps for measuring body temperature using a variety of thermometers at different sites.

PROCEDURE 3-1

MEASURING ORAL TEMPERATURE WITH GLASS NONMERCURY THERMOMETER

ABHES VII.MA.A.1 9(C)   CAAHEP I.P (1)

OBJECTIVE: To measure oral temperature accurately, performing all steps of procedure.

STANDARD: This task takes 5 minutes (for cleaning, preparing, shaking down thermometer, measuring the temperature, and waiting 3 to 5 minutes to read thermometer, then cleaning again).

EQUIPMENT AND SUPPLIES: Oral glass nonmercury thermometers; disposable plastic sheath; watch with second hand; biohazard waste container; patient's chart; paper and pencil; nonsterile gloves.

STEPS:

1. Check physician's orders, and check for patient allergies.
2. Perform hand hygiene.
3. Apply gloves.
4. Identify patient.

5. Ask if patient has taken hot or cold drink or smoked in previous 15–30 minutes. If yes, then wait 15 minutes before proceeding.
6. Take thermometer out of container. If stored in disinfectant, rinse thoroughly under cool water.
7. Read thermometer (Figure 3-1A). If it is not at 95°F, shake down to that reading while firmly holding the end of the glass shaft with thumb and index finger (Figure 3-1B).
8. Place plastic sheath on thermometer.
9. Place sheathed thermometer bulb end in patient's mouth sublingually on either side of the **frenulum linguae** (fold of tissue beneath tongue that anchors tongue to bottom of mouth).
10. Ask patient to close mouth, hold thermometer with lips, and not talk (Figure 3-1C).
11. Leave thermometer in place 3 minutes.

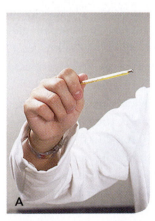
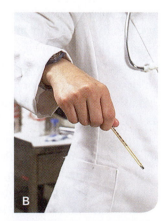
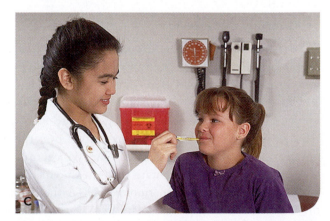

FIGURE 3-1   (A) Inspect the thermometer; (B) shake down the thermometer; (C) place thermometer under tongue after inserting it into thermometer sheath.

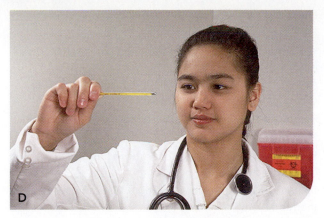 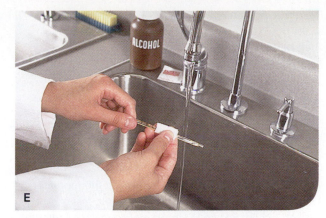

FIGURE 3-1 (Continued) (D) read the thermometer; (E) wash the thermometer with soap and warm water.

12. Remove from patient's mouth and read. If reading is below 97°F, reinsert for several minutes (Figure 3-1D).

13. Take sheath off and discard in biohazard waste container. Read thermometer accurately, and write down the results.

14. Follow procedure for temporary storage of thermometers.

15. Remove gloves and discard in biohazard waste container.

16. Perform hand hygiene.

17. Record reading in patient's chart (O).

18. Follow Procedure 3-3 for cleaning and storage of thermometers (Figure 3-1E).

CHARTING EXAMPLE: 2/14/XX 10:02 A.M. T 99.2°F (O) · · · ·
· A. Martinez, CMA (AAMA)

PROCEDURE 3-2

MEASURING RECTAL TEMPERATURE USING GLASS NONMERCURY THERMOMETER

ABHES VII.MA.A.1 9(C)   CAAHEP I.P (1)

OBJECTIVE: To measure rectal temperature accurately by performing all the procedural steps properly.

STANDARD: This task takes 5–10 minutes.

EQUIPMENT AND SUPPLIES: Rectal nonmercury glass thermometer; disposable thermometer sheaths; disposable gloves; patient's record; paper and pencil; tissue; watch with second hand; water-soluble lubricant; and biohazard waste container.

STEPS:

1. Check physician's orders, and check for patient allergies.
2. Perform hand hygiene.
3. Apply gloves.
4. Identify patient.
5. Explain procedure. If patient is child, explain to both parent and child.
6. Instruct patient to remove appropriate clothing so that rectal area is exposed while providing privacy for patient.
7. Assist patient onto exam table, and drape patient for privacy.
8. Place a small amount of lubricant on tissue.
9. Remove rectal thermometer from packaging, holding firmly by end, and inspect for defects.

WHY? Why and when would you measure rectal temperature rather than oral or aural? Rectal temperature is measured for an unconscious patient, one who is nauseous, a small child, or a patient who has had oral surgery. Glass nonmercury thermometers are not used rectally for the most part because of the availability of other thermometers that are easier to use, require less time, and are less dangerous.

10. Read thermometer. If it is not 95°F, firmly snap wrist to shake down to that point while holding the end of glass shaft between thumb and index finger.

11. Place plastic sheath on thermometer, and apply lubricant by rolling bulb end in lubricant on tissue.

12. Instruct patient to lie on left side with right leg bent (Sims' position).

13. With one hand, raise patient's upper buttock to expose anal opening. If unable to see anal opening, ask patient to bear down slightly, which will expose it.

14. With other hand, gently insert lubricated thermometer 1½ inches into anal canal if patient is adult. Insert ½ inch if patient is child. Rotate thermometer to make penetration easier.

15. Hold in place 3 minutes.

16. Withdraw thermometer, and dispose of sheath in biohazard waste container.

17. Read thermometer, and write result on piece of paper.

18. Place thermometer back on tissue until procedure finished.

19. Wipe anus from front to back to remove excess lubricant.

20. Assist patient from exam table, and instruct patient to dress; offer assistance if necessary.

21. Remove gloves, and place in biohazard waste container.

22. Perform hand hygiene.

23. Record temperature in patient's record using "(R)" to indicate rectal.

24. Follow Procedure 3-3 for cleaning and disinfecting soiled thermometers.

CHARTING EXAMPLE: 2/14/XX 7:00 A.M. T 99.8°F (R) · A. Martinez, CMA (AAMA)

NOTE: Rather than glass thermometers, other available rectal thermometers should be used if possible to avoid risk of breakage.

PROCEDURE 3-3

CLEANING AND STORING GLASS NONMERCURY THERMOMETER

ABHES VII.MA.A.1 9(k)   CAAHEP I.P (10)

OBJECTIVE: Correctly clean, inspect, disinfect, and store glass nonmercury thermometers to prevent spread of pathogens.

STANDARD: This task takes about 30 minutes.

EQUIPMENT AND SUPPLIES: 70% isopropyl alcohol or other disinfectant for thermometer use; container with soiled thermometers; cotton balls; soap; utility or disposable gloves; water; biohazard waste container.

STEPS:

1. Perform hand hygiene.

2. Apply gloves.

3. Take soiled thermometers to sink.

4. Liberally apply soap and water to cotton balls, and wipe each thermometer from stem to bulb with friction while rotating the glass stem.

5. Discard cotton balls in biohazard waste container.

6. Rinse thermometers under cool running water while holding the stem.

7. Inspect for cleanliness and defects. If still soiled, wash again.

8. While holding by stem, shake down thermometer to at least 95°F with quick snapping motion of wrist.

9. Place thermometer in a container filled with disinfectant, covering completely.

10. Set timer for 20 minutes.

11. Wash thermometer storage container, which previously held dirty thermometers, with soap, water, and disinfectant.

12. Remove gloves, and perform hand hygiene.

13. After 20 minutes, remove thermometers, rinse under cool water, and place in disinfected storage container for next use.

PROCEDURE 3-4

MEASURING ORAL TEMPERATURE USING ELECTRONIC OR DIGITAL THERMOMETER

ABHES VII.MA.A.1 9(c)   CAAHEP I.P (1)

OBJECTIVE: To accurately measure patient's body temperature by performing all steps of procedure.

STANDARD: This task takes 5 minutes.

EQUIPMENT AND SUPPLIES: Electronic or digital thermometer (rechargeable); probe cover; biohazard waste container; pen; patient's record.

STEPS:

1. Check physician's orders, and check for patient allergies.
2. Perform hand hygiene.
3. Assemble equipment.
4. Identify patient, and explain procedure.
5. Remove thermometer unit from base and attach probe (blue for oral thermometer).
6. Remove thermometer probe from holder.
7. Insert thermometer probe into disposable tip box (Figure 3-2A).

8. Insert thermometer into patient's mouth on either side of frenulum linguae, and instruct patient to close mouth.
9. When thermometer signal is seen or heard, remove thermometer from patient's mouth and read the result in the LED window.
10. Dispose of the thermometer tip in biohazard waste container (Figure 3-2B). Return thermometer probe to storage place (Figure 3-2C).
11. Replace unit on rechargeable base.
12. Perform hand hygiene.
13. Document results.

CHARTING EXAMPLE: 2/14/XX 12:30 P.M. T 100.2°F (O)
. . . . H. Martinez, CMA (AAMA)

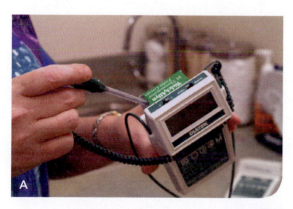

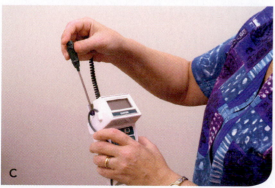

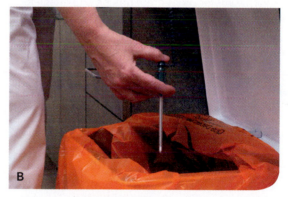

FIGURE 3-2   Using the electronic thermometer. (A) Insert probe into probe cover; (B) after measuring the temperature, press to eject the probe cover into hazardous waste container; (C) replace the probe in the holder.

PROCEDURE 3-5

MEASURING RECTAL TEMPERATURE USING ELECTRONIC OR DIGITAL THERMOMETER

ABHES VII.MA.A.1 9(c)   CAAHEP I.P (1)

OBJECTIVE: To accurately measure patient's rectal temperature, performing all steps of procedure.

STANDARD: This task takes 5 minutes.

EQUIPMENT AND SUPPLIES: Electronic or digital thermometer (rechargeable); probe cover; lubricating jelly; biohazard waste container; pen; patient's record; tissue.

STEPS:

1. Check physician's orders, and check for patient allergies.
2. Perform hand hygiene.
3. Assemble equipment.
4. Identify patient, and explain procedure.
5. Place disposable plastic-lined drape or pad on table to prevent contamination.
6. Ask patient to remove clothing from waist down. Assist patient into Sims' position, and drape patient to protect privacy.
7. Remove thermometer probe from holder, and attach red probe for measuring rectal temperature.
8. Insert thermometer probe into disposable-tip box to secure tip.
9. Put on gloves.
10. Lubricate thermometer probe (see Procedure 3-2) for easier insertion.
11. Spread buttocks, and insert thermometer 1½ inches for an adult (½ inch for child).
12. Hold buttocks together until thermometer beeps.
13. Read results on digital display.
14. Remove thermometer from rectum, and discard probe in biohazard waste container.
15. Replace thermometer in holder base.
16. Offer patient tissue to wipe rectum, or offer assistance if needed.
17. Assist patient off table and with dressing if needed.
18. Remove gloves, and discard in biohazard waste container.
19. Perform hand hygiene.
20. Record results in patient's record.

CHARTING EXAMPLE: 2/13/XX 9:00 A.M. T 102.4°F (R) · H. Campo, CMA (AAMA)

PROCEDURE 3-6

MEASURING TEMPERATURE USING AURAL (TYMPANIC MEMBRANE) THERMOMETER

ABHES VII.MA.A.1 9(c)   CAAHEP I.P (1)

OBJECTIVE: To accurately measure aural temperature by performing all steps of procedure.

STANDARD: This task takes 3 minutes.

EQUIPMENT AND SUPPLIES: Tympanic membrane thermometer; disposable protective probe covers; paper and pen; patient's record; biohazard waste container.

STEPS:

1. Check physician's orders, and check for patient allergies.
2. Perform hand hygiene.
3. Identify patient.
4. Explain procedure to patient.

5. Remove thermometer from base. Display should read "Ready."

6. Gently straighten ear canal by pulling up and back for adult, down and back for child.

7. Press scan button to activate thermometer.

8. Wait until temperature is displayed on screen.

9. Remove from ear.

10. Eject probe cover into biohazard waste container.

11. Perform hand hygiene.

12. Record temperature using the designation (Tym) to indicate tympanic membrane thermometer.

NOTE: Tympanic membrane thermometers can be set to correlate with either an oral or rectal reading. Check manufacturer's directions.

CHARTING EXAMPLE: 2/14/XX 7:05 P.M. T 98.4°F (Tym) · · · ·
· L. Brown, RMA

PROCEDURE 3-7

MEASURING DERMAL TEMPERATURE USING DISPOSABLE THERMOMETER

ABHES VII.MA.A.1 9(c)   CAAHEP I.P (1)

OBJECTIVE: To accurately measure temperature using disposable thermometer, performing all steps of procedure.

STANDARD: This task takes 3 minutes.

EQUIPMENT AND SUPPLIES: Dot-matrix single-use thermometer; watch; biohazard waste container; paper and pen; patient's record.

STEPS:

1. Check physician's orders, and check for patient allergies.

2. Perform hand hygiene.

3. Assemble equipment.

4. Identify patient.

5. Explain procedure.

6. Carefully unwrap the dermal strip without touching the chemical dots and place it on the forehead.

7. Leave the strip on the forehead for the length of time recommended by the manufacturer, usually about 15 seconds.

8. Note the temperature of the last color-changed dot (Figures 3-3A and 3-3B).

9. Record temperature in patient's chart.

10. Remove the thermometer from the patient's forehead.

11. Dispose of used thermometer in biohazard waste container.

12. Perform hand hygiene.

CHARTING EXAMPLE: 2/14/XX 9:15 A.M. T 100.2°F (dermal)
· T. Antonelli, RMA

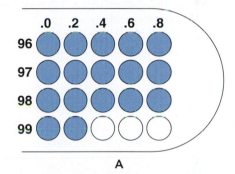

A

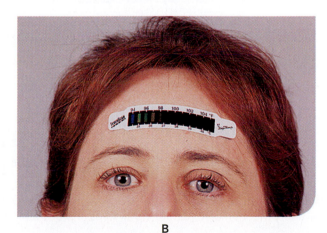

B

FIGURE 3-3   (A) Disposable thermometer with chemical dots. Read the temperature by looking at the last colored dot; (B) temperature-sensitive tape on patient's forehead.

PROCEDURE 3-8

MEASURING AXILLARY TEMPERATURE

ABHES VII.MA.A.1 9(c)   CAAHEP I.P (1)

OBJECTIVE: To accurately measure axillary temperature, performing all steps of procedure.

STANDARD: This task takes 10 minutes.

EQUIPMENT AND SUPPLIES: Mercury-free glass thermometer or electronic thermometer; paper and pen; watch with second hand; thermometer sheaths; tissues; patient's record.

STEPS:

1. Check physician's orders, and check for patient allergies.
2. Perform hand hygiene.
3. Identify patient.
4. Explain procedure.
5. Take glass thermometer out of container and rinse in cool water if stored in disinfectant. Inspect thermometer for defects and discard if damaged.
6. For electronic thermometer, attach probe as indicated in Procedure 3-5.
7. Read glass thermometer and shake down to 95°F, holding the stem end securely between thumb and index finger.
8. Ask patient to expose axilla. Provide gown for privacy if necessary.
9. Using tissues, pat axilla dry of perspiration.
10. Place plastic sheath on glass thermometer.
11. Place thermometer under armpit, making sure it contacts patient's skin.
12. Ask patient to hold still and hold arm tightly against body, taking care not to break glass thermometer.
13. Leave thermometer in place for 6 to 9 minutes or until electronic thermometer beeps. Do not leave patient unattended.
14. Remove glass thermometer after designated minutes elapsed. Read, and if lower than 96°F reinsert for several more minutes. Read electronic thermometer after beeping.
15. Remove sheath or eject probe, and discard in biohazard waste container.
16. Read and record results in patient's record.
17. Follow procedure for soiled glass thermometers (see Procedure 3-3).
18. Perform hand hygiene.

NOTE: Axillary temperature also may be assessed using dot-matrix or digital thermometer. Manufacturers' recommendations for timing should be followed.

CHARTING EXAMPLE: 2/14/XX 8:00 A.M. T 99.0°F (A) · · · · · ·
· C. Blardo, CMA (AAMA)

PROCEDURE 3-9

MEASURING TEMPERATURE WITH TEMPORAL ARTERY THERMOMETER

ABHES VII.MA.A.1 9(c)   CAAHEP I.P (1)

OBJECTIVE: To accurately measure temperature using a temporal artery thermometer, performing all steps of procedure.

STANDARD: This task should take less than 5 minutes.

EQUIPMENT AND SUPPLIES: Temporal artery thermometer; paper and pen; watch with second hand; tissues; patient's record.

STEPS:

1. Check physician's orders, and check for patient allergies.
2. Perform hand hygiene.
3. Assemble equipment.
4. Identify patient.
5. Explain procedure.

6. Using exposed side of head (not resting on pillow), brush hair aside. If forehead is damp, dry with tissue.

7. Place probe flush on the center of the forehead, and depress the red button.

8. Keep the button depressed, and slowly slide the probe on the midline across the forehead to the hairline.

9. Lift the probe from the forehead, and touch it on the neck just behind the earlobe.

10. Release the button and read.

11. Record the results in the patient's record.

12. Perform hand hygiene.

CHARTING EXAMPLE: 12/18/XX 10:00 A.M. T 100°F (TA)
. . . . L. Cohen, CMA (AAMA)

Pulse

Each pulse beat represents one heartbeat or cardiac cycle. The pulse beat is caused by the blood exerting pressure on the arterial walls during the contraction (systole) phase of the cardiac cycle. Each wave of contraction, or beat, can be felt in areas of the body where arteries are closest to the surface. When the heart rests, the pressure on the arterial wall decreases (known as diastole). The wave of expansion and contraction is felt as a pulse beat. Figure 3-4 illustrates the nine pulse locations in the body. Table 3-2 explains in more detail the pulse sites and their locations.

Normal pulse rate in an adult is 60–100 beats per minute. Many factors influence pulse rates such as illness, exercise, temperature, age, medications, and mood. In addition to counting the number of pulse beats per minute, other pulse qualities should be noted: volume (strength of pulse beat), rhythm (regularity or spacing of beats), and compliance of the arterial wall (elastic, soft or hard and ropelike). The radial artery in adults is most commonly used to obtain pulse rate. Procedure 3-10 provides the method for measuring patient's pulse rate at the wrist. The pulse is measured for one full minute unless office policy states otherwise.

The apical heart rate is the number of beats per minute measured at the apex of the heart. It is measured by placing a stethoscope over the apex. The apex of the heart is located at the fifth intercostal space on the left at the midclavicular line. The stethoscope is placed between the fifth and sixth ribs in a line down from the middle of the clavicle or collar bone (Figure 3-6). Apical pulse (AP) is used on infants and young children and on some cardiac patients. The method for measuring apical pulse is given in Procedure 3-11.

Apical–radial pulse rate is measured to determine if the two rates differ. It is measured for 1 full minute. Normally the pulse rates should be the same. The radial pulse is never greater than the apical pulse. The difference between the two is called the **pulse deficit**. Two people are necessary to perform this procedure. One takes the radial pulse, and simultaneously the other takes the apical pulse. Refer to Procedure 3-12 for taking an apical–radial pulse.

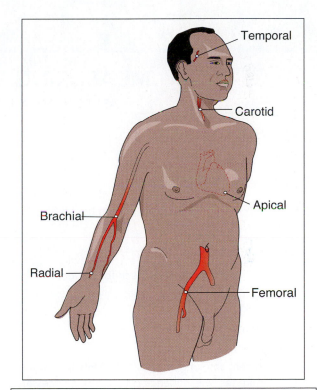

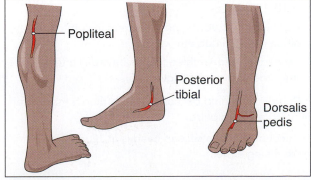

FIGURE 3-4 **Nine sites for measuring pulse.**

TABLE 3-2 Location of Common Pulse Sites

Site	Location
Apical	At apex of heart, left of sternum, 4th–5th intercostal space below nipple
Brachial	Inner (antecubital fossa/space) aspect of elbow (pulse heard when taking BP)
Carotid	At side of neck between larynx and sternocleidomastoid muscle (pulse used in CPR; pressing both carotids at same time can cause a reflex drop in BP and pulse)
Dorsalis pedis	On top of foot, slightly lateral to midline; helps assess adequate circulation to foot
Femoral	In groin where femoral artery passes to leg
Popliteal	Behind knee; pulse is located deeply behind knee and can be felt when knee slightly bent
Posterior tibial	On medial surface of ankle near ankle bone
Radial	Thumb side of wrist, about 1 inch below base of thumb (most frequently used site)
Temporal	At side of head just above ear

PROCEDURE 3-10

MEASURING RADIAL PULSE

ABHES VII.MA.A.1 9(c)   CAAHEP I.P (1)

OBJECTIVE: To accurately measure radial pulse, performing all steps of procedure.

STANDARD: This task takes 3–5 minutes.

EQUIPMENT AND SUPPLIES: Paper; pen; patient's record; watch with second hand.

STEPS:

1. Check physician's orders, and check for patient allergies.
2. Perform hand hygiene.
3. Identify patient.
4. Explain procedure.
5. Ask about recent smoking or physical activity during preceding 15 minutes (will influence pulse rate). If necessary wait 10–15 minutes.
6. Ask patient to sit down and place arm in comfortable position on lap or table.
7. Place pads of middle three fingers on radial artery on the thumb side of the wrist (Figure 3-5).

NOTE: Do not use thumb because pulse in thumb may be felt in addition to patient's pulse.

8. Start counting when second hand is at 12, 3, 6, or 9 to make timing easier.

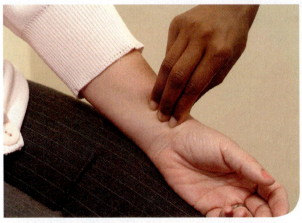

FIGURE 3-5 Palpate radial pulse by using pads of middle three fingers, not thumb, for accurate results.

9. Count pulse for 1 full minute. If facility policy permits, count for 30 seconds unless pulse is irregular, in which case 1 minute is required.
10. Note quality of pulse.
11. Write pulse rate and quality on piece of paper.
12. Perform hand hygiene.
13. Record pulse beats per minute in patient's chart.

CHARTING EXAMPLE: 2/14/XX 9:00 A.M. P 78 · · · · · · · · · ·
· A. Martinez, CMA (AAMA)

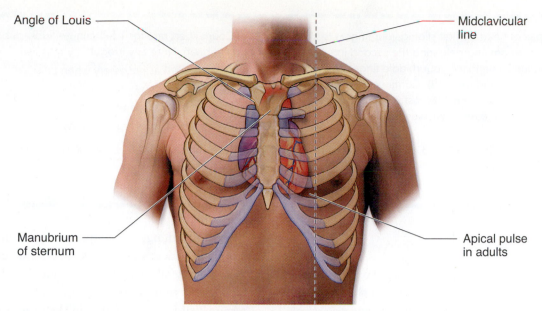

Angle of Louis

Midclavicular line

Manubrium of sternum

Apical pulse in adults

FIGURE 3-6 Apical pulse site in adult.

PROCEDURE 3-11

MEASURING APICAL PULSE

ABHES VII.MA.A.1 9(c)   CAAHEP I.P (1)

OBJECTIVE: To accurately perform apical pulse measurement, performing all the steps of the procedure.

STANDARD: This task takes 3–5 minutes.

EQUIPMENT AND SUPPLIES: Stethoscope; alcohol wipe/cotton ball with 70% isopropyl alcohol; watch with second hand, patient's record; pen.

STEPS:

1. Check physician's orders, and check for patient allergies.

2. Perform hand hygiene.

3. Prepare stethoscope by cleaning the diaphragm and earpieces with alcohol.

4. Identify patient.

5. Explain procedure thoroughly.

6. Uncover left side of patient's chest, providing privacy with drape if necessary.

7. Place earpieces in ears.

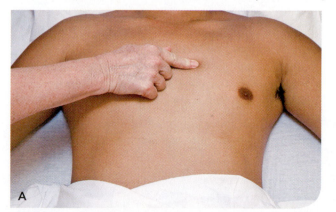

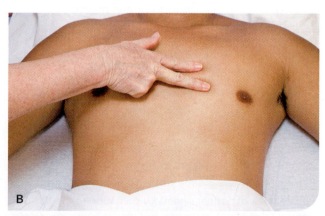

FIGURE 3-7 (A) Slide index finger to left of sternum and palpate 2nd intercostal space; (B) place middle and index finger at third intercostal space and continue palpating downward to the fifth intercostal space and on to the midclavicular line (MCL), where apical pulse is heard.

8. Locate apex of heart by first sliding your fingers to the left of the sternum and palpating the second intercostal space (Figure 3-7A). Place your middle finger on the third intercostal space (Figure 3-7B). Continue palpating downward to the left fifth intercostal space (between fifth and sixth ribs) at the midclavicular line (just below left nipple).

9. Warm diaphragm by holding in palm of hand before placing on patient's chest at apex of heart.

10. Count heart rate for 1 full minute (lubb-dubb sound is one beat). Note any irregularity to pulse.

11. Assist patient as necessary when finished.

12. Clean stethoscope.

13. Perform hand hygiene.

14. Record apical pulse rate and rhythm.

CHARTING EXAMPLE: 2/14/XX 10:00 A.M. Apical Pulse 82
· A. Martinez, CMA (AAMA)

Respiration

Respiration or breathing is the exchange of oxygen and carbon dioxide between the atmosphere and the body cells. One respiration consists of one inhalation and one exhalation. When counting a patient's respiratory rate, watch the rise and fall of the chest. Each rise and fall together equals one respiration. Because patients have voluntary control over their breathing, it is important to count respirations without the patient's awareness. The pulse and respiratory rate are usually taken at the same time. While holding the patient's wrist to measure the pulse rate, count the number of respirations for 30 seconds and then count the pulse rate for the remaining 30 seconds. Multiply each value by 2, and document accurately. The normal adult respiratory rate is 12 to 20 cycles per minute. Children have a much more

PROCEDURE 3-12

MEASURING APICAL–RADIAL PULSE (TWO PERSON)

ABHES VII.MA.A.1 9(c)   CAAHEP I.P (1)

OBJECTIVE: To accurately perform all steps of procedure and provide an accurate apical–radial pulse.

STANDARD: This task takes 5–10 minutes.

EQUIPMENT AND SUPPLIES: Watch with second hand; stethoscope; alcohol wipes; paper and pen; patient's record; additional trained staff person to assist with procedure.

STEPS:

1. Check physician's orders, and check for patient allergies.

2. Perform hand hygiene.

3. Clean stethoscope earpieces and diaphragm with alcohol.

4. Identify patient.

5. Explain procedure.

6. Place patient in supine position, and uncover left side of patient's chest, providing privacy with drape if necessary.

7. Place watch where clearly visible to both caregivers.

8. Locate apex of patient's heart by palpating to the fifth left intercostal space at midclavicular line just below the nipple.

9. Warm chest piece by holding in palm of hand before placing on patient's chest.

10. First person places earpieces of stethoscope in ears.

11. Second person locates radial pulse on thumb side of wrist.

12. First person places chest piece of stethoscope at apex of heart. When heartbeat is heard, a nod is made to the second person, and simultaneous counting begins. Begin counting if possible when the second hand is at 12, 3, 6, or 9 on watch.

13. Count for 1 full minute (lubb-dubb counts as one beat).

14. Remove stethoscope and earpieces.

15. Record rate and quality of apical and radial rates, using AP designation. Calculate pulse deficit by subtracting radial pulse rate from apical pulse rate.

NOTE: A pulse deficit may indicate that heart contractions are not strong enough to produce a palpable radial pulse.

16. Assist patient as needed.

17. Clean stethoscope.

18. Perform hand hygiene.

CHARTING EXAMPLE: 2/14/XX 1:00 P.M. Apical Pulse 84; Radial P 82; Pulse Deficit = 2 · · · · · · · · · · · · S. Martin, RMA

TABLE 3-3 Abnormal Breath Sounds and Respiratory Patterns

Abnormal Breath Sounds	Description
Bubbling	Gurgling sounds as air passes through moist secretions in airways
Friction rub	Dry rubbing or grating sound
Rales	Crackling sound usually at inspiration as air passes through moist secretions in airways
Rhonchi	Low-pitched continuous sound as air moves past thick mucus or through narrowed air passages
Stertor	Snoring sound on inspiration or expiration; possible partial airway obstruction
Stridor	Shrill, harsh inspiratory sound; indicates laryngeal obstruction
Wheeze	High-pitched sound on inspiration or expiration; indicates partial airway obstruction

Abnormal Respiratory Patterns	Description
Apnea	No respirations
Bradypnea	Slow respirations
Cheyne-Stokes	Rhythmic cycles of dyspnea or hyperpnea, subsiding gradually into brief apnea
Dyspnea	Difficult or labored respirations
Hypopnea	Shallow respirations
Hyperpnea	Deep respirations
Orthopnea	Inability to breathe except while sitting or standing
Tachypnea	Fast respirations

rapid respiratory rate than adults with an average of 30 to 50 cycles per minute. As with other vital signs, many factors may influence respiratory rate, including exercise, emotion, and high altitude. The quality of the respirations should be noted for rate, rhythm, depth, and abnormal characteristics. Table 3-3 lists terms associated with abnormal breath sounds and respiratory patterns. These terms and conditions are important when documenting patients' results. Procedure 3-13 indicates the method for measuring respirations.

PROCEDURE 3-13

MEASURING RESPIRATIONS

ABHES VII.MA.A.1 9(c)   CAAHEP I.P (1)

OBJECTIVE: Accurately perform all steps of the procedure and obtain accurate respiration rate.

STANDARD: This task takes 3–5 minutes.

EQUIPMENT AND SUPPLIES: Watch with second hand; pen and paper.

STEPS:

1. Check physician's orders, and check for patient allergies.

2. Perform hand hygiene.

3. Identify patient.

4. Place your hand on patient's wrist in position to take pulse. Arm may be placed across patient's chest to make it easier to notice the rise and fall of the chest.

5. Count each breathing cycle by observing the rise and fall of the chest without indicating to the patient what you are doing.

NOTE: Patients may alter breathing cycle by laughing or talking if they are aware of what you are doing.

6. Count for 1 full minute using watch unless facility policy differs.

NOTE: It is convenient to take respiratory rate and pulse one following the other so patient is unaware.

7. Record respiratory rate and any abnormality in rate, rhythm, and depth.

8. Perform hand hygiene.

CHARTING EXAMPLE: 2/14/XX 8:00 A.M. R 16 · · · · · · · · ·
· S. Martin, RMA

Blood Pressure

Blood pressure, another of the vital signs, is caused by the action of blood pressing on the walls of arteries. It is an important indication of cardiac function. Blood pressure measurements or readings indicate the pressure in the arteries when the heart is contracting. This is represented by the upper reading in the blood pressure fraction (systole). The second reading represents the pressure on the arteries when the heart is at rest. This is the lower reading in the blood pressure fraction (diastole). An example would be systole/diastole, or 120/80 mm Hg. **Pulse pressure** is the difference between the systolic and diastolic readings. A pulse pressure greater than 50 mm Hg or less than 30 mm Hg is considered abnormal. Blood pressure is affected by many factors, among which are weight, elasticity of arterial walls, blood volume, condition of heart muscle, viscosity of blood, and body position. When a patient's blood pressure reading is taken in recumbent position and then in standing position, the systolic can fall as much as 10 to 15 points, and diastolic may rise 5 points.

Blood pressure is measured by listening to the changes of sounds with a stethoscope when the blood pressure cuff (sphygmomanometer) is inflated and then the pressure is slowly released. These sounds are known as Korotkoff sounds and represent the sounds from the arterial walls. Box 3-1 lists the Korotkoff sounds and the phases they represent.

The three main types of equipment used in ambulatory care facilities for measuring blood pressure are mercury, digital, and aneroid sphygmomanometers. Many institutions are phasing out the mercury sphygmomanometers; however, this is not happening as quickly as the replacement of mercury thermometers. As a result, information regarding mercury sphygmomanometers is included in this text. The aneroid and digital instruments are more widely used. Figure 3-8 provides examples of both mercury and aneroid sphygmomanometers and cuffs.

Cuff size is important. Three sizes are available: adult for average adult arm, pediatric for children younger than age 13 years and large for patients with obese arms or for thigh readings.

Procedure 3-14 provides the steps for measuring systolic pressure using the palpatory method. This method of feeling the radial pulse while inflating the blood pressure cuff can be used to measure the systolic pressure only. The

BOX 3-1 Five Phases of Korotkoff Sounds

Phase I	This is the first faint sharp tapping sound heard as the cuff is deflated. Record this reading as the systolic reading.
Phase II	The second phase occurs as the cuff continues to deflate and blood flows through the artery. It has a swishing quality. The cuff has to be slowly deflated to hear this sound.
Phase III	During this phase the sound will become less muffled and will develop a crisp tapping sound as blood flow moves easily through the artery. If the BP cuff was not inflated enough to hear the Phase I sounds, then the Phase III sound may be interpreted as the systolic reading.
Phase IV	The blood is now passing through the arteries easily as the cuff continues to be deflated. The sounds will be muffled fading or tapping sounds. This phase is used as the diastolic reading in a child and for those patients for whom tapping sounds continue to zero.
Phase V	Sound disappears at this phase. The disappearance of sound is the diastolic reading. Some physicians prefer that both Phase IV and Phase V be recorded (for example, 120/78/74).

MERCURY SPHYGMOMANOMETER

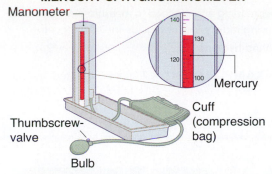

Manometer

Mercury

Thumbscrew-valve

Cuff (compression bag)

Bulb

ANEROID SPHYGMOMANOMETER

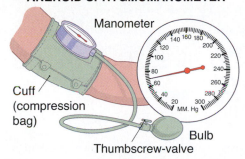

Manometer

Cuff (compression bag)

Thumbscrew-valve

Bulb

FIGURE 3-8 Sphygmomanometers are used to measure blood pressure and may be either mercury or aneroid.

TABLE 3-4 Average Blood Pressure Readings

Newborn	75/55
6–9 years of age	90/55
10–15 years of age	100/65
16–18 years of age	118/76
18 years and older (adult)	120/80

palpatory method is useful to ascertain that the pressure is high enough to exceed the patient's systolic pressure and is useful while training students to evaluate blood pressures. Procedure 3-15 lists the steps for measuring systolic/diastolic blood pressure with a sphygmomanometer.

The normal blood pressure for an adult should be no higher than 120/80 mm Hg based on the 2003 guidelines established by the *Seventh Report of the Joint National Committee* (*JCN7*) published by the National Institute of Health (NIH). Refer to Table 3-4 for average normal blood pressure readings.

This reading is not usually recorded since it is only an estimate of the systolic BP.

PROCEDURE 3-14

MEASURING SYSTOLIC BLOOD PRESSURE USING PALPATORY METHOD

ABHES VII.MA.A.1 9(c)   CAAHEP I.P (1)

OBJECTIVE: To accurately measure systolic blood pressure following all steps in procedure.

STANDARD: This task takes 5 minutes.

EQUIPMENT AND SUPPLIES: Sphygmomanometer (monometer and BP cuff); stethoscope; 70% isopropyl alcohol; alcohol sponges or cotton balls; paper; pen.

STEPS:

1. Check physician's orders, and check for patient allergies.
2. Perform hand hygiene.
3. Assemble equipment. Thoroughly cleanse earpieces, bell, and diaphragm of stethoscope with alcohol.
4. Place the monometer within 3 feet for easy viewing.
5. Uncover patient's arm by rolling sleeve 5 inches above the elbow.
6. Place arm in comfortable position at heart level, and have patient straighten arm.

NOTE: If arm is below the heart, the reading may be higher than normal; if above the heart, it may be higher than normal.

7. Apply cuff 1 to 2 inches above the brachial artery (see Figure 3-4 for location of artery) above the antecubital space. Locating the brachial artery before placing the diaphragm on the arm improves the ability to hear the sounds. (Many cuffs are marked with an arrow or circle to mark placement over artery.
8. Palpate with fingers for the brachial artery where pulse felt.
9. Place earpieces in ears and diaphragm over brachial artery and hold in place with fingers, not thumb. Make sure tubing is hanging freely.
10. Locate radial pulse on thumb side of wrist on same arm.

11. Inflate blood pressure cuff until pulse disappears, and note reading on monometer.

12. Reinflate cuff until pulse once again disappears, and inflate another 30 mm above that point.

13. Slowly deflate cuff while feeling radial pulse. The point at which radial pulse can be felt is systolic pressure.

14. Remember reading and proceed to measure brachial blood pressure using radial pulse as a guide for inflating cuff.

15. Perform hand hygiene.

CHARTING EXAMPLE: 07/24/XX 7:00 P.M. Palpated systolic pressure 170 mm Hg · · · · · · · · · · · H. Martinez, CMA (AAMA)

PROCEDURE 3-15

MEASURING SYSTOLIC/DIASTOLIC BLOOD PRESSURE USING SPHYGMOMANOMETER

ABHES VII.MA.A.1 9(c)   CAAHEP I.P (1)

OBJECTIVE: To accurately measure blood pressure following all steps in procedure.

STANDARD: This task takes 5 minutes.

EQUIPMENT AND SUPPLIES: Sphygmomanometer (manometer and BP cuff); stethoscope; 70% isopropyl alcohol; alcohol sponges or cotton balls; paper; pen; patient's record.

STEPS:

1. Check physician's orders, and check for patient allergies.

2. Perform hand hygiene.

3. Assemble equipment. Thoroughly cleanse earpieces, bell, and diaphragm of stethoscope with alcohol.

4. Identify patient.

5. Explain procedure. Ask about recent exercise or smoking during preceding 15 minutes. If response is positive, allow patient to rest several minutes before beginning. Remind patient not to cross legs.

6. Place the manometer within 3 feet for easy viewing.

7. Uncover patient's arm by rolling sleeve 5 inches above elbow.

8. Place arm in comfortable position at heart level, and have patient straighten arm.

NOTE: If arm is below the heart, the reading may be higher than normal; if above the heart, it may be lower than normal.

9. Apply cuff 1 to 2 inches above the brachial artery above the antecubital space. (Many cuffs are marked with an arrow or circle to mark placement over artery.

10. Palpate with fingers for the brachial artery where pulse felt.

11. Place earpieces in ears and diaphragm over brachial artery, and hold in place with fingers, not thumb. Make sure tubing is hanging freely.

12. Close thumbscrew on hand bulb, turning it clockwise just enough so no air leaks.

13. Palpate the radial artery.

14. Pump air into cuff until radial pulse is no longer felt (palpatory systolic reading). Inflate 20 to 30 mm Hg above this number.

15. Slowly release air by turning thumbscrew counterclockwise, allowing pressure to fall 2 to 3 mm/second.

16. Listen for first distinct sound (phase I Korotkoff sound). This is systolic reading.

17. Continue to deflate at the same rate listening for phases II, II, and IV of Korotkoff sounds. (The point where sound becomes muffled is phase IV.)

18. Continue to deflate until there is a complete absence of sound (phase V), the diastolic reading. Some physicians require reporting of both phase IV and V.

19. Quickly open thumbscrew and deflate completely.

20. Wait 1 to 2 minutes, and repeat if you are unsure of reading. (Never take more than two readings in one arm; an inaccurate reading may result.)

21. Remove cuff.

22. Clean stethoscope.

23. Perform hand hygiene.

24. Record result in patient's chart. Be sure to record patient's position if it is other than sitting.

CHARTING EXAMPLE: 2/05/XX 11:08 A.M. B/P 132/82/78 left arm · C. Blardo, CMA (AAMA)

BOX 3-2 How to Measure Pain

Location	Ask patient to indicate location of pain on or in body such as diffuse, localized, and radiating.
Intensity	Determine strength, power, and force of pain using numeric pain scales or face pictures. (*Scale:* 0–10, where 0 = no pain, 10 = worst pain ever.)
Quality	Determine characteristics of pain, such as dull, searing, throbbing, sharp, burning, cramping, suffocating, stabbing, knifelike, and viselike.
Pattern	Ask patient how pain changes and when it changes, such as intermittent, continuous, steady, transient.

Pain

Pain, the fifth vital sign, is a symptom most people have experienced. It is subjective and personal, and no two individuals experience pain in the same way. According to the Joint Commission, pain should be considered the fifth vital sign, and it must be assessed and documented when other vital signs are measured. The U.S. Department of Veterans Affairs also has incorporated pain into the vital signs records. Caregivers must ask about pain when interviewing the patient. Any description of pain by the patient should be recorded in his or her own words in the chart. Many individuals will not bring up pain unless they are asked about it by the health care provider.

Pain is difficult to describe; therefore, medical assistants and other providers must have a vocabulary to assist the patient in describing pain. Box 3-2 describes some terms used to describe pain.

Nonverbal signs of pain, such as grimacing or clutching an area are important also. Numerical pain measurement scales, with 1 being no pain and 10 being extreme pain, are useful in gathering information. For children, scales with happy and sad faces are useful. (Figures 3-9A and 3-9B illustrate

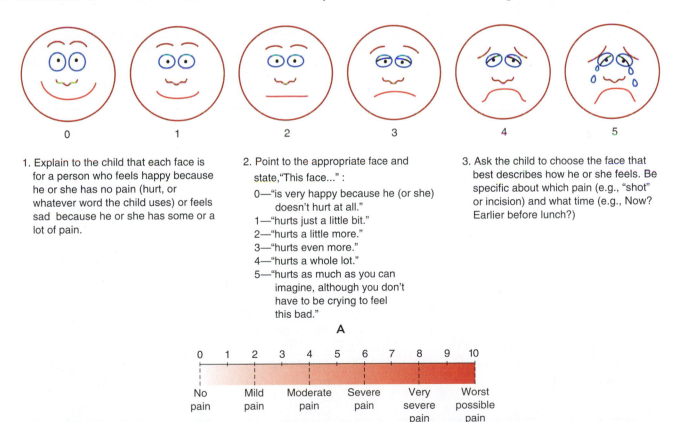

1. Explain to the child that each face is for a person who feels happy because he or she has no pain (hurt, or whatever word the child uses) or feels sad because he or she has some or a lot of pain.

2. Point to the appropriate face and state,"This face..." :

  0—"is very happy because he (or she) doesn't hurt at all."
  1—"hurts just a little bit."
  2—"hurts a little more."
  3—"hurts even more."
  4—"hurts a whole lot."
  5—"hurts as much as you can imagine, although you don't have to be crying to feel this bad."

3. Ask the child to choose the face that best describes how he or she feels. Be specific about which pain (e.g., "shot" or incision) and what time (e.g., Now? Earlier before lunch?)

A

0	1	2	3	4	5	6	7	8	9	10

No pain   Mild pain   Moderate pain   Severe pain   Very severe pain   Worst possible pain

B

FIGURE 3-9 (A) Ask the patient to choose the face that best describes the level of pain; (B) pain intensity scale.

two examples of pain scales.) Pain is influenced by the ethnic and cultural background of the patient. How one behaves when in pain is learned in the cultural environment. These factors must all be considered when interacting with patients.

Oxygen Saturation Measurement

Oxygen saturation measurements provide important data related to the general well-being of the patient. A pulse oximetry is a noninvasive method of measuring the arterial oxygen saturation of a patient's functional hemoglobin (oxygen carrying molecules in blood). An oximeter is a photoelectric device that measures oxygen saturation by recording the amount of light transmitted or reflected by venous blood (deoxygenated blood) versus oxygenated arterial blood. (Refer to Figure 3-10 for an example of a pulse oximeter.) Procedure 3-16 provides the steps for measuring oxygen saturation using a pulse oximeter. Normal values for oxygen saturation are 95% to 100%, while below 70% is considered life threatening.

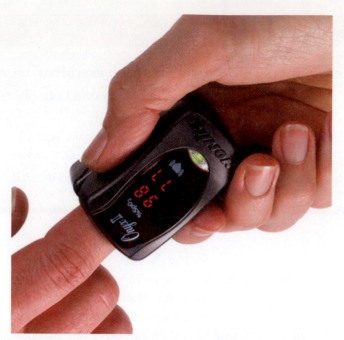

FIGURE 3-10 **Sensor probe placed on finger for hemoglobin oxygen saturation analysis and microprocessing unit with digital display.**

PROCEDURE 3-16

MEASURING OXYGEN SATURATION USING A PULSE OXIMETER

ABHES VII.MA.A.1 9(o)(2)   CAAHEP I.P (4)

OBJECTIVE: To accurately measure arterial blood oxygen saturation following all steps of procedure.

STANDARD: This task takes 5 minutes.

EQUIPMENT AND SUPPLIES: Pulse oximeter; alcohol wipe; towel; nail polish remover as needed; patient's record.

STEPS:

1. Check physician's orders, and check for patient allergies.
2. Perform hand hygiene.
3. Identify patient, and explain procedure.
4. Select appropriate size sensor (pediatric, small, and large).
5. Clean site with alcohol.

6. Remove nail polish if present. It interferes with accuracy of results.
7. Apply sensor and connect to pulse oximeter, making sure to align correctly.
8. Turn on machine according to manufacturers' directions. Ask patient to remain still, as patient movement may be interpreted as arterial pulsations. A beep will indicate each arterial pulsation.
9. Take reading and document.
10. Perform hand hygiene.

CHARTING EXAMPLE: 02/05/XX 7:05 A.M. (SaO_2) Blood oxygen saturation 86% · · · · · · · · · · C. Blardo, CMA (AAMA)

Anthropometry

Anthropometry is the science of size, proportion, weight, and height. Although not considered vital signs, height and weight measurements are often taken along with vital signs. These measurements can provide indications of a patient's general well-being. Procedure 3-17 lists the steps to measure the height and weight of an adult. Measuring the height and weight of infants and small children is considered in Chapter 6. Monitoring of weight and height provides valuable information when following patients with conditions such as diabetes, cardiac problems, pregnancy, and eating disorders and when evaluating growth patterns of infants and children. Body fat measurements are useful in individuals with eating disorders and hormonal imbalance.

Many methods are available to measure body fat. Two relatively easy methods are calculating body mass index (Procedure 3-18) and determining fat fold measurement in an adult (Procedure 3-19).

PROCEDURE 3-17

MEASURING ADULT HEIGHT AND WEIGHT

ABHES VII.MA.A.1 9(m)   CAAHEP I.P (10)

OBJECTIVE: To accurately weigh and measure height following all procedural steps and performing math conversions.

STANDARD: This task takes 5 minutes.

EQUIPMENT AND SUPPLIES: Balance scale with height bar; paper towel; pen; patient's record.

> ## HIPAA Alert!
> In some facilities patients are weighed in a hallway or other less-than-private place. Be sure that any measurements are not observed by other patients.

STEPS:

1. Check physician's orders, and check for patient allergies.
2. Perform hand hygiene.
3. Identify patient.
4. Explain procedure.
5. Balance scale, and place paper towel on scale.
6. Ask patient to remove shoes and heavy objects such as keys from pockets. Place paper towel or other protection on the scale to prevent spread of pathogens.
7. Assist patient onto scale, and ask patient to stand still.
8. Move large weight to weight closest to your estimation. Move small weight to a point at which pointer floats without touching.
9. Leave weights in place.
10. Ask patient to turn so back is to the scale and to look straight ahead.
11. Raise height bar in collapsed position to a point over patient's head to avoid hitting patient's head.
12. Open horizontal bar and bring it down to touch top of patient's head.
13. Assist patient off scale.
14. Read the weight by adding together to the nearest ¼ pound the number at the large weight and the number at the small weight. Record this amount. Read in kilograms if required by facility.
15. Read height as marked, and record to nearest ¼ inch. (Convert to feet by dividing by 12). Read in centimeters as required.
16. Return weights to zero and height bar to normal position.
17. Discard paper towel.
18. Perform hand hygiene.

CHARTING EXAMPLE: 2/5/XX 2:00 P.M. Wt 179½ lbs w/o shoes; Ht 5'7¼" (67¼") · · · · · · · · · · · · · · · · · · · A. Allen, RMA

PROCEDURE 3-18

CALCULATING ADULT BODY MASS INDEX

ABHES VII.MA.A.1 9(m)   CAAHEP I.P (10)

OBJECTIVE: To accurately calculate adult body mass index following all steps in procedure.

STANDARD: This task takes 5 minutes.

EQUIPMENT AND SUPPLIES: Patient's record; paper; pen; scale for height and weight; BMI formula; nomogram for BMI.

STEPS:

1. Check physician's orders, and check for patient allergies.
2. Perform hand hygiene.
3. If recent height and weight measurements are not available, follow steps in Procedure 3-16 to obtain values needed.

4. Insert patient's height and weight into formula using pounds and inches or kilograms and meters according to office policy.

$$\text{Formula BMI} = \frac{\text{Weight in pounds} (\times 703)}{\text{Height in inches} \times \text{Height in inches}}$$

Example:

Wt 175 lbs; Ht 64 inches

$$\frac{175 \times 703}{64 \times 64} = 0.0427 \times 703 = 30.0181 = 30 \text{ BMI}$$

5. Record the result in patient's chart.

CHARTING EXAMPLE: 03/18/XX 1:00 P.M. Ht 64 in Wt 175 lb; BMI = 30.0 · C. Moran, RMA

PROCEDURE 3-19

DETERMINING FAT FOLD MEASUREMENT IN ADULTS

ABHES VII.MA.A.1 9(m)   CAAHEP I.P (10)

OBJECTIVE: To accurately determine and record body fat measurement.

STANDARD: This task takes 5 to 10 minutes.

EQUIPMENT AND SUPPLIES: Fat-fold body calipers; patient's record; pen; paper.

STEPS:

1. Check physician's orders, and check for patient allergies.
2. Perform hand hygiene.
3. Gather equipment and supplies.
4. Read caliper directions.
5. Identify patient, and explain procedure.
6. Grasp the triceps in the upper arm with thumb and index finger. (Do not pinch too hard or grasp muscle tissue).

7. Place calipers over fold and measure.
8. Record measurement.
9. Grasp the subscapular region beneath shoulder blade, and obtain and record a reading.
10. At the suprailiac area (located posterior and immediately superior to the fanning of the hip bone), obtain a reading and record.
11. Determine total percentage of body fat using appropriate table. (Table 3-5 provides an example of body fat classification using fat fold measurements.)
12. Perform hand hygiene.
13. Document results in patient's record.

CHARTING EXAMPLE: 2/14/XX 2:00 P.M. Triceps 9 mm; Scapula 12 mm; Abdomen 40 mm; within acceptable ranges (7%–15%) · S. Lopez, CMA (AAMA)

TABLE 3-5 Body Fat Percentages and Guidelines

Sex	Triceps	Scapular	Abdomen	Total
Male				
Lean < 7%	< 7 mm	< 8 mm	< 10 mm	< 25 mm
Acceptable 7%–15%	7–13 mm	8–15 mm	10–20 mm	25–48 mm
Obese > 15%	> 13 mm	> 15 mm	> 20 mm	> 48 mm
Female				
Lean < 12%	< 9 mm	< 7 mm	< 7 mm	< 23 mm
Acceptable 12%–25%	9–17 mm	7–14 mm	7–15 mm	23–46 mm
Obese > 25%	> 17 mm	> 14 mm	> 15 mm	> 46 mm

4 Assisting with Physical Examination

PROCEDURES

Procedure 4-1 Cleaning the Examination Room

Procedure 4-2 Interviewing a New Patient to Obtain Medical History to Prepare for Physical Examination

Procedure 4-3 Documenting a Chief Complaint During a Patient Interview

Procedure 4-4 Positioning Patient in Supine Position

Procedure 4-5 Positioning Patient in Fowler's Position

Procedure 4-6 Positioning Patient in Dorsal Recumbent Position

Procedure 4-7 Positioning Patient in Lithotomy Position

Procedure 4-8 Positioning Patient in Prone Position

Procedure 4-9 Positioning Patient in Sims' Position

Procedure 4-10 Positioning Patient in Knee–Chest Position

Procedure 4-11 Assisting with Complete Physical Examination

Procedure 4-12 Performing Scoliosis Screening

Procedure 4-13 Assisting Vomiting Patient

Procedure 4-14 Communicating with Patients from Other Cultures

Procedure 4-15 Communicating Effectively with the Elderly

TERMS TO LEARN

inspection
palpation
percussion
auscultation
mensuration
manipulation

problem-oriented medical record (POMR)
SOAP charting
electronic medical records (EMR)
scoliosis
lordosis

kyphosis
scapula
vomitus
gerontology

One of the main roles of medical assistants and other health care providers is to assist the physician with the physical examination of a patient. Assisting with physical examinations includes preparing the examination room prior to patient appointments, interviewing the patient, documenting information, positioning and draping the patient, and cleaning the room after the examination. Other duties include maintaining supplies and equipment, ensuring patient safety, respecting confidentiality, and providing comfort and privacy. Before presenting the procedures associated with this chapter, a review of patient positioning is presented. A list of equipment and supplies accompanied by photographs of equipment used in a health examination is shown in Figure 4-1.

Positioning and Methods of Examination

Eleven standard positions are used for a variety of medical and surgical examinations: sitting, supine, dorsal recumbent, lithotomy, Fowler's, semi-Fowler's, prone, Sims', knee–chest, proctological, and Trendelenburg. Figures 4-2A through 4-2D illustrate some of these positions. The rest of the positions are shown with their procedures. In addition, the jack-knife position involves the patient lying on the back with shoulders elevated, legs flexed at knees, and thighs at right angles to the abdomen. This procedure is used to introduce urethral sound. It is essentially a supine position with legs flexed as described. In the Trendelenburg position, or head-down position, the patient is on the back with arms straight along sides of the body, with the head of the bed lowered so the head is lower than the hips and the legs are elevated at approximately 45 degrees. This position is used to increase blood flow to the head in case of shock. Procedures for assisting patients into some of these positions follow later in this chapter.

It is important to explain to the patient the position you would like him or her to assume and why. Some of the positions are embarrassing and uncomfortable. Every effort must be made to use proper draping to protect the privacy of the patient. Never leave a patient in an uncomfortable position any longer than is necessary.

The six methods of examination used during a physical examination are **inspection** (Figure 4-3), **palpation** (Figures 4-4A and 4-4B), **percussion** (Figures 4-5A and 4-5B), **auscultation** (Figure 4-6), **mensuration** (Figure 4-7) and **manipulation** (Figure 4-8). Some of these methods require the use of specific pieces of equipment. Other methods such as inspection are performed with the patient unaware, as when the physician inspects the patient while engaging him or her in conversation.

Cleaning the Examination Room

Prior to seeing each new patient, the examination room must be cleaned. All evidence of previous patients must be removed. The exam table is covered with new paper, and a quick check of supplies is done to prevent running out of anything during the examination. All soiled items must be disposed of in the appropriate waste containers. Procedure 4-1 lists the steps to be taken to clean an examination room prior to patient examination.

Interviewing Patient for Physical Examination

Once the examination room is clean and ready, the patient is greeted with a smile and escorted to the prepared room. Usually the patient has completed the patient data portion of the intake form. Once in the examination room, introduce yourself, make eye contact, shake hands, and ask how patient wants to be addressed. It is important to put patient at ease and build rapport and to build patient's confidence in you and the physician. Explain that you will be asking some questions prior to the examination. After reviewing what the patient has completed on the form, ask any questions that help shed light on the patient's past and present health. Next, explain what you would like the patient to do—what clothes to remove, whether the gown is to open in the back or front and ask if the patient needs assistance. If no assistance is needed, leave the room and knock before reentering. The patient history includes the following sections:

- **Patient database.** Demographic information: name, address, date of birth, sex, race, marital status, phone number; next of kin name, address, phone number; employer name, address, phone number; insurance company and phone number.
- **Chief complaint (CC).** Reason for office visit today. What? When? Where?
- **Present illness (PI).** Provides more complete description of the chief complaint recorded in patient's own words.
- **Past medical history (PH).** All diseases, medical problems experienced in past; immunizations, allergies; hospitalizations, surgeries.
- **Family history (FH).** Health status of patient's parents, siblings, grandparents; if any are deceased, cause of death.

Supplies		Purpose
Flashlight or penlight	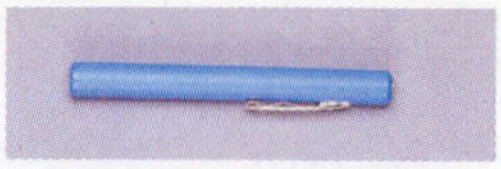	To assist viewing of the pharynx and cervix or to determine the reactions of the pupils of the eye
Laryngeal or dental mirror	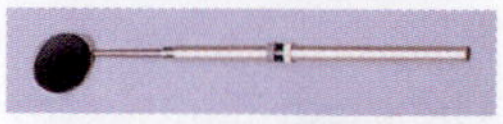	To observe the pharynx and oral cavity
Nasal speculum	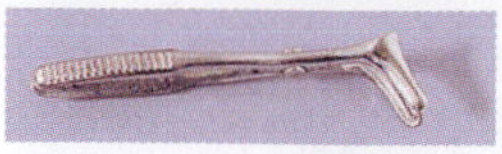	To permit visualization of the lower and middle turbinates; usually, a penlight is used for illumination
Ophthalmoscope	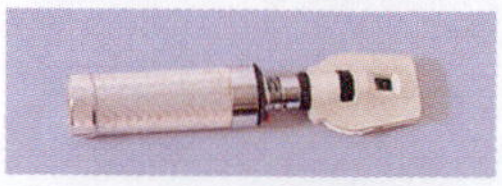	A lighted instrument to visualize the interior of the eye
Otoscope	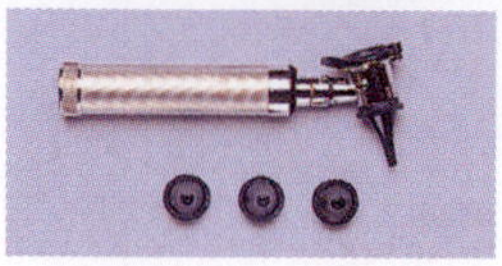	A lighted instrument to visualize the eardrum and external auditory canal (a nasal speculum may be attached to the otoscope to inspect the nasal cavities)
Percussion (reflex) hammer	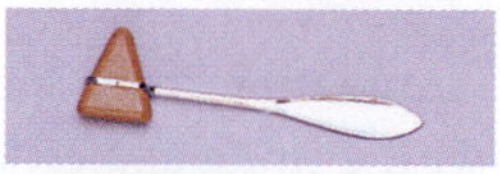	An instrument with a rubber head to test reflexes
Tuning fork	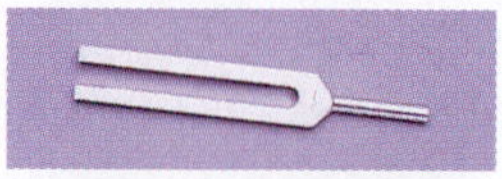	A two-pronged metal instrument used to test hearing acuity and vibratory sense
Vaginal speculum	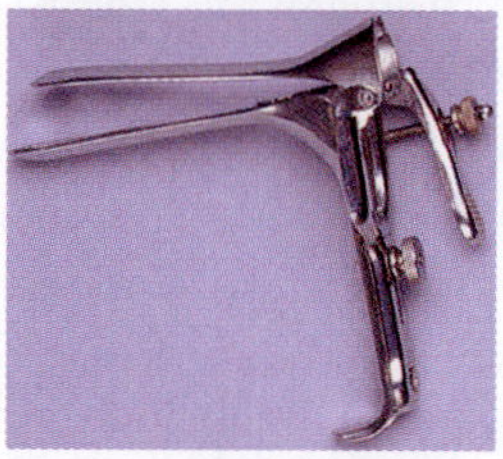	To assess the cervix and the vagina
Cotton applicators	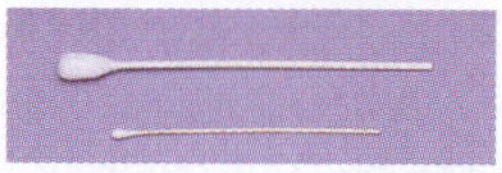	To obtain specimens
Disposable pads	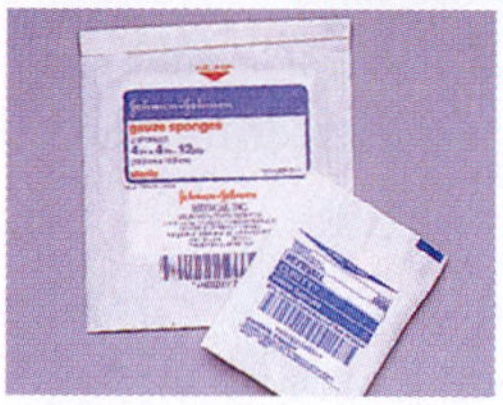	To absorb liquid
Gloves	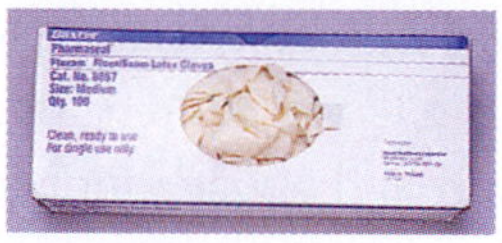	To protect the nurse
Lubricant	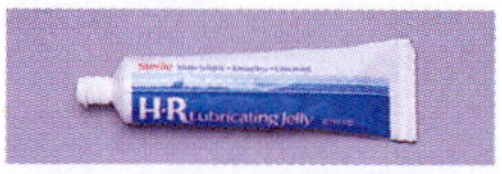	To ease insertion of instruments (e.g., vaginal speculum)
Tongue blades (depressors)	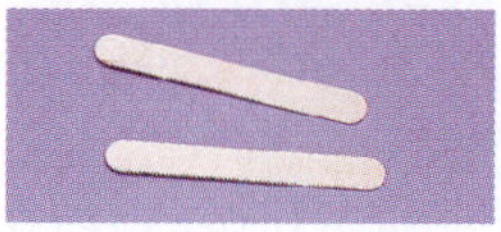	To depress the tongue during assessment of the mouth and pharynx

FIGURE 4-1 Equipment and supplies used for physical examination.

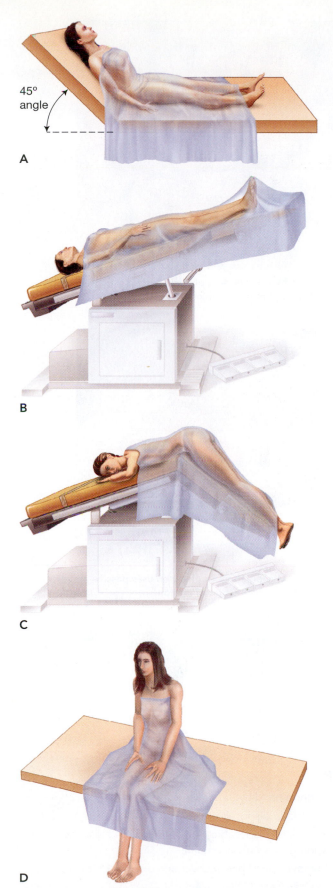

FIGURE 4-2 (A) Semi-Fowler's position; (B) Trendelenburg position; (C) proctological (jackknife) position; (D) sitting position.

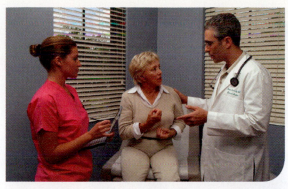

FIGURE 4-3 Inspection is one method of examination used in a health examination.

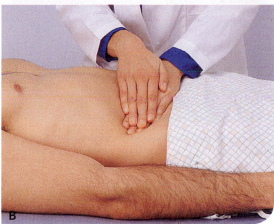

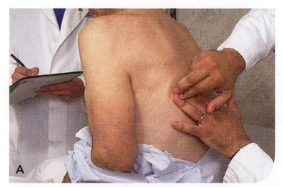

FIGURE 4-4 (A) An example of light palpation of the abdomen; (B) the physician uses two hands for deep bimanual palpation.

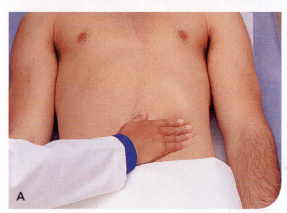

FIGURE 4-5 (A) The physician uses percussion—tapping—to detect sound or vibration.

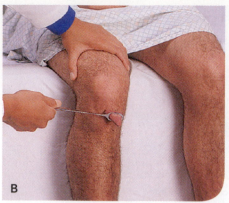

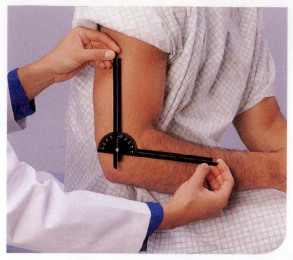

FIGURE 4-5 (Continued) (B) testing patellar reflex with percussion hammer.

FIGURE 4-7 Mensuration—a physician uses a goniometer to measure range of motion in a joint.

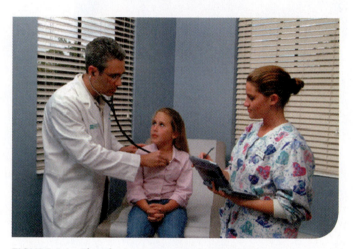

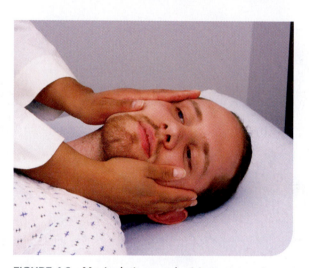

FIGURE 4-6 The physician uses auscultation to listen to a patient's heart.

FIGURE 4-8 Manipulation—a physician uses passive movement of patient's neck to check range of motion.

PROCEDURE 4-1

CLEANING THE EXAMINATION ROOM

ABHES VII.MA.A.1 9(k)   CAAHEP I.P (10)

OBJECTIVE: To clean an examination room prior to patient examination to prevent spread of pathogens.

STANDARD: This task takes 5–10 minutes.

EQUIPMENT AND SUPPLIES: Disinfectant; paper towels; disposable gloves; examination table; pillow; disposable gown.

STEPS:

1. Perform hand hygiene.
2. Don clean disposable gloves.
3. Roll soiled disposable gown into ball and dispose of it in appropriate waste container.
4. Remove soiled pillow cover and dispose of it in appropriate waste container.

5. Remove other soiled items or equipment from the examination room.

6. Wipe down examination table and counter surfaces with disinfectant and paper towels.

7. Dispose of soiled paper towel and gloves in appropriate waste container.

8. Perform hand hygiene.

9. Place clean paper on examination table and a new pillow covering over pillow.

10. Make sure examination room is clean and odor and clutter free (Figure 4-9).

11. Check amounts of frequently used supplies and resupply as needed.

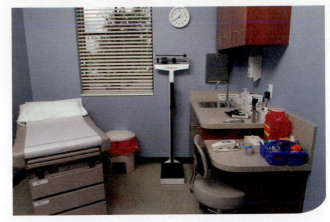

FIGURE 4-9 Examination room cleaned and ready for next patient.

- **Social history (SH).**   Patient's lifestyle, occupation, education, hobbies, use of alcohol, drugs, tobacco, sexual preferences, sleep habits.
- **Review of systems (ROS).**   Review of each body system, beginning at head and working toward feet.

Many formats are used for recording medical information. The chronological format follows patient over time, with each entry corresponding to date rather than to symptoms or diagnosis. The **problem-oriented medical record (POMR)** is based on identifying patient problems and charting by problems. **SOAP charting** is used in POMR format, with the acronym derived from the following:

- **Subjective (S).**   Information from patient relative to why being seen by physician.
- **Objective (O).**   Information gathered during the visit, such as vital signs, weight, and height.

- **Assessment (A).**   Physician's preliminary diagnosis.
- **Plan (P).**   Plan of care for the patient, established by physician.

It is important to be thoroughly familiar with the charting format used in your facility. All personnel in a facility must utilize the same format system. **Electronic medical records (EMRs)** are becoming more widely used. Handheld computer devices are used to input information during patient visits. Confidentiality must be maintained regardless of the type of record format.

Procedure 4-2 presents the steps for interviewing a patient to obtain medical history and to prepare for a physical examination.

Procedure 4-3 lists the steps necessary to correctly document a chief complaint and present illness during a patient interview.

PROCEDURE 4-2

INTERVIEWING A NEW PATIENT TO OBTAIN MEDICAL HISTORY TO PREPARE FOR PHYSICAL EXAMINATION

ABHES VII.MA.A.1 9(a); VII.MA.A.1 9(ff)   CAAHEP IV.P (1)

OBJECTIVE: To complete various sections of medical history form while interviewing patient to prepare patient for physical examination.

STANDARD: This task takes 10 minutes.

EQUIPMENT AND SUPPLIES: Medical history form; clipboard; black or blue pen; red pen; scale; vital sign equipment; urine container; exam table paper; gown; drape.

STEPS:

1. Check physician's orders.
2. Identify patient, greet warmly, and identify yourself.
3. Explain what you are going to do and why.
4. Provide a private area to conduct interview.
5. Check to see that the patient has filled in patient data portion of history form. Assist if patient is unable to complete on own.
6. Review data portion, and ask for any additional necessary information.
7. Ask for the reason for the visit: chief complaint (CC).
8. Record CC in patient's own words.
9. Ask open-ended questions to gather more information, and record under in "Present Illness" (PI) section. Record in patient's own words.
10. Gather information on past history, social history, and family history, and document in patient's record.
11. Ask about allergies. Record in red ink, usually on first page of medical history, or follow other office policy.
12. Note any other relevant information.
13. Ask the patient to disrobe, and explain how the gown, if needed, is to be worn and where to be seated. Leave the room to provide privacy, and knock before reentering.
14. Provide any draping that is needed.
15. Perform vital signs, plus height and weight, and record.
16. Correct any errors, using one line through the error and then date and initial. Record correct information.
17. Ask patient either to provide and label a urine specimen (and explain how; see Chapter 11) or, if specimen not required, to empty bladder.
18. Explain what procedures physician will perform and how long the wait may be.
19. Place medical history in designated location outside room for physician.

CHARTING EXAMPLE: 03/02/XX 3:15 P.M. CC new patient exam. MH form completed and in chart. Pt. states "No health problems at present." · · · · · · · · · · A. Martinez, CMA (AAMA)

PROCEDURE 4-3

DOCUMENTING A CHIEF COMPLAINT DURING A PATIENT INTERVIEW

ABHES VII.MA.A.1 9(a); VII.MA.A. 4(a)   CAAHEP IV.P (2); IX.P (7)

OBJECTIVE: To accurately document the chief complaint, using correct charting format and abbreviations while interviewing a patient.

STANDARD: This task takes 10 minutes or less.

EQUIPMENT AND SUPPLIES: Problem list or progress notes form; black or blue pen.

NOTE: Instructor may provide a variety of patient scenarios for students to role-play for this procedure.

STEPS:

1. Check physician's orders. Check for patient allergies.
2. Gather supplies, including medical record with problem list or progress note form.
3. Review briefly patient's medical history form before greeting patient.
4. Greet and identify patient and escort into examination room.
5. Ask open-ended questions to gather information about why patient is being seen today. Maintain eye contact, and actively listen to patient responses.
6. Gather information about PI by asking questions such as, What makes problem better or worse? When did it start? Where does it hurt? Ask patient to rate pain on scale of 1–10.
7. Document CC and PI correctly on the correct form in patient's own words where necessary.
8. Thank patient, and explain that physician will be in shortly to perform examination.
9. Make sure patient is comfortable, and inform patient that physician will be in shortly.

10. Place medical record in designated location outside room, and inform physician that patient is ready.

CHARTING EXAMPLE: 03/03/XX 11:00 A.M. CC: Pt. c/o N&V × 3 days. "Pounding headache not relieved by Tylenol. Unable to eat or drink." PI: Pt states N&V started after eating fried clams at home. T 101 × 2 days. "Has pain all over belly." T 99.8°F (O), P 84, R 20, BP 110/68 (L) Sitting. · · · · · · · · · · · · ·
· A. Martinez, CMA (AAMA)

Assisting with Complete Physical Examination

Individual physicians have a preference about the order of the examination. Typically the physician asks about past history, chief complaint, and history of the current illness first and then performs a review of systems (ROS), beginning with the head and progressing to the feet. Figure 4-10 is an example of a medical history sheet used by a physician to record the review of systems. Procedures 4-4 through 4-10 list steps to assist patients to assume various positions. Procedure 4-11 provides the steps for assisting with complete physical examination.

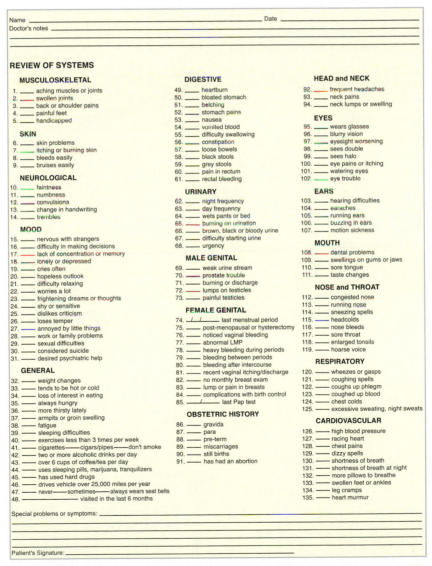

Name _____ Date _____
Doctor's notes _____
_____

REVIEW OF SYSTEMS

MUSCULOSKELETAL
1. ____ aching muscles or joints
2. ____ swollen joints
3. ____ back or shoulder pains
4. ____ painful feet
5. ____ handicapped

SKIN
6. ____ skin problems
7. ____ itching or burning skin
8. ____ bleeds easily
9. ____ bruises easily

NEUROLOGICAL
10. ____ faintness
11. ____ numbness
12. ____ convulsions
13. ____ change in handwriting
14. ____ trembles

MOOD
15. ____ nervous with strangers
16. ____ difficulty in making decisions
17. ____ lack of concentration or memory
18. ____ lonely or depressed
19. ____ cries often
20. ____ hopeless outlook
21. ____ difficulty relaxing
22. ____ worries a lot
23. ____ frightening dreams or thoughts
24. ____ shy or sensitive
25. ____ dislikes criticism
26. ____ loses temper
27. ____ annoyed by little things
28. ____ work or family problems
29. ____ sexual difficulties
30. ____ considered suicide
31. ____ desired psychiatric help

GENERAL
32. ____ weight changes
33. ____ tends to be hot or cold
34. ____ loss of interest in eating
35. ____ always hungry
36. ____ more thirsty lately
37. ____ armpits or groin swelling
38. ____ fatigue
39. ____ sleeping difficulties
40. ____ exercises less than 3 times per week
41. ____ cigarettes——cigars/pipes——don't smoke
42. ____ two or more alcoholic drinks per day
43. ____ over 6 cups of coffee/tea per day
44. ____ uses sleeping pills, marijuana, tranquilizers
45. ____ has used hard drugs
46. ____ drives vehicle over 25,000 miles per year
47. ____ never——sometimes——always wears seat belts
48. ____ visited in the last 6 months

DIGESTIVE
49. ____ heartburn
50. ____ bloated stomach
51. ____ belching
52. ____ stomach pains
53. ____ nausea
54. ____ vomited blood
55. ____ difficulty swallowing
56. ____ constipation
57. ____ loose bowels
58. ____ black stools
59. ____ grey stools
60. ____ pain in rectum
61. ____ rectal bleeding

URINARY
62. ____ night frequency
63. ____ day frequency
64. ____ wets pants or bed
65. ____ burning on urination
66. ____ brown, black or bloody urine
67. ____ difficulty starting urine
68. ____ urgency

MALE GENITAL
69. ____ weak urine stream
70. ____ prostate trouble
71. ____ burning or discharge
72. ____ lumps on testicles
73. ____ painful testicles

FEMALE GENITAL
74. __/__/__ last menstrual period
75. ____ post-menopausal or hysterectomy
76. ____ noticed vaginal bleeding
77. ____ abnormal LMP
78. ____ heavy bleeding during periods
79. ____ bleeding between periods
80. ____ bleeding after intercourse
81. ____ recent vaginal itching/discharge
82. ____ no monthly breast exam
83. ____ lump or pain in breasts
84. ____ complications with birth control
85. __/__ last Pap test

OBSTETRIC HISTORY
86. ____ gravida
87. ____ para
88. ____ pre-term
89. ____ miscarriages
90. ____ still births
91. ____ has had an abortion

HEAD and NECK
92. ____ frequent headaches
93. ____ neck pains
94. ____ neck lumps or swelling

EYES
95. ____ wears glasses
96. ____ blurry vision
97. ____ eyesight worsening
98. ____ sees double
99. ____ sees halo
100. ____ eye pains or itching
101. ____ watering eyes
102. ____ eye trouble

EARS
103. ____ hearing difficulties
104. ____ earaches
105. ____ running ears
106. ____ buzzing in ears
107. ____ motion sickness

MOUTH
108. ____ dental problems
109. ____ swellings on gums or jaws
110. ____ sore tongue
111. ____ taste changes

NOSE and THROAT
112. ____ congested nose
113. ____ running nose
114. ____ sneezing spells
115. ____ headcolds
116. ____ nose bleeds
117. ____ sore throat
118. ____ enlarged tonsils
119. ____ hoarse voice

RESPIRATORY
120. ____ wheezes or gasps
121. ____ coughing spells
122. ____ coughs up phlegm
123. ____ coughed up blood
124. ____ chest colds
125. ____ excessive sweating, night sweats

CARDIOVASCULAR
126. ____ high blood pressure
127. ____ racing heart
128. ____ chest pains
129. ____ dizzy spells
130. ____ shortness of breath
131. ____ shortness of breath at night
132. ____ more pillows to breathe
133. ____ swollen feet or ankles
134. ____ leg cramps
135. ____ heart murmur

Special problems or symptoms: _____
_____
_____
_____

Patient's Signature: _____

FIGURE 4-10 Example of a medical history sheet used by the physician to record the review of systems (ROS) during a physical examination.

PROCEDURE 4-4

POSITIONING PATIENT IN SUPINE POSITION

ABHES VII.MA.A.1 9(I)   CAAHEP IV.P (6)

OBJECTIVE: To safely assist patient into supine position for examination of anterior surface of body.

STANDARD: This task takes 1 minute.

EQUIPMENT AND SUPPLIES: Examination table; gown; drape.

STEPS:

1. Check physician's orders. Check for patient allergies.
2. Perform hand hygiene.
3. Provide gown, and assist patient if necessary.
4. Assist patient onto table. If separate step stool is used, stabilize it with your feet to prevent it from sliding as the patient steps up.
5. Ask patient to lie back on table while you pull out foot extension. Support patient's back.
6. Place a pillow under patient's head.
7. Cover patient with drape from chest to ankles.
8. Make sure patient is comfortable, and inform patient that physician will be in shortly.
9. Place medical record in designated location outside room, and inform physician that patient is ready.
10. After examination, assist patient to sitting position and allow to remain seated to prevent dizziness.
11. Push foot extension into place while supporting patient's feet.
12. When patient stable and examination complete, assist patient to standing position and hold arm while patient steps down. Stabilize step stool with your feet as before. Give further instructions as needed.
13. Clean examination room for next patient (follow steps of Procedure 4-1).
14. Perform hand hygiene.

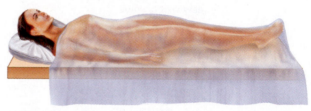

FIGURE 4-11   The supine or horizontal recumbent position.

PROCEDURE 4-5

POSITIONING PATIENT IN FOWLER'S POSITION

ABHES VII.MA.A.1 9(I)   CAAHEP IV.P (6)

OBJECTIVE: To safely assist patient into Fowler's position for examination of upper body and head.

STANDARD: This task takes 1 minute.

EQUIPMENT AND SUPPLIES: Examination table; gown; drape.

STEPS:

1. Check physician's orders, and check for patient allergies.
2. Perform hand hygiene.
3. Provide gown and assist patient as necessary.
4. Assist patient up step to sit on end of table. Stabilize step stool if used.
5. Cover legs with drape.
6. Assist patient to slide back and lean on raised end of table.
7. Pull out foot extension while supporting patient's feet.
8. Raise head of table to 90° angle for Fowler's position (45° angle for semi-Fowler's position).
9. Place pillow under patient's knees to relieve strain on lower back. Adjust drape as needed.

10. Make sure patient is comfortable, and inform patient that physician will be in shortly.

11. Place medical record in designated location outside room, and inform physician that patient is ready.

12. When examination is complete, push in foot extension. Ask patient to remain seated at end of table to avoid dizziness.

NOTE: Inform patient before lowering table. Ask patient to lean forward while you support patient's back as you lower table.

13. Assist off table, stabilizing step stool as needed. Give further instructions as needed.

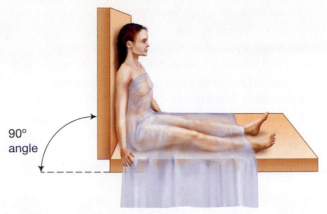

FIGURE 4-12   Fowler's position.

14. Clean examination room for next patient (follow steps in Procedure 4-1).

15. Perform hand hygiene.

PROCEDURE 4-6

POSITIONING PATIENT IN DORSAL RECUMBENT POSITION

ABHES VII.MA.A.1 9(I)   CAAHEP IV.P (6)

OBJECTIVE: To safely assist patient into dorsal recumbent position for examination of anterior surface of body, catheterization, or pelvic examination.

STANDARD: This task takes 1 minute.

EQUIPMENT AND SUPPLIES: Examination table; gown; drape.

STEPS:

1. Check physician's orders, and check for patient allergies.

2. Perform hand hygiene.

3. Have patient disrobe as appropriate for examination and don gown; assist as needed.

4. Assist patient onto end of table, stabilizing step stool as needed.

5. Assist patient to lie back while you support patient's back while pulling out foot extension.

6. Ask patient to bend knees and place feet flat on table. Push in foot extension.

7. Cover patient with drape with point of drape between patient's legs.

8. Place pillow under head if needed.

9. Place light and stool in place for examiner.

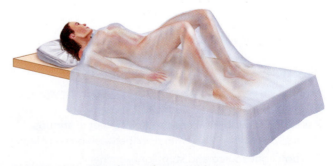

FIGURE 4-13   Dorsal recumbent position.

10. Make sure patient is comfortable, and inform patient that physician will be in shortly.

11. Place medical record in designated location outside room, and inform physician that patient is ready.

12. After procedure is complete, assist patient to sitting position using foot extension to support patient's feet.

13. Ask patient to remain seated a few moments to prevent dizziness.

14. Assist off table, stabilizing step stool as needed.

15. Give other instructions as necessary.

16. Clean examination room for next patient (follow steps in Procedure 4-1).

17. Perform hand hygiene.

PROCEDURE 4-7

POSITIONING PATIENT IN LITHOTOMY POSITION

ABHES VII.MA.A.1 9(I)   CAAHEP IV.P (6)

OBJECTIVE: To safely assist patient into and out of lithotomy position for pelvic examination or catheterization.

STANDARD: This task takes 1 minute.

EQUIPMENT AND SUPPLIES: Examination table with stirrups; gown; drape.

STEPS:

1. Check physician's orders, and check for patient allergies.
2. Perform hand hygiene.
3. Ask patient to disrobe and don gown, and provide assistance as needed.
4. Assist patient to sit on end of table, and brace step stool as needed.
5. Cover legs with drape.
6. Ask patient to lie back on table while you support feet and pull out foot extension.
7. Position stirrups level with height of table about 1 foot from side of table. Lock stirrups.
8. Ask patient to slide down on table until buttocks are on edge of table end.

WHY? The lithotomy position is used to perform vaginal examination using a vaginal speculum.

9. Assist patient to bend knees and place feet in stirrups. Position drape for privacy with point between patient's legs.
10. Position light source and stool for examiner.

11. Place pillow under patient's head as needed.
12. Make sure patient is comfortable, and inform patient that physician will be in shortly.
13. Place medical record in designated location outside room, and inform physician that patient is ready.
14. When examination complete, pull out foot extension and help patient remove feet from stirrups, if needed, and place them on foot extension.
15. Ask patient to slide up on table, and assist as needed. Keep drape in place to ensure privacy.
16. Assist patient to sitting position, and push in foot extension. Allow time to prevent dizziness.
17. Assist from table, stabilizing step stool if necessary, and provide further instructions.
18. Clean examination room for next patient (follow steps in Procedure 4-1).
19. Perform hand hygiene.

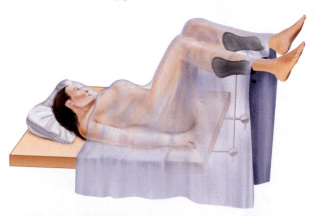

FIGURE 4-14   Lithotomy position.

PROCEDURE 4-8

POSITIONING PATIENT IN PRONE POSITION

ABHES VII.MA.A.1 9(I)   CAAHEP IV.P (6)

OBJECTIVE: To safely assist patient into prone position for examination of the posterior of the body.

STANDARD: This task takes 1 minute.

EQUIPMENT AND SUPPLIES: Examination table; gown; drape.

STEPS:

1. Check physician's orders, and check for patient allergies.
2. Perform hand hygiene.
3. Provide a gown, ask patient to disrobe, and provide assistance as needed.
4. Assist patient onto end of table, bracing step stool as needed. Cover patient's legs with drape.
5. Ask patient to lie back on table while you support patient's back and pull out foot extension.

WHY? The prone position is used for back examinations and is unsuitable for women in late stages of pregnancies.

6. Ask patient to turn toward you onto side, then onto abdomen. Position yourself against table to prevent patient from falling.

7. Place pillows as needed for comfort under patient's head and feet. Cover patient with drape from shoulders to ankles.
8. When examination complete, ask patient to turn toward you and help to a sitting position.
9. Have patient stay seated a few moments to prevent dizziness.
10. Assist from table, stabilizing step stool if needed, and provide further instructions.
11. Clean examination room for next patient (follow steps in Procedure 4-1).
12. Perform hand hygiene.

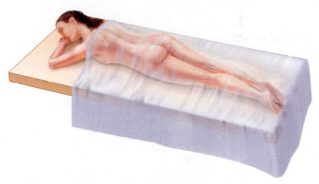

FIGURE 4-15   **Prone position.**

PROCEDURE 4-9

POSITIONING PATIENT IN SIMS' POSITION

ABHES VII.MA.A.1 9(I)   CAAHEP IV.P (6)

OBJECTIVE: To safely assist patient into Sims' position for possible rectal exam, proctological exam, sigmoidoscopic exam, vaginal exam, rectal temperature measurement, or enema.

STANDARD: This task takes 1 minute.

EQUIPMENT AND SUPPLIES: Examination table; gown; drape.

STEPS:

1. Check physician's orders, and check for patient allergies.
2. Perform hand hygiene.
3. Ask patient to disrobe, and provide gown and assist as needed.
4. Ask patient to sit on end of table and stabilize step stool as needed.
5. Place drape over patient's lap and legs.
6. Assist patient to lie back, while you support patient's back and extend foot of table.

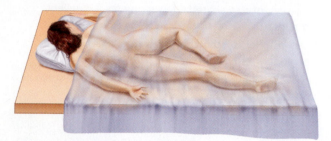

FIGURE 4-16   Sims' or lateral position.

7. Ask patient to turn toward you onto their left side with body weight on chest, left knee flexed slightly.
8. Ask patient to flex right knee to a 90° angle. Bend right arm at elbow with hand toward head. Adjust drape to cover from shoulders to ankles.

WHY? The Sims' position is used for colonoscopies, enemas, and rectal temperatures.

9. When procedure is complete, ask patient to turn toward you and onto back. Assist patient to sitting position. Ask patient to remain seated at end of table a few moments to prevent dizziness.
10. Assist patient from table, stabilize step stool as needed, and provide further instruction.
11. Clean examination room for next patient (follow steps in Procedure 4-1).
12. Perform hand hygiene.

PROCEDURE 4-10

POSITIONING PATIENT IN KNEE–CHEST POSITION

ABHES VII.MA.A.1 9(I)   CAAHEP IV.P (6)

OBJECTIVE: To safely assist patient into knee–chest position for examination of rectum, sigmoid colon, or vagina.

STANDARD: This task takes 1 minute.

EQUIPMENT AND SUPPLIES: Examination table; gown; drape.

STEPS:

1. Check physician's orders, and check for patient allergies.
2. Perform hand hygiene.
3. Ask patient to disrobe, provide gown, and assist as needed.
4. Ask patient to sit on end of table, and stabilize step stool as needed.
5. Cover patient's legs with drape.

6. Ask patient to lie back while you support back and pull out foot extension.
7. Ask patient to turn toward you onto abdomen, and provide assistance as needed. Position yourself against table to prevent patient from falling. Adjust drape.
8. Assist patient onto knees with hips bent and chest on table. Buttocks will be raised, arms bent, head turned to side, hands next to head. Patient may rest weight on elbows if more comfortable.

WHY? The knee–chest position is used for proctological examinations and is uncomfortable for elderly patients and pregnant women.

9. Adjust drape so point of drape is between legs.

10. When examination is complete, help patient lie flat on abdomen. When patient is ready, ask patient to turn toward you and lie on back. Help patient to sit up. Have patient remain seated a few moments to prevent dizziness.

11. Assist from table, stabilize step stool as needed, and provide further instructions.

12. Clean examination room for next patient (follow steps in Procedure 4-1).

13. Perform hand hygiene.

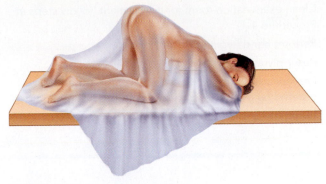

FIGURE 4-17 Knee–chest position.

PROCEDURE 4-11

ASSISTING WITH COMPLETE PHYSICAL EXAMINATION

ABHES VII.MA.A.1 9(m)   CAAHEP IV.P (10)

OBJECTIVE: To assist physician with complete physical examination and assist patient as needed while ensuring safety and privacy during procedure.

STANDARD: This task takes 15–20 minutes.

EQUIPMENT AND SUPPLIES: Scale; gown; drape; thermometer; sphygmomanometer; alcohol wipes; tongue depressors; otoscope; ophthalmoscope; penlight; nasal speculum; tape; tuning fork; percussion hammer; safety pin; stethoscope; measuring tape; cotton balls; gloves; tissues; lubricant; emesis basin; gauze sponges; specimen bottles; slides; request forms; visual acuity chart; regular waste and biohazard waste containers; pen; paper.

STEPS:

1. Check physician's orders, and check for patient allergies.

2. Perform hand hygiene.

3. Assemble all equipment in examination room.

4. Identify patient, and explain procedure.

5. Ask patient to provide urine specimen, if needed, or to empty bladder for comfort during examination.

6. Take vital signs, height, and weight, and measure visual acuity if ordered. Document all results immediately.

7. Ask patient to disrobe, provide a gown, and offer assistance as needed.

8. Explain where you want patient to sit and where gown opening should be. Knock before reentering.

9. Assist patient onto exam table, and stabilize step stool if necessary. Have patient sit on side of exam table, and provide drape for lap and legs.

10. Make sure patient is comfortable, and inform patient that physician will be in shortly.

11. Place medical record in designated location outside room, and inform physician that patient is ready.

12. Assist physician as needed by handing instruments and assisting patient to change positions.

13. As physician moves through ROS, provide draping as needed, exposing only the area of patient being examined at the moment. (Use gloves when handling specimens or equipment that may be contaminated such as tongue depressor, mirror.)

14. Immediately label all specimens.

15. When examination is complete, assist patient to sit up slowly, allowing time to prevent dizziness.

16. Assist patient off examination table while ensuring safety.

17. Ask patient to dress, and provide assistance as needed. Provide privacy.

18. Clean examination room for next patient (follow steps in Procedure 4-1).

19. Perform hand hygiene.

20. Resupply examination room.

21. Prepare specimens for transport; perform other tasks ordered by physician, such as scheduling appointments.

22. Complete any documentation on patient's record.

CHARTING EXAMPLE: 02/03/XX 11:30 A.M. CC: Annual PE by Dr. Fox. ECG results given to Dr. Fox. Blood drawn for profile and sent to Smith Lab. Pt. told to schedule a follow-up appointment for 2 weeks to review PE findings. Confirmed appointment made. · H. Martinez, CMA (AAMA)

Performing Scoliosis Examination

Three abnormal curvatures of the spine are possible: scoliosis, lordosis, and kyphosis (see Figure 4-18). **Scoliosis**, an abnormal lateral curvature, usually appears during periods of rapid growth. Screening for scoliosis may be performed in a number of different types of facilities. In some locations, only licensed personnel may perform this screening. **Lordosis** is an abnormal increase in the forward curvature of the spine and is also known as swayback. **Kyphosis** is an abnormal increase in the outward curvature of the thoracic spine and is also known as

hunchback or humpback. (Procedure 4-12 lists steps for performing scoliosis screening.)

Caring for Vomiting Patient

Vomiting is a common situation that may arise in any type of facility and may occur more frequently in medical facilities. Assistive personnel must be prepared to deal with a vomiting patient and take measures to prevent choking and aspiration of **vomitus**. Procedure 4-13 provides the steps for assisting a vomiting patient.

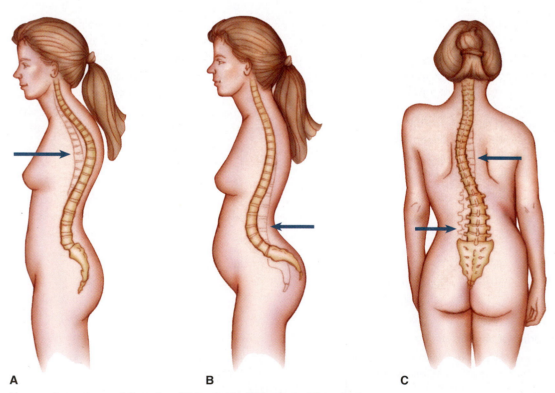

A **B** **C**

FIGURE 4-18 **Abnormal curvatures of the spine: (A) kyphosis; (B) lordosis; (C) scoliosis.**

PROCEDURE 4-12

PERFORMING SCOLIOSIS SCREENING

ABHES VII.MA.A.1 9(m)   CAAHEP IV.P (10)

OBJECTIVE: To observe patient for possible scoliosis.

STANDARD: This task takes 5 minutes.

EQUIPMENT AND SUPPLIES: Patient's record; pen.

STEPS:

1. Check physician's orders, and check for patient allergies.
2. Perform hand hygiene.
3. Identify patient, and introduce yourself.
4. Explain procedure.
5. Ask patient to remove shirt or blouse and to stand up straight.
6. Observe whether one shoulder is higher than the other or one **scapula** (shoulder blade) is more prominent than the other.
7. Have patient hang arms loosely at sides, and check to see if one hip is higher than the other or whether patient tilts more to one side or the other; or whether one arm swings away from body more than the other when patient takes a few steps.
8. Ask patient to bend forward at waist, arms hanging down with palms together at knee height. Check for a hump on the back at ribs near waist.
9. Document findings in patient's record.
10. Instruct patient to dress, and provide assistance as needed.

CHARTING EXAMPLE: 01/19/XX 4:00 P.M. Scoliosis examination performed. (L) scapula slightly more prominent than right. Dr. Izzo to recheck. · · · · · · · · · · · · · · · · · D. Martin, RMA

PROCEDURE 4-13

ASSISTING VOMITING PATIENT

ABHES VII.MA.A.1 9(m)   CAAHEP IV.P (10)

OBJECTIVE: To assist vomiting patient and prevent aspiration while providing comfort and safety.

STANDARD: The time this task takes is dependent on patient circumstances.

EQUIPMENT AND SUPPLIES: Emesis basin; gloves; cup of water; paper towels; tissues.

STEPS:

1. Check physician's orders, and check for patient allergies.
2. Perform hand hygiene.
3. Don necessary PPE (gown, goggles, gloves, mask).
4. Give patient emesis basin, and observe amount, color, odor, consistency of vomitus. If lying down, have patient turn onto side to prevent aspiration of vomitus. Wipe mouth, and place cool compress on forehead. Offer water and clean emesis basin to permit mouth rinsing.
5. Check for such signs of dehydration as dry skin, flushing, confusion, irregular pulse. When appropriate, ask patient when vomiting began, how often it occurs, and if in pain.
6. Follow up with any other orders physician may have given.
7. Clean patient as needed, and make comfortable.
8. Clean area, and dispose properly of vomitus in toilet. Dispose of anything used to wipe up area in biohazard waste container.
9. Remove gloves, discard in biohazard waste container, and perform hand hygiene.
10. Document in patient's record.

CHARTING EXAMPLE: 03/05/XX 12:03 P.M. Pt. complained of N while on exam table. Provided emesis basin. Pt. vomited approx. 200 cc clean odorless vomitus one time. T 99.6., R 20, BP 130/80 · I. Lopez, CMA (AAMA)

Communicating Effectively with Elderly and Culturally Diverse Patients

Health care providers find they are responsible for working with and delivering care to patients of a wide variety of ages and racial, ethnic, cultural, religious, and socioeconomic backgrounds. In every instance, it is important to treat each person as an individual and to treat them as you would like to be treated: with respect and dignity. Patients from other cultures may be completely unfamiliar with the Western model of medicine, and language barriers may exist. Prejudging patients or generalizing about a group of people should be avoided. Routine behaviors such as reaching out to touch a patient's arm in comfort may be an affront to the patient from some cultures. Although it is impossible to know all the customs and traditions of every group of people, we must be sensitive caregivers. Procedure 4-14 provides guidelines for communicating with non-English-speaking patients as well as those who are culturally diverse and speak some English.

PROCEDURE 4-14

COMMUNICATING WITH PATIENTS FROM OTHER CULTURES
ABHES VII.MA.A.1 5(g)   CAAHEP IV.A (3); IV.A (10); IV.C (7)

OBJECTIVE: To effectively communicate with patients from other cultures while being sensitive to their need for privacy.

STANDARD: The time this task takes will vary with needs of patient.

EQUIPMENT AND SUPPLIES: Pen; paper; patient's health record; gown; drape; translator or family member who understands English.

STEPS:

1. Check physician's orders, and check for patient allergies.
2. Greet the patient warmly with a smile in the front office. Determine if the patient understands English. Check if family member who can translate for you is present.
3. If no family member is present, locate a translator if possible.

NOTE: If possible, determine language barrier prior to patient's appointment so you have time to locate translator.

4. If using a translator, direct your conversation to that individual.
5. If you have to demonstrate your wishes, direct the demonstrations to the patient (e.g., donning gown, sitting on table). Use illustrations to further comprehension.
6. Confirm with the translator that he or she and the patient understand the instructions you gave.
7. If the patient understands some English, speak slowly, in simple terms, and demonstrate or use pictures to make your point.

8. Patients from other cultures may be more modest and reluctant to disrobe in the presence of another person, especially someone of the opposite sex. Make arrangements to comply with patient's wishes as much as possible.
9. At this stage in the examination, be certain the person translating understands why patient needs to disrobe and that you will protect privacy as much as possible.
10. Leave the room, and provide enough time for disrobing.
11. Knock before reentering. Provide extra drapes if patient will feel more comfortable.
12. If patient refuses to disrobe, politely excuse yourself, leave room, and explain situation to physician. (A physician may be more successful in obtaining patient compliance.) Before leaving the room, make sure patient is comfortable, and inform patient that physician will be in shortly.
13. Place medical record in designated location outside room, and inform physician of patient's hesitancy about disrobing or that patient is ready.
14. Smile at patient during procedure, and speak in soothing tones. Empathy is felt even though words may not be understood. Be aware that extra time is needed to assist patients from other cultures.
15. Perform hand hygiene, and clean room for the next patient (following steps in Procedure 4-1).
16. Document patient's record.

Special needs patients, such as children and the elderly, also require more time at each encounter. **Gerontology** is the study of the aging process and its effects on people. The number of elderly is increasing in the United States for a variety of reasons; by 2020 the elderly will comprise 20% of the population. Health care providers must be aware of the special needs of the elderly and how to interact effectively with them at each encounter. (Communicating with children is covered in Chapter 6. Procedure 4-15 lists some steps to help you communicate effectively with the elderly.)

PROCEDURE 4-15

COMMUNICATING EFFECTIVELY WITH THE ELDERLY

ABHES VII.MA.A.1 5(f)   CAAHEP IV.C (7); IV.A (10)

OBJECTIVE: To ensure effective communication with elderly patient preparing for a physical examination.

STANDARD: The time this task takes depends on the needs of the patient.

EQUIPMENT AND SUPPLIES: Pen; paper; patient's record; history form; gown; drape; other examination equipment as needed.

STEPS:

1. Check physician's orders, and check for patient allergies.
2. Welcome the patient in front office warmly and with a smile.
3. Face the patient and speak clearly and directly to him or her.
4. Introduce yourself with sincerity.
5. Address the patient as Mr. or Mrs. unless instructed otherwise by them.
6. Observe carefully for cues to indicate comprehension by patient.
7. If it appears that the patient has difficulty understanding you, paraphrase and use other words and simple directions.
8. Ask the patient to follow you to exam room, and allow extra time for patient to comply.
9. Observe patient's overall ability to comply with your requests. If patient seems confused during preparation for exam, note it so physician will be alerted.

10. Offer assistance if needed, but allow patient as much autonomy as possible.
11. Ask patient to be seated, and gather information for health history.
12. Never assume patient is incompetent solely because of age.
13. If patient's replies to your questions become too lengthy, gently interrupt and bring patient back to the topic.
14. If some replies seem inappropriate, do not correct but rather gently guide patient to another topic. Proceed with examination procedures.
15. If patient is confused, do not leave unattended.
16. Do not argue with patient's version of reality.

NOTE: Relaxed body gestures, facial expressions, and caring touch are most important when caring for a confused patient.

17. Perform hand hygiene.
18. Document all your findings and impressions.
19. Place medical record in designated location outside room, and inform physician of patient's hesitancy about disrobing or that patient is ready.

CHARTING EXAMPLE: 03/05/XX 1:30 P.M. Pt. appeared confused. Unable to follow directions or to undress w/o help. Cheerful attitude. · · · · · · · · · · · · · · · M. Blardo, CMA (AAMA)

5 Assisting with Medical Specialties

PROCEDURES

Procedure 5-1 Performing Scratch Testing

Procedure 5-2 Performing Patch Testing

Procedure 5-3 Taking a Wound Culture

Procedure 5-4 Administering Disposable Enema

Procedure 5-5 Assisting with Sigmoidoscopy Examination

Procedure 5-6 Assisting with Colonoscopy

Procedure 5-7 Instructing Patient in Collecting Stool Specimens

Procedure 5-8 Testing for Occult Blood

Procedure 5-9 Performing a Pupil Check

Procedure 5-10 Assisting with Neurologic Screening Examination

Advanced Procedure 5-11 Assisting with Lumbar Puncture

Procedure 5-12 Instructing a Patient on Breast Self-Examination

Procedure 5-13 Assisting with Pelvic Examination and Pap Test (Conventional and ThinPrep Methods)

Procedure 5-14 Preparing Wet Mount/Wet Prep and KOH Slides

Procedure 5-15 Obtaining Material for Amplified DNA Probe Test for Chlamydia and Gonorrhea

Procedure 5-16 Assisting with Routine Prenatal Visit

Procedure 5-17 Assisting with Postpartum Examination

Procedure 5-18 Assisting with Colposcopy and Cervical Biopsy

Procedure 5-19 Performing Urinary Catheterization on a Female

Procedure 5-20 Instructing Male Patient on Testicular Self-Examination

Procedure 5-21 Performing Urinary Catheterization on a Male

Procedure 5-22 Screening Distance Visual Acuity with Snellen Chart

Procedure 5-23 Screening for Near-Vision Acuity

Procedure 5-24 Screening for Color-Vision Acuity

Procedure 5-25 Irrigating the Eye

Procedure 5-26 Instilling Eye Medications

Procedure 5-27 Applying Eye Patch Dressing

Procedure 5-28 Assisting with Audiometry

Procedure 5-29 Irrigating the Ear

Procedure 5-30 Instilling Ear Medication

Procedure 5-31 Instilling Nasal Medication

Procedure 5-32 Assisting with Treatment of Epistaxis

Procedure 5-33 Obtaining a Throat Culture

TERMS TO LEARN

hypersensitivity

allergen

anaphylactic shock

rhinorrhea

dyspnea

papules

vesicles

desensitization injections

excision

punch biopsy

squamous cell carcinoma

obturator

anoscope

insufflator

Romberg test

stat

Queckenstedt test

puerperium

menses

menarche

gravida

para

abortion

dysplasia

carcinoma in situ

fundal height

fetal heart rate

abdominal ultrasound

amniocentesis

chorionic villi sampling (CVS)

alpha-fetoprotein (AFP)

lochia

electrocautery

catheterization

urinary meatus

epididymis

lavage

strabismus

cerumen

pinna

epitaxis

Chapter 4 presented information on assisting with general physical examinations. This chapter deals with examinations and procedures relating to specific body systems. The most commonly performed examinations include neurologic, gynecologic, prenatal, proctoscopic, sigmoidoscopic, cardiovascular, and pulmonary. Cardiology and pulmonology examinations are presented in Chapter 21. Examinations and procedures differ from practice to practice; however, you may be expected to perform these common procedures wherever you are employed. Additional specialty procedures such as those associated with dermatology, immunology, ophthalmology, and otorhinolaryngology also are presented in this chapter.

A thorough understanding of anatomy and physiology of each system and the diseases related to each is beyond the scope of this text. Medical assistants and other health care providers should review one of the many available texts before considering this chapter.

Allergy

Allergists specialize in diagnosing and treating allergies. An allergy is an abnormal reaction or **hypersensitivity** to an **allergen**. Allergens are antigenic (capable of inducing the productions of antibodies) substances, such as pollen, insect bites, molds, and dust mites. Allergens may enter the body through inhalation, injection, swallowing, or contact with the skin. Allergic or hypersensitivity (exaggerated) reactions may be localized, such as a mosquito bite, or systemic and life threatening, such as asthma or anaphylactic shock.

Anaphylactic shock (a life-threatening reaction, including respiratory distress, tachycardia, convulsions, and death) can occur from bee or wasp stings, allergies to drugs such as penicillin, or food allergies to nuts, food, or food preservatives. Patients with this type of hypersensitivity should carry an anaphylactic shock kit containing a self-injecting dose of epinephrine. Table 5-1 describes common types of allergies.

Allergy testing methods include scratch or skin testing, intradermal tests, patch tests, and radioallergosorbent test (RAST). Procedures for scratch testing (Procedure 5-1) and patch testing (Procedure 5-2) follow. Allergy testing may produce a severe reaction in the patient and should never be performed unless a physician is on site. Box 5-1 lists safety guidelines for allergy testing.

Performing Scratch Testing

A scratch test is performed to determine which specific allergens are causing reactions in the patient. The skin on the patient's arms or back is scratched, and extracts of suspected allergens are applied to that area. A negative control solution containing no allergens but made with the same base material as the other extracts is applied in the same manner. This is done to rule out a reaction to the solution itself.

Always ask patients to refrain from taking antihistamines prior to allergy testing. The patient should be made aware that the procedure may cause discomfort and itching. To check reaction site again, the physician may require the patient to return 24 hours after testing.

TABLE 5-1 Common Types of Allergies

Allergy	Description
Allergic rhinitis	Inflammation of the nasal mucosa resulting in nasal congestion, **rhinorrhea** (runny nose), sneezing, itching of nose. Seasonal allergic rhinitis such as hay fever occurs during certain seasons of the year. Children suffering from this type of allergy may rub their noses in an upward movement called "allergic salute."
Asthma	A condition seen most frequently in childhood in which wheezing, coughing, and **dyspnea** (difficulty breathing) are the major symptoms. Asthmatic attacks may be caused by allergens inhaled from air or ingested from food or drugs. The patient's airway is affected by constriction of the bronchial passages. Treatment consists of medication and control of causative factors.
Contact dermatitis	Inflammation and irritation of the skin due to contact with an irritating substance such as soap, perfume, cosmetics, plastics, dyes, and plants such as poison ivy. Treatment consists of topical and systemic medications and removal of the causative agent.
Eczema	A superficial dermatitis accompanied by **papules** (small bump or pimple), **vesicles** (blister), and crusting. The condition may be acute or chronic.
Urticaria	Hives: a skin eruption of pale reddish wheals (circular elevations of the skin) with severe itching usually associated with a food allergy, stress, or drug reactions.

PROCEDURE 5-1

PERFORMING SCRATCH TESTING

ABHES VII.MA.A.1 10(b)(4)   CAAHEP I.P (15)

OBJECTIVE: To determine specific substances that cause an allergic reaction in the patient.

STANDARD: This task takes 15 minutes.

EQUIPMENT AND SUPPLIES: Allergen extracts; control solution; cotton balls; alcohol; disposable sterile needles or lancets; timer; tape; ruler; cold packs or ice bag; patient's record; disposable gloves; biohazard waste containers, including sharps container.

STEPS:

1. Check physician's orders, and check for patient allergies.
2. Perform hand hygiene.
3. Identify patient, introduce yourself, and explain procedure.
4. Assist patient onto examination table if necessary.
5. Don gloves and swab test site (either upper arm or back) with alcohol, and allow to air-dry.
6. Label skin with adhesive tape and name of allergen applied in rows about 1½ to 2 inches apart.
7. Place a drop of allergen above or below correct label. Be consistent.
8. Using a separate sterile lancet or needle for each extract, make a small scratch (no more than ⅛ inch deep) on skin below each drop.
9. Set timer for specified reaction time (usually 10–30 minutes).

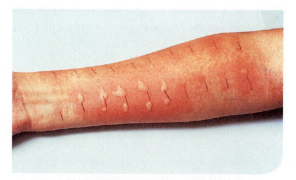

FIGURE 5-1 Allergy Skin Testing. This patient's arm shows a number of wheals after introduction of a variety of antigens. The size of the wheal corresponds to the degree of allergy to that antigen.

10. After time elapses, clean each site with alcohol applied to cotton ball, taking care not to remove labels.

11. Examine and measure each site, and record results in patient's record. (Figure 5-1 shows examples of wheals resulting from allergy testing.)

12. Have physician check patient.

13. If necessary, apply cold packs to sites to relieve itching.

14. Dispose properly of used material.

15. Assist patient off examination table, allow time and privacy for patient to dress, and offer aid as needed.

16. Clean examination room. Record any additional data in patient's record.

17. Perform hand hygiene.

CHARTING EXAMPLE: 03/13/XX Scratch testing performed. No positive reactions. Checked by Dr. Rosen. · M. Dennehey, CMA (AAMA)

PROCEDURE 5-2

PERFORMING PATCH TESTING

ABHES VII.MA.A.1 10(b)(4)   CAAHEP I.P (15)

OBJECTIVE: To determine patient's sensitivity to a suspected allergen.

STANDARD: This task takes 15 minutes.

EQUIPMENT AND SUPPLIES: Gloves; alcohol; cotton balls; patches; allergen extracts; droppers; control solution; adhesive tape; ruler; plastic wrap; and biohazard waste containers.

STEPS:

1. Check physician's orders, and check for patient allergies.

2. Perform hand hygiene.

3. Identify and greet patient.

4. Introduce yourself, and explain procedure.

5. Assist patient onto examination table.

6. Don gloves and clean anterior surface of patient's forearm with alcohol. Let air-dry.

7. Place allergen-soaked patch on forearm in area free of any sign of skin irritation. Take care to label appropriately. Place as many patches as physician's order requires.

8. Cover patches with plastic wrap, and ask patient to keep area dry for 24 hours.

9. Assist patient off examination table and provide further instructions.

10. Review instructions with patient, and set appointment time for next day.

11. Clean examination room. Remove gloves.

12. Document patient's record.

13. Perform hand hygiene.

CHARTING EXAMPLE: 03/13/XX 9:00 A.M. Patches for Tide detergent, Calgon bathing gel, Jergens body cream applied. Pt. to return 9:00 A.M. 3/14/XX. · · · · · · · · · · · · · C. Poke, RMA

BOX 5-1 Safety Guidelines for Allergy Testing

Observe Patient	Observe patients for sign of severe reaction for 30 minutes after allergy desensitizing injection or allergy skin testing.
Emergency Cart	Have readily available an emergency cart containing injectable epinephrine with syringes and needles; airways of various sizes; oxygen masks and bag mask devices; tourniquet; defibrillator; tracheotomy equipment; ECG machine; and intravenous setup.

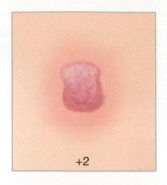
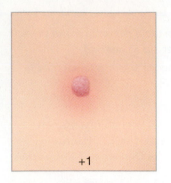

+1

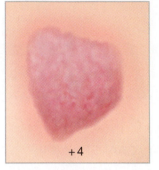

+2

+3

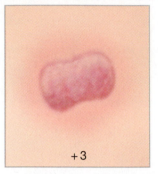

+4

FIGURE 5-2 Classifications of reactions to allergy testing: wheals.

Reactions are classified as negative (no reaction: same size or smaller than negative control), positive reactions are rated on a scale of 1+ (5 mm), 2+ (10 mm), 3+ (15 mm), and 4+ (20 mm) as shown in Figure 5-2. If no conclusive results are found, other testing may be necessary. (Procedure 5-1 describes how to perform scratch testing.)

Patch Testing

Patch testing consists of placing a small patch soaked with allergen onto the anterior surface of the forearm and covering it with plastic wrap. After 24 hours, the patient returns to have each site observed for positive reaction or wheal formation. Patch testing is usually done to discover the source of contact dermatitis. If necessary, several different patch tests may be performed at the same time. Care must be taken to label each correctly.

Intradermal Allergy Testing

Intradermal allergy testing is performed by injecting 0.01 to 0.02 mL of an allergen extract into the anterior surface of the forearm, and 10 to 18 tests can be performed on each arm. A red wheal is a positive result. The intradermal test is considered to be more accurate than the scratch test. The procedure for intradermal injections is covered in Chapter 18.

Radioallergosorbent (RAST) Testing

Radioallergosorbent testing, or RAST testing, may be performed when direct skin testing is impossible. The RAST test detects the presence of allergen-specific immunoglobulin E (IgE) antibodies in the blood. There is no need for the patient to stop antihistamines prior to RAST testing.

RAST testing requires a venipuncture, which makes it easier on the patient and perhaps less dangerous than other tests, which introduce allergens that may possibly cause severe reactions. (The procedure for venipuncture is found in Chapter 13.) Follow laboratory protocol for type and number of tubes required.

Desensitizing Allergy Injection Treatment

Treatment for allergies consists of medications (e.g., antihistamines such as Benadryl), allergy testing, and desensitization injections. **Desensitization injections** involve administering minute amounts of the allergen into the patient's system over an extended period of time to build up a tolerance for the allergen. Figure 5-3 shows a young patient receiving an allergy injection. (The procedure for administering subcutaneous injection is covered in Chapter 18.)

Dermatology

The skin is the largest organ in the body. It consists of three layers. The outermost layer is the epidermis, the middle layer is the dermis, and the innermost is the subcutaneous layer. The skin provides a boundary separating us from the outside world, regulates body temperature, prevents infection, and provides sensory receptors to respond to

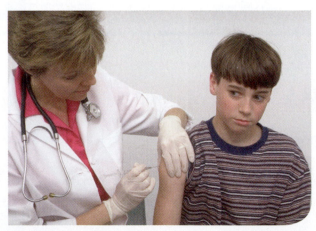

FIGURE 5-3 An allergy injection is used to desensitize an allergen.

BOX 5-2 Guidelines for Assisting with Tissue Biopsy

- Observe strict surgical asepsis throughout the procedure.
- Assemble all supplies needed for procedure.
- Prepare patient by explaining procedure, including possibility of some discomfort.
- Follow office protocol for preparing skin site, and document.
- Assist physician as needed, observing standard precautions and using PPE.

- Immediately and thoroughly label any specimen removed.
- Clean procedure area and properly dispose of all waste materials.
- Document thoroughly in patient's record, including where specimen sent and patient education regarding care of biopsy site.
- Perform hand hygiene.

heat, pain, and pressure. Many conditions affect the skin and its accessory structures: hair, nails, and sweat glands.

A wide variety of diagnostic procedures are associated with treating disorders of the integumentary system. A dermatologist examines the outer layer of skin over the entire body, beginning with scalp, including the genital area, and continuing to the soles of the feet and between the toes. Inspection may include using a magnifying glass and bright light to closely evaluate a lesion or growth. Wood's light, a type of ultraviolet light, is used in a darkened room to treat and evaluate certain dermatologic conditions. Photographs of suspicious areas may be taken. Skin biopsies, cultures for bacteria, viruses or fungi also may be required. Allergy testing may be necessary. The procedure for taking a wound culture follows.

ASSISTING WITH SKIN BIOPSY

There are several methods for obtaining a small piece of tissue for examination. **Excision** refers to the removal of the entire lesion, such as a mole, wart, or tumor. A **punch biopsy** involves removing a small section from a specific location in the lesion. A shave biopsy involves using a scalpel to cut or shave off the growth or lesion just above the skin line, as is done to examine for **squamous cell carcinoma**, a type of skin cancer. Regardless of the type of biopsy, strict surgical asepsis must be observed. (Chapter 8 covers sterile asepsis and assisting with needle biopsy. Box 5-2 provides guidelines for tissue biopsy.)

TAKING A WOUND CULTURE

A wound culture is ordered to determine the causative agent of an infection. Wound cultures may be obtained from any surface of the body and from any body orifice. A sensitivity test is often ordered at the same time. This test helps the physician select the appropriate antibiotic based on the test results.

PROCEDURE 5-3

TAKING A WOUND CULTURE

ABHES VII.MA.A.1 10(d)(3)   CAAHEP III.P (7)

OBJECTIVE: To obtain a sample from a wound using swab technique without contamination or error.

STANDARD: This task takes 10 minutes.

EQUIPMENT AND SUPPLIES: Gloves; culture tube with sterile swab and aerobic and anaerobic transport media; tape for dressing; sterile water for cleansing wound; sterile 4 × 4 gauze dressing; biohazard waste container; bag for

soiled dressing; prepared label for culture; pen; patient's record.

STEPS:

1. Check physician's orders, and check for patient allergies.
2. Perform hand hygiene.
3. Assemble equipment.
4. Identify patient, and explain procedure.

5. Apply gloves.

6. Remove dressing, noting amount and type of **exudate** (oozing matter), and place soiled dressing in bag.

7. Observe wound for redness, crusting, swelling, and odor.

8. Using a sterile swab, place it in wound and use a wiping motion in area of most exudate. Obtain anaerobic swab first if so directed. Place swab in sterile culture tube. Crush ampule of preservative in the culture tube, then seal tube. Repeat for aerobic culture if required.

9. Label the culture tube with patient's name, identification number, date, and source of specimen.

10. Remove gloves and dispose of them in biohazard waste container.

11. Perform hand hygiene, and apply sterile gloves.

12. Clean wound using sterile water and sterile 4 × 4 gauze squares.

13. Apply sterile dressing over wound.

NOTE: Chapter 8 deals with the specifics of sterile asepsis.

14. Instruct patient on wound care.

15. Remove gloves, and dispose of them properly.

16. Clean area.

17. Perform hand hygiene.

18. Document procedure.

CHARTING EXAMPLE: 03/14/XX 10:10 A.M. Open wound on (L) ankle approximately 1 inch in diameter. Small amount greenish exudate. Aerobic wound culture obtained per Dr. Fleiss. Sent to Marymount Hospital. Applied sterile dressing. Instructed pt. to apply warm compresses 2×/day for 2 days and redress wound. Instructed pt. to call for lab results on 3/17. · · · · · · · · · · · · · · S. Mendoza, CMA (AAMA)

Legal Alert! Only licensed personnel may give test results to a patient unless assistive personnel are specifically instructed to do so by the physician.

Gastroenterology

Gastroenterology is the study of the digestive system. The digestive system involves many organs, and therefore symptoms of digestive disorders are numerous and varied. Many of the examinations associated with the digestive system may be uncomfortable or embarrassing for the patient. Every effort must be made to ensure the patient's privacy.

In an office setting, fecal occult blood is among the most common tests performed. Sigmoidoscopy or proctosigmoidoscopy may be performed; they are useful in the detection of polyps, cancer of the colon, ulcerations, and diverticulitis. A flexible metal or plastic instrument with a light source and magnifying lens is used to perform this procedure.

Patient preparation prior to the examination is important. This includes having the patient empty bowel and bladder ahead of the procedure. A commercially prepared enema may be required 2 hours before the test. Patients should be advised to drink plenty of clear liquids and eat sparingly the day before testing. It is critical that the patient follow bowel preparations, or testing may need to be postponed.

It is uncommon to have to administer a disposable enema in a physician's office. However, if the patient has not complied with preparation instructions, the physician may order administration of an enema to complete the examination. Clear instructions to the patient may ensure better compliance and comfort. (Procedure 5-4 lists the steps for administering a disposable enema.)

PROCEDURE 5-4

ADMINISTERING DISPOSABLE ENEMA

ABHES VII.MA.A.1 9(m)   CAAHEP I.P (10)

OBJECTIVE: To assist in cleansing bowel of fecal material in preparation for a diagnostic examination.

STANDARD: This task takes 10 minutes.

EQUIPMENT AND SUPPLIES: Examination table; disposable enema; lubricant; Mayo tray; towel; gloves; tissues; drape; pen; patient's record.

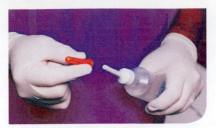

FIGURE 5-4 Removing the cap on a disposable enema container.

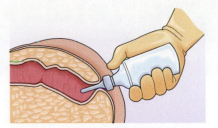

FIGURE 5-5 Insert the enema tip through the anus and 2 inches into the rectum.

STEPS:

1. Check physician's orders, and check for allergies.

2. Assemble equipment. Warm disposable enema container prior to using (to avoid causing abdominal cramping).

3. Identify patient, and explain procedure.

4. Perform hand hygiene.

5. Instruct patient to disrobe from waist down. Assist onto examination table as needed.

6. Ask patient to assume Sims' position (left side with right knee at 90° angle). Drape patient for comfort and privacy.

7. Don gloves.

8. Remove tip from enema container. Apply small amount of lubricant. (See Figure 5-4.)

9. Separate buttocks to expose anus. Gently insert the lubricated tip into the anus about 2 inches, with tip pointing toward patient's navel. (See Figure 5-5.)

10. Instruct patient to take deep breaths while you slowly empty contents of container.

11. Ask patient to retain liquid as a long as possible to ensure good results (5–10 minutes should be sufficient).

12. After withdrawing the tip, gently wipe anal area with tissue to remove excess lubricant.

13. Provide bedpan, or direct patient to restroom with instructions not to flush the toilet until you have checked results.

14. Instruct patient as necessary for test procedure.

15. Discard disposable enema equipment in appropriate waste containers. Clean room.

16. Remove gloves, and perform hand hygiene.

17. Document patient's record.

CHARTING EXAMPLE: 03/21/XX 2:15 P.M. Pt. to have sigmoidoscopy. Bowel preparation at home not entirely successful. Administered disposable cleansing enema per Dr. Chang. Enema returned small amount of dark brown, hard stool. Pt. complained of stomach cramps but tolerated procedure. · R. Negri, CMA (AAMA)

ASSISTING WITH SIGMOIDOSCOPY

Sigmoidoscopy is the visual examination with an endoscope of the sigmoid colon. Many physicians prefer that patients have a colonoscopy instead of a sigmoidoscopy because the latter covers a greater length of the colon and may offer more diagnostic information. (Colonoscopies are discussed later in this chapter.) Procedure 5-5 describes the steps in assisting with sigmoidoscopy.

ASSISTING WITH COLONOSCOPY

Colonoscopy procedures are performed in an office or hospital outpatient area. An IV sedative is administered prior to the procedure. Colonoscopy allows the physician to examine more of the large intestine than the sigmoidoscopy. The American Cancer Society recommends all individuals over the age of 50 have a colonoscopy to screen for cancer.

Preparation the day prior to colonoscopy involves the following:

- Cathartic administered at home at various intervals the day before the procedure

- High intake of water or other clear liquids to avoid dehydration

- No dairy products or solid foods or juices with pulp

- No red or purple liquids

Sometimes the patient will not have complied with preparation instructions, in which case the physician may order an enema in the office prior to the examination. Procedure 5-4 lists the steps for administering a disposable enema to a patient.

After a colonoscopy the patient should restrict activities, including heavy lifting and driving, for 12 to 24 hours. The patient should be encouraged to drink plenty of fluid,

PROCEDURE 5-5

ASSISTING WITH SIGMOIDOSCOPY EXAMINATION

ABHES VII.MA.A.1 9(m)   CAAHEP I.P (10)

OBJECTIVE: Set up the examination room for a flexible sigmoidoscopy and assist the physician during the procedure while ensuring patient comfort and safety.

STANDARD: This task takes about 30 minutes.

EQUIPMENT AND SUPPLIES: Sigmoidoscope with light source (Figure 5-6 shows a flexible sigmoidoscope and its parts); **obturator** (device used to close the end of an instrument to allow easier penetration); **anoscope** (instrument used to examine anal area); rectal speculum; **insufflator** (device used to blow air, powder, or gas into a body cavity); suction equipment; sterile specimen container with preservative for biopsy specimen; sterile transport forceps; cotton applicators; lubricating jelly; basin of warm water; patient drape; gloves; patient gown; small towel or examination table pad; tissue; biohazard waste container.

STEPS:

1. Check physician's orders, and check for patient allergies.
2. Perform hand hygiene.
3. Prepare equipment and supplies. Ensure that all lights and lightbulbs in equipment are working. Prepare a basin of warm water to receive used instruments.
4. Test suction equipment. Place obturator in sigmoidoscope.

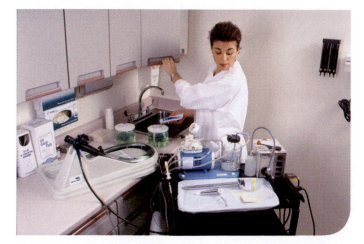

FIGURE 5-6 Flexible sigmoidoscope.

5. Identify patient, and explain procedure. Confirm that patient has followed all bowel preparation and dietary instructions.
6. Confirm consent form signed.
7. Ask patient to empty bladder, then undress and put on a gown.
8. Assist patient onto table and into Sims' position, lateral position, or knee–chest position.
9. Drape patient and place a towel or disposable pad under perineal area.
10. Don gloves.
11. Place lubricant for digital examination on physician's gloved fingers.
12. Lubricate tip of sigmoidoscope.
13. Attach inflation bulb and light source. Turn on scope just before ready to use it.
14. Remind patient to take deep breaths to relax abdominal muscles. Observe patient for any undue reactions.
15. Assist the physician by handing instruments and equipment such as suction and cotton-tipped applicators. Place used equipment, including suction tubing, into basin of water.
16. Assist with biopsy by holding open specimen container to receive specimen while maintaining sterility of container.
17. Following procedure, clean around patient's anal opening with tissue. Discard tissue in biohazard waste container.
18. Remove gloves, and perform hand hygiene.
19. Assist patient to slowly sit up.
20. Ask patient to dress. Provide assistance as needed.
21. Label specimen container.
22. Apply gloves, and clean and sterilize equipment as needed.
23. Clean room.
24. Remove gloves, and perform hand hygiene.
25. Document procedure.

CHARTING EXAMPLE: 03/02/XX 2:00 P.M. Assisted Dr. Rowe with sigmoidoscopy. Pt. tolerated procedure well. No biopsies obtained. · · · · · · · · · · · N. Blardo, CMA (AAMA)

rest, and refrain from drinking alcoholic beverages during the first 24 hours. (Procedure 5-6 lists the steps for assisting with a colonoscopy.)

COLLECTING STOOL SPECIMEN

Stool specimens (feces) may be collected to detect bacteria, viruses, parasites, and occult blood. The first three topics are discussed in Chapter 12: Microbiology. Occult or hidden blood in feces may be an indication of bleeding in the gastrointestinal (GI) tract. Instructing patients to collect a fecal specimen either at the office or at home may be embarrassing and difficult for the patient.

Fecal bleeding may be intermittent; therefore, fecal specimens should be obtained on 3 separate days. Patients who have daily bowel movements should not find this a problem. Those who have bowel movements less regularly may take more than 3 days to collect specimens. Procedure 5-7 lists the steps for instructing patients to collect stool specimens.

PROCEDURE 5-6

ASSISTING WITH COLONOSCOPY

ABHES VII.MA.A.1 9(m)   CAAHEP I.P (10)

OBJECTIVE: Set up an examination room for a colonoscopy and assist the physician during the procedure while ensuring patient comfort and safety.

STANDARD: This task takes 45 to 60 minutes.

EQUIPMENT AND SUPPLIES: Colonoscope; gloves; water-soluble lubricant; patient gown and drapes; sterile cotton-tipped applicators for specimen collection; suction device; sterile biopsy forceps; sterile rectal speculum; specimen containers with lab requisition form and labels; tissues; biohazard waste container; patient's record; pen.

NOTE: The physician administers a sedative or anesthetic to patient for this procedure.

STEPS:

1. Check physician's orders, and check for patient allergies.
2. Perform hand hygiene.
3. Assemble equipment and supplies.
4. Check all equipment for proper functioning.
5. Identify the patient, and explain procedure. Verify that pre-exam instructions were followed. Ask patient to empty bladder.
6. Provide instructions for gown opening, and ask patient to disrobe. Provide privacy by leaving room unless assistance needed.
7. Assist patient onto examination table, and drape appropriately.
8. Measure and record vital signs.
9. Don gloves.
10. Assist physician by handing instruments and supplies as requested.
11. After physician has collected specimens, place them in sterile specimen containers.
12. When procedure is completed, wipe patient's anal area with tissues.
13. Monitor patient as directed by physician.
14. Remove gloves, and discard in hazardous waste container. Perform hand hygiene.
15. Retake vital signs and record.
16. Complete laboratory forms. Label specimens. Seal specimen containers in biohazard specimen transport bag.
17. Assist patient with dressing once stable.
18. Provide postprocedure instructions, and verify that patient or caregiver understands.
19. After patient is released, perform hand hygiene, don new gloves, and clean and disinfect the exam room. Sanitize and prepare instruments for autoclaving.
20. Document procedure in patient's record.

CHARTING EXAMPLE: 05/08/09 9:00 A.M. Assisted with colonoscopy. Patient's vital signs stable before and after procedure. Pt. reports not feeling dizzy or in discomfort after procedure. After-care instructions given to patient and verified understanding by having instructions repeated. Specimens sent to Memorial Lab. · · · · · · · · · · · · C. Collins CMA (AAMA)

PROCEDURE 5-7

INSTRUCTING PATIENT IN COLLECTING STOOL SPECIMENS

ABHES VII.MA.A.1 10(f)   CAAHEP III.P (7)

OBJECTIVE: To instruct patients to obtain an adequate stool specimen for laboratory testing.

STANDARD: This task takes 5–10 minutes.

EQUIPMENT AND SUPPLIES: Specimen container with lid (for culture or ova and parasite testing); three occult blood slides with envelopes and applicator sticks (for testing for occult blood); lab request form; pen; patient's record; label; printed instructions; tongue depressor; biohazard transport bag; notepad.

STEPS:

1. Check physician's orders.
2. Assemble needed items next to patient.
3. Label specimen cup/occult blood slides, and fill in lab request form.
4. Identify patient, and explain physician orders. Give patient copy of printed instructions.
5. Instruct patient how to obtain a small amount of stool.

NOTE: Three to four tablespoons are needed for culture/ova and parasites, small amount on applicator stick for occult

blood. For the culture, nothing else may be placed in container (no toilet paper, tissues, urine, or menses). To maintain sterility, patient should not touch inside cup or cover. Patient may use a sterile tongue depressor to obtain larger samples of stool from toilet bowel. Patient compliance is difficult to obtain, so you must put patient at ease as much as possible.

6. Instruct patient to label each collection device with date and time of specimen, place it in biohazard transport bag, and bring it to lab or office with lab request form as soon as possible. Larger specimens should be refrigerated if not dropped off at office within 2 hours. It is unnecessary to refrigerate occult blood smears. (See Procedure 5-8 for further instructions for collecting and testing for occult blood.)
7. To verify comprehension, have patient or caregiver repeat instructions to you.
8. Document that instructions were given to patient.

CHARTING EXAMPLE: 03/21/XX 9:00 A.M. Verbal & printed instructions given to Pt. for collection of stool specimen for lab testing. Pt. seemed to understand. · · · · · M. Blardo, CMA (AAMA)

TESTING FOR OCCULT BLOOD

To collect occult blood, patients must be instructed to follow guidelines listed by manufacturer of testing kits. Guidelines should be observed 2 days prior to collecting specimens and continued until all three samples have been obtained. The guidelines are as follows:

- Drink plenty of fluids.
- Do not collect samples during menses.

PROCEDURE 5-8

TESTING FOR OCCULT BLOOD

ABHES VII.MA.A.1 10(b)(5)   CAAHEP III.P (8)

OBJECTIVE: To test feces for occult blood.

STANDARD: This task takes 5 minutes.

EQUIPMENT AND SUPPLIES: Three occult blood slides; applicators; envelope; timer; patient's record; pen; gloves; color developer.

NOTE: Many occult blood test kits are available on the market. Each one has its own set of directions, color developer, slides, and control monitors. The test kit directions should be followed exactly.

STEPS:

1. Perform hand hygiene, and don gloves.
2. Place paper towel on area to hold slides.

3. Check name and date on occult blood slides.
4. Check expiration date on color developer.
5. Open window flap on back of slide, and apply two drops of developer to Box A and Box B.
6. Interpret the results in 30 to 60 seconds or according to manufacturer's directions. A positive result will have blue color around the edge of the specimen. A negative result will have no color change visible. Any amount of blue color is positive for occult blood.
7. Perform test on positive and negative controls as required by manufacturer.

NOTE: This ensures that test system is working appropriately and is a method of quality control.

8. Test remaining slides in same manner.
9. Dispose of all materials in biohazard waste container. Clean work area.
10. Remove gloves, and perform hand hygiene.
11. Document results in patient's record.

CHARTING EXAMPLE: 03/21/XX 10:30 A.M. 3 occult blood rec'd. All tested neg. for occult blood. Dr. Chang notified of results. Pt. notified per Dr. Chang. · · · · B. Negri, CMA (AAMA)

- Avoid red meats, liver, processed meats.
- Avoid turnips, broccoli, cauliflower, and melons.
- Avoid aspirin, iron supplements, and large doses of vitamin C for 7 days before collecting specimens (unless otherwise instructed by physician).
- Eat a high-fiber diet. Store slides at room temperature and away from sun and heat.

Neurology

Neurology is the study of the nervous system. Patients with conditions of the nervous system exhibit wide varieties of physical and mental symptoms. A neurological examination focuses on the patient's state of consciousness, reflex responses, motor responses, speech patterns, and patterns of behavior. A neurological examination requires the following equipment:

- Otoscope
- Ophthalmoscope
- Percussion hammer
- Penlight

- Tuning fork
- Cotton ball or feather
- Pin
- Tongue depressor
- Small vials containing hot/cold liquids; vials with different scents; vials with different tasting liquids as ordered by physician

Assisting with a neurological examination entails handing equipment to the physician and monitoring patients for unusual patterns of behavior or speech. (The procedures for performing evaluation of patient's pupils and assisting with lumbar puncture follow.)

The pupils of the eyes often display signs relevant to the functioning of the brain and nervous system. Observation is a straightforward, noninvasive, simple, and quick procedure. (Procedure 5-9 lists the steps to perform to evaluate patients' pupils.) The pupils are checked for the following:

- Equality in size
- Equal dilation in both eyes in darkness or dim light

PROCEDURE 5-9

PERFORMING A PUPIL CHECK

ABHES VII.MA.A.1 9(m)   CAAHEP I.P (10)

OBJECTIVE: To correctly check patient's pupils for size, dilation, constriction, accommodation, and equal reaction to light.

STANDARD: This task takes 5 minutes.

EQUIPMENT AND SUPPLIES: Penlight or flashlight; patient's record; pen.

STEPS:

1. Identify patient and introduce yourself.
2. Observe patient for responsiveness to your introduction.
3. Explain procedure. (It may help to partially darken the room).
4. Ask patient to look straight ahead.
5. Using a penlight or flashlight, approach from the side and shine light on one pupil at a time. Observe for constriction of pupil.
6. Shine light on pupil again, and observe other pupil for constriction.
7. Hold open eyes, and observe pupils for size. (They should be equal in size.)
8. Hold an object, penlight, or pen about 10 cm (4 in.) from bridge of patient's nose. Ask patient to look at top of object and then at an object on wall across room. Observe for pupil response. (Pupil should constrict when looking at close object and dilate when looking across room.)
9. Move pen toward the patient's nose. Pupils should converge toward patient's nose.
10. Observe pupils for shape. (They should be equal or similar in shape.)
11. Explain to patient what other tests will be performed.
12. Document patient's record. If "Pupils Equal, Round, Reactive to Light and Accommodation," use abbreviation PERRLA; if not, document whatever result obtained.

CHARTING EXAMPLE: 03/21/XX 11:00 A.M. BP 168/80; T 99°F; P 82; R 18; PERRLA. HT 68″ WT 182 lb. · · · · · · · · · · ·
· T. Blardo, CMA (AAMA)

- Rapid constriction to light in both eyes
- Equal reaction to light
- Accommodation to objects near or far

ASSISTING PHYSICIAN WITH NEUROLOGICAL EXAMINATION

In evaluating neurologic disorders, the physician uses all methods of examination previously described. Vision and hearing tests may be required and are covered elsewhere in this chapter.

ASSISTING WITH LUMBAR PUNCTURE

A lumbar puncture is performed when the physician wishes to examine the cerebral spinal fluid (CSF) for the presence of red cells, white cells, or pathogenic microorganisms, or to administer pain control medication. Examination of cerebral

PROCEDURE 5-10

ASSISTING WITH NEUROLOGIC SCREENING EXAMINATION

ABHES VII.MA.A.1 9(m)   CAAHEP I.P (10)

OBJECTIVE: To assist physician with neurologic screening examination.

STANDARD: This task takes 5–10 minutes.

EQUIPMENT AND SUPPLIES: Percussion hammer; safety pin; tongue depressor; Mayo tray; penlight; cotton ball; tuning fork; neurological wheel; ophthalmoscope; otoscope; hot and cold water; materials with different odors.

STEPS:

1. Check physician's orders.
2. Perform hand hygiene.
3. Assemble and cover equipment on tray.
4. Identify patient, and explain procedure.
5. Evaluate patient's mental status while taking medical history while paying attention to responses, memory, and coherence of thought, overall mood, and awareness.
6. If ordered, perform visual acuity test.
7. Assist patient onto examination table, and drape as needed for comfort.
8. Physician will test reflexes with percussion hammer.
9. Sensory abilities and skin sensations are tested using safety pin, neurological wheel, cotton ball, and

patient's recognition of simple objects by touch (key, pen, coin).

10. Physician will check cranial nerves by having patient touch finger to nose, touch heel to shin, and move heel down opposite shin.

11. Assist physician as needed during remainder of examination by handing equipment.

12. Assist patient off table if physician wants to evaluate gait, or to perform **Romberg test** (patient closes eyes and attempts to stand without swaying with feet together).

13. Assist patient off table and instruct to dress. Provide assistance and privacy as needed.

14. Clean examination room.

15. Document patient's record.

16. Perform hand hygiene.

CHARTING EXAMPLE: 03/21/XX 11:00 A.M. Assisted Dr. Young with neurologic screening. Scheduled Pt. to see Dr. Black, neurologist, on 04/04/XX at 11:00 A.M. · C. Negri, CMA (AAMA)

spinal fluid is an important tool in diagnosing conditions such as stroke, brain hemorrhage, meningitis, encephalitis, polio, and tumors. CSF is normally clear, colorless, and free of microorganisms. Generally three tubes of specimen are collected using sterile technique and are sent to the laboratory for cell count, culture, and chemical testing for glucose and protein.

This is an invasive procedure; therefore, sterile techniques must be used, and special care must be taken in handling specimens. (See Chapter 8 for sterile technique procedures.) All CSF tests should be treated as **stat** (without delay) procedures. A needle is inserted into the subarachnoid space at L 4–5 below the level of the spinal cord (Figure 5-7). Intracranial pressure may be evaluated with the **Queckenstedt test**, which involves having the assistant press on the patient's jugular vein (right, left, or both, in the neck) while the physician monitors the CSF pressure. The pressure should increase when the jugular vein is compressed. If pressure does not increase, it signifies blockage of CSF flow. (The procedure for assisting with lumbar puncture follows.)

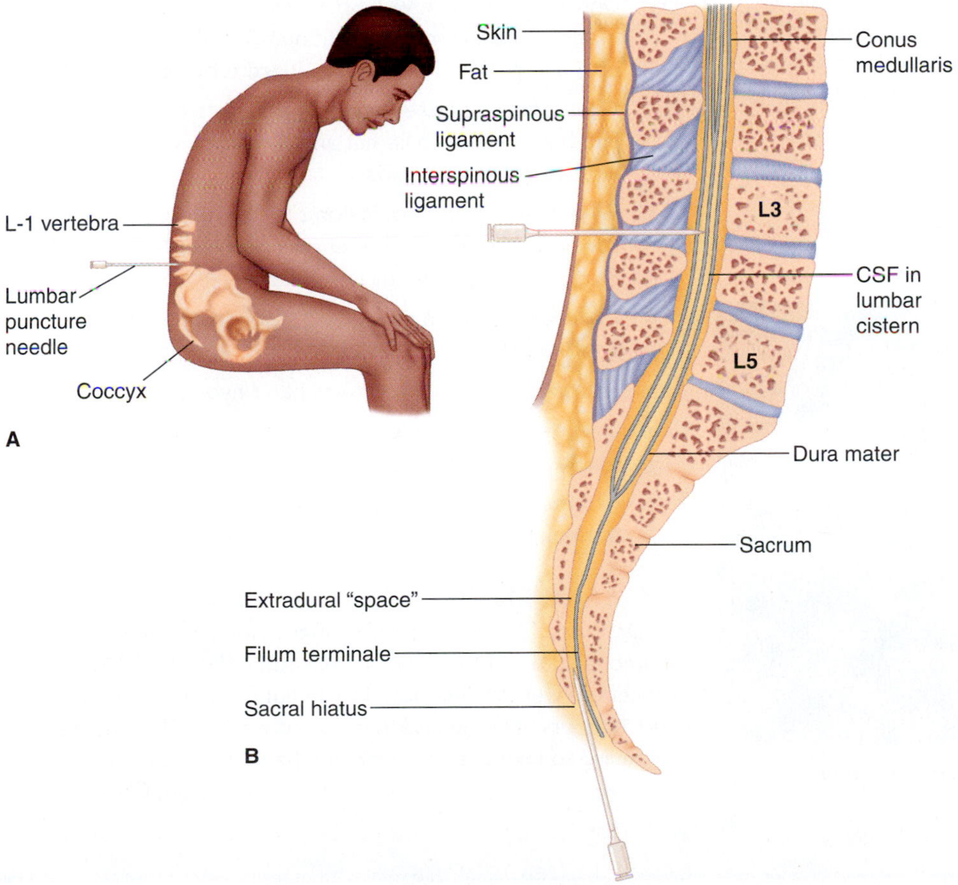

Headaches are common following a lumbar puncture. Headaches may be diminished by having the patient remain prone for some time (6 to 12 hours) after the procedure. Thus a clinic setting for this procedure may be more appropriate than a medical office. In some states, only licensed personnel assist with lumbar punctures.

FIGURE 5-7   Place client in Sims' position to facilitate needle insertion for lumbar puncture.

Obstetrics and Gynecology

Obstetrics (OB) is the study of women's health during pregnancy, childbirth, and the **puerperium**, a period of 4 to 6 weeks after

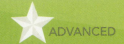
ASSISTING WITH LUMBAR PUNCTURE
ABHES VII.MA.A.1 9(m) CAAHEP I.P (10)

OBJECTIVE: To set up and assist with a lumbar puncture while maintaining sterile technique.

STANDARD: This task takes about 20 minutes.

EQUIPMENT AND SUPPLIES: Sterile gloves; Xylocaine 1%–2%; syringe and needle for anesthetic; disposable lumbar puncture tray, including skin antiseptic with applicator; adhesive bandage; spinal puncture needle; three or four sterile tubes with stoppers; drape; manometer; light; gauze sponges; patient's record; pen.

STEPS:

1. Check physician's orders, and check for patient allergies.

2. Perform hand hygiene.

3. Assemble equipment, and check that consent form was signed and in chart. (Figure 5-8 is an example of a lumbar puncture tray.)

4. Explain procedure, and stress that patient must remain still during procedure. Be clear when explaining that patient will receive something to numb area but will feel pressure during procedure.

5. Ask patient to empty bowels and bladder and to don gown with opening in back. Assist onto examination table as needed.

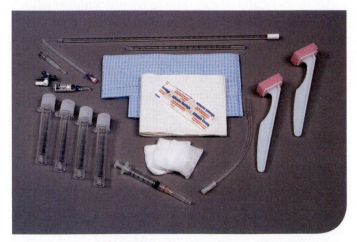

FIGURE 5-8 A preassembled lumbar puncture set. Note the manometer at top of set.

6. Assist patient to assume the Sims' position with back at edge of table, and cover with drape.

7. When physician is ready, expose only patient's back. Open sterile tray on Mayo stand, and pour antiseptic into sterile medicine cup if needed. Observe sterile techniques as explained in Chapter 8.

8. Help patient to pull knees up to abdomen and chin to chest to widen space between lower lumbar vertebrae for easier needle insertion. Place pillow between knees to prevent upper leg from sliding off lower leg.

9. Encourage patient to relax and take deep slow breaths through mouth. Offer comfort to patient, and observe closely for signs of nausea, dyspnea, or cyanosis. Monitor pulse at intervals and record after procedure.

10. When needle in place, assist with Queckenstedt test if requested by applying pressure to patient's jugular vein with fingers while physician monitors CSF pressure.

11. Don gloves to receive CSF specimen vials, labeling tubes in sequence as received with number of tube (1, 2, 3, etc.) and patient information. Place tubes safely aside.

12. After removal of needle, apply adhesive bandage to site and help patient to lie flat and remain in supine position until instructed otherwise.

13. Fill out laboratory requisition slip for ordered tests. Route specimens as required to ensure accurate test results. Process CSF specimens immediately.

14. Clean examination room, and dispose of equipment appropriately.

15. Remove gloves, and perform hand hygiene.

16. Document patient's record.

17. When patient is ready for discharge after lying flat for required time as ordered by physician, encourage patient to drink fluids to reduce chances of headache.

CHARTING EXAMPLE: 03/27/XX 10:00 A.M. LP performed by Dr. Russo. Approx. 20 cc of clear colorless CSF sent to Memorial Lab at 11:00 A.M. No leakage at LP site. Pt. tolerated procedure well. Pt. instructed to lie flat for 2 hours in office and 12 hours at home and to drink extra fluids. Pt. instructed by Dr. Russo to take acetaminophen if headache develops. · · · · · ·
· B. Negri, CMA (AAMA)

childbirth. Gynecology (Gyn) is the study of the female reproductive organs and conditions and diseases that affect them. To assist a physician with procedures associated with the female reproductive system, one should be familiar with the anatomy and physiology of the system and review it before proceeding.

Examination of the female reproductive organs includes a breast examination and a pelvic examination. A Pap test may be performed for early detection of cancer of the cervix. Many gynecologists perform a digital rectal examination as part of the routine pelvic examination. Prenatal care for obstetrical patients requires frequent office visits as pregnancy progresses.

The following are the OB/Gyn procedures covered in this chapter:

- Instructing a patient on breast self-examination
- Assisting with a pelvic examination and Pap test
- Preparing wet mount/wet prep and KOH slides
- Performing an amplified DNA test for chlamydia and gonorrhea

- Obtaining cultures for sexually transmitted diseases (STDs)
- Assisting with routine prenatal visit
- Assisting with postpartum examination
- Assisting with colposcopy and cervical biopsy
- Performing urinary catheterization on a female

BREAST EXAMINATION

The physician performs a breast examination as part of a complete pelvic examination. Assisting personnel may be called on to instruct a patient on the importance and steps needed to perform breast self-examination. Early detection of lumps in the breast means earlier treatment and a greater rate of success. The American Cancer Society advises a monthly self-examination of the breasts at the same time each month, about 7 to 10 days after **menses** (menstrual flow). Posters, brochures, and breast self-examination models are available to assist in patient instruction. (Procedure 5-12 lists the steps for teaching a patient how to perform breast self-examination.)

PROCEDURE 5-12

INSTRUCTING A PATIENT ON BREAST SELF-EXAMINATION

ABHES VII.MA.A.1 9(r)   CAAHEP IV.P (5)

OBJECTIVE: To instruct patient to correctly perform breast self-examination.

STANDARD: This task takes about 5 minutes.

EQUIPMENT AND SUPPLIES: Breast model; pamphlets on breast self-examination.

STEPS:

1. Check physician's orders, and check for patient allergies.
2. Perform hand hygiene.
3. Assemble equipment.
4. Identify patient, and explain procedure while stressing importance of performing the examination monthly, 7 to 10 days after period, and in three different positions (in front of mirror, in shower, and lying down).
5. *In front of mirror,* Explain that patient should disrobe from waist up.

6. Inspect breasts for any irregularity in shape with arms at sides.
7. Look for swelling, pimpling or puckering of skin, lumps, or changes in nipples, such as retracting. Squeeze nipples, and look for discharge.
8. Raise arms overhead, and look for size, shape, and contour changes in each breast.
9. With palms on hips, flex chest muscles to observe for any obvious differences in breasts.
10. *Lying down:* To examine right breast, place a towel under right shoulder and raise right arm, placing hand behind head. Using left hand, examine right breast, using small circular motions beginning at outermost top of right breast and working clockwise around breast toward nipple while feeling for lumps or abnormal changes in breast tissue.
11. Repeat with right hand examining left breast.

12. *In shower:* Raise right arm. Using left hand, examine right breast. Then use right hand to examine left breast, feeling with flat fingertips for any lump or thickening, including underarm areas.

13. Instruct patient to promptly report any abnormalities to physician.

14. Ask patient to verbally repeat instructions to you to verify comprehension of instruction.

15. Document education.

CHARTING EXAMPLE: 03/37/XX 1:00 P.M. Provided patient instruction using breast model. Pt. able to verbally repeat procedure steps. · · · · · · · · · · · · · · A. Martinez, CMA (AAMA)

PELVIC EXAMINATION AND PAP TEST

The pelvic examination begins with a taking the patient's reproductive history, which provides basic important information, including menstrual history, age of **menarche** (first menstruation), menstrual cycle intervals and regularity, duration of period, amount of flow, menstrual cycle problems, methods of contraception used (if any), and date of last menstrual period (LMP). Obstetrical history includes number of times pregnant (**gravida**), number of births after 20 weeks of gestation (**para**), and number of fetuses not reaching viability (**abortion**).

Patients should be reminded to refrain from douching and sexual intercourse for 24 to 48 hours before a Pap test. The Pap test should be done 2 weeks after the first day of the last period or whenever the physician deems it necessary. A female is usually present, for legal reasons, to assist with a gynecological examination performed by a male physician.

The Pap smear is a thin scraping of exfoliated cells taken from the cervix, vagina, and endocervical canal for cytological screening. Two methods are used to prepare the Pap specimen. In the older direct method, or dry method, three separate slides are made by the physician of cervical, vaginal, and endocervical areas; sprayed with a fixative to preserve the cells; and sent for cytological evaluation. This method often resulted in false negatives. The newer wet method, or ThinPrep, obtains cervical cells with a cytology broom or brush. The broom is then swished around in a vial of liquid preparation, the entire specimen is deposited, and the vial is recapped and transported to a laboratory. The better specimen obtained with the wet method can also be used to evaluate for human papillomavirus (HPV), gonorrhea, and chlamydia.

With either method of evaluation, the slides are examined by a cytologist for **dysplasia**, signs of infection, or cancerous (tumor) cells. Cellular changes are graded using the cervical intraepithelial neoplasia (CIN) classification.

CIN 1 = mild dysplasia

CIN II = moderate dysplasia

CIN III = severe dysplasia, or **carcinoma in situ** (no invasion of surrounding tissues)

Procedure 5-13 describes the procedure for assisting with pelvic examination and Pap test.

PROCEDURE 5-13

ASSISTING WITH PELVIC EXAMINATION AND PAP TEST (CONVENTIONAL AND THINPREP METHODS)

ABHES VII.MA.A.1 9(m)   CAAHEP I.P (10)

OBJECTIVE: To set up and assist with a gynecologic examination, including collection of dry and wet prep methods.

STANDARD: This task takes about 15 minutes.

EQUIPMENT AND SUPPLIES: Vaginal speculum; water-soluble lubricant; cotton-tipped applicator; drape; gown; urine specimen container; dry Pap smear materials (cervical spatula, brush, glass slides, fixative spray or liquid slide preservative identification label); Liquid Pap test materials (ThinPrep vial, plastic spatulas, and endocervical brush or cytology broom identification label); laboratory request form; cleansing tissue; gloves; container for contaminated instruments; light; stool for examiner; biohazard waste container.

STEPS:

1. Check physician's orders, and check for patient allergies.
2. Perform hand hygiene.
3. Assemble equipment.
4. Ask patient to empty bladder.

NOTE: If urine specimen required, provide a specimen container and label).

5. Measure patient's vital signs, height, and weight.
6. Instruct patient to remove all clothing, don gown with opening in front, and sit on examination table. Provide drape, privacy, and assistance as needed.
7. Ask patient to assume a supine position for breast and abdominal examination.
8. Assist patient into lithotomy position, draping to provide as much privacy as possible. Knees should be relaxed and rotated outward. Adjust the examination light and stool.
9. Warm vaginal speculum before procedure to lessen patient discomfort. Hand speculum to physician, either moistened with warm water (dry prep method) or water-soluble lubricant (wet prep method), depending on which method of Pap preparation is to be used.
10. Remind patient to take deep breaths to help relax abdominal muscles.
11. Apply gloves, and assist with collection of specimen as follows.
12. *Dry Prep Method:* Hold prelabeled slides so physician can smear specimen on appropriate slide (V–vaginal; C–cervical, E–endocervical).
13. Fix each slide immediately after collection, either by spraying evenly with cytology fixative from a distance of 5 to 6 inches or flooding with 95% ethyl alcohol.
14. Allow slides to air-dry, and place them in appropriate container.

15. *Wet Prep Method:* Open vial of wet prep solution to allow physician to place collection device used (cytology brush or spatula or broom) into vial, and mix at least 10 times. Discard collection device, and recap vial.
16. Make available container to receive used speculum when physician is finished.
17. Apply lubricant to gauze, and hold for physician to lubricate fingers for digital examination of vagina. (For vaginal exam, middle and index fingers of gloved hand are lubricated and inserted into vagina while other hand presses on abdomen to palpate uterus and ovaries. For rectal exam, one lubricated and gloved finger is inserted into vagina and one lubricated and gloved finger of other hand is inserted into rectum.) Collect specimen for occult blood if requested. (See Procedure 5-8.)
18. Help patient remove feet from stirrups and sit up. Offer tissues.
19. Remove gloves, and perform hand hygiene
20. Request patient to dress, offering assistance and ensuring privacy as needed. Provide further instructions.
21. Don gloves. Clean examination room, dispose of soiled materials in biohazard waste container, and remove instruments to area for later sterilization.
22. Complete all lab slips, including the following information: LMP; pregnant, postpartum, perimenopausal, or postmenopausal; type of hormone therapy begin taken, if any; previous Pap smear results; cervical cancer or surgery, if any. Prepare pathology and paperwork for transportation.
23. Remove gloves. Perform hand hygiene.
24. Document patient's record.

CHARTING EXAMPLE: 04/01/XX 2:00 P.M. Provided BSE instruction. Pap specimen sent to Memorial Laboratory. · · · · · ·
· R. Mendoza, RMA

OBTAINING SPECIMENS FOR SEXUALLY TRANSMITTED DISEASES

If during the procedure for pelvic examination the physician suspects a sexually transmitted disease (STD), a culture will be performed. All states require that confirmed cases of HIV/AIDS be reported. In many states other diseases such as gonorrhea and syphilis are reportable diseases. Confidentiality of patient information is extremely important. Gathering information from the patient regarding past sexual history and providing education about symptoms of STDs are vital parts of the office visit. Table 5-2 lists some sexually transmitted diseases and their symptoms in males and females.

If the physician determines cultures or slides must be prepared during a pelvic examination, equipment and supplies should be readily available. (Procedure 5-14 describes how to prepare wet mount slides for yeast, bacteria, and trichomonas.)

AMPLIFIED DNA PROBE TEST FOR CHLAMYDIA AND GONORRHEA

This test is performed on males and female and uses separate kits. The male test kit is blue, and the female test kit is pink. The test on females is performed as part of the pelvic examination but must be performed before any lubricating

TABLE 5-2 Sexually Transmitted Diseases/Symptoms/Tests

Disease	Male Symptoms	Female Symptoms	Diagnosis
Acquired immune deficiency syndrome (AIDS)	Symptoms appear from several months to several years after acquiring virus; reduced immunity to other diseases; heavy night sweats; fatigue; weight loss; enlarged lymph glands in neck axillae, or groin; persistent diarrhea; skin rashes; headache; cough; gray-white coating on tongue	Same as male	Direct antigen detection; ELISA and nucleic probes; Antibody detection; Western blot; ELISA and latex agglutination tests
Candidiasis	Itching; irritation; discharge; cheesy material under foreskin	Red irritated ovular area; intense itching of vaginal and vulvar area; thick white, cheesy or curdlike discharge	Microscopic examination of vaginal discharge with KOH, or culture
Chlamydia	Urinary frequency; watery mucoid urethral discharge	May be asymptomatic; vaginal discharge; frequently a carrier; dysuria; and urinary frequency	DNA probe test; ThinPrep Pap test
Genital herpes	Painful sores or large vesicles lasting for weeks; may be itchy in recurrent cases	Same as male	Culture with special transport media; antibody testing; DNA probe test
Genital warts	Caused by human papilloma virus (HPV); single lesions or clusters of lesions beneath foreskin or on penis; on dry skin areas, lesions hard, yellow-gray; moist areas pink to red, cauliflowerlike	Lesions appear at bottom part of vaginal opening, vaginal lips, perineum, inner walls of vagina and cervix; some strains linked to cervical cancer	DNA test on cells scraped from cervix; Pap smear; colposcopy or biopsy of tissue
Gonorrhea	Painful urination; urethritis with watery white discharge; may become purulent	May be asymptomatic or vaginal discharge; pain in abdomen; urinary frequency may occur	DNA probe test or culture; Gram stain slide for direct identification
Syphilis	Chancre on glans penis painless; heals in 4–6 weeks; secondary symptoms: skin eruptions; low-grade fever; inflammation of lymph glands 6 weeks to 6 months later	Chancre on cervix or genital areas that heals in 4–6 weeks; other symptoms same as for male	Antibody tests such as VDRL or RPR; fluorescent treponemal antibody absorbed (FTA-ABS) test
Trichomoniasis	Slight itching; moisture on top of penis; may be asymptomatic	Itching; redness of vulva and skin inside of thighs; abundant watery, frothy discharge	Wet mount slide preparation

jelly is used. The pink test kit for females contains a large and small swab. (Procedure 5-15 describes the steps in assisting with this test.)

ASSISTING WITH PRENATAL EXAMINATIONS

Prenatal care takes place before delivery and includes tests and office visits to promote the health of mother and child.

The first prenatal visit is scheduled after the woman has missed her second menstrual period. This visit is longer because a complete history and physical examination is performed. The physical examination includes a pelvic exam, Pap smear, and cultures if needed. Blood tests are ordered, and a complete urinalysis is performed. These tests provide a baseline for comparison at later visits. Time also is required for patient prenatal education about what to expect in the

PROCEDURE 5-14

PREPARING WET MOUNT/WET PREP AND KOH SLIDES

ABHES VII.MA.A.1 10(b)(5)   CAAHEP III.P. (7)

OBJECTIVE: To prepare wet mount preparations to detect cause of vaginitis using wet mount tests for yeast, bacteria, and *Trichomonas* and potassium hydroxide (KOH) prep test for yeast.

STANDARD: This task takes 5–10 minutes.

EQUIPMENT AND SUPPLIES: Normal saline; test tubes; 10% potassium hydroxide (KOH); microscope slides; cover slips; microscope; vaginal speculum; drape; sterile cotton-tipped applicator sticks; gloves; other pelvic examination equipment (see Procedure 5-13).

STEPS:

1. Check physician's orders, and check for patient allergies.
2. Assemble equipment and follow Procedure 5-13 for setup of pelvic examination.
3. Place several drops of normal saline into small test tube.
4. Using sterile technique, hand physician sterile cotton-tipped applicator to obtain sample of vaginal discharge.
5. Don gloves, and receive applicator stick from physician. Rinse swab well in test tube containing saline to obtain entire specimen.
6. Dispose of swab in biohazard waste container.
7. Using dropper, place a drop on slide and cover with coverslip. Give prepared slide to physician for examination. (According to Clinical Laboratory Improvement Amends, or CLIA, regulations, only a physician may perform the Physician Performed Microscopy Procedure, or PPMP.)
8. Assist patient into sitting position, and request she dress and wait for physician.
9. Physician will view slide under microscope.

NOTE: The slide will be examined for budding yeast (candidiasis), clue cells (bacterial infection), and motile protozoa (*Trichomonas* infection, or trichomoniasis).

10. After wet mount is completed, add a few drops of 10% KOH solution to remaining test tube, and make another slide.
11. Physician will examine second slide for fungus and yeast. (KOH destroys other cells and leaves fungal cells.)
12. Dispose of all slides and test tubes in sharps container.
13. Clean and disinfect examination area.
14. Remove gloves, and perform hand hygiene.
15. Return to patient, and assist as needed.
16. Physician will document findings.
17. Document patient's record.

CHARTING EXAMPLE: 04/01/XX 4:00 P.M. Pelvic exam of Pt. performed by Dr. Ames. Wet mount and KOH prep done. Candidiasis confirmed by Dr. Ames. RX for Gyne-Lotrimin vaginal supp. 200 mg each night at bedtime × 3. · · · · · · · · · ·
· F. Kyle, RMA

PROCEDURE 5-15

OBTAINING MATERIAL FOR AMPLIFIED DNA PROBE TEST FOR CHLAMYDIA AND GONORRHEA

ABHES VII.MA.A.1 10(d)   CAAHEP III.P (7)

OBJECTIVE: To obtain vaginal specimen and properly prepare it for transportation to laboratory for testing.

STANDARD: This task takes 5 minutes.

EQUIPMENT AND SUPPLIES: Equipment and supplies for pelvic examination (Procedure 5-13); Amplified DNA test kit (pink); transport tube with media; swabs (large, small); gloves; pen; patient's record.

STEPS:

1. Check physician's orders, and check for patient allergies.
2. Assemble equipment and supplies.
3. Perform hand hygiene, and don gloves.
4. Prepare patient for pelvic examination (Procedure 5-13).
5. Hand large swab to physician to clean cervix and allow for better specimen collection.
6. Discard large swab in biohazard waste container. Hand small swab to physician. This swab is inserted into the cervical os and rotated for 15 to 20 seconds to collect adequate sample.
7. Receive swab from physician and immediately place swab into transport tube to preserve sample. Break off shaft of swab at score line, and recap tube.
8. Confirm labeling (patient's name, date, time of collection, identification number, physician's name and phone number). Attach laboratory requisition to tube, and place in transport bag for lab pickup.
9. Assist patient as needed.
10. Remove gloves, and perform hand hygiene.
11. Document patient's record.

> **HIPAA Alert!** All patient information is considered confidential. Telling a friend that Mrs. So-and-So was in your office to be tested for STD violates HIPAA regulations.

CHARTING EXAMPLE: 04/02/XX 9:00 A.M. DNA probe test done by Dr. Walsh & sent to Memorial Lab. · K. Allen, RMA

---

coming months, including dietary guidelines, vitamin and mineral requirements, and what substances must be avoided, such as alcohol and over-the-counter medications. The estimated date of delivery (EDD, formerly "estimated date of confinement," or EDC) is determined using Naegele's rule or a gestational wheel and plugging in the first day of the last menstrual period (LMP). Box 5-3 illustrates the formula for Naegele's rule.

Follow-up prenatal visits are scheduled approximately every 4 weeks until the seventh month, every 2 weeks until the final month, and then weekly until delivery. The patient should be instructed to bring in a first morning urine specimen at each visit. Vaginal examination are performed during the last visits before delivery or based on individual patient circumstances. Each follow-up visit requires the following:

- Setting up examination room
- Measuring weight
- Measuring blood pressure
- Testing urine sample for glucose and protein
- Testing blood sample for hemoglobin or hematocrit
- Asking patient about any signs and symptoms

The physician will measure the **fundal height** (top of uterus to top of pubic bone) on the first and subsequent visits and will monitor the **fetal heart rate** (different from maternal heart rate) from the tenth week on. Other tests may be ordered, such as **abdominal ultrasound**, **amniocentesis**, **chorionic villi sampling (CVS)**, and **alpha-fetoprotein (AFP)**.

ASSISTING WITH POSTPARTUM VISIT

The puerperium is the 4- to 6-week period of time following delivery when body systems return to their pre-pregnancy state. The postpartum visit is scheduled for 4 to 6 weeks after delivery. **Lochia** is the vaginal discharge consisting of

---

BOX 5-3 Naegele's Rule

- LMP + 7 days − 3 months + 1 year

  Example:
  LMP = June 10, 2006
  + 7 days
  = June 17

  − 3 months
  = March 17
  + 1 year = 2007
  Thus, EDD is March 17, 2007.

PROCEDURE 5-16

ASSISTING WITH ROUTINE PRENATAL VISIT

ABHES VII.MA.A.1 9(m)   CAAHEP I.P (10)

OBJECTIVE: To assist patient during routine follow-up prenatal visit to monitor progress of pregnancy.

STANDARD: This task takes about 15 minutes.

EQUIPMENT AND SUPPLIES: Gown; drape; scale; tape measure; stethoscope; sphygmomanometer; Doppler fetoscope and coupling agent; vaginal speculum; urine specimen container; urine testing supplies; testing equipment for hemoglobin/hematocrit; watch with second hand; patient's record; pen.

STEPS:

1. Check physician's orders, and check for patient allergies.
2. Assemble equipment and supplies.
3. Perform hand hygiene.
4. Identify patient.
5. Provide a urine specimen container if patient did not bring a first morning sample; if urine specimen received, ask patient to empty her bladder.
6. Put on gloves.
7. Use reagent test strips to test urine for glucose, ketones, and protein, and record results. (See Chapter 11.) Dispose of equipment in biohazard waste container. Remove gloves, and perform hand hygiene.
8. Weigh patient.
9. Measure blood pressure. If blood pressure is elevated, allow patient to rest and repeat. Record results.
10. Ask patient about any symptoms, such as bleeding, nausea, and vomiting.
11. Measure hemoglobin or hematocrit levels (if this test is done in the office; patient may be referred to outside laboratory). Record results.
12. Ask patient to disrobe from waist down. Provide a gown and privacy. Instruct patient to sit on table and assist as necessary. Drape appropriately.
13. Assist physician by handing tape measure to measure fundal height. Hand physician Doppler fetal pulse detector, and spread coupling gel onto patient's abdomen to detect fetal heart tones (FHT).
14. If vaginal examination is to be done at this visit, assist patient into lithotomy position. Proceed as with pelvic examination (Procedure 5-13).
15. When examination is completed, assist patient to sit up. Allow time to prevent dizziness. Ask patient to dress, and provide privacy and assistance as necessary.
16. Provide appropriate patient education, and clarify physician's orders as needed.
17. Clean examination room. Remove gloves, and perform hand hygiene.
18. Document any other results and education provided.

CHARTING EXAMPLE: 04/03 XX 1:15 P.M. Wt 167 lbs. BP 122/70 sitting. Urine neg for glucose and protein. Fundal height/20 wks at umbilicus; FHR 114/min. Pt. complains of A.M. nausea. · N. Lopez, CMA (AAMA)

---

blood, mucus, and white blood cells that occurs during this approximately 3-week-long period. The postpartum visit includes family planning advice, hemoglobin and hematocrit tests for anemia, weight, vital signs, breast and pelvic examinations, and rectal examination. Allow time for questions about breast feeding and contraception. Resumption of sexual activities should be allowed.

ASSISTING WITH COLPOSCOPY AND CERVICAL BIOPSY

Patients with atypical Pap smear results may be required to have a colposcopy performed to determine the origin and extent of abnormal cells. Colposcopy is also performed to evaluate effectiveness of treatment for cervical cancer. A colposcopy is a visual examination by the physician of the vaginal and cervical areas with a colposcope (a lighted instrument with binocular microscopy). A biopsy often is done at the same time and requires prior written consent of the patient.

This procedure is performed in the office and requires sterile field setup as well as regular setup for pelvic examination. (Chapter 8 covers sterile techniques.) The procedure is usually performed 1 week after the end of the last menstrual period. The patient should be instructed not to douche, use vaginal creams, or have sexual intercourse for 2 days prior to this procedure. Inform the patient that a

PROCEDURE 5-17

ASSISTING WITH POSTPARTUM EXAMINATION

ABHES VII.MA.A.1 9(m)   CAAHEP I.P (10)

OBJECTIVE: To assist physician in postpartum examination, performance of any tests ordered, and requests for information.

STANDARD: This task takes about 15 minutes.

EQUIPMENT AND SUPPLIES: Supplies and equipment for vital signs and weight (see Chapter 3); supplies and equipment for measuring hemoglobin and hematocrit (see Chapter 14); supplies and equipment for pelvic examination (see Procedure 5-13); biohazard waste containers; pen; patient's record; gloves.

STEPS:

1. Check physician's orders, and check for patient allergies.
2. Assemble equipment and supplies.
3. Identify and greet patient.
4. Perform hand hygiene.
5. Ask patient to remove shoes. Obtain patient weight (Procedure 3-17).
6. Measure pulse, respiration, and blood pressure. (See Chapter 3).
7. Document results.
8. Don gloves.
9. If office policy requires, measure hemoglobin and hematocrit and document results.
10. Instruct patient to disrobe completely. Provide gown and drape. Assist as needed.
11. Assist patient onto table and cover with drape. Instruct patient to assume supine position for breast examination. Assist patient to assume lithotomy position for pelvic examination. Hand physician vaginal speculum and other equipment.

NOTE: Pap smear is not usually done at this visit since cervical cells are still healing from delivery.

12. Once examination is completed, assist patient to sitting position and allow time to prevent dizziness. Provide tissues to remove lubricant as needed. Instruct patient to dress. Provide postexamination instructions per order of physician.
13. Clean examination room.
14. Remove gloves. Perform hand hygiene.
15. Document any other information not already recorded.

CHARTING EXAMPLE: 04/03/XX Wt. 177 lbs. P 70, R 14, BP 124/68, Hgb 12.4 gm. Hct 38%, Pt. to con't prenatal vitamins for 2 months per Dr. Schwartz. · · · · · · · · L. Chin, RMA

PROCEDURE 5-18

ASSISTING WITH COLPOSCOPY AND CERVICAL BIOPSY

ABHES VII.MA.A.1 9(m)   CAAHEP I.P (10)

OBJECTIVE: To prepare examination room and assist with colposcopy and cervical biopsy.

STANDARD: This task takes 20–30 minutes.

EQUIPMENT AND SUPPLIES: *Items on side of sterile field:* colposcope; sterile gloves; normal saline; 3% acetic acid; Lugol's iodine solution; Monsel's solution; specimen container with label and preservative; laboratory request form; sanitary pad; nonsterile gloves; gown; drape; examination light; tissues; biohazard waste container; container for contaminated instruments; pen; patient's record. *Items on sterile field:* vaginal speculum; long, sterile, cotton-tipped applicators; cervical punch biopsy forceps; uterine dressing forceps; uterine tenaculum; 4 × 4 sterile gauze.

STEPS:

1. Check physician's orders, and check for patient allergies.
2. Perform hand hygiene.

3. Assemble nonsterile equipment and supplies. Check light on colposcope.

4. Assemble sterile equipment and supplies without contamination, and cover field as required prior to use to preserve sterility.

5. Identify patient, explain procedure, and verify signed consent form is in chart.

6. Ask patient to disrobe from waist down and sit on table. Cover with drape.

7. When physician is ready, assist patient into lithotomy position.

8. Remove cover from sterile field. Pour normal saline into sterile container without spilling or contaminating. Pour acetic acid into second sterile container, observing sterile techniques as before. If Lugol's iodine is to be used, pour this solution into another sterile container.

9. Don sterile gloves.

10. Hand physician sterile vaginal speculum.

11. Hand physician sterile applicator dipped in normal saline to wipe cervix and remove mucus film.

12. Physician will focus colposcope on cervix.

13. Hand physician applicator stick dipped in acetic acid for removal of cervical mucus and other secretions to allow for easier visualization of area.

14. If requested, hand physician applicator stick dipped in Lugol's iodine. This provides better identification of unhealthy epithelium.

15. If abnormal area observed, a cervical punch biopsy will be performed. Remove sterile gloves, and put on non-sterile gloves to receive biopsy specimen.

16. If bleeding occurs, physician will control it with sterile gauze packing, Monsel's solution, or **electrocautery** (cauterization by electric current).

17. When procedure completed, assist patient to sit up. Provide patient with sanitary napkin.

18. Label specimen container with patient's name and date, prepare laboratory request form, and package specimen for transportation.

19. Request patient to dress, assisting as needed. Provide privacy. When patient is ready, review physician instructions and inform patient to expect a small amount of bleeding for a few days and gray-green foul-smelling discharge for 3 to 4 weeks. Remind patient to schedule follow-up appointment if ordered by physician.

20. Clean examination room, properly disposing of equipment and supplies.

21. Remove gloves. Perform hand hygiene.

22. Document results as needed. (The physician will also document results.)

CHARTING EXAMPLE: 04/03/XX 10:00 A.M. Colposcopy performed with cervical biopsy by Dr. DeNegri. Biopsy specimen sent to Memorial Lab. Pt. given sanitary pad, written and oral instructions. Pt. verbalized understanding. · M. Wasserman, RMA

minimum amount of bleeding may occur and a foul-smelling gray-green discharge may occur for several days after the procedure for a period of up to 3 weeks.

URINARY CATHETERIZATION ON A FEMALE

This procedure is usually associated with urology, not gynecology; however, it will be considered here, and the procedure for catheterizing a male will be considered in this chapter's section on conditions of the male reproductive system. If a patient cannot urinate to provide a sample for testing or has urinary retention, catheterization (which required a physician's order) may be performed.

Catheterization is the process of introducing a sterile tube into the urinary bladder to obtain urine. In outpatient facilities, a straight catheter usually is used. Hospitalized patients may have indwelling catheters that are left in place over a longer time. Catheterization requires sterile equipment and sterile technique. Figure 5-9 is an example of a catheterization kit.

Team Approach to the Male Reproductive System

Traditionally, urologists were tasked with treatment of male reproductive issues. Today, urologists, neurologists, endocrinologists, and physicians from various other disciplines comprise a team approach, as dictated by the patient's needs.

The male reproductive system is a combination of reproductive and urological organs. A number of conditions and diseases have an impact on both systems. As with females, cultures for STDs are performed on males, and amplified DNA probe tests for chlamydia and Gonorrhea may be ordered. Two additional competencies encountered in an

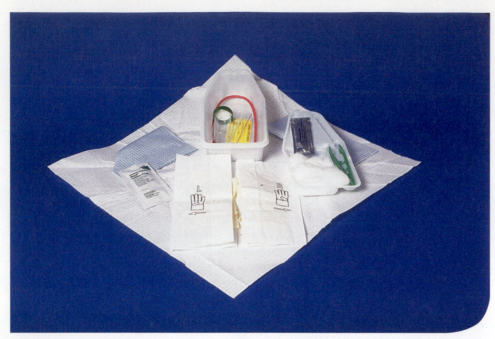

FIGURE 5-9 Catheter kit.

office setting are instructing the patient in testicular self-examination and, less frequently, assisting with male urinary catheterization. These are covered in the following sections.

INSTRUCTING MALE PATIENT ON TESTICULAR SELF-EXAMINATION

Testicular cancer is primarily a disease of young men between 20 and 35 years of age. It is important that young boys from puberty on be taught to perform testicular self-examination. Procedure 5-20 outlines instructing male patients about testicular self-examination.

PROCEDURE 5-19

PERFORMING URINARY CATHETERIZATION ON A FEMALE

ABHES VII.MA.A.1 9(m)   CAAHEP I.P (10)

OBJECTIVE: To successfully perform urinary catheterization on a female patient while maintaining sterile aseptic technique.

STANDARD: This procedure takes about 15 minutes.

EQUIPMENT AND SUPPLIES: Disposable urinary catheterization tray; 14 or 16 French catheter; sterile drapes; light; lubricant; sterile gloves; cotton balls; sterile forceps; cleansing solution or povidone-iodine (e.g., Betadine); specimen container with label; nonsterile gloves; biohazard waste container; pen; patient's record; female torso model.

STEPS:

1. Check physician's orders, and check for patient allergies.
2. Perform hand hygiene.
3. Assemble equipment and supplies.
4. Identify patient, and explain procedure. Ask patient to disrobe from waist down. Provide privacy, and assist if necessary. Drape patient to prevent unnecessary exposure.
5. Ask about allergies to latex or iodine. If patient has such allergies, use nonlatex gloves and alternative cleansing agent.
6. Assist patient into dorsal recumbent position with feet flat on table. Pull out table extension to provide more work space, or place Mayo stand between patient's legs.
7. Adjust light.
8. Use sterile aseptic technique to open disposable sterile kit. Remove sterile drape, and hold by corners. Place on area chosen to be sterile field. Remove fenestrated drape by corners, and place over exposed genital area.
9. Don sterile gloves. Set up remainder of kit. Pour cleansing solution over cotton balls.
10. Open lubricant, and apply to 2 to 3 inches of catheter tip (leave on tray). Place container near patient to drain urine.
11. Inform patient you are going to touch her.
12. Spread labia as wide as possible with nondominant hand to expose urethra. Maintain this position until procedure complete.
13. With other gloved hand, use moistened cotton ball to cleanse one side of **urinary meatus** (where urine is discharged) in one motion from top to bottom, then discard. Repeat with another moistened cotton ball on other side,

then discard. Repeat down middle, and discard. Repeat these steps if area is heavily soiled.

14. Pick up lubricated catheter with dominant gloved hand, and tell patient you are going to insert the catheter.

15. Insert catheter 2 to 3 inches into urethral opening until urine begins to flow into the kit tray (Figure 5-10). If resistance at end of catheter is great, do not force it. Notify physician or other licensed personnel.

16. Catch some urine in sterile specimen container. Allow remaining urine to drain into kit tray (not to exceed more than 750 to 1000 mL of urine at one time).

17. Remove catheter when drainage (step 16) is finished. Place top on specimen container.

18. Discard all supplies in biohazard waste containers.

19. Clean patient. If Betadine was used for cleansing solution, explain that genital area may be yellow.

20. Assist patient to sitting position, and allow time to prevent dizziness.

21. Place and secure specimen and completed lab requisition in laboratory transport bag. Ask patient to dress, and provide privacy and assistance as needed.

22. Provide further instructions to patient per physician's orders.

23. Clean examination room. Remove and dispose of gloves in biohazard waste container. Perform hand hygiene.

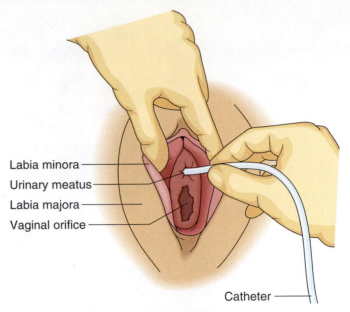

Labia minora
Urinary meatus
Labia majora
Vaginal orifice

Catheter

FIGURE 5-10 **Inserting a urinary catheter into a female.**

24. Document procedure in patient's record, including color and amount of urine.

CHARTING EXAMPLE: 04/05/XX 1:15 P.M. Pt. catheterized w/o difficulty. 200 mL clear, colorless urine obtained, sent to Memorial Lab for UA, C&S. · · · · · · · J. Kennedy, CMA (AAMA)

PROCEDURE 5-20

INSTRUCTING MALE PATIENT ON TESTICULAR SELF-EXAMINATION

ABHES VII.MA.A.1 9(r)   CAAHEP IV.P (5)

OBJECTIVE: To instruct a male patient to perform testicular self-examination.

STANDARD: This task takes about 10 minutes.

EQUIPMENT AND SUPPLIES: Instruction sheet; testicular examination model or illustrations.

STEPS:

1. Identify the patient, and introduce yourself.

2. Explain procedure to patient, noting that patient should perform it in shower or right after warm shower, which causes scrotal tissue to relax.

3. Using testicular model or illustration, explain how to place middle and index fingers underneath scrotum, with thumb on top, and to use a gentle motion to roll testes between fingers.

4. On model or illustration, indicate location of **epididymis**, a soft tubular cord behind the testis that stores and carries sperm. Patient should know what the epididymis feels like so as not to confuse it with a lump. (See Figure 5-11.)

5. Tell patient to repeat entire procedure on second testis.

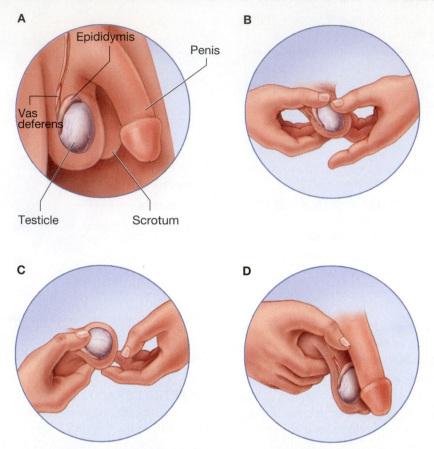

FIGURE 5-11 (A) Male reproductive system; (B) begin by examining the testicles. Roll the testicle gently between the thumb and fingers, applying very slight pressure while attempting to feel any hard or pain less lumps; (C) next, examine the cord behind each testicle (epididymis). This may be tender and is the location of most noncancerous conditions; (D) continue the examination by gently feeling the tube that runs up from the epididymis (vas deferens). It is normally a smooth, firm tube.

6. Encourage patient to immediately report to physician any lumps or thickening. (Early testicular cancer cases have a high cure rate.)

7. Document instruction in patient's record.

CHARTING EXAMPLE: 04/06/XX 3:30 P.M. Pt. given verbal and written instructions on testicular self-examination. Pt. verbalized understanding. · · · · · · · · · · · · · J. Holloran, RMA

URINARY CATHETERIZATION ON A MALE

In urology offices, it may be necessary for the physician to perform male catheterization. In this situation you would be called upon to assist. In other types of facilities, assisting personnel may perform the procedure per physician's orders.

Ophthalmology

Several competencies relate to vision and conditions of the eye. Screening for visual acuity and testing for color vision acuity are common procedures often performed as part of a physical examination. Administering eye medications and irrigating the eye to remove foreign objects are also performed frequently. Competencies for each of these procedures follow. In addition, procedures for measuring near-vision acuity and assisting vision-impaired patients are covered.

SCREENING FOR VISUAL ACUITY WITH SNELLEN EYE CHART

Distance visual acuity is measured by asking the patient to recognize letters on a chart placed 20 feet away. Children and non-English-speaking patients are asked to identify the

PROCEDURE 5-21

PERFORMING URINARY CATHETERIZATION ON A MALE

ABHES VII.MA.A.1 9(m)   CAAHEP I.P. (10)

OBJECTIVE: To perform urinary catheterization on a male using sterile technique.

STANDARD: This task takes 15 minutes.

EQUIPMENT AND SUPPLIES: Sterile catheter tray with sterile gloves; fenestrated drape; povidone-iodine (e.g., Betadine) solution or swabs; lubricant; cotton balls; sterile urine container with label; sterile 2 × 2 gauze squares; disposable forceps; absorbent pad; 14 or 16 French catheter; examination light; Mayo stand; anatomically correct model; waste bag near exam table; biohazard waste container; pen; patient's record.

STEPS:

1. Check physician's orders, and check for patient allergies.
2. Identify patient, and introduce yourself. Explain procedure.
3. Perform hand hygiene, and assemble equipment and supplies.
4. Ask patient to disrobe below waist. Provide gown and privacy, assisting as needed.
5. Instruct patient to sit on table. Assist into dorsal recumbent position, draping to expose external genitalia.
6. Open sterile tray. Holding sterile absorbent pad by corners, place under patient's penis. Empty contents of sterile tray onto absorbent pad, which is now the sterile field.
7. Don sterile gloves. Place fenestrated drape over patient's penis.
8. Open antiseptic. Pour solution over cotton balls. Lubricate end of catheter.
9. With nondominant hand, hold penis just below glans to expose urinary meatus. If patient is uncircumcised, pull foreskin back to expose meatus.
10. With dominant hand, use forceps and pick up cotton ball saturated with antiseptic solution or pick up povidone-iodine swab. Cleanse meatus with circular stroke, using cotton ball or swab, and discard into waste bag.
11. Repeat circular cleaning motion around tip of penis. Cleanse three times using new cotton ball or swab each time.
12. Continue holding penis with nondominant hand. Discard forceps into waste bag.
13. With sterile, gloved, dominant hand, pick up catheter about 3 to 4 inches (8–10 cm) from catheter tip. Lift penis at a 90° angle (perpendicular to body) to straighten urethra. Insert catheter about 8 inches (20 cm) until urine begins to flow into tray.
14. If catheter meets resistance, decrease angle to 45° and tell patient to take a deep breath. If catheter still meets resistance, remove and notify physician.
15. Allow initial urine to flow into tray. Using sterile specimen container, continue collecting urine as ordered. Allow urine to drain into tray until it stops. No more than 750 to 1000 mL of urine should be removed at one time.
16. Remove catheter. Place lid on specimen container.
17. Dry penis. Remove drapes.
18. Discard equipment in appropriate containers.
19. Label and bag specimen for transport with laboratory requisition.
20. Assist patient to sit up, allowing time to prevent dizziness. Assist patient from examination table, and ask patient to dress, assisting as needed.
21. Clean examination room. Remove gloves, and perform hand hygiene.
22. Document procedure in patient's record.

CHARTING EXAMPLE: 04/06/XX 11:00 A.M. Straight catheterization performed with 14 Fr cath. Per Dr. Wokowski. 250 mL of cloudy yellow urine obtained. Specimen sent for UA & C&S to Memorial Lab. Pt. told to call in office on 4/10 for results. · K. Leahy, CMA (AAMA)

---

direction in which the capital letter E is pointing. An individual with normal vision can see at 20 feet what a normal eye would see at 20 feet.

Distance visual acuity (DVA) is reported in a fraction format. The upper number indicates the distance from the eye chart and is always 20 feet. The lower number indicates the visual acuity of the patient compared to a normal eye's vision. Thus a patient with 20/50 reading in left eye means that the normal eye would see this at 50 feet.

work appears blurry. This is done by having the patient read a card with print sizes ranging from newspaper headlines down to small print, as in a telephone directory. The patient holds the card a distance of 14 to 16 inches and is asked to read the smallest line possible with no errors. Procedure 5-23 provides steps for performing this competency.

SCREENING FOR COLOR-VISION ACUITY

The Ishihara method is used to test color deficits. The Ishihara book or series of cards consists of a series of polychromatic plates of primary colors and shades of colors arranged to form a number on a background of similar dots of contrasting colors. Figure 5-12 is an example of one plate from the Ishihara book. Patients with normal vision are able to identify the numbers in at least 10 of the 14 plates. Patients with deficient color perception are unable to

Patients should be screened according to the preference of the physician, either with or without their corrective lens. Some physicians prefer screening for DVA both with and without corrective lenses.

SCREENING FOR NEAR-VISION ACUITY

Near-vision acuity (NVA) testing is performed when the patient is complaining of difficulty reading or when close

---

PROCEDURE 5-22

SCREENING DISTANCE VISUAL ACUITY WITH SNELLEN CHART

ABHES VII.MA.A.1 9(m)   CAAHEP I.P (10)

OBJECTIVE: To measure and document distance visual acuity using Snellen chart.

STANDARD: This task takes about 5 minutes.

EQUIPMENT AND SUPPLIES: Snellen chart placed at a distance of 20 feet, eye shield or occluder; pen; patient's record; alcohol; gauze.

STEPS:

1. Assemble equipment, and perform hand hygiene.
2. Identify patient, and explain procedure.
3. Determine patient's ability to recognize letters. If patient is unable to read, is a child, or is a non–English speaker, use necessary chart to accommodate patient's abilities.
4. Position patient either seated or standing 20 feet from chart in a well-lighted area. Place chart at eye level. Observe patient for glasses or ask if wearing contacts and record.
5. Follow facility's policy for testing with or without corrective lenses. (Many physicians prefer corrective lenses or glasses, except reading glasses, be worn.)
6. Ask patient to cover left eye with occluder but to leave eye open. If wearing glasses, instruct patient to hold occluder so normal position of glasses is not disturbed.
7. Starting with the 20/70 line, ask patient to identify each line and proceed down chart to last line patient can read without error. Observe for signs of squinting or tilting head, which can indicate difficulty identifying letters.
8. For one error in a line, record the numerical fraction next to the line with –1 after it (e.g., Left eye (OS): 20/40 –1).
9. Repeat procedure with other eye and record results (e.g., Right eye (OD): 20/20 –1).
10. Some facilities repeat procedure with both eyes open.
11. Clean occluder with alcohol and gauze.
12. Perform hand hygiene.
13. Document results in patient's record.

CHARTING EXAMPLE: 04/07/XX 9:00 A.M. Snellen eye test performed w/o correction per Dr. Luc. Right eye (OD) 20/30, left eye (OS) 20/20 –1, both eyes (OU) 20/20 –1. · · · · · · · · · ·
· P. Rosen, RMA

PROCEDURE 5-23

SCREENING FOR NEAR-VISION ACUITY

ABHES VII.MA.A.1 9(m)   CAAHEP I.P (10)

OBJECTIVE: To screen near-vision acuity.

STANDARD: This task takes 5 minutes.

EQUIPMENT AND SUPPLIES: Near-vision acuity chart; patient's record; pen; occluder or eye shield; alcohol; gauze pad or cotton ball.

STEPS:

1. Perform hand hygiene.
2. Assemble equipment.
3. Identify patient and explain procedure. Ask patient to leave glasses on or contact lenses in place for this test.
4. In a well-lighted room, have patient hold near-vision acuity card 14 to 16 inches away, covering first one eye with occluder and then the other. Both eyes should remain open during testing. The occluder should be held in such a way as not to interfere with normal position of patient's glasses.
5. Ask patient to read aloud smallest paragraph or line possible without error. Note any squinting or other signs of difficulty seeing the print.
6. Record value of line patient could read comfortably at a distance of 14 inches. Value will depend on type of card used.
7. Clean eye occluder with alcohol.
8. Document results in patient's record.

CHARTING EXAMPLE: 04/07/XX 1:00 P.M. Near-vision acuity checked. Pt. had no trouble reading card at 14 inches.
.... L. Fox CMA (AAMA)

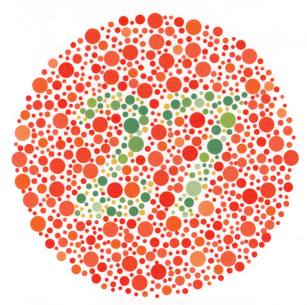

FIGURE 5-12   Color plate from Ishihara color vision test.

discern the numbers of some of the plates depending on their color deficiency.

IRRIGATION OF THE EYE

Lavage, or irrigation, of the eye is performed to remove foreign substances or chemicals. Eye irrigation requires sterile technique and equipment. Never try to remove a foreign object with a cotton applicator stick as this may cause corneal abrasions.

INSTILLING EYE MEDICATIONS

Only ophthalmic or optic medication may be used in the eye. Medicated eye ointments and eye drops are used to treat infection, to dilate the pupil for retinal examination, or to apply anesthetic for testing.

Teaching patients how to instill eye medications at home is frequently required. When teaching this to patients, it is important to reinforce the need for both sterile medications and sterile technique. Medications should never be shared with others or even used again or on the other eye if treatment is needed at another time. Medications should be discarded at the end of the treatment period to prevent cross-infection and contamination.

ASSISTING VISION-IMPAIRED PATIENT

To be declared legally blind, an individual must see at 20 feet what a person with normal vision would see at 200 feet. If a vision-impaired patient is scheduled for an appointment

PROCEDURE 5-24

SCREENING FOR COLOR-VISION ACUITY

ABHES VII.MA.A.1 9(m)   CAAHEP I.P (10)

OBJECTIVE: To assess color vision using Ishihara method.

STANDARD: This task takes 5 minutes.

EQUIPMENT AND SUPPLIES: Ishihara screening book/card; paper; pen; patient's record.

STEPS:

1. Perform hand hygiene.
2. Assemble equipment.
3. Identify patient, and explain procedure.
4. Seat patient in a room with daylight for better testing results. Hold Ishihara book 30 inches from patient, and ask patient to identify practice page. All patients will be able to read this page successfully. Explain that 3 seconds will be given for identification of each plate.
5. Record number patient sees for each plate in order. Ten or more plates identified correctly are regarded as normal color acuity.

CHARTING EXAMPLE: 04/07/XX 9:00 A.M. Ishihara color-vision test performed. 11 identified correctly. · B. Diane, CMA (AAMA)

PROCEDURE 5-25

IRRIGATING THE EYE

ABHES VII.MA.A.1 9(m)   CAAHEP I.P (10)

OBJECTIVE: To cleanse or irrigate the eye while using sterile technique.

STANDARD: This task takes about 10 minutes.

EQUIPMENT AND SUPPLIES: Nonpowdered gloves; irrigating solution (normal saline or whatever physician ordered); emesis basin; sterile irrigating syringe; sterile gauze; towel; tissues; pen; patient's record.

STEPS:

1. Check physician's orders, and check for patient allergies.
2. Perform hand hygiene.
3. Assemble equipment and supplies. Check label of irrigating solution three times to be sure it is in date and is the solution ordered by physician. Solution should be brought to room temperature by wrapping bottle in dry heating pad or standing it in warm water bath.
4. Identify patient, and explain procedure.
5. Ask patient which position he or she prefers: sitting or lying down. Assist patient with getting into position.
6. Don gloves.
7. Place towel on shoulder of patient on side to be irrigated.

NOTE: If both eyes are to be irrigated, two separate sets of equipment must be used to prevent cross-infection.

8. Open irrigating solution, and pour into sterile container.
9. If seated, ask patient to tilt head to side of affected eye and hold emesis basin. If lying down, position emesis basin on table with patient lying on same side as affected eye.
10. Using index finger and thumb of nondominant hand, open affected eye. Ask patient to look up and stare at specific object.

11. Fill syringe with irrigating solution, and irrigate affected eye with solution from inner to outer canthus with tip of syringe about ½ inch from eye and aimed at conjunctiva, not cornea.

12. Continue irrigation until debris is returned, or as ordered by physician.

13. Dry area around eye with sterile gauze.

14. Discard waste in biohazard waste container.

15. Remove gloves, and perform hand hygiene.

16. Document procedure in patient's record.

CHARTING EXAMPLE: 04/10/XX 11:30 A.M. Right eye (OD) irrigated with 50 mL of 100° normal saline. Eye slightly red. Pt. says "Eye feels fine." · · · · · · · · · · · · · E. Zandri, CMA (AAMA)

PROCEDURE 5-26

INSTILLING EYE MEDICATIONS
ABHES VII.MA.A.1 9(m)   CAAHEP I.P (10)

OBJECTIVE: To instill eye medication as ordered by physician.

STANDARD: This task takes 5 minutes.

EQUIPMENT AND SUPPLIES: Sterile medication; sterile eyedropper (if needed); tissues; sterile gauze squares; nonsterile gloves; drape or towel; pen; patient's record.

STEPS:

1. Perform hand hygiene.

2. Identify patient, and explain procedure.

3. Check physician's orders and check for patient allergies.

4. Check type of medication, dose, and expiration date three times to prevent medication error.

5. Ask patient about allergies to medications. (Obviously, if patient is allergic to a specific medication, it cannot be given.)

6. Don gloves.

7. Position patient with head tilted back. Ask patient to look up. Give patient tissue to blot cheek.

8. Uncap medication, placing cap on its side.

9. Pull down lower eyelid to expose the conjunctiva.

10. a. *If no ointment is ordered:* With dominant hand, place dropper about ½ inch above eyeball. Do not touch dropper or ointment tube to eye. Instill prescribed number of eyedrops onto center of conjunctiva. Ask patient to close eye and rotate eyeball to disperse medication.
    b. *If ointment is ordered:* Ask patient to look up. Place medication tube tip about ½ inch above exposed conjunctival sac. (See Figure 5-13.) Squeeze a ribbon

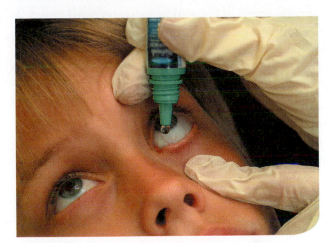

FIGURE 5-13   Instilling eye medication.

of ointment along middle third of inside edge of lower lid without touching with tip of ointment tube. Ask patient to close eye and rotate eyeball (as in preceding steps).

11. Using sterile gauze, remove excess medication from inner canthus or outer canthus. Explain to patient that vision may be blurry for a few minutes.

12. Clean area, and dispose of equipment and used medication.

13. Remove gloves, and perform hand hygiene.

14. Document procedure in patient's record.

CHARTING EXAMPLE: 04/10/XX 3:00 P.M. Instilled 2 gtt of 1% atropine sulfate both eyes (OU). Pt. complained of stinging and blurry vision. · E. Garcia, RMA

BOX 5-4 Guidelines for Assisting the Vision-Impaired Patient

- Ask patient how you can help. Follow patient's suggestions.
- Face the patient when speaking, and speak slowly and carefully (not more loudly).
- Identify yourself when you enter the room.
- Explain why you are in the room.
- Do not touch the patient unless you ask permission first.
- Describe the room.
- Identify others in the room as well as their purpose and location in the room.
- Provide step-by-step instructions for procedures as you perform them.
- To assist patient with walking, walk slightly ahead, ask which arm patient would prefer to grasp, and then offer that arm.
- Walk at a normal pace.
- Describe obstacles such as stairs or steps.
- Keep hallways and rooms free of clutter and obstacles.
- Treat the vision-impaired patient with respect.

in the facility, examine the patient's record to determine the level of impairment in order to be better prepared. Box 5-4 lists some general guidelines to assist in caring for the visually impaired patient.

EYE PATCH DRESSING

Injuries, infections, and vision disorders may require application of an eye patch ordered by the physician. Sterile dressings are applied after some eye surgeries and infections. An eye patch also is used in cases of **strabismus**, or lazy eye, in which case the patch is worn over the good eye for a period of months to strengthen the weaker eye.

Otorhinolaryngology

Otorhinolaryngology is the study of the ear, nose, and throat. Every general physical examination includes examination of the ear, nose, and throat. Infection of the nose and throat often affect the ear, which is the organ of balance and hearing. Reviewing the structures of the ear, nose, and throat will help with comprehension of the competencies presented in this section.

The steps for the following procedures follow:

- Assisting with audiometry
- Irrigation of ear

PROCEDURE 5-27

APPLYING EYE PATCH DRESSING

ABHES VII.MA.A.1 9(m)   CAAHEP I.P (10)

OBJECTIVE: To apply a sterile eye patch.

STANDARD: This task takes 5 minutes.

EQUIPMENT AND SUPPLIES: Sterile eye patch; sterile gloves; tape; pen; patient's record.

STEPS:

1. Check physician's orders.
2. Perform hand hygiene.
3. Assemble equipment.

4. Identify patient, explain procedure, and inquire whether patient has transportation home. (Eye patch restricts the field of vision and impairs driving ability.) Each facility will decide what to do if transportation is a problem.
5. Position patient either in supine or sitting position.
6. Open sterile packet, and use inside of packet as sterile field.
7. Don sterile gloves.
8. Ask patient to close both eyes, and place sterile eye patch over affected eye.

9. Secure patch with transparent tape placed diagonally from mid forehead to below ear.

10. Assist patient off table as needed.

11. Provide further instruction, both verbal and written, per physician's orders. Confirm patient understanding of instructions.

12. Remove gloves, and perform hand hygiene.

13. Document patient's record.

CHARTING EXAMPLE: 04/11/XX 2:00 P.M. Sterile patch left eye (OS). Pt. complains of "pain and itching in eye." No exudate present. Brother to drive Pt. home. Pt. verbalized understanding of instructions. · · · · · · · F. James, CMA (AAMA)

- Instillation of ear medications
- Instilling nasal medications
- Assisting with treatment of epistaxis
- Obtaining a throat culture

During a physical examination, the physician examines the ear with an otoscope and tests the patient's hearing acuity with a simple instrument, the tuning fork. The physician strikes the tuning fork on the palm of her hand, causing it to vibrate. The tuning fork is then held on the top of the head (Weber test: Figure 5-14) and against the mastoid bone behind the ear (Rinne test: Figure 5-15). The patient is asked whether he or she can hear or feel the vibrations of the tuning fork. Gross assessment can also be done by holding a ticking watch 4 to 6 inches from the ear to determine if the patient can hear the ticking.

Damage to nerve receptors in the ear or to the auditory nerve can result in sensorineural hearing loss. Conduction hearing loss is due to obstruction of the sound waves reaching the nerve receptors in the ear. This type of hearing loss can be caused by foreign material or **cerumen** in the ear canal or calcification of the bones of the inner ear, infection of the ear, fluid buildup in the middle ear, or a combination of these problems.

ASSISTING WITH AUDIOMETRY

The audiometer is an electronic device that emits sounds of varying frequencies and decibels. The patient is asked

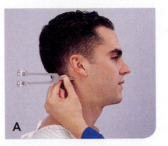 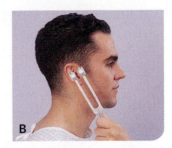

FIGURE 5-15 Placement of tuning fork for Rinne test: (A) Base of tuning fork on mastoid process; (B) tuning fork prongs in front of client's ear.

to push a button in response to each sound heard. The decibel levels vary from very high to very low. An audiogram is recorded, indicating each of the patient's responses, and then evaluated by the physician. Hearing is considered within normal limits if the patient can hear sounds up to 15 decibels, depending on environmental noise. Before operating an audiometer, assisting personnel should receive training by an audiologist and follow manufacturer's directions.

IRRIGATING THE EAR

Irrigation of the ear consists of rinsing the external auditory canal with a solution per physician's orders. It is ordered to remove impacted earwax, to relieve inflammation with an antiseptic solution, or to remove foreign matter from the external ear canal. The abbreviation *AD* indicates right ear, *AS* is left ear, and *AU* is both ears. The Joint Commission now recommends that the words for each be used, not the abbreviations, to avoid errors.

INSTILLING EAR MEDICATION

Ear medications are used to soften cerumen, to treat infection, and to relieve pain. They are usually liquid placed by dropper into the external auditory canal. Ear medications are designated by words "For Otic Use" on the label.

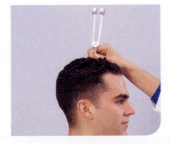

FIGURE 5-14 Place the base of a tuning fork on the client's skull (Weber test).

PROCEDURE 5-28

ASSISTING WITH AUDIOMETRY

ABHES VII.MA.A.1 9(m)   CAAHEP I.P (10)

OBJECTIVE: To perform audiometric testing as ordered by the physician.

STANDARD: This task takes 10 minutes.

EQUIPMENT AND SUPPLIES: Audiometer with headphones; quiet room or small enclosed cubicle; patient's record; pen.

STEPS:

1. Check physician's orders.
2. Perform hand hygiene.
3. Prepare equipment and examination room for patient.
4. Test equipment and make sure power is on.
5. Identify patient, and explain procedure.
6. Establish response signal patient will give if automatic button is not available. (Nodding head or holding up one finger is an acceptable signal).
7. Seat patient comfortably in room.
8. Place headphones snugly over patient's ears. (Signals will be given to each ear separately.)
9. Begin with low frequency, and watch patient for agreed-upon response signal.
10. Gradually increase frequency until test is completed in first ear. Repeat procedure on other ear.
11. Remove headphones and give patient further instructions per physician's orders.
12. Clean equipment following manufacturers' directions.
13. Perform hand hygiene.
14. Document procedure in patient's record.

CHARTING EXAMPLE: 04/11/XX 4:30 P.M. Audiometry test administered; results given to Dr. Fu. · · · · · · · · · · · · · ·
· M. Dennehey, RMA

PROCEDURE 5-29

IRRIGATING THE EAR

ABHES VII.MA.A.1 9(m)   CAAHEP I.P (10)

OBJECTIVE: To perform ear irrigation as directed by physician.

STANDARD: This task takes 10 minutes.

EQUIPMENT AND SUPPLIES: Irrigating syringe; sterile basin; ear or emesis basin; irrigation solution; gloves; towel; gauze pads; cotton ball; pen; patient's record.

STEPS:

1. Check physician's orders, and check for patient allergies.
2. Perform hand hygiene.
3. Assemble equipment.
4. Check irrigating solution label three times for name of solution per physician's order, concentration, and expiration date. Warm solution to body temperature.
5. Identify patient, and explain procedure.
6. Assist patient into Fowler's position, and place absorbent towel over shoulder. Ask patient to tilt head slightly toward affected ear. Ask patient to hold basin below ear, if possible.
7. Pour warmed solution into sterile basin, fill syringe with 50 mL of solution, and expel air.
8. Straighten ear canal by pulling **pinna** (projecting portion of the external ear) up and back for adult and down and back for children under age three.
9. Insert tip into ear canal, aiming stream of flow toward roof of canal. Note return flow during procedure, continuing until desired results are obtained.
10. Dry outside of ear, and repeat if ordered for other ear.

11. Place cotton ball in ear to absorb excess fluid. Provide further directions as needed for home care.
12. Clean examination room, and dispose of waste materials properly.
13. Perform hand hygiene.
14. Document procedure, describing type of results achieved by irrigation and noting any patient symptoms.

CHARTING EXAMPLE: 04/11/XX 9:15 A.M. AU irrigated with 250 mL sterile water @ 98.6 °F. Yellowish-brown cerumen plug returned from AD. Clear liquid return AS. No pain or dizziness reported. Cotton ball inserted AU × 10 min. Pt. states "Hearing better." · · · · · · · · · · · · · · · · T. Roberts, CMA (AAMA)

Patients may require instruction about administering ear medication at home. (Procedure 5-30 covers the steps for instilling ear medications.)

NOSE AND THROAT

Examination of the nose with a nasal speculum is a regular part of a physical examination. The physician also palpates the sinuses for tenderness. A nasal swab may be collected to evaluate for allergic rhinitis. Nasal irrigation is occasionally performed to remove foreign objects, assist drainage, or reduce inflammation. Treating patients with nosebleed (epistaxis) by cauterization or nasal packing is fairly common.

Using a tongue depressor, the throat is inspected for enlarged tonsils, signs of infection, and other abnormalities of the oral cavity and tongue. A throat culture is obtained to determine the cause of infections. The procedures for instilling nasal medications assisting with treatment of epistaxis and obtaining a throat culture follow.

Instillation of nasal medication is ordered for sinusitis, treatment of allergic rhinitis, and treatment of infection. Patient instruction for home instillation may be required. Patients should be cautioned about overuse of over-the-counter (OTC) nasal spray. If dosage is exceeded, the nasal passages may dry out and make congestion worse due to rebound effect.

PROCEDURE 5-30

INSTILLING EAR MEDICATION

ABHES VII.MA.A.1 9(m)   CAAHEP I.P (10)

OBJECTIVE: To instill ear medication as ordered by physician.

STANDARD: This task takes 5 minutes.

EQUIPMENT AND SUPPLIES: Prescribed otic medication; dropper for instilling medication; cotton balls; gloves; pen; patient's record.

STEPS:

1. Check physician's orders, and check for patient allergies.
2. Assemble equipment.
3. Perform hand hygiene.
4. Identify patient, and explain procedure.
5. Check medication label three times for correct name per physician order, expiration date, and concentration. Warm by rolling medication between hands.
6. Don gloves.
7. Position patient either lying on side with affected ear facing up or seated with head tilted away from the affected ear.
8. Fill dropper with prescribed amount of medication, and pull pinna up and back for adult (Figure 5-16) or down and back for child under age three (Figure 5-17). Instill ear drops, holding dropper slightly above ear without touching sides of ear canal.
9. Instruct patient to remain in position for 3 to 5 minutes. If ordered by physician, place a slightly moistened cotton ball in ear canal to prevent medication from running out of the ear.
10. Assist the patient off table as needed.

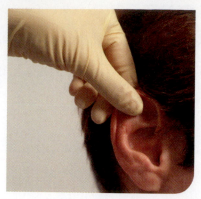

FIGURE 5-16 Straightening the ear canal of an adult to instill ear drops.

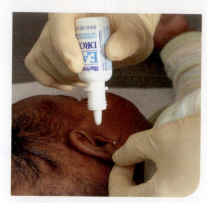

FIGURE 5-17 Straightening the ear canal of a child to instill ear drops.

11. Provide instructions for home care as ordered. Confirm understanding of instructions by having patient verbally repeat or demonstrate.

12. Dispose of equipment, and clean area.

13. Remove gloves, and perform hand hygiene.

14. Document procedure in patient's record.

CHARTING EXAMPLE: 04/11/XX 7:00 P.M. 2 gtt Neosporin otic solution instilled right ear (AD) as ordered. Pt. verbally confirmed instruction for home instillation 2×/day for 7 days. Appointment made for 4/18 recheck. · · · · · · · · · · · · · · · · ·
· C. Lynch, CMA (AAMA)

PROCEDURE 5-31

INSTILLING NASAL MEDICATION

ABHES VII.MA.A.1 9(m)   CAAHEP I.P (10)

OBJECTIVE: To instill nasal medication as ordered by the physician.

STANDARD: This task takes 5 minutes.

EQUIPMENT AND SUPPLIES: Physician's order; patient's record; nasal medication; medicine dropper (sterile); tissues; gloves.

STEPS:

1. Check physician's orders, and check for patient allergies.
2. Perform hand hygiene.
3. Assemble equipment.
4. Identify patient, and explain procedure.
5. Position patient with head lower than shoulders. Place patient in supine position with pillow under neck to lower head below shoulders. Make patient as comfortable as possible.
6. Check medication three times for correct name based on physician's order, dosage, and expiration date. Draw

medication into dropper and hold over center of affected nostril, taking care not to touch dropper to inside of nostril. Repeat in other nostril if ordered.

7. Tell patient to stay in that position for 5 minutes to prevent medication from running out of nostril.
8. Provide tissues for patient to wipe excess from skin.
9. Discard dropper in biohazard waste container. Recap medication, and return it to storage place.
10. Clean area, and remove gloves.
11. Provide home instruction if needed. Verify patient understanding.
12. Perform hand hygiene.
13. Document procedure in patient's record.

CHARTING EXAMPLE: 04//11/XX 5:00 P.M. Afrin nasal spray 3 gtt instilled each nostril per Dr. Schwartz. · · · · · · · · · ·
· N. Lynch, CMA (AAMA)

ASSISTING WITH TREATMENT FOR EPISTAXIS

Epistaxis, or nosebleed, is a fairly common occurrence in children from ages 2 to 10. Individuals with high blood pressure or injuries to the face and nose may have nosebleeds as well. The common at-home treatment is to sit patient upright (not with head tilted backward) to keep blood from running down the throat, then to pinch the sides of the nose together for 10 to 15 minutes. Ice may then be applied. If bleeding continues after these measures have been tried, the individual should seek medical assistance. The nose may be chemically cauterized or packed with sterile gauze. If neither of these causes bleeding to stop, heat cauterization is performed.

THROAT CULTURE

Throat culture is one of the most frequently requested laboratory tests in an outpatient facility. Throat cultures are performed to determine the cause of pharyngitis and to determine the most suitable treatment. Confirmation of *Streptococcus pyogenes*, the primary cause of pharyngitis in North America, is important because of the pathogen's virulence and possible complications. Further discussion of microbiology is found in Chapter 12.

PROCEDURE 5-32

ASSISTING WITH TREATMENT OF EPISTAXIS

ABHES VII.MA.A.1 9(m)   CAAHEP I.P (10)

OBJECTIVE: To assist with treatment of epistaxis.

STANDARD: This procedure takes about 20 minutes.

EQUIPMENT AND SUPPLIES: Sterile gloves; nonsterile gloves; epinephrine; syringe and needles; silver nitrate sticks; sterile cotton balls; sterile medicine cup; sterile cotton-tipped applicator sticks; local anesthetic; Vienna nasal speculum; light source; bayonet forceps; biohazard waste container; patient's record; pen.

STEPS:

1. Check physician's orders, and check for patient allergies.
2. Perform hand hygiene.
3. Assemble equipment and supplies.
4. Identify patient, and explain procedure.
5. Assist physician as needed to visualize area.
6. If you will be handling sterile items, don sterile gloves. (If not, nonsterile gloves are worn.)

NOTE: Each physician has individual preferences for the role of assistants during such procedures.

7. Assist physician with applying anesthetic. Remove appropriate amount of anesthetic from vial, and dispense into sterile medicine cup. Soak sterile cotton-tipped applicator in anesthetic, and apply to nasal membranes.
8. Assist physician during cauterization, packing, or both.
9. When procedure is concluded, assist patient and provide clear written and verbal instructions for home care. Explain that patient must refrain from blowing and picking nose to avoid disturbing scab or clot.
10. Clean equipment, and dispose of contaminated supplies.
11. Perform hand hygiene.
12. Document procedure in patient's record.

CHARTING EXAMPLE: 04/14/XX 6:00 P.M. Epistaxis treated with cauterization by Dr. Luc. Written and verbal instructions given to refrain from blowing nose or disturbing clot. Call and come in ASAP if bleeding reoccurs. · · · · · · · · · · · · · · · · ·
· A. Campo, CMA (AAMA)

PROCEDURE 5-33

OBTAINING A THROAT CULTURE

ABHES VII.MA.A.1 10(d)(4)   CAAHEP III.P (7)

OBJECTIVE: To collect a throat culture without contamination and process correctly.

STANDARD: This task takes 5 minutes.

EQUIPMENT AND SUPPLIES: Gloves; tongue depressor; light; sterile swab; sterile culture medium; transport tube; laboratory requisition; patient's record; pen; biohazard waste container.

STEPS:

1. Check physician's orders, and check for patient allergies.
2. Gather equipment.
3. Identify patient, and explain procedure.
4. Perform hand hygiene and don gloves.
5. Remove sterile swab from culture tube by rotating cap to break seal.
6. Ask patient to tilt head back and open mouth.
7. Use a tongue depressor to hold down tongue, and swab the throat in the tonsillar area from right side of throat to left. Take care not to contaminate swab on teeth or lips. Discard tongue depressor in biohazard waste container.
8. Place swab into tube, and immerse in culture medium.

NOTE: Culture swab must be cultured immediately or kept moist for later testing. With some tubes, the internal vial of media must be crushed first.

9. Tell patient to assume a comfortable position.
10. Remove gloves. Label specimen tube, and prepare for transport.
11. Perform hand hygiene.
12. Document procedure in patient's record.

CHARTING EXAMPLE: 04/16/XX 11:05 A.M. Throat culture obtained and sent to Memorial Lab. · · · · · · M. Dennehey, RMA

6 Assisting with Pediatrics

PROCEDURES

Procedure 6-1 Wrapping an Infant or Small Child

Procedure 6-2 Measuring Pediatric Vital Signs

Procedure 6-3 Measuring the Weight and Length of Infants

Procedure 6-4 Measuring Infant Head Circumference

Procedure 6-5 Measuring Circumference of Child's Chest

Procedure 6-6 Calculating Growth Percentiles

Procedure 6-7 Documenting and Maintaining Patient Immunization Record

Procedure 6-8 Applying Pediatric Urine Collection Device

TERMS TO LEARN

fontanels

vertex

genitalia

mons pubis

Pediatrics is the branch of medicine dealing with the care and development of children and the diagnosis and treatment of childhood diseases and conditions. Pediatricians, primary care physicians, and osteopaths treat pediatric patients. Establishing trust and good rapport with each child encourages a more cooperative, compliant patient. Each child should be greeted warmly with a smile. Simple terms should be used without lying when explaining to children what to expect in discomfort from an injection or procedure.

The two types of pediatric visits are well-child visits and sick-child visits. Well-child visits include measuring growth and assessing development, providing childhood immunizations, and providing health information. Sick-child visits include examination to diagnose and recommend treatment for an illness or injury. To avoid spreading infection, sick children are separated from well children in many offices.

Pediatricians usually treat patients until they reach eighteen years of age or have completed high school. Each practice sets its own standards based on the needs of individual patients. After leaving a pediatric practice, adolescents or young adults are then referred to family or internal medicine practices. In addition, female adolescents are referred to obstetrics and gynecology practices.

Legal Alert! In some states caregivers other than parents must have signed legal permission to bring a pediatric patient into a medical facility for treatment. In California, carrying and undressing a pediatric patient is the responsibility of the parent.

Apgar Scoring

Immediately after birth the newborn is assessed using the Apgar scoring system. This is a method of evaluating a newborn's condition at 1 and 5 minutes after birth. If a score is under 7 for a newborn at 5 minutes after birth, reevaluation

must be done every 5 minutes for 20 minutes more. Physicians may intubate an infant if two or more scores are not 7 or higher. Table 6-1 illustrates Apgar scoring.

- Newborns scoring 7–10 are considered out of immediate danger.
- Newborns scoring 4–6 are considered moderately depressed.
- Newborns scoring of 0–3 are severely depressed.

Patient Safety

The safety of each pediatric patient is a primary concern. No child should ever be left alone on an examination table, scale, toilet, or anywhere else that could pose a danger.

When carrying an infant, it is helpful to notice the way the parent or guardian holds the child. This position is most likely preferred by the infant. Three positions are used to carry an infant: the cradle hold (Figure 6-1A), football hold (Figure 6-1B), and upright or shoulder hold (Figure 6-1C). Support for the infant's head is necessary, especially in the upright position.

Wrapping the Infant

At times it may be necessary to restrict the movement of the infant or small child to perform a procedure. A small sheet or receiving blanket may be used to wrap the child (mummy restraint) and bind the arms to the sides. If head movement must be restricted, hands should be placed on either side of the head, avoiding sealing of the ears or touching the soft spot or **fontanels** on the baby's head. Encourage the parent or guardian to assist with restraining the child if necessary. Demonstrate the manner in which you would like the child held. Restraint policies usually do not apply when restriction is for security, is procedure related, uses protective devices such as bed rails, or is done with voluntary consent of the patient.

Steps for wrapping and restraining a small pediatric patient are found in Procedure 6-1.

TABLE 6-1 Apgar Scoring

Sign	0	1	2
Heart rate (pulse)	Absent	Slow (less than 110)	Over 100
Breathing (respiratory rate and effort)	Absent	Slow, irregular	Good crying
Activity (muscle tone)	Flaccid	Some flexion of extremities	Active motion
Grimace (responsiveness or "reflex irritability")	No response	Cry	Vigorous cry
Appearance (skin color)	Blue; pale	Body pink, extremities blue	Completely pink

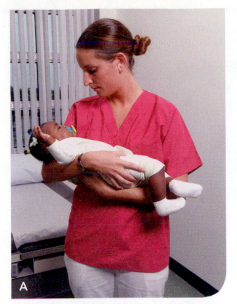 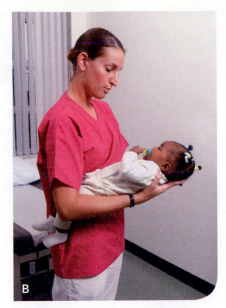 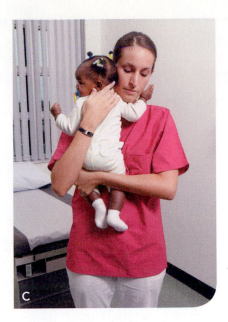

FIGURE 6-1   (A) The cradle hold; (B) the football hold; (C) the shoulder or upright hold.

Pediatric Vital Signs

Vital signs are covered in Chapter 3. A review of the procedures is suggested at this point. Pediatric vital signs differ somewhat from those of an adult. Table 6-2 indicates vital sign ranges and averages for children newborn to 10 years of age.

Temperature, pulse, and respiration are routinely measured at each visit. Blood pressure is measured annually from age three years on unless cardiac disorders warrant more regular evaluation. A pediatric cuff should be used for small patients. Temperature is measured in a child using any of the types of thermometers mentioned in Chapter 3. The oral route is used for older children who can follow directions. Tympanic or temporal artery measurements are quick and easy to obtain on the pediatric patient. Rectal temperature may be assessed; however, close monitoring of the patient during the procedure is necessary. Glass thermometers should not be used if other types are available. Pulse in a child under age 5 years is done by measuring the

PROCEDURE 6-1

WRAPPING AN INFANT OR SMALL CHILD

ABHES VII.MA.A.1 9(l)   CAAHEP I.P (10)

OBJECTIVE: To wrap an infant or small child securely to restrain movement.

STANDARD: This task takes less than 5 minutes.

EQUIPMENT AND SUPPLIES: Small sheet or receiving blanket; examination table; patient's record; pen.

STEPS:

1. Perform hand hygiene.
2. Speak to child in soft soothing tones, and explain what you are going to do.

3. Place child on table. Have parent or guardian undress child as needed.
4. Place receiving blanket or small sheet on table. Fold down top corner. Fold bottom corner up.

NOTE: Size of sheet or blanket depends on age and size of child.

5. Place child diagonally on blanket while keeping one hand on abdomen to ensure safety. See Figure 6-2.
6. Wrap right corner across torso, covering right arm, and tuck snugly under left arm.

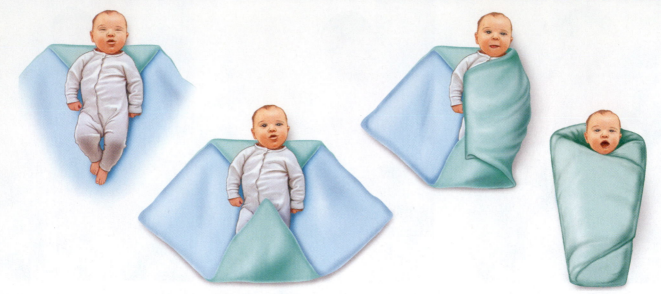

FIGURE 6-2 How to wrap a baby and secure arms.

7. Wrap left corner across torso, covering left arm, and tuck snugly under torso.

8. To restrain head, place yourself at end of table where infant's head is located and place one hand on either side of head. Avoid sealing ears or touching fontanels.

9. Speak soothingly to comfort child and allay fears as much as possible.

10. When procedure is completed, pick up child and offer comfort for a few moments. Then proceed to redress, or continue with examination as directed.

11. Clean examination room.

12. Perform hand hygiene.

13. Document if necessary.

apical pulse. Because young children breathe so rapidly, it is important to measure respiration with the child lying in the supine position and you placing your hand on the chest. Procedure 6-2 lists the steps for measuring pediatric vital signs.

Height, Weight

An infant's height and weight are measured at each visit to monitor growth patterns and to calculate medication dosages if needed. An infant may be weighed with or without

TABLE 6-2 Vital Sign Chart for Children

Age	Pulse Range	Pulse Average	Blood Pressure Average	Respiration Average
Newborn	110–180	140	90/55	30–50
1 Year	80–150	120	90/60	20–40
2 Years	80–130	110	95/60	20–30
4 Years	80–120	100	99/65	20–25
6 Years	75–115	100	100/56	20–25
8 Years	70–110	90	105/56	15–20
10 Years	70–110	90	110/58	15–20

PROCEDURE 6-2

MEASURING PEDIATRIC VITAL SIGNS

ABHES VII.MA.A.1 9(c)   CAAHEP I.P (1)

OBJECTIVE: To measure and record temperature, pulse, respiration, and blood pressure accurately on a pediatric patient.

STANDARD: This task takes 5–10 minutes.

EQUIPMENT AND SUPPLIES: Gloves; tympanic thermometer; nonglass nonmercury thermometer; digital thermometer; temporal artery thermometer; watch with second hand; stethoscope and pediatric blood pressure cuff; patient's record; pen; biohazard waste container.

STEPS:

1. Perform hand hygiene.
2. Assemble equipment and supplies.
3. Identify patient, and explain procedures to the parent or caregiver. Speak reassuringly to the child to win his or her trust.
4. Explain to the parent how she or he can assist you.

Obtaining temperature with tympanic thermometer

1. Remove thermometer from base and note that it reads "Ready."
2. Attach disposable probe cover to earpiece.
3. Gently pull pinna downward to straighten ear canal on a child under age 3 years, up and back for older children.
4. Insert probe into ear canal.
5. Press scan button.
6. Observe temperature reading.
7. Gently withdraw the thermometer and eject probe cover into biohazard waste container.
8. Record temperature reading "T" to denote tympanic reading.
9. Return thermometer to base.

Obtaining temperature reading using axillary method

1. Remove nonmercury thermometer from container and rinse with cool water. Inspect for defects.
2. Shake down thermometer to 95°F/35°C.
3. Place thermometer in the infant's armpit and hold arm across chest for required time (10 minutes).
4. Read thermometer and record by designating reading with AX for axillary.

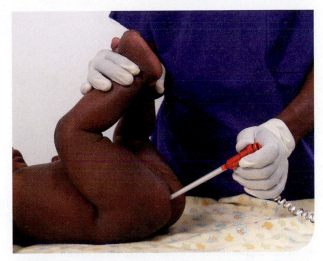

FIGURE 6-3 Obtaining a temperature reading rectally on an infant.

Obtaining temperature reading rectally using a digital thermometer (Figure 6-3)

1. Don gloves.
2. Attach disposable tip to the top of the (red for rectal) probe.
3. Lubricate tip of probe to provide easy insertion.
4. Place child on bed or exam table in supine or prone position.
5. Insert thermometer ½ inch into rectum, and hold in place with hand to prevent expelling.
6. Hold the child securely to restrict movement.
7. Leave the thermometer in required time until it beeps.
8. Remove thermometer, remove probe cover, and dispose in biohazard waste container. Take the reading.
9. Record the reading using "R" to indicate rectal.
10. Replace thermometer in base.

Measure temperature with temporal artery thermometer

1. Perform hand hygiene.
2. Assemble equipment.
3. Identify patient.
4. Explain procedure.
5. Using side of head exposed (not resting on pillow), brush hair aside. Dry forehead with tissue if damp.

6. Place probe flush on the center of the forehead, and depress the red button.

7. Keep probe button depressed, and slowly slide the probe on the midline across the forehead to the hairline.

8. Lift the probe from the forehead, and touch it on the neck just behind the earlobe.

9. Release the button and read.

10. Record the results in the patient's record.

11. Perform hand hygiene.

Measure pulse/heart rate by apical method

1. Remove or lift up child's shirt. Distraction may be necessary to have the child lie still to obtain apical pulse.

2. Place the child in sitting or supine position. Place stethoscope on the child's chest at the midpoint between the sternum and the left nipple (Figure 6-4). Some facilities do not use a stethoscope. Apical pulse is performed by simply placing a hand on the child's chest and counting the beats.

3. Listen for apical beat. Using a watch with second hand, count apical pulse for 1 full minute. Note count at 30 seconds in case child becomes too restless to continue.

4. Record apical pulse (AP) using "AP" before pulse to indicate apical reading.

Measure respiration as follows

1. Place child in supine position on bed or exam table.

2. Have parent or caregiver distract patient so respirations may be counted.

3. Place your hand on the child's chest and count each rise and fall as 1 respiration.

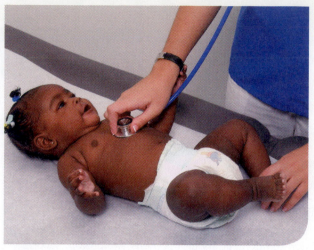

FIGURE 6-4 Measuring apical pulse of an infant.

4. Count for 1 minute, noting count at 30 seconds in case child is too restless to continue.

Measure child or infant's blood pressure using pediatric cuff as follows

1. Place child on exam table or bed and place cuff on upper arm.

2. Feel for brachial pulse.

3. Place earpieces of stethoscope in your ears and diaphragm over pulse site.

4. Pump up cuff until pulse no longer heard and listen for systolic/diastolic sounds.

5. Record results.

CHARTING EXAMPLE: 05/23/XX 4:00 P.M. T.99°F (T); AP 92; R 20; BP 100/78. · M. Ford, RMA

a diaper, depending on the facility policy. Weight charts for infants are based on weight measured without clothing. If the infant is to be measured with diaper, a clean diaper must be weighed first and then placed on the child during weighing. The weight of the diaper is then subtracted from the total weight of the baby.

The length of an infant is measured in the supine position from the **vertex** (top, highest point) of the head to the heel with knees straight. Measurement is done on the examining table until the child is old enough to stand on an adult scale at about age 24 months. The child is placed on the examination table with the head up against the measuring bar and legs stretched out until straight. The procedure is easier to accomplish with a second person holding the

child's head still or straightening out the knees. A tape measure is used to find the distance between the two bars, or the tape is held on the side of the head and stretched to the heel. The procedures for measuring height and weight using an adult scale are provided in Chapter 3, Procedure 3-17. Procedure 6-3 lists the steps for measuring the weight and length of infants.

Head and Chest Circumference

Head circumference is measured as part of every well-child visit until age 6 years. Infancy is a time of rapid brain growth; therefore, this is a vital measurement. Normal head

MEASURING THE WEIGHT AND LENGTH OF INFANTS

ABHES VII.MA.A.1 9(m)   CAAHEP I.P (10)

OBJECTIVE: To measure the weight and length of an infant accurately.

STANDARD: This task takes 5 minutes.

EQUIPMENT AND SUPPLIES: Infant scale; tape measure; examination table; paper; patient's record; pen.

STEPS:

1. Perform hand hygiene.
2. Identify infant by stating the name to parent or caregiver.
3. Explain procedure to parent or caregiver.
4. Prepare pediatric scale by placing paper protector on it and balancing scale for accuracy.
5. Remove infant's clothing and diaper according to facility policy. Weigh clean diaper, then use to rediaper. (Hold another clean diaper over infant boys while you weigh them.)

NOTE: Never leave any child unattended at any time.

6. Keeping one hand over infant, slide large pound weight into groove closest to estimated weight (Figure 6-5). Move smaller ounce weight by tapping gently until it reaches weight at which pointer floats in center of balance area. Distract infant by speaking in soothing tones.
7. Read results in pounds and ounces while infant is still. Remove infant from scale and place on examination table under parent or caregiver's care before recording results.
8. Return scale to resting position. Record results. (If weighed with diaper on, subtract diaper weight from total weight before recording).
9. Place infant on examination table in supine position with head against headboard at zero mark. If possible, have parent hold child's head still. Straighten child's knees and place footboard against child's foot, or mark examination table paper where heel reaches, and measure total length with measuring tape (Figure 6-6). Record measurement to nearest ¼ inch. While parent redresses child, offer to answer any questions.
10. Perform hand hygiene.

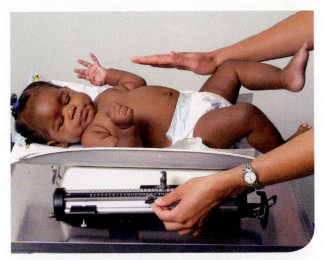

FIGURE 6-5 Weighing a baby on infant scale.

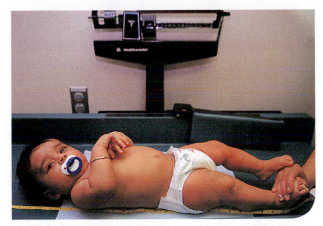

FIGURE 6-6 Measuring length of an infant from top of head to base of heel with knees straight.

CHARTING EXAMPLE: 05/25/XX 11:15 A.M. Parent brought 13-month-old in for well-child visit. Wt: 26 lbs 2 oz. Ht: 32 inches. · A. Rashid, RMA

circumference at birth should be between 12.5 and 14.5 inches (31.75–38.0 cm). The head and chest circumferences are generally equal at about 1 to 2 years of age.

The circumference of the chest is measured if there is suspicion of over- or underdevelopment of the heart and lungs. Procedure 6-4 lists the steps for measuring head

PROCEDURE 6-4

MEASURING INFANT HEAD CIRCUMFERENCE

ABHES VII.MA.A.1 9(m)   CAAHEP I.P (10)

OBJECTIVE: To correctly measure circumference of an infant or child's head.

STANDARD: This task takes 1–2 minutes.

EQUIPMENT AND SUPPLIES: Disposable tape measure; examination table; patient's record; pen.

STEPS:

1. Perform hand hygiene.
2. Identify patient, and explain procedure to caregiver.
3. Talk to patient soothingly to gain trust.
4. Position infant on table, or have caregiver hold infant.
5. Hold end of tape (0) on forehead over patient's eyebrows (Figure 6-7).
6. Bring tape around head over ears, without pulling or twisting, to meet in front.
7. Take measurement to nearest fraction of inch or centimeter as per facility policy. Repeat if in doubt.

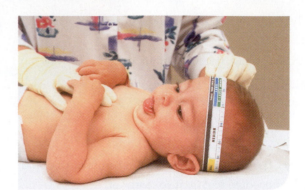

FIGURE 6-7 Measuring the head circumference of an infant.

8. Document results.
9. Perform hand hygiene.

CHARTING EXAMPLE: 05/25/XX 11:15 A.M. Well-child visit for 13-month-old. Head circumference 40 cm. · A. Rashid, RMA

---

circumference, and Procedure 6-5 lists the steps for performing measurement of chest circumference.

Growth and Development

The child is measured and weighed during each well-child visit, and measurements are plotted on growth chart, which becomes part of the child's permanent record. Head and chest circumference are measured up to age 3 years to provide parameters for monitoring growth patterns. Once measurement values are obtained, they are plotted on National Center for Health Statistics (NCHS) growth charts (www.cdc.gov/growthcharts). The value is plotted according to the child's age, and a percentile is determined. The percentile is then used to identify children with growth or nutritional abnormalities. The type of growth chart utilized depends on the physician and facility. Body mass index (BMI) also may be calculated for children over age 2 years. The same procedure is used. (See Procedure 3-18.)

PROCEDURE 6-5

MEASURING CIRCUMFERENCE OF CHILD'S CHEST

ABHES VII.MA.A.1 9(m)   CAAHEP I.P (10)

OBJECTIVE: To accurately measure child's chest circumference.

STANDARD: This task takes 1–2 minutes.

EQUIPMENT AND SUPPLIES: Disposable tape measure; examination table; patient's record; pen.

STEPS:

1. Perform hand hygiene.
2. Identify patient, and explain procedure to caregiver.
3. Talk soothingly to patient to gain trust.
4. Position infant on table in supine position. A child over 2 years old may sit on table for this procedure.
5. Place end of tape (0) in center of child's chest in line with child's nipples. Slip tape under child's body, and bring it to meet other end of tape. Take measurement in inches to nearest ½ inch (or in centimeters to nearest 0.01).
6. Place child in caregiver's care.
7. Record results.
8. Perform hand hygiene.

CHARTING EXAMPLE: 05/25/XX 11:15 A.M. Well-child visit for 13-month-old. Chest circumference: 18 inches. ········· ································· A. Rashid, RMA

The following are examples of types of growth charts available:

- **Girls: Birth to 36 months.** Length-for-age and weight-for-age percentiles
- **Girls: Birth to 36 months.** Head circumference-for-age and weight-for-length percentiles
- **Girls: 2 to 20 Years.** Stature-for-age and weight-for-age percentiles
- **Boys: Birth to 36 months.** Length-for-age and weight-for-age percentiles
- **Boys: Birth to 36 months.** Head-circumference-for-age and weight-for-length percentiles
- **Boys: 2–20 Years.** Stature-for-age and weight-for-age percentiles

Procedure 6-6 lists the steps to calculate growth percentiles using Birth to 36 Months: Girls/Length-for-Age and Weight-for-Age Percentiles chart.

Immunizations

Childhood immunizations are administered during well-child visits. Immunizations or vaccines are given to individuals to decrease their susceptibility to disease. Vaccines are produced by altering infectious agents to lessen their virulence and then injecting the vaccine into the body to encourage the production of antibodies. Children have underdeveloped immune systems during their first year; therefore, immunizations must be given several times during this period to ensure the development of antibodies to specific diseases. Some immunizations cause the child to develop slight fever or irritability and discomfort at the site of the immunization. Protocols of the physician, the facility, or both designate what steps parents should take to relieve postimmunization symptoms.

A recommended schedule of childhood and adolescent immunizations is issued each year by the American Academy of Pediatrics, the Advisory Committee on Immunization

PROCEDURE 6-6

CALCULATING GROWTH PERCENTILES

ABHES VII.MA.A.1 9(m)   CAAHEP I.P (10); II.P (3)

OBJECTIVE: To plot age, weight, and height of a patient and obtain correct percentiles.

STANDARD: This task takes 5 minutes or less.

EQUIPMENT AND SUPPLIES: Patient's record with weight and height values; pen; growth chart.

STEPS:

1. Select proper growth chart for patient. (See Figure 6-8 for an example.)
2. Locate child's age along horizontal axis at bottom of chart. Draw imaginary vertical line on chart.
3. Locate proper growth value (in this case, weight and height). Draw an imaginary horizontal line on chart.
4. Find point at which these two imaginary lines intersect on graph, and place a dot there.
5. Follow curved line closest to dot upward. Read percentile located on right side of chart.

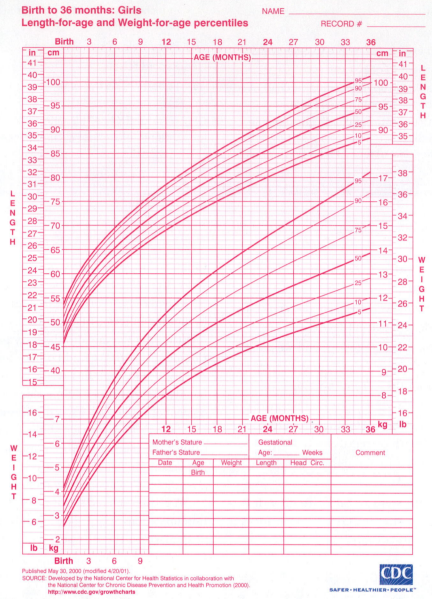

Birth to 36 months: Girls
Length-for-age and Weight-for-age percentiles

NAME _____

RECORD # _____

FIGURE 6-8   Calculating growth percentiles: Birth to 36 months: Girls/Length-for-age and Weight-for-age percentiles.

6. If dot falls between two curved lines, interpolate or estimate percentile that falls between two closest percentile lines.

NOTE: For example, if the dot you placed based on the correct age and weight were halfway between 10 and 25 percentile lines, the difference between 25 and 10 is 15, and half of 15 is 7.5. Therefore, the percentile would be 17.5. The child would weigh more than 17.5% of children of the same age do, which is below normal.

7. Record results in patient's chart.

CHARTING EXAMPLE: 05/25/XX Length 34¾ inches, 95th percentile. Wt. 31 lbs, 95th percentile. · · · · · · · · · · · · · · · · · · ·
· A. McGrath, CMA (AAMA)

Practices of the CDC, and the American Academy of Family Physicians. The schedule indicates recommended ages for immunization administration of childhood vaccines (Figure 6-9). The National Childhood Vaccine Injury Act (NCVIA) was enacted in 1988 and requires that parents be provided with information about the benefits and risks of childhood immunizations in lay terms. A set of vaccine information statements (VIS) was developed by the CDC to accompany each vaccine. The correct VIS statement should be provided to parents for each dose of each vaccine

7 Assisting with Therapeutic Modalities and Rehabilitation

PROCEDURES

Procedure 7-1 Performing and Instructing Range-of-Motion Exercises

Procedure 7-2 Applying a Hot Compress

Procedure 7-3 Performing a Hot Soak Procedure

Procedure 7-4 Applying a Heating Pad

Procedure 7-5 Applying a Cold Compress

Procedure 7-6 Applying an Ice Bag

Procedure 7-7 Applying a Cold Chemical Pack

Advanced Procedure 7-8 Administering an Ultrasound Treatment

Procedure 7-9 Instructing a Patient to Use a Cane Correctly

Procedure 7-10 Measuring a Patient for Axillary Crutches

Procedure 7-11 Instructing a Patient to Use Crutches Correctly

Procedure 7-12 Instruct a Patient on Correct Use of Walker

Procedure 7-13 Performing Patient Wheelchair Transfer to Chair or Examination Table

Procedure 7-14 Transferring Patient from Examination Table or Bed to Wheelchair

Procedure 7-15 Ambulating Patient with One Assistant

Procedure 7-16 Assisting the Falling Patient

Procedure 7-17 Assisting with Cast Application

Procedure 7-18 Assisting with Cast Removal

Procedure 7-19 Applying an Arm Sling

Procedure 7-20 Applying a Spiral Bandage

Procedure 7-21 Applying a Figure-Eight Bandage

Procedure 7-22 Applying a Cervical Collar

TERMS TO LEARN

rehabilitation

restoration

goniometer

Sitz baths

aquathermic pads

cryotherapy

gait belt

orthostatic hypotension

periosteum

Physical agents and assistive devices are employed to help individuals who have experienced disability due to injury or disease. Treatments are prescribed by physicians who specialize in physical medicine, including physiatrists and orthopedists, and other medical specialists. Physical therapists and occupational therapists treat patients as ordered by physicians. Means and methods of physical therapy include **rehabilitation** (the process of returning a patient as close as possible to the person's normal physical condition after injury or disease), **restoration** (to bring back to the former state), and prevention of disabilities. A physical therapist uses treatments including heat, cold, massage, exercise, traction, electricity, ultraviolet radiation, ultrasonic diathermy, hydrotherapy, hot paraffin, and instruction on the correct use of assistive devices such as canes, walkers, crutches, and artificial limbs or prostheses. In turn those licensed professionals may delegate certain duties to other health care workers. These procedures or tasks are described later in this chapter.

Range of Motion

Patients who have suffered temporary or permanent loss of mobility need assistance with and instruction on performing range-of-motion (ROM) exercises. These activities help maintain muscle tone and flexibility. Range of motion is the degree of movement in a specific joint that can occur without causing pain. It is measured with a special type of protractor, a **goniometer**.

Once the physician has made an assessment of the patient and recommended ROM exercises based on the patient's ability, the exercises fall into the following categories:

- **Active range of motion (AROM).** Patient able to move all limbs through entire ROM unassisted.
- **Passive range of motion (PROM).** Patient must have someone else move his or her limbs through ROM because he or she is unable to do it.
- **Active assist range of motion (AAROM).** Patient participates to a limited extent in ROM but requires some assistance.

Procedure 7-1 lists and illustrates the steps for performing passive ROM exercises on a patient.

Heat Therapies

The application of heat to a body part causes dilation of blood vessels and allows more blood to circulate to injured tissues. The increased circulation assists in providing the body with oxygen and nutrients necessary for repair and healing. Heat can also relieve pain and hasten pus formation. Moist

PROCEDURE 7-1

PERFORMING AND INSTRUCTING RANGE-OF-MOTION EXERCISES

ABHES VII.MA.A.1 2(c); VII.MA.A.1 9(r)   CAAHEP I.P (10); IV.P (5); I.A (2)

OBJECTIVE: To assist a patient to perform range-of-motion exercises.

STANDARD: This task takes 15–30, minutes depending on patient's condition.

EQUIPMENT AND SUPPLIES: Examination table or bed; drape; illustrations of range-of-motion exercises; patient's record; pen.

STEPS:

1. Perform hand hygiene.
2. Check physician's orders.
3. Explain procedure. Instruct caregiver to actively watch as you and patient perform exercises.
4. Position patient in supine position.
5. Provide draping as needed to ensure privacy.
6. Put all joints through ROM exercises starting at head (following sequence in Table 7-1 and Table 7-2).
7. Protect against detrimental movement, and watch patient for indications of discomfort. At any sign of discomfort, stop that particular exercise. Support limbs against gravity. Use a cradling support above and below joint while patient performs exercises.
8. As you proceed through each exercise, explain to caregiver what you are doing and, if possible, allow caregiver to demonstrate understanding. Answer questions posed by patient and caregiver as needed.
9. Encourage patient to participate as much as possible with each exercise, and offer words of encouragement.

TABLE 7-1 Performing Passive Range of Motion: Upper Body

Movement	Neck	Shoulder	Elbow	Forearm	Wrist	Finger & Thumb	Figures
Flexion	Move head forward 90° with chin on chest	Raise arm 180° from side to above head	Bend elbow so arm moves up toward shoulder		Bend hand 90° toward inner arm	Make a fist so fingers are all bent inward	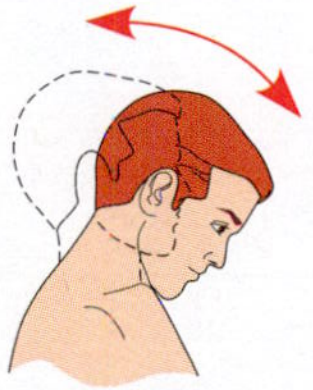
Extension	Move head up from chest 90° to erect position	Move arm to side of body	Straighten elbow and return to position		Move hand pointed straight out	Move fingers 90° to straight position	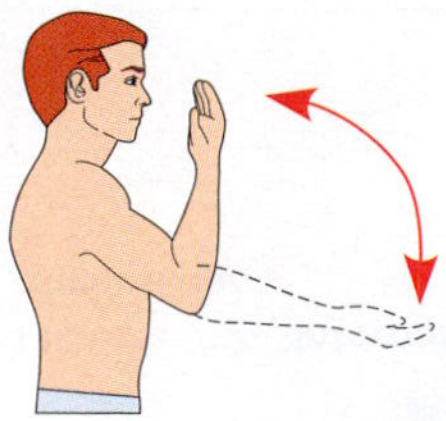 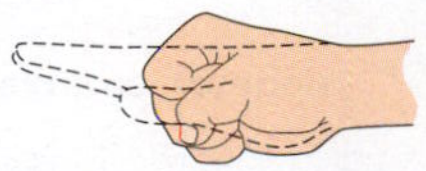
Hyper-extension	Move head backward 90°	Move arm to back of body at 50° angle			Bend hand up and back 90° toward arm	Move fingers up toward back of hand	
Abduction		Hold arm away from side 180° to above head			Bend wrist out and away from arm	Spread fingers as much as possible	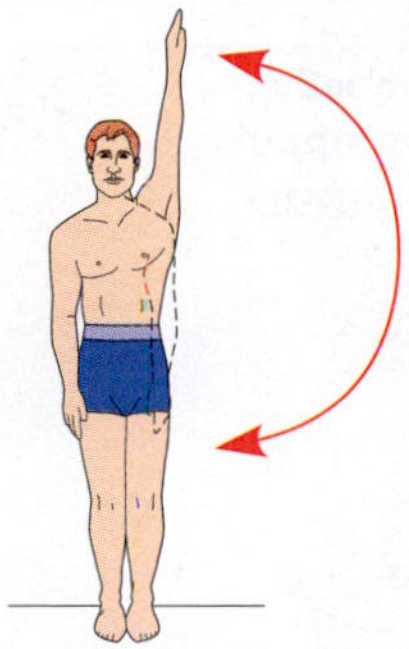

FIGURE 7-1 Flexion (movement 90° toward chest) and extension (movement up 90° from chest) of head.

FIGURE 7-2 Flexion and extension of elbow.

FIGURE 7-3 Flexion and extension of finger joints.

FIGURE 7-4 Abduction of shoulder.

(continued)

TABLE 7-1 (continued)

Movement	Neck	Shoulder	Elbow	Forearm	Wrist	Finger & Thumb	Figures
Adduction		Move arm from side and across chest			Bend wrist inward toward radius	Move fingers and thumb together	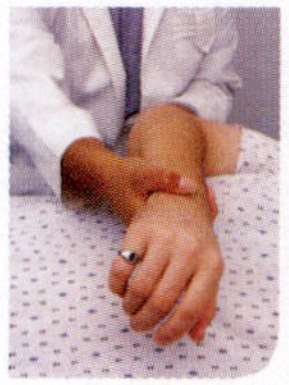 FIGURE 7-5 Adduction of shoulder. 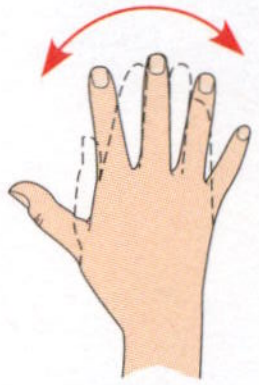 FIGURE 7-6 Adduction–abduction finger exercises.
External Rotation		Hold arm out to side with elbow bent 45°; move forward so palm faces forward					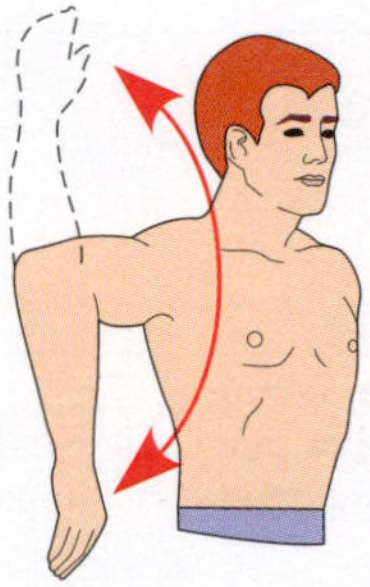
Internal Rotation		Move arm to side at shoulder level with elbow bent 45°; lower arm so palm faces back					FIGURE 7-7 Internal and external rotation of shoulder.
Rotation	Move head in circular motion 90° left, then 90° right						
Circumduction		Move arm in full circle					
Supination				Rotate forearm 90° so palm is up			
Pronation				Rotate forearm 90° so palm is down			

TABLE 7-2 Performing Passive Range of Motion: Lower Body

Movement	Trunk	Hip	Knee	Ankle	Toe	Figures
Flexion	Bend forward 90°	Move leg forward and up 90°	Bend knee 90°; foot moves back and up		Point down 90°	FIGURE 7-8 Flexion of hip and knee.
Extension	Stand in straight position	Move leg in straight alignment with trunk	Move foot 90° with knee straight and leg in line with body		Straight out from foot	
Hyper-extension	Bend backward 30°	Move leg backward 50°			Point up to 45°	
Lateral flexion	Bend to both sides 45°					
Internal Rotation		Turn leg and foot inward 90°				
External Rotation		Turn leg and foot outward 90°				
Circum-duction		Move leg in circle 360°				
Abduction		Move leg away from body 45°			Spread apart 15°	FIGURE 7-9 Abduction of leg (movement away from midline of body).
Adduction		Move leg toward body 45°			Bring together in normal position	FIGURE 7-10 Adduction of leg (movement toward midline of body).

(continued)

TABLE 7-2 (*continued*)

Movement	Trunk	Hip	Knee	Ankle	Toe	Figures
Plantar flexion				Point toes downward		FIGURE 7-11 Plantar flexion (movement of foot or toes down and away from leg).
Dorsiflexion				Point toes upward		FIGURE 7-12 Dorsiflexion (movement up and toward leg) of toes.
Rotation	Move in circle 360° from waist	Move leg 90° from hip				
Eversion				Move sole of foot lateral to outside		
Inversion				Move sole of foot medial to inside		

10. After exercises are completed, provide time for caregiver to revisit any exercise for review.
11. Make patient comfortable.
12. Perform hand hygiene.
13. Document patient's record.

CHARTING EXAMPLE: 06/01/XX 4:00 P.M. ROM exercises performed and instruction provided to pt's. husband. Handout sheet containing ROM to be done 2×/day for 1 wk. 5 reps each exercise per Dr. Allen. Pt. tolerated ROM well. · · · · · · · · ·
· E. Corso, RMA

heat application uses heated water, as in a tub or on a wet compress, **Sitz baths**, tub baths, warm soaks, hydrotherapy or whirlpool, and paraffin treatments. Dry heat treatments (heat without water) include heating pad, infrared radiation (heat lamps), hot water bottles, **aquathermic pads**, and chemical hot packs. Procedures for applying a hot compress, hot soaks, heating pads, and aquathermic pads follow.

APPLYING HOT SOAKS

Hot soaks involve having the patient put the affected part of the body into a container of water with or without medication for 15 to 20 minutes. The water temperature should be no more than 110°F (44°C). Procedure 7-3 provides the steps for hot soak application.

PROCEDURE 7-2

APPLYING A HOT COMPRESS

ABHES VII.MA.A.1 2(c); VII.MA.A.1 9(r)   CAAHEP I.P (10); IV.P (5)

OBJECTIVE: To apply a hot compress according to physician's orders and document correctly.

STANDARD: This task takes 15–20 minutes.

EQUIPMENT AND SUPPLIES: Soaking solution (or water) as ordered by physician; PPE; basin; bath thermometer; absorbent cloths such as washcloths or gauze squares; waterproof cover such as plastic wrap; patient's record; pen; watch or timer.

STEPS:

1. Check the patient's record for physician's orders.
2. Perform hand hygiene.
3. Assemble the equipment. If an open wound is present, use sterile equipment, Standard Precautions, and PPE.
4. Identify patient, and explain procedure.
5. Fill basin half full of water or medicated solution prepared according to order.
6. Ask patient to remove any clothing necessary to expose area to be treated. Assist as needed.
7. Check temperature of solution with bath thermometer. Temperature range for an adult is between 105°F and 110°F (41°C and 44°C).
8. Place patient in a comfortable, well-supported position.
9. Place cloths in basin of heated solution. Wring out one cloth at a time so it is damp but not dripping. Gradually place compress on patient's body part (Figure 7-13). Ask patient if temperature is tolerable (should be hot but not uncomfortable).
10. Cover compress with waterproof covering to retain heat.
11. Repeat application every 2–3 minutes for length of time ordered.
12. Frequently check temperature of solution, removing cooled solution and replacing it with hot solution. Check temperature.

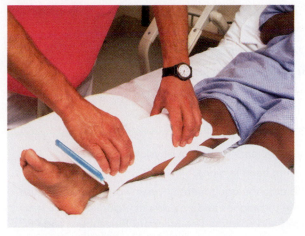

FIGURE 7-13   Applying a hot compress to a patient's leg.

13. Check patient for localized signs of redness, swelling, or pain.
14. When time for hot compress is completed, dry affected body part.
15. Provide instruction for home care, both written and by demonstration.
16. Clean area and care for equipment. (If an open wound was present, handle soiled linens according to Standard Precautions.)
17. Perform hand hygiene.
18. Document patient's record.

CHARTING EXAMPLE: 06/08/XX 10:00 A.M. Hot compress at 105°F applied to right shin for 20 min. Redness of skin noted after application. Pt. stated "some pain relief." Instruction, written and verbal, for home application of hot compress given. Verified understanding. · C. Lynch, RMA

APPLYING HEATING PAD OR AQUATHERMIC PAD

Heating and aquathermic pads are dry heat applications. Electric heating pads, like those used at home, are flat, covered electrical pads that are used to provide dial-controlled and localized heat. Skin must be protected by a towel from direct contact with heating devices, unless otherwise ordered.

Patients should be warned to avoid burns by never lying on heating pads. Aquathermic pads are filled with water and used in the same way as the previously mentioned electric heating pads. To avoid piercing pad elements and causing electric shocks, safety pins must not be used to hold either type of pad in place. Procedure 7-4 lists the steps for application of a heating pad.

PERFORMING A HOT SOAK PROCEDURE

ABHES VII.MA.A.1 2(c); VII.MA.A.1 9(r)   CAAHEP I.P (10); IV.P (5)

OBJECTIVE: To perform and document a hot soak procedure and document procedure correctly.

STANDARD: This task takes 15–20 minutes.

EQUIPMENT AND SUPPLIES: Soaking solution or water as ordered by physician; PPE; basin or tub; pitcher; bath thermometer; patient's record; pen.

STEPS:

1. Check patient's record for physician's orders.
2. Perform hand hygiene.
3. Assemble the equipment. If open wound is present use sterile techniques and equipment including sterile basin, towels and solution. Use Standard Precautions and PPE.
4. Identify patient, and explain procedure.
5. Ask patient to remove any obstructing clothing. Soaking involves placing affected area into soaking solution.
6. Check temperature of solution with bath thermometer. (Temperature range for an adult is between 105°F and 110°F [41°C and 44°C].)
7. Position patient in comfortable well-supported position.
8. Pad side of basin or tub with towel to prevent patient's body from rubbing on edge.
9. Gradually immerse patient's body part (Figure 7-14) into solution. Ask patient if temperature is tolerable.
10. Frequently test temperature of solution. Using a pitcher, remove some liquid every 5 minutes and replace with hot water or designated solution. Pour hot solution near edge of basin or tub while protecting patient's body part with your hand. Swirl water while pouring to mix hot and cool fluid together.
11. Time procedure according to physician's orders. Check patient periodically for any signs of pain, swelling, and redness.
12. Gently dry affected body part.
13. Instruct patient on any aftercare, such as further soaks at home. Provide both written and verbal instructions and verify understanding.

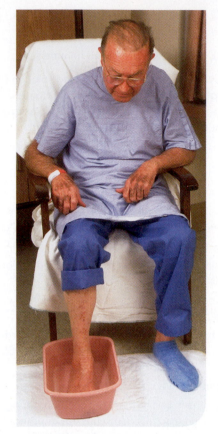

FIGURE 7-14 **Place a basin where the patient can easily dip a foot into the water for a hot soak.**

14. Place towels in laundry. If open wound is present, handle items according to Standard Precautions.
15. Clean equipment and examining room.
16. Perform hand hygiene.
17. Document procedure in patient's record,

CHARTING EXAMPLE: 06/08/XX 5:00 P.M. Hot soak at 105°F applied to right foot for 20 minutes. Skin sl. pink after soak. Pt. tolerated procedure well. Instruction, written and verbal, provided with understanding verified. · · · · · · · · · · L. Lynch, RMA

Cold Therapies

Cold applications result in constriction of blood vessels, which is the opposite effect of warm applications. Constriction of blood vessels helps to reduce swelling, as in cases of ankle sprain. In addition, cold reduces pain and helps control bleeding. **Cryotherapy** is the practice of using cold for therapeutic purposes. Cold applications may be applied to a body part or to the entire body to reduce an elevated body

APPLYING A HEATING PAD

ABHES VII.MA.A.1 2(c); VII.MA.A.1 9(r)   CAAHEP I.P (10); IV.P (5)

OBJECTIVE: To apply heating pad per physician's orders and document procedure.

STANDARD: This task takes 15–20 minutes, based on physician's order.

EQUIPMENT AND SUPPLIES: Heating pad or aquathermic pad with protective covering; PPE; patient's record; pen; watch.

STEPS:

1. Check physician's orders.
2. Perform hand hygiene.
3. Assemble equipment, and check for safety factors such as leaks in aquathermic pads and frayed cords.
4. Identify patient, and explain procedure. Instruct patient about safety issues: protecting skin by applying towel below heating device, not using safety pins to secure pad, not lying on pad, and so on.

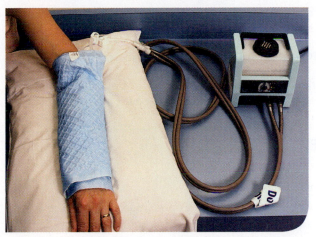

FIGURE 7-15 Aquathermic pad and heating unit provide dry heat treatment to a patient's arm.

> **Safety Alert!** Remind patients not to lie on a heat source because it may cause burns to tissues in the area.

- Aquathermic pad (Figure 7-15) is filled prior to use with distilled water. The pad is connected to pump hoses (male, female fittings) and the reservoir is filled 2/3 full with room temperature distilled water. Pump should be placed above level of pad to avoid having water drain back into pump when shut off. Set key on reservoir to temperature as ordered. Remove key to avoid temperature being changed. Plug pump into grounded wall outlet.
- Aquathermic pad is applied with its coiled surface over patient's extremity or over moist pad on area to be treated.
- If open wound exists, use sterile technique, PPE, and cover wound with sterile gauze.

5. Place heating pad in protective cover or pillowcase as needed.

6. Connect heating pad to wall plug and select temperature setting. Place heating pad over affected area. Protect skin by placing a towel below heating pad. Secure with tape if necessary. Ask patient if temperature is comfortable and not too hot.
7. Remind patient not to change setting and to notify you if temperature is uncomfortable.
8. Leave heating pad in place for length of time ordered by physician.
9. Remove heating pad when indicated time is reached. Instruct patient on aftercare and home application of heat by providing written and verbal instruction. Confirm understanding of instructions.
10. Place pad covering in laundry, and return equipment to designated place.
11. Perform hand hygiene.
12. Document procedure in patient's record.

CHARTING EXAMPLE: 06/08/XX 4:00 P.M. Heating pad on medium setting applied to (L) elbow for 20 min. Pt. states "some pain relief and increased movement" in elbow joint.
· E. Lenhardt, CMA (AAMA)

---

temperature, as with hypothermia blankets. Other examples of cold applications include cold compresses, ice bags, cold soaks, and chemical packs. The procedures for use of cold compresses, ice bags, and chemical packs follow.

Ultrasound Therapy

Ultrasound therapy uses sound energy from high-frequency sound waves that penetrate deeply through tissue layers.

PROCEDURE 7-5

APPLYING A COLD COMPRESS

ABHES VII.MA.A.1 2(c); VII.MA.A.1 9(r)   CAAHEP I.P (10); IV.P (5)

OBJECTIVE: To apply cold compress as ordered by physician and document correctly.

STANDARD: This task takes 15–20 minutes.

EQUIPMENT AND SUPPLIES: Water; absorbent cloths or gauze squares; waterproof cover or plastic wraps; basin; ice; patient's record; pen; watch.

STEPS:

1. Check physician's orders.
2. Perform hand hygiene.
3. Assemble equipment. If open wound present, use sterile equipment and Standard Precautions.
4. Identify patient, and explain procedure.
5. Fill basin half full of cold water. Add ice cubes and compresses.
6. Wring out compress until it is wet but not dripping. Gently place compress on patient's affected body part. Ask patient if comfortable with application. Wrap compress with plastic or waterproof covering to prevent dripping.

> **Safety Alert!** Keep in mind that skin sensations may be decreased; thus careful monitoring is essential.

7. Check compress every 3 to 5 minutes, and replace with another cold compress. Add ice as needed as water becomes warm.
8. Leave compress in place for time specified (usually 15–20 minutes).
9. Gently dry affected body part. Instruct patient, using written and verbal instruction, on home care. Verify understanding of instructions.
10. Place linens in proper container. Clean all equipment.
11. Perform hand hygiene.
12. Document procedure in patient's record.

CHARTING EXAMPLE: 06/08/XX 11:00 A.M. Cold compresses applied to R ankle for 20 minutes. Erythema noted over application site. Instruction provided, written and verbal, on home application. Understanding verified. · B. Smith, CMA (AAMA)

PROCEDURE 7-6

APPLYING AN ICE BAG

ABHES VII.MA.A.1 2(c); VII.MA.A.1 9(r)   CAAHEP I.P (10); IV.P (5)

OBJECTIVE: To apply an ice bag as ordered by physician and document correctly.

STANDARD: This task takes 15–20 minutes.

EQUIPMENT AND SUPPLIES: Ice bag with protective cover or small hand towel; ice chips or crushed ice; patient's record; pen; watch.

STEPS:

1. Check physician's orders.
2. Perform hand hygiene.
3. Identify patient, and explain procedure.
4. Fill ice bag with ice ½ to ⅔ full (Figure 7-16A). Expel air by squeezing empty half of bag (Figure 7-16B). Replace cap (Figure 7-16C).
5. Dry bag, then place in protective covering or wrap in small hand towel (Figure 7-16D).
6. Gently place ice bag on affected body part and ask for patient feedback on comfort level.
7. Refill bag with ice as needed.
8. Leave ice bag in place for specified time (usually 15–20

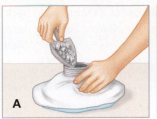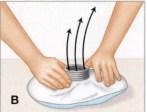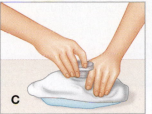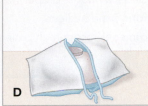

FIGURE 7-16 (A) Preparing an ice bag; (B) press on the ice bag after ice is added to remove air; (C) recap ice bag after removing air; (D) cover the ice bag with protective covering before placing on patient.

minutes) as ordered by physician. Check patient periodically for comfort level.

9. Clean equipment. Allow bag to air-dry.

10. Perform hand hygiene.

11. Document procedure in patient's record.

CHARTING EXAMPLE: 06/08/XX 9:00 A.M. Ice bags applied on right forehead. Swelling reduced some after 20 minutes. Erythema noted in treatment area. Pt. instructed on home application and verified verbally understanding. · · · · · · · · · · · ·
· J. Caruso, RMA

PROCEDURE 7-7

APPLYING A COLD CHEMICAL PACK

ABHES VII.MA.A.1 2(c)   CAAHEP I.P (10)

OBJECTIVE: To apply cold chemical pack per physician's orders and document correctly.

STANDARD: This task takes 15–20 minutes.

EQUIPMENT AND SUPPLIES: Cold chemical pack; soft cloth or small towel; patient's record; pen; watch.

STEPS:

1. Check physician's orders.
2. Perform hand hygiene.
3. Assemble equipment (Figure 7-17).

NOTE: Commercial chemical packs, both hot and cold, are available in a variety of sizes and shapes. Once activated they are good for 30 to 60 minutes, depending on type. They are disposable and should be stored at room temperature before use.

4. Identify patient, and explain procedure.
5. Agitate bag to allow crystals to fall to bottom. Compress pack until inner bag ruptures. Shake again to mix contents. The chemical bag immediately should feel cold and should remain cold for about 30 minutes.

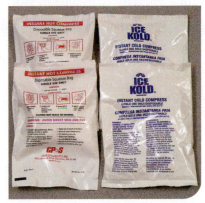

FIGURE 7-17 Examples of disposable hot and cold packs before activation.

6. Wrap bag in soft cloth or small towel.
7. Place cloth-protected bag over patient's affected body part.
8. Check patient every 3 to 5 minutes.
9. Leave cold pack in place for time specified by physician (usually 15–20 minutes).

10. Discard ice pack in proper waste container after use.

11. Perform hand hygiene.

12. Document procedure in patient's record.

Ultrasound waves vibrate at the rate of one million times per second; they cannot be heard by the human ear but produce a mechanical and heating effect. This mechanical effect works on connective tissue, such as ligaments and tendons. The heat effect works on all body tissues. Ultrasound should be used carefully and not near bony tissues to avoid causing injury from concentration of waves.

Ultrasound treatments are used to treat pain, relax muscle spasms, stimulate circulation in patients with vascular disorders, and break up calcium deposits and scar tissue. Ultrasound is administered via a machine with an applicator head containing a quartz crystal that vibrates rapidly when an electric current passes through it. Since these waves do not travel through air, they must be used in contact with a coupling gel or oil placed on the skin to aid conduction. Treatments are applied for 10 minutes or less, according to physician's orders.

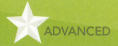 ADVANCED

PROCEDURE 7-8

ADMINISTERING AN ULTRASOUND TREATMENT

ABHES VII.MA.A.1 2(c); VII.MA.A.1 9(r)   CAAHEP IV.P (5); IV.A (7); I.A (2)

OBJECTIVE: To administer an ultrasound treatment per physician's orders and document correctly.

STANDARD: This task takes 10 minutes or less.

EQUIPMENT AND SUPPLIES: Ultrasound machine; coupling gel; tissues; patient's record; pen; watch.

STEPS:

1. Check physician's orders.

2. Perform hand hygiene.

3. Assemble equipment.

4. Identify patient, and explain procedure, noting that no discomfort or pain should be felt from the treatment. Pain or discomfort indicates that the intensity is set too high.

5. Ask patient to disrobe and expose area of treatment. Provide privacy and assistance as needed. Drape appropriately.

6. Apply room-temperature coupling agent to treatment area with head of ultrasound applicator. Cover area of treatment completely and evenly.

7. Turn on machine. Set ultrasound intensity level to minimum position and set timer for prescribed time of treatment per physician's orders.

8. Increase intensity level (watts) to prescribed level. Holding applicator head at right angle to coupling agent on body surface, press firmly and begin to move head either in circular motion for small areas or in back-and-forth motion for larger areas.

9. Use short strokes approximately 1 inch in diameter or length at the rate of 1 to 2 inches per second. Gradually overlap previous strokes by about ½ inch.

10. Do not remove applicator head from patient's skin until treatment is completed. Overheating of head will result if it is held too long in one spot or is held in the air.

11. Stop treatment immediately if patient complains of discomfort or pain, and notify physician.

12. Machine will automatically shut off when set time has ended. Remove applicator head from patient's skin.

13. Wipe excess coupling agent off with tissues or paper towels.

14. Ask patient to don clothes, and assist as needed.

15. Clean treatment area.

16. Perform hand hygiene.

17. Document procedure in patient's record.

Adaptive Equipment and Devices

Adaptive equipment (e.g., walkers, crutches, canes) and special furniture (e.g., shower chairs or geriatric chairs) are used to assist recovery from physical disorders and disabilities. Mobility aids (e.g., casts, braces, prostheses) and adaptive equipment (e.g., eating utensils, special toothbrushes, reaching sticks) help individuals with disabilities perform activities of daily living (ADL). (See Figure 7-18 for examples of assistive devices.) Procedures for instructing a patient to use a cane or single crutch, instructing a patient to use crutches, and instructing a patient to use a walker follow.

CANES

Canes are used by patients who have muscle or bone weakness on one side or need assistance with balance. Two common types of canes are shown in Figure 7-19. Four-point canes provide the most stability. The correct height for a cane is determined when the patient is standing tall: the hand grip of the cane should then be level with the hip joint, and the elbow should be flexed at a 25- to 30-degree angle. The handle must fit the patient's hand comfortably.

A **gait belt** is sometimes used when assisting a patient using a cane. The device is worn around a patient's waist and helps caregivers to transfer people from one position to another or from one thing to another. The gait belt is customarily made of cotton webbing with a durable metal buckle on one end.

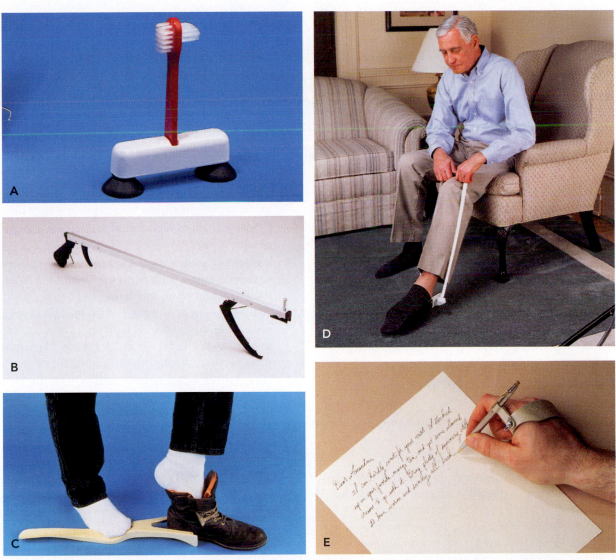

FIGURE 7-18 (A) Adaptive device: toothbrush; (B) adaptive device: reaching stick; (C) adaptive device: shoe holder; (D) adaptive device: stocking helper; (E) adaptive device: writing aid.

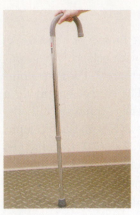 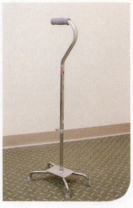

FIGURE 7-19 Two types of canes.

CRUTCHES

Crutches allow the patient to walk without putting weight on the affected leg. Weight is transferred to the arm and hands. Crutches are made of metal or wood and should have rubber tips to prevent slipping on a smooth floor surface. The following are the three most common types of crutches:

- **Axillary crutch.** Reach from ground to axilla with padded shoulders and hand rests. Used for stronger patients on short-term basis. Weight borne on hands, not under axilla. Should be fitted correctly based on patient's height. (Measurements for axillary crutches must be taken carefully to prevent pressure damage to the brachial plexus, comprised of the nerves running under the axilla and down the arm.)
- **Forearm or Lofstrand crutch.** A single aluminum tube with an arm cuff that fits snugly around the patient's forearm and has a hand grip for weight bearing. Used for patients with good upper body strength and coordination who need long-term use of an assistive device.

PROCEDURE 7-9

INSTRUCTING A PATIENT TO USE A CANE CORRECTLY

ABHES VII.MA.A.1 9(r); VII.MA.A.1 8(cc)   CAAHEP IV.P (5); IV.A (7); I.A (2)

OBJECTIVE: To instruct and assist the patient to use a cane correctly.

STANDARD: This task takes about 15 minutes, depending on patient's condition.

EQUIPMENT AND SUPPLIES: Cane suited to patient's needs, gait belt, patient's record, pen.

STEPS:

1. Assemble equipment according to physician's order.
2. Check height of cane and condition of cane tip.
3. Identify patient, and explain procedure.
4. Perform hand hygiene.
5. Check to see that patient is wearing sturdy nonskid shoes.
6. Demonstrate correct position.
7. Demonstrate gait.
8. Instruct patient to hold cane on side opposite affected limb (adjacent to strong leg). As affected leg moves forward, cane will move forward to provide support.
9. Place cane 6 inches in front of and slightly to side of strong leg. Make sure cane tip is firmly on floor and weight is supported on strong leg and cane. Patient's elbow should be slightly flexed during weight bearing.
10. Instruct patient to look straight ahead, not down at ground or feet.
11. Instruct patient to move cane forward 6 to 12 inches and to bring affected leg forward even with cane. Weight should be placed on strong foot and leg.
12. Instruct patient to move strong leg forward past cane and weaker leg. As unaffected foot moves forward, weight shifts to weak or affected foot and cane. Thus, cane provides support for weight bearing on affected leg.
13. Have patient repeat walking pattern. Evaluate his or her balance and endurance. Correct as needed until both you and patient feel comfortable with level of ability.
14. Perform hand hygiene.
15. Document procedure in patient's record.

CHARTING EXAMPLE: 06/09/XX 9:00 A.M. Four-point cane adjusted to patient's hip joint. Pt. ambulated 75 yds. Slightly fatigued. Repeated after 5 min. rest for another 25 yds. · L. Fox, CMA (AAMA)

- **Platform crutch**—Used for patients who cannot grip handles or bear weight on wrists and hands. Includes a platform and attached hand grip so patient places entire forearm on platform with hand in hand grip with weight borne on the forearm.

Patients use several types of gaits to ambulate with crutches. The type of crutch and gait are determined and ordered by the physician. Box 7-1 indicates and illustrates types of gaits. Table 7-3 offers home safety suggestions for patients using crutches, canes, and walkers. Procedures for

BOX 7-1 Types of Crutch Walking Gaits

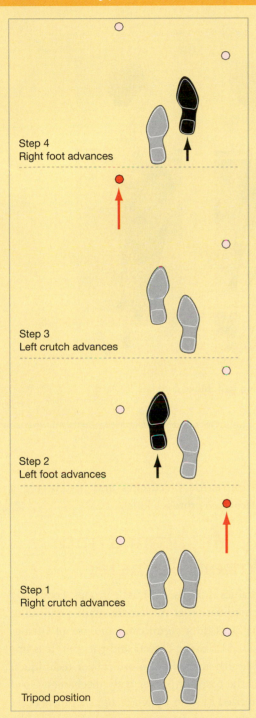

Step 4
Right foot advances

Step 3
Left crutch advances

Step 2
Left foot advances

Step 1
Right crutch advances

Tripod position

FIGURE 7-20   Four-point gait.

Four-Point Gait.   Safest gait when patient can bear some weight on both legs (Figure 7-20).
- Right crutch moved forward followed by left foot
- Then left crutch moved forward followed by right foot

Three-Point Gait.   Used when one leg is stronger than the other or no weight is borne on one of the legs (Figure 7-21).
- Both crutches and affected leg move forward
- Balance weight on both crutches and move stronger leg forward

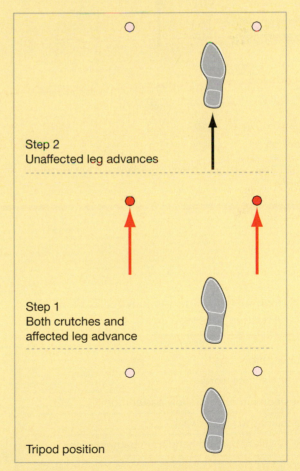

Step 2
Unaffected leg advances

Step 1
Both crutches and
affected leg advance

Tripod position

FIGURE 7-21   **Three-point gait. Both crutches and affected leg move forward.**

Two-Point Gait. Faster-moving gait. Some weight is borne on both feet for good balance (Figure 7-22).
- Right crutch and left foot moved forward together
- Then left crutch and right foot moved forward together

Swing Gait. Used by patients with severe leg disabilities. Both legs swing forward together (Figure 7-23).
- Crutches move forward
- Legs swing to or past crutches/faster movement

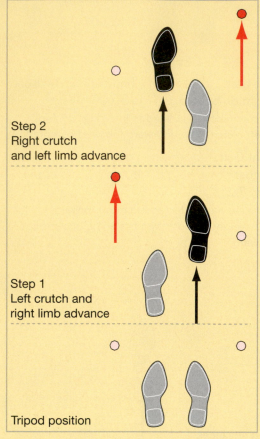

Step 2
Right crutch
and left limb advance

Step 1
Left crutch and
right limb advance

Tripod position

FIGURE 7-22 Two-point gait. Move right foot and left crutch simultaneously.

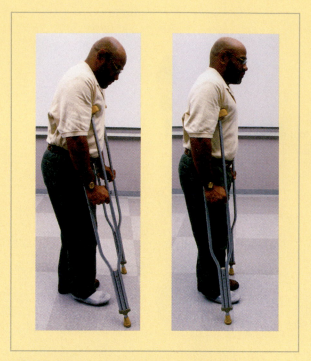

FIGURE 7-23 Swing gait. Move crutches forward.

TABLE 7-3 Home Safety Suggestions for Patients Using Assistive Devices.

1. Remove throw rugs.
2. Secure electrical cords.
3. Reposition furniture to allow easier mobility.
4. Add railings to all stairways.
5. Provide safety bar and handles in bathing area.
6. Keep floors clear of obstacles, such as toys and stacks of books or newspapers.

correctly measuring axillary crutches and instructing a patient to ambulate with crutches follow.

Body Mechanics and Patient Transfer

Proper body mechanics is the use of muscle groups, good body alignment, and coordination of movement while performing daily tasks. Caregivers do a significant amount of lifting, bending, carrying, and moving objects and patients. It is important for their health and safety to use proper techniques. Correct posture is the basis for proper body mechanics. Good posture is characterized by chin up, chest up, shoulders back, pelvis tilted slightly inward, feet straight and about shoulder

PROCEDURE 7-10

MEASURING A PATIENT FOR AXILLARY CRUTCHES

ABHES VII.MA.A.1 9(m)   CAAHEP I.P (10)

OBJECTIVE: To accurately measure and fit a patient for axillary crutches.

STANDARD: This task takes 10 minutes.

EQUIPMENT AND SUPPLIES: Axillary crutches with tips; pads for the axillae; hand rests; tools to loosen/tighten bolts; patient's record; pen.

STEPS:

1. Check physician's orders.
2. Perform hand hygiene.
3. Assemble proper size crutch for patient. (Children should have pediatric crutches.)
4. Identify patient, and explain procedure.
5. Check patient's shoes for low heels and nonskid soles.
6. Have patient stand erect, holding crutches with tips 2 inches in front and 4 to 6 inches to sides of feet.

NOTE: This position is used to begin all crutch gaits and is known as the tripod position (Figure 7-24).

7. Adjust central support in base so that, when held upright, axillary pad is two fingers' breadth below axillae (Figure 7-25).
8. Tighten bolts at proper height, and test for safety.

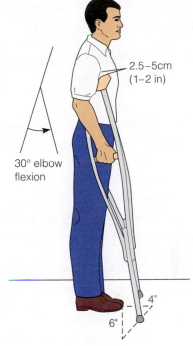

FIGURE 7-25 **Two fingers' width from axilla to crutch pad is the correct measurement for fitting axillary crutches.**

Labels on figure: 2.5–5cm (1–2 in); 30° elbow flexion; 4"; 6"

9. Adjust hand grips by raising or lowering bar. Patient's elbow should be at 30° angle when hand is on bar. Tighten bolts and test for safety.
10. Have patient stand erect with crutches in tripod position, and recheck both crutches. Place two fingers beneath each axilla and check angle of hand. Recheck bolts.
11. If extra padding is required, tape gauze squares to axillary or hand grips as needed.
12. Perform hand hygiene
13. Document procedure in patient's record.

CHARTING EXAMPLE: 06/10/XX 1:00 P.M. Pt. fitted with axillary crutches. No pressure on axillae, elbows at 30° angles. Instruction on crutch safety given in writing and verbally. Pt. able to walk with crutches safely 25 ft. · · · · · · · · · · · · ·
· S. Cohen, CMA (AAMA)

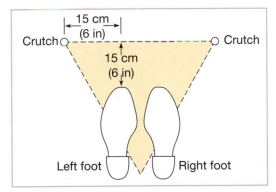

Labels on figure: 15 cm (6 in); Crutch; Crutch; 15 cm (6 in); Left foot; Right foot

FIGURE 7-24 **Tripod crutch stance for balance in crutch walking.**

PROCEDURE 7-11

INSTRUCTING A PATIENT TO USE CRUTCHES CORRECTLY

ABHES VII.MA.A.1 9(r); VII.MA.A.1 8(cc)   CAAHEP IV.P (5); IV.A (7); I.A (2)

OBJECTIVE: To teach a patient to use crutches correctly.

STANDARD: This task takes 15–20 minutes.

EQUIPMENT AND SUPPLIES: Crutches per order of physician; gait belt; patient's record; pen.

STEPS:

1. Assemble equipment ordered by physician.
2. Check crutches to determine they are in good working condition.
3. Perform hand hygiene.
4. Identify patient, and explain procedure.
5. Check to see if patient is wearing sturdy nonskid shoes.
6. Demonstrate correct position and gait ordered by physician.
7. Have patient stand against wall or near chair for support.
8. Adjust crutch length to appropriate height as in Procedure 7-10. Check for two finger breadths' space under axillae.
9. Instruct patient to keep head up and stand erect with abdomen in, feet straight, and knees slightly bent (5 degrees). Remind patient to look ahead for obstacles, not at feet.
10. Instruct to support weight with hands, not underarms.
11. Have patient practice standing still while maintaining balance on hands. Remind patient that resting body weight on axillary bars for more than 1 to 2 minutes could cause injury to brachial plexus.
12. Ask patient to assume basic crutch tripod position (Figure 7-24).
13. Instruct patient to take small steps (about 9 to 12 inches forward) to prevent crutches from slipping.
14. Have patient practice an orderly gait (Box 7-1 explains various gaits and includes diagrams), and correct as needed.
    - **Four-Point Gait.** Move right crutch, then left foot; move left crutch, then right foot.
    - **Three-Point Gait.** Two crutches support weaker extremity. Balance weight on crutches. Move both crutches and affected leg forward. Move unaffected leg forward.
    - **Two-Point Gait.** Advance right foot and left crutch simultaneously, then left foot and right crutch.
    - **Swing Gait.** Move both crutches forward. *Swing-to-gait:* Lift and swing body to crutches. *Swing-through-gait:* Lift and swing body past crutches; bring crutches in front of body; and repeat.
15. Remind patient to report any numbness or tingling in arms. Explain that hands and underarms should feel comfortable and that you can add more padding if needed. Remind patient to recheck bolts to maintain tightness and to check rubber tips for cracks. (Tips can be replaced if needed.)
16. Once patient is comfortable with performing designated gait, have patient practice going up and down stairs. Secure gait belt around patient's waist, tucking in ends securely under belt.

    Down Stairs (Figure 7-26A):
    - Start with weight on uninjured leg and crutches on same level.
    - Put crutches on first step.
    - Put weight on crutch handles and transfer stronger leg to step where crutches are located.
    - Repeat until patient understands procedure and performs it comfortably.

    Up stairs (Figure 7-26B):
    - Start with crutches and unaffected extremity on same level.
    - Put weight on crutch handles and lift stronger leg onto first step of stairs.
    - Put weight on unaffected extremity, and lift other extremity and crutches to step.
    - Repeat until patient understands and is comfortable performing procedure.
    - Once you and patient feel comfortable with instruction and confident that patient can manage crutches safely, patient may leave. Provide written instructions for home use.
17. Perform hand hygiene.
18. Document procedure in patient's record.

CHARTING EXAMPLE: 06/10/XX Crutches adjusted for patient. Pt. instructed on use of crutches. Demonstrated three-point gait with no weight on right leg. Practiced 10 min. written instructions given to pt. Pt. verbalized understanding. · A. Kim, RMA

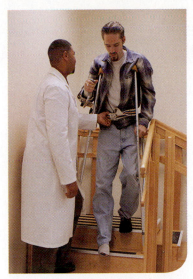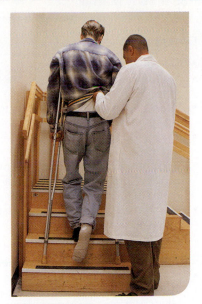

FIGURE 7-26 (A) Teaching ambulation on stairs. Put crutches on first stair, place weight on crutch handles, transfer unaffected leg to stair with crutches, then repeat; (B) starting with crutches and legs on same level, put weight on crutch handles and lift unaffected leg onto first stair. Put weight on stronger leg, then lift crutches and other leg to same stair. Repeat.

PROCEDURE 7-12

INSTRUCT A PATIENT ON CORRECT USE OF WALKER

ABHES VII.MA.A.1 9(r); VII.MA.A.1 8(cc)   CAAHEP IV.P (5); IV.A (7); I.A (2)

OBJECTIVE: To instruct patient to correctly use a walker and document properly.

STANDARD: This task takes 15–20 minutes.

EQUIPMENT AND SUPPLIES: Walker as ordered by physician; gait belt; patient's record; pen.

STEPS:

1. Assemble equipment according to physician's order.
2. Check condition of walker.
3. Perform hand hygiene.
4. Identify patient, and explain procedure.
5. Check to see if patient is wearing sturdy nonskid shoes.
6. Demonstrate correct stance and gait with walker.
7. Answer any questions patient or caregiver may have.
8. Evaluate walker for proper height and fit. (Top of walker should reach patient's hip bone; patient's hands should be on handgrip with elbow flexed at 30° angle).
9. Instruct patient to distribute weight evenly between walker and both legs.
10. Instruct patient to move walker 6 to 8 inches ahead with all four legs of walker hitting floor at same time.
11. Instruct patient to bring affected foot into walker, then to bring stronger foot forward and even with affected foot.
12. Have patient continue walking with walker while you evaluate balance and endurance.
13. Make any corrections on use of walker as needed.
14. Provide patient with written instructions for home use. Verify understanding.
15. Perform hand hygiene.
16. Document procedure in patient's record.

CHARTING EXAMPLE: 06/10/XX 10:00 A.M. Evaluated walker height and fit. Pt. instructed on proper use of walker. Pt. practiced 10 min. w/o difficulty. · R. Schwartz, CMA (AAMA)

TABLE 7-4 Principles of Proper Body Mechanics.

Movement	Description
Stoop	• Do not bend from your back. • Stand close to the object you are moving. • Keep your feet 6–8 inches apart to create a base of support. • Place one foot slightly ahead of the other. • Bend at the hips and knees, keeping the back straight, and lower the body and hands to the object (Figure 7-27). • Use the large leg muscles to assist in returning to a standing position (Figure 7-28). FIGURE 7-27 Correct position when lifting a heavy object off the floor. FIGURE 7-28 When lifting, use strong leg muscles, keeping back straight.
Lift firmly and smoothly	• If you think you cannot move a heavy or awkward load, get help. • Grasp the load by using the large leg muscles. • Keep the load close to the body.
Use the center of gravity for carrying a load	• Keep your back as straight as possible • Keep the weight of the load close to your body and centered over the hips. • Put the load down by bending at the hips and knees. • When two or more people carry the load, have one person give the commands to lift or move the object.
Pull or push, rather than lift, a load	• Remain close to the object you are moving. • Keep feet apart with one slightly forward. • Have a firm grasp on the object. • Crouch down with feet apart if the object is on the floor. • Bend your elbows and place hands on the load at chest level. • Keep your back straight. • Push up with your legs in order to stand up with the load.
Avoid reaching	• Evaluate the distance before reaching too far for an object. • Stand close to the object. • Do not reach to the point of straining. • To change direction point your feet in the direction you wish to go. • Keep the object close to your body as you lower it.
Avoid twisting	• Do not twist your body.

width apart, knees slightly bent, and weight evenly distributed on both legs. Table 7-4 describes the principles of proper body mechanics and illustrates proper lifting techniques.

TRANSFERRING PATIENTS

Transferring or moving patients who cannot move themselves may be necessary. Patient safety is critical in every encounter. Before beginning any transfer, explain to the patient what you are going to do and what they should do to help you. Other points to keep in mind are these:

• Always use a gait belt to assist in lifting. Never lift patient under armpit or by the arms.

• Determine ahead of time whether help is needed to be better prepared.

• Practice good body mechanics.

• Get close to the patient so you can lift with your legs.

• Make certain that the equipment to be used is stable and firmly placed.

• Keep surfaces used in transfer fairly level (chair and wheelchair at same height).

• Remove all obstructions in area.

• Place transfer equipment on the patient's strong side.

Procedures for transferring a patient from a wheelchair to a chair or examination table, transferring patient from examination table or bed to wheelchair, ambulating patient with one assistant, and assisting falling patient follow.

PROCEDURE 7-13

PERFORMING PATIENT WHEELCHAIR TRANSFER TO CHAIR OR EXAMINATION TABLE

ABHES VII.MA.A.1 9(l); VII.MA.A.1 9(m)   CAAHEP IV.P (6); I.P (10)

OBJECTIVE: To safely transfer patient from wheelchair to chair or examination table.

STANDARD: This task takes 5 minutes.

EQUIPMENT AND SUPPLIES: Chair or examination table; gait belt; step stool if needed.

STEPS:

1. Perform hand hygiene.
2. Identify patient, and explain procedure. Explain what patient must do to assist you.
3. Place wheelchair at 45-degree angle to chair or examination table. Lock brakes on wheelchair. This shortens distance to pivot patient from wheelchair. Patient's strongest side should be closest to examination table or chair.
4. Place gait belt snugly around patient's waist, and tuck in excess under belt.
5. Make sure examination table or chair is stable before attempting any transfer.
6. Lift patient's legs off footrest by supporting ankles and lower leg. Gently place feet on floor. Have patient move forward slightly in chair if possible. Move foot pedals up and out of way.
7. Position yourself in front of patient with feet slightly apart. Be ready to provide support on patient's affected side. Patient can use stronger side as much as possible. Patient will move toward stronger side.
8. Stabilize patient's foot by placing your foot at outside edge of patient's foot. Establish firm base of support for your body.
9. Bend at hips and knees and grasp gait belt. Ask patient to place hands on arm supports of wheelchair.
10. Ask patient to lean forward on count of three and then push up with arms and stronger leg as much as possible as you assist patient to standing position.
11. Position yourself so patient's affected limb is between your knees. Support this limb with your knees to avoid having leg slip as patient stands.

12. Allow patient to stand for a moment before attempting to move to chair or examination table.
13. Help patient pivot toward stronger side by pivoting your own body while holding gait belt firmly. Turn as one unit.
14. *To lower patient into chair,* gently lower patient by bending your knees with back straight. *To move patient onto examination table,* have patient place stronger limb onto step stool, then pivot as a unit and turn so patient can sit on edge of table; to have patient assume supine position, support affected limb gently onto table.
15. Ask patient to move away from edge to prevent a fall.
16. If patient is unable to assist you, ask a co-worker to assist on other side, count aloud, and lift on three.
17. Move wheelchair, and stool if used, out of way.
18. Never leave a physically or mentally challenged patient unattended.

Two-Person Transfer

1. Place gait belt snugly around patient's waist, tucking in ends under belt.
2. Position one person in front of patient and one to side closest to examination table.
3. Both persons grasp gait belt underneath while patient places hands on arm support of wheelchair.
4. One caregiver gives signal, and both persons lift patient up to standing position while patient pushes up, if possible, with hands. If patient's upper body strength is diminished, have patient dangle arms in front.
5. Person nearest examination table moves wheelchair out of way.
6. Other person pivots patient around so buttocks are at edge of table.
7. On signal, both caregivers lift patient onto table while holding gait belt.
8. Position patient as needed for examination.
9. Never leave a physically or mentally challenged patient unattended.

PROCEDURE 7-14

TRANSFERRING PATIENT FROM EXAMINATION TABLE OR BED TO WHEELCHAIR

ABHES VII.MA.A.1 9(m)   CAAHEP I.P (10)

OBJECTIVE: To transfer a patient safely from examination table or bed to wheelchair.

STANDARD: This task takes 5 minutes.

EQUIPMENT AND SUPPLIES: Gait belt; stool; wheelchair.

STEPS:

1. Perform hand hygiene.
2. Identify patient, and explain procedure.

3. Lock examination table or bed in place.
4. Place wheelchair at head of bed and lock wheels. If possible, have someone hold chair as you move patient (Figure 7-29A).
5. If possible, lower table or bed to lowest position.
6. Move patient to edge of bed, and instruct patient to bend knees. (This allows patient to move legs and feet over side of bed onto floor.)

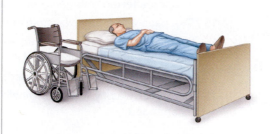

A Position the chair with the back even with the head of the bed.

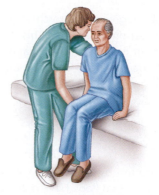

B Assist the patient to dangle.

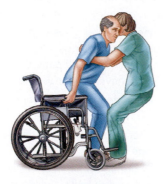

C Bend your knees as you lower the patient to the chair.

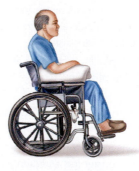

D Use pillows as needed to position the patient in correct body alignment.

FIGURE 7-29 (A) Position the chair with the back even with the head of the bed and wheels locked; (B) help the patient to dangle his or her legs over the side of the bed; (C) stand at client's hip with feet spread apart for support, and pivot patient around to chair; (D) place pillows to provide comfort for patient.

7. Have patient turn onto side with knees flexed, or place bed or table in semi-Fowler's position with head raised at 45° angle. (This may make it easier for caregiver to assist patient to pivot to sitting position.)

8. Stand at patient's hip level with feet apart to provide broad base of support with forward foot closest to patient.

9. Flex knees, hips, and ankles, and place one of your arms under patient's shoulders and other arm beneath patient's thighs near knees. (This keeps patient from falling backward.)

10. Lift patient's thighs slightly, and pivot on balls of your feet as you move patient to sitting position.

11. Allow patient to dangle legs until stable (Figure 7-29B).

12. Make sure patient is wearing nonskid slippers or shoes.

13. Have patient reach across chair and grasp chair arm to provide stability, if possible.

14. Grasp patient by placing your hands underneath gait belt with feet planted shoulder width apart and knees bent. On signal, pull patient to standing position and pivot on stronger leg with back toward wheelchair. Have patient place hands on chair's arm support.

15. Bend your knees and lower patient to chair. (Figure 7-29C).

16. Lower foot pedals and place patient's feet on them. Use pillows to pad areas of pressure and provide comfort (Figure 7-29D).

PROCEDURE 7-15

AMBULATING PATIENT WITH ONE ASSISTANT
ABHES VII.MA.A.1 9(m)   CAAHEP I.P (10)

OBJECTIVE: To help patient to ambulate safely.

STANDARD: This task takes 5–10 minutes per physician's orders.

EQUIPMENT AND SUPPLIES: Gait belt; shoes or slippers with nonskid soles.

STEPS:

1. Check patient's record for physician's orders and for history of **orthostatic hypotension** (a sudden drop in blood pressure when moving from sitting to standing).

2. Perform hand hygiene.

3. Identify patient, and explain procedure.

4. Assist patient to dangle legs (as in Procedure 7-14, steps 5–11).

5. Allow time to prevent dizziness.

6. Place gait belt around patient's waist, and tuck in ends under belt.

7. Grasp gait belt from underneath with palm up and elbow bent, and assist patient to stand. Assess skin color, balance, and stability.

8. Standing slightly behind and off to patient's affected side, grasp gait belt with one hand and place other hand on patient's bent arm.

9. Starting on same foot as patient, proceed slowly, keeping in step with patient.

10. Encourage patient to maintain good posture and look straight ahead, not at feet. Remind patient not to shuffle but to lift each foot for each step.

11. Walk as far as patient is capable, following physician's orders. If patient is fatigued, allow patient to sit and rest briefly before resuming.

12. Return patient to examination table or bed, assisting as needed.

13. Document procedure in patient's record.

14. Perform hand hygiene.

CHARTING EXAMPLE: 06/15/XX 7:00 P.M. Pt. walked w assistance 5 min., rested 5 min., and repeated walk. No dizziness reported. · · · · · · · · · · · · · · · · · · F. Collins, CMA (AAMA)

PROCEDURE 7-16

ASSISTING THE FALLING PATIENT

ABHES VII.MA.A.1 9(m)   CAAHEP I.P (10); IX.P (6)

OBJECTIVE: To assist falling patient to prevent injury.

STANDARD: This task takes 1–2 minutes.

EQUIPMENT AND SUPPLIES: Gait belt on patient.

STEPS:

1. While assisting patient, always keep one hand on safety or gait belt. It is unsafe to grab patient's robe or clothing because material moves, and instability may result.

2. If patient falls to side, try to guide back to stable position on feet. Provide stability by moving your foot in direction patient is falling. Once stable, inquire whether patient wants to continue with activity or end session (Figure 7-30). Call for assistance as needed. Check blood pressure and pulse.

3. If patient falls backward, spread your feet to establish stable base for patient to lean against. Guide patient to floor if necessary, call for assistance, and take patient's pulse and blood pressure.

4. If patient falls forward, hold around waist. Step forward, and use outermost leg to gently lower patient to floor. Call for assistance, and take pulse and blood pressure.

5. Have patient examined by physician or other licensed staff before moving.

6. Document fall in an incident report as soon as patient is stable.

7. Perform hand hygiene.

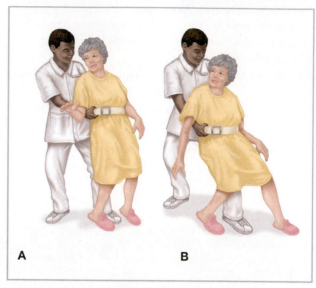

FIGURE 7-30 **(A) If patient begins to fall, pull him or her close to your body with gait belt; (B) ease the patient to the floor by letting him or her slide down your leg.**

CHARTING EXAMPLE: 06/13/XX 10:50 A.M. Assisting with ambulation per physician's orders. After 5 steps Pt. stated "knees gave out and I feel faint." Gently guided Pt. to floor without striking any body parts. Dr. Mench notified. BP 106/58, P 102 lying on floor. Rechecked after patient seated in chair. BP 130/70, P 88. · · · · · · · · · · · · · · · · · · M. Linn, CMA (AAMA)

Cast Care

A fracture is a break or disruption in the continuity of a bone. Each fracture is different and presents its own set of problems. Several different types of fractures are illustrated in Figure 7-31. Box 7-2 describes different types of fractures and related information.

Casts are applied to maintain proper alignment of the bone once the fracture has been reduced, and they generally remain on until healing is completed. Casts are made of plaster of Paris or synthetic materials such as fiberglass, plastic, or polyester. Air casts are a type of inflatable immobilizer; they use air to stabilize a limb. Synthetic casts weigh less and dry easily but are costly.

After casts are applied, they should be allowed to dry uncovered while the patient is kept immobilized. Drying time depends on the type of casting material used. Once casts are in place, the patient's extremities should be monitored for the four P's: pain, pallor, pulse, and paresthesia (numbness). A cast that is too tight can cause tissue, nerve, and vascular damage, so always check tightness and circulation. (Procedure 7-17 and Procedure 7-18 describe cast application and removal.)

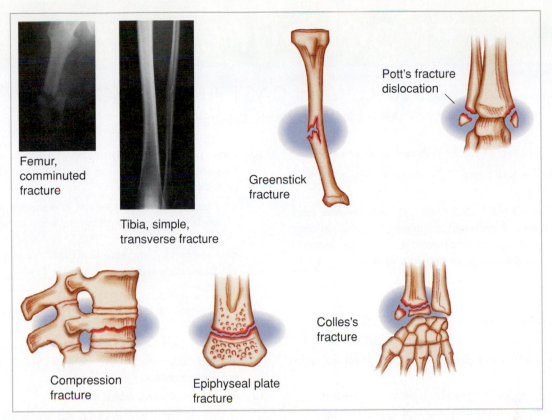

Femur, comminuted fracture

Tibia, simple, transverse fracture

Greenstick fracture

Pott's fracture dislocation

Compression fracture

Epiphyseal plate fracture

Colles's fracture

FIGURE 7-31 **Types of bone fractures.**

BOX 7-2 Types of Fractures

GREENSTICK
- A crack, or the bending of a bone with incomplete fracture that only affects one side of the **periosteum**.
- Common in children or in skull fractures when bones are pliable.

COMMINUTED
- Bone completely broken in a transverse, spiral, or oblique direction (indicates the direction of the fracture in relation to the long axis of the fracture bone).
- Bone broken into several fragments.

OPEN OR COMPOUND
- Bone is exposed to the air through a break in the skin.
- Also can be associated with soft tissue injury.
- Infection is common complication due to exposure to bacterial invasion.

CLOSED OR SIMPLE
- Skin remains intact.
- Chances are greatly decreased for infection.

COMPRESSION
- Frequently seen with vertebral fractures.
- Fractured bone has been compressed by other bones.

COMPLETE
- Bone is broken with a disruption of both sides of the periosteum.

IMPACTED
- One part of fractured bone is driven into another.

DEPRESSED FRACTURE
- Usually seen in skull or facial fractures.
- Bone or fragments of bone are driven inward.

PATHOLOGIC
- Break caused by disease process.

PROCEDURE 7-17

ASSISTING WITH CAST APPLICATION

ABHES VII.MA.A.1 9(m)   CAAHEP I.P (10)

OBJECTIVE: To assist physician with cast application.

STANDARD: This task takes 15–30 minutes, depending on patient.

EQUIPMENT AND SUPPLIES: Cast material to be used; stockinette to fit extremity or body part; sheet wadding (cast padding); basin for warm water; container of warm water; gloves; bandages; scissors; sponge rubber for padding; patient's record; pen.

STEPS:

1. Perform hand hygiene.
2. Check patient's record for physician's orders.
3. Assemble equipment and supplies needed.
4. Identify patient, and explain procedure. Answer questions as needed.
5. Position patient as required by type of cast needed. Alignment of body part is important during casting.
6. Don gloves, and drape patient for privacy and comfort as needed.
7. Clean and thoroughly dry area to be cast as directed by physician. Observe skin condition and signs of bruising and cuts. Remove and dispose of gloves and wash hands.
8. Prepare appropriate size stockinette, leaving 2 inches above and below designated area to be cast. (This will be applied by physician to ensure that all creases made are smooth. Excess length will be used after casting to protect skin from edges of cast.)
9. Prepare cast padding per physician's orders. (Padding will be applied by physician with extra padding over bony prominences.)

10. When physician is ready to apply cast, don gloves and prepare material (plaster or fiberglass), then hand it to physician.
    - **Plaster.** Place plaster roll in water for about 5 seconds. Remove and gently squeeze to remove excess water.
    - **Fiberglass.** Immerse fiberglass in warm water for 10 seconds and gently squeeze to remove excess water.

11. Assist physician by holding body part in specified position.
12. Repeat steps 10 and 11 until cast is complete. Physician will fold excess stockinette material over edges of cast to provide protection.
13. Provide comforting words to patient.
14. Once cast application is complete, clean any plaster off patient and review cast care with patient and caregiver. Provide written and verbal instructions for cast care and for isometric exercises if so ordered. Review complications. Verify understanding.
15. Clean equipment and examination room.
16. Remove gloves, and perform hand hygiene.
17. Document procedure in patient's record.

CHARTING EXAMPLE: 06/14/XX 12:30 P.M. R arm plaster cast applied by Dr. Riaz. Pt. instructed about cast care, exercises. Verbally returned understanding to call office to report signs of infection, numbness, and excess pain. Fingers on R hand warm to touch. Sling applied. · · · · · · · · · · · · · · · · · F. Murray, RMA.

PROCEDURE 7-18

ASSISTING WITH CAST REMOVAL

ABHES VII.MA.A.1 9(m)   CAAHEP I.P (10)

OBJECTIVE: To assist with cast removal.

STANDARD: This takes 10–15 minutes.

EQUIPMENT AND SUPPLIES: Cast cutter; cast spreader; bandage scissors; drape; bag for cast disposal; patient's record; pen.

STEPS:

1. Perform hand hygiene.
2. Review physician's orders.
3. Identify patient, and explain procedure. Explain that cast cutter vibrates to separate material and patient may feel vibration and warmth as spreader is used to separate cast, then bandage scissors are used to cut stockinette material (Figure 7-32).

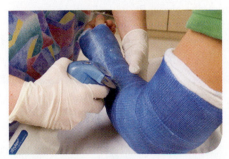

FIGURE 7-32 Cast is split with a vibrating blade. Underlying padding is cut with bandage scissors.

4. Inform patient that skin below cast may be pale and flaky, muscle tissue may be flabby from disuse, and foul odor may be present. Reassure patient that this is normal.
5. Assist physician by handing requested instruments.
6. Don gloves.
7. After cast removed, gently wash area where cast removed. Skin will be tender, so avoid scrubbing.
8. Provide written and verbal instructions for home care, including any exercises ordered by physician. Confirm patient understands.
9. Clean equipment and area, and properly dispose of cast and bandaging material.
10. Perform hand hygiene.
11. Document procedure in patient's record.

CHARTING EXAMPLE: 06/14/XX 6:00 P.M. Cast removed from R arm by Dr. Riaz. Muscles slightly atrophied, skin flaky and pale. Instructions for skin care and PT appointment for next day given. · · · · · · · · · · · · · · · · · · B. Archer, CMA (AAMA)

Applying Immobilizing Devices

Immobilizing devices are used to maintain body alignment, limit harmful movement, reduce pain, and promote healing. Devices such as a sling, spiral bandage, splint, spiral-eight bandage, cervical collar, and certain types of back braces may be ordered by the physician. (Procedures for applying some of the previously mentioned devices follow.)

PROCEDURE 7-19

APPLYING AN ARM SLING

ABHES VII.MA.A.1 9(m)   CAAHEP I.P (10)

OBJECTIVE: To correctly apply an arm sling and document correctly.

STANDARD: This task takes 5 minutes.

EQUIPMENT AND SUPPLIES: Commercial arm sling; triangular arm sling; safety pins; patient's record; pen.

STEPS:

1. Check physician's orders for sling.
2. Perform hand hygiene.
3. Identify patient, and explain procedure.
4. Check distal pulse, sensation in hands.
5. Commercial sling:
   - Ask patient to sit or stand and place affected arm across chest with thumb pointing up.
   - Carefully place arm in sling so elbow fits snugly in corner of sling.
   - Bring sling strap around neck of patient and through metal loops. Adjust as needed with wrist raised

slightly above elbow to improve circulation. Check position of arm and pad neck area if needed to avoid pressure and chaffing.

6. Triangular cloth sling:

- Position sling over chest with point toward affected side extending beyond elbow. Upper end should be over shoulder on unaffected side.
- Bring lower end up and over affected arm, keeping hand elevated above elbow.
- Tie two ends together at side of neck (not at back of neck). Pad knot as needed to avoid pressure.

- Secure point of sling by folding neatly and fastening with safety pin or tape.

7. Reassess distal pulse and sensation.

8. Provide written instructions for home care as ordered by physician. Confirm understanding.

9. Perform hand hygiene.

10. Document procedure in patient's record.

CHARTING EXAMPLE: 06/18/XX Triangular sling applied to R arm. Written instructions given. Pt. verbalized understanding. No swelling in hand, fingers warm to touch. · · · · · · ·
· P. Price, CMA (AAMA)

PROCEDURE 7-20

APPLYING A SPIRAL BANDAGE

ABHES VII.MA.A.1 9(m)   CAAHEP I.P (10)

OBJECTIVE: To properly apply spiral bandage to forearm and document.

STANDARD: This task takes 1–2 minutes.

EQUIPMENT AND SUPPLIES: Nonsterile gloves; bandaging material as prescribed by physician; bandage scissors; tape; patient's record; pen.

STEPS:

1. Check physician's orders.
2. Perform hand hygiene.
3. Assemble equipment.
4. Identify patient, and explain procedure.
5. Check pulse and fingers for sensation.
6. Don nonsterile gloves.
7. Have patient sit or stand with forearm elevated. Hold bandage material several inches below site of injury.
8. Anchor bandage by wrapping two times around extremity, then proceed to wrap from distal to proximal, using some tension to apply evenly.
9. Use spiral or angled turns (Figure 7-33) with bandage turns overlapping one half of previous turn.

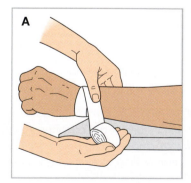
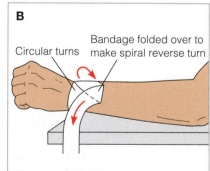
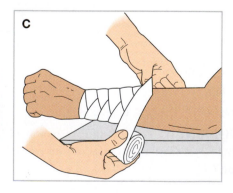

FIGURE 7-33 **Wrap bandage two times around wrist to anchor.**

10. Complete wrapping with two turns directly over each other, and secure with tape or tie.
11. Check for any blood flow restriction.
12. Provide written and verbal instruction for home care. Ask patient to repeat instruction to ensure comprehension.
13. Remove gloves, and dispose of them properly.
14. Document procedure in patient's record.

PROCEDURE 7-21

APPLYING A FIGURE-EIGHT BANDAGE
ABHES VII.MA.A.1 9(m)   CAAHEP I.P (10)

OBJECTIVE: To correctly apply a figure-eight bandage to a patient's ankle.

STANDARD: This task takes 2–3 minutes.

EQUIPMENT AND SUPPLIES: Roller bandage; safety pin; tape; patient's record; pen.

STEPS:

1. Check patient's record for physician's orders.
2. Identify patient, and explain procedure.
3. Assemble equipment and supplies.
4. Position ankle in neutral position (not overflexed or overextended).
5. Hold bandage roll with outer part next to patient's skin.
6. Anchor bandage with a circular turn around instep.
7. Make circular turn around ankle and over heel, and bring back to starting area.
8. Make spiral turn down over ankle and around foot. Continue making turns over ankle and around foot, overlapping preceding turn by two-thirds over previous layer (Figure 7-34).
9. Wrap area below and above ankle to immobilize affected area.
10. Check foot and toes for circulation and sensation. Check patient comfort level.
11. Instruct patient to keep foot elevated to promote venous return.

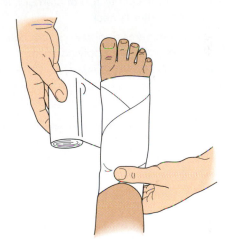

FIGURE 7-34 A figure-eight turn is used to support and limit joint movement.

12. Provide written and verbal instruction for home care. Ask patient to verbalize directions to ensure comprehension.
13. Perform hand hygiene.
14. Document procedure in patient's record.

PROCEDURE 7-22

APPLYING A CERVICAL COLLAR

ABHES VII.MA.A.1 9(m)   CAAHEP I.P (10)

OBJECTIVE: To apply correct size of cervical collar per physician's orders.

STANDARD: This task takes 10 minutes, depending on patient condition.

EQUIPMENT AND SUPPLIES: Patient's record; two semi-rigid collars of appropriate size; pen.

STEPS:

1. Check patient's record for physician's order.
2. Perform hand hygiene.
3. Identify patient, and explain procedure.
4. If measurements not included in orders, measure patient's neck from bottom of chin to top of sternum. Measure circumference of patient's neck.
5. Use these measurements to obtain proper collar. Follow manufacturer's direction for applying collar.
6. Place back half of collar on patient's neck, making sure it is centered directly over spine with arrow pointing up.
7. Center front half of collar on neck so chin fits into indentation on collar (neutral alignment).
8. Overlap front collar piece over back collar piece, and secure after adjusting fasteners on sides.
9. Check patient for any discomfort.
10. Provide patient with written and verbal instructions, as well as extra collar. Instruct patient to use soap and water to clean collar and allow collar to air-dry as needed.
11. Remind patient that collar is to be used for prescribed number of hours per day. Warn patient to walk with caution because objects on floor and stairs may not be visible while wearing collar.
12. Perform hand hygiene.
13. Document procedure in patient's record.

CHARTING EXAMPLE: 06/18/XX 10:00 A.M. Cervical collar applied per physician's order and measurements. Pt. verbalized home instructions. Pt. tolerated collar well. · · · · · · · · · · ·
· M. McCue, CMA (AAMA)

8 Assisting with Minor Surgery

PROCEDURES

Procedure 8-1 Performing Surgical Hand Scrub/Sterile Scrub

Procedure 8-2 Donning and Removing Sterile Gloves

Procedure 8-3 Opening a Sterile Packet

Procedure 8-4 Dropping a Sterile Item onto a Sterile Field

Procedure 8-5 Transferring Sterile Items with Sterile Transfer Forceps

Procedure 8-6 Pouring from a Sterile Container onto a Sterile Field

Procedure 8-7 Assisting with Minor Surgery

Procedure 8-8 Preparing a Patient's Skin for Minor Surgery

Procedure 8-9 Cleaning a Minor Wound

Procedure 8-10 Assisting with Suturing

Procedure 8-11 Changing a Sterile Dressing

Procedure 8-12 Removing Sutures and Staples

Procedure 8-13 Applying and Removing Sterile Adhesive Skin Closures

Procedure 8-14 Irrigating a Wound

Procedure 8-15 Packing a Wound

Procedure 8-16 Assisting with Excision of a Sebaceous Cyst

Procedure 8-17 Assisting with Aspiration of Joint Fluid

Procedure 8-18 Assisting with a Hemorrhoid Thrombectomy

Procedure 8-19 Preparing a Patient for Laser Surgery

TERMS TO LEARN

thrombectomy

specula

trocars

exudate

serous

purulent

sanguineous

serosanguineous

purosanguineous

approximated

Ringer's solution

debridement

autolytic

biopsy

thoracentesis

vertigo

abdominal paracentesis

ascites

Minor surgery procedures are performed in diverse settings in today's changing health care world. Ambulatory care centers handle an increasing number of minor surgery procedures that were previously done in hospitals. The types of surgical procedures vary with the category of medical specialty in which the health care assistant is employed. The basic guidelines and procedures are similar in each situation. The primary concern in all cases is reducing the risk of infection regardless of the surgical procedure performed. Hand washing is the most important action that can be taken to reduce the risk of infections. In Chapter 2, hand washing for medical asepsis and standard precautions were covered. In this chapter, the principles of surgical asepsis are presented. Surgical asepsis means that practices such as surgical scrub or sterile technique are utilized to maintain areas free of all forms of microorganisms. The following procedures are presented in this chapter: surgical hand scrubbing; donning and removing surgical gloves; opening a sterile packet; dropping a sterile item on a sterile field; transferring sterile items with sterile transfer forceps; pouring from a sterile container onto a sterile field; assisting with minor surgery; preparing a patient's skin for minor surgery; cleaning minor wounds; assisting with suturing; changing a sterile dressing; removing sutures and staples; applying and removing adhesive skin closures; irrigating a wound; packing a wound; assisting with excision of a sebaceous cyst; assisting with aspiration of joint fluid; assisting with hemorrhoid **thrombectomy** (removal of a blood clot or thrombus); and utilizing safety precautions for laser surgery.

Surgical Asepsis, Surgical Instruments, and Supplies

When practicing surgical asepsis, the guidelines presented in Box 8-1 should be followed. Each facility may have additional guidelines to follow for specific surgical procedures.

BOX 8-1 Surgical Asepsis Guidelines

A sterile item can only touch another sterile item.

- If a sterile item touches a nonsterile item, the sterile item is contaminated.
- If a clean item touches a sterile item, the sterile item is contaminated.
- If a sterile packet is torn, wet, or punctured, it is contaminated.
- A sterile packet is contaminated after the date on the packet has passed. If unsure of sterility, consider the item contaminated.
- Skin is always considered to be contaminated. It cannot be sterilized, only disinfected.

A sterile item on a sterile field must be within your field of vision and above your waist.

- If you cannot see an item, it is contaminated.
- If items or your hands are below your waist, they are contaminated.
- If you turn your back on a sterile field, it is contaminated.
- If you leave a sterile field, it is contaminated.

Airborne microorganisms contaminate sterile fields.

- Do not place sterile fields in a draft.
- Avoid extra movements near the sterile field.
- Do not talk, cough, sneeze, or laugh over a sterile field.
- Wear a mask if you need to talk during a procedure.

- Do not reach over a sterile field.
- A wet field is contaminated. Avoid spills on a sterile field.

The edges of a sterile field are contaminated.

- If an item touches any part of the 1-inch border around the sterile field, it is contaminated.

Sterile gloves must only touch sterile items.

- Do not touch the outside of sterile gloves with bare hands.
- Sterile gloves are contaminated if punctured. Remove and dispose of the item and gloves, rescrub, and reglove.

Sterile packets may be touched on the outside with bare hands.

- Outer wrappings are considered contaminated.
- Open sterile packets away from you to avoid contaminating the packet by touching your clothing.
- Never rewrap an unused sterile packet. The unused items must be resanitized, rewrapped, and reautoclaved.

Be honest if you make an error or suspect you have made an error.

- Remove the contaminated item and correct the error.
- Report contamination to your superior.

Before presenting specific procedures in this chapter, supplies and instruments used in association with minor surgeries must be mentioned.

Instruments are divided among four basic categories:

- Cutting instruments, such as scalpels and knives, used to make incisions.
- Dissecting instruments, such as scissors, used to cut or dissect tissues.
- Grasping and clamping instruments, used to grasp tissues or objects such as blood vessels or towels.
- Probing and dilating instruments, such as scopes (used to visualize internal structures); **specula** (used to spread apart a body cavity for ease of visualization); probes (used to explore wounds and cavities); **trocars** (used to withdraw fluids from cavities); punches (used to remove tissue for examination and biopsy).

Several categories of supplies are utilized, including suture materials and needles (Figure 8-1), dressings, band-

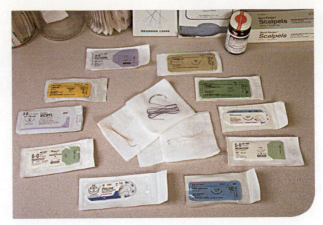

FIGURE 8-1 Types of suture material.

ages, anesthetics, solutions, sponges and wicks. Box 8-2 lists and describes supplies associated with minor surgery procedures. Procedure 8-1: Performing Surgical Hand Scrub/Sterile Scrub follows.

BOX 8-2 Supplies/Equipment Used in Minor Surgical Procedures

Anesthetics

- Substances used to cause loss of feeling—may be inhaled, topical, sprayed on, or injected, such as lidocaine.

Creams/Ointments

- Antibacterial/antifungal materials used to treat infection and promote healing. Creams are water based, and ointments are oil based.

Dressings

- Sterile gauzelike materials applied directly on a wound or surgical site that are absorbent and will cover the area.

Bandages

- Nonsterile materials applied over dressings to hold dressing in place, such as rolled gauze elastic bandages.

Solutions

- Liquid substances used as skin cleansers, preoperative scrubs, antiseptics such as povidone-iodine, isopropyl alcohol, or soaps.

Sponges

- Folded gauze squares of various sizes used to cleanse wounds, as dressings, and as coverings

Sutures

- Threadlike materials used to approximate (bring together) incisions or wounds. May be made of various materials such as silk, catgut and are absorbable or nonabsorbable. Size or thickness of suture materials is stated in terms of 0s with more 0s equaling thinner sutures material. (See Figure 8-1 for examples of suture materials.)

Needles

- Used to penetrate tissues with either a cutting or noncutting point and available in a variety of shapes: straight, curved, or swaged (suture material attached).

Sterile strips and staples

- Used to approximate wounds (Steri-Strips); available in various widths and materials; staples of stainless steel applied with a surgical stapler.

Wicks

- Made of narrow stripes of sterile gauze in varying lengths packaged in glass containers and used to keep a wound open to provide drainage.

PERFORMING SURGICAL HAND SCRUB/STERILE SCRUB

ABHES VII.MA.A.1 9(b)   CAAHEP III.P (4)

OBJECTIVE: To correctly perform surgical hand scrub/sterile scrub on hands and arms.

STANDARD: This procedure takes 8–10 minutes.

EQUIPMENT AND SUPPLIES: Antimicrobial solution in a dispenser; plastic or orangewood stick; scrub brush; sterile towels; sink.

STEPS:

1. Remove all jewelry (rings, watch, bracelets).
2. Without allowing your body to touch the sink, turn on water with hand, foot, or knee lever so water is tepid temperature.
3. Wet your hands thoroughly with arms raised so water flows from tips of fingers to elbows.

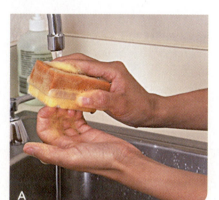
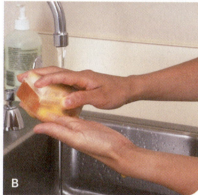
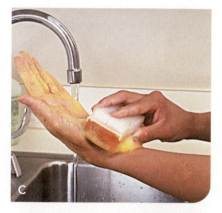
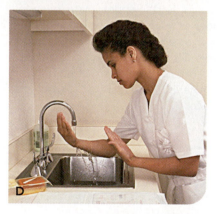
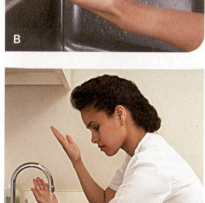
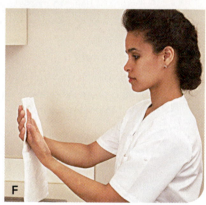
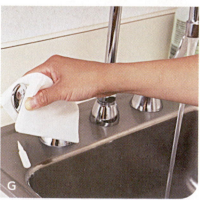

FIGURE 8-2 (A) Sterile scrub hand hygiene; (B) scrub for 5 minutes on each hand; (C) continue scrubbing toward elbows; (D) rinse hands while bending at elbows to rinse off soap; (E) allow water to flow from fingertips to elbows; (F) after rinsing, hold hands above waist; (G) dry hands, and use paper towel used to dry hands to turn off faucets.

4. With arms raised and hands above elbows, begin by using plastic or orangewood stick to clean fingernails.

5. Scrub hands for 10 strokes (or time dictated by facility policy) with 2 to 4 mL of antimicrobial solution. Scrub may be done with brush or by rubbing hands together.
   a. Start at fingertips with circular motion and work around and between each finger (Figure 8-2A).
   b. Next scrub back and front of hands with circular motion (Figure 8-2B).
   c. Move 3 inches up wrist up to elbow with circular scrubbing motion for 10 more strokes, keeping hands raised above wrists (Figure 8-2C)
   d. Repeat with second hand and arm.

6. Place arms under faucet with fingertips pointed upward. Rinse thoroughly with water flowing toward elbows (Figures 8-2D and 8-2E).

7. Dry hands from fingertips toward elbows with dry paper towel (Figure 8-2F).

8. If hand levers are used for water control, use paper towel used to dry hands to turn off faucets. *Do not touch sink or faucets with hands* (Figure 8-2G).

9. Glove immediately, and keep hands above waist and folded together until procedure begins.

WHY? The rule is that hands must not go below the waist after surgical scrub or when wearing sterile gloves. If they do, they are considered contaminated.

STERILE GLOVES

Once a surgical scrub has been performed, it is necessary to don sterile gloves to continue with the procedure. It is important to have sterile gloves of different sizes available to accommodate personnel. If a sterile glove is punctured or you touch the outside of the glove with your hand, it is contaminated, and you must reglove. (The steps for donning and removing sterile gloves are listed in Procedure 8-2.)

PROCEDURE 8-2

DONNING AND REMOVING STERILE GLOVES

ABHES VII.MA.A.1 9(i)   CAAHEP III.P (2)

OBJECTIVE: To don and remove sterile gloves without contamination.

STANDARD: This task takes 1 minute or less.

EQUIPMENT AND SUPPLIES: Packaged sterile gloves.

STEPS:

To don gloves

1. Wash and dry hands.
2. Place glove packet on clean, dry, flat surface.
3. Open outside wrapper by peeling apart tabs laterally to expose internal glove package. Do this over a flat surface to prevent accidentally contaminating gloves.
4. Place glove packet on firm surface, touching only outside of wrapper.
5. Open inner wrapper without reaching over pack or touching inside of wrapper. Spread wrapper edges up and away from gloves (Figure 8-3A).

6. Using thumb and fingers of nondominant hand, pick up opposite glove by folded inside edge of cuff. Lift glove up and away from wrapper (Figure 8-3B).
7. Insert dominant hand into glove while pulling glove on with nondominant hand, touching only inside of cuff (Figure 8-3C).
8. Remove second glove from wrapper by placing gloved fingers under cuff (touching outside of glove) and lifting glove up and away from wrapper (Figure 8-3D).
9. Place ungloved fingers into second glove. Holding gloved thumb away from area to prevent touching skin, pull glove over hand (Figure 8-3E).
10. Keeping hands above waist, adjust both gloves by touching only sterile surfaces of gloves. Continue to keep hands in front and raised above waist to prevent contamination.

To remove gloves

11. Grasp outside of left glove with right gloved hand 2 inches from top of glove. Pull glove down hand. It will

turn inside side out as it is removed (Figures 8-3F, 8-3G, and 8-3H). Pull glove free, and either make a ball of it in remaining gloved hand or discard in biohazard waste container

12. Insert two fingers in glove and pull second glove off. It will turn inside out and cover balled up first glove. Take care not to touch outside of contaminated glove.

13. Discard gloves in biohazard waste container and perform hand hygiene.

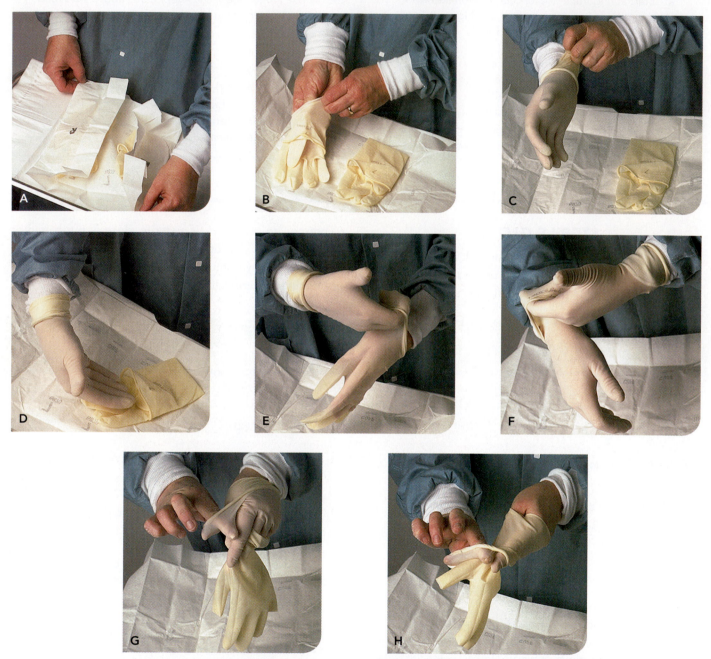

FIGURE 8-3 (A) Pull inner wrapper edges to each side without touching the inside of the pack; (B) using thumb and fingers of nondominant hand, pick up the glove on the side of the pack nearest the dominant hand by grasping the folded inside edge of the glove; (C) pull the glove onto the dominant hand, using only the thumb and fingers of the other hand; (D) place the fingers of the gloved hand under the cuff of the other glove, pick up, and pull; (E) with gloved dominant hand, place fingers under the cuff of the second gloved hand and pull up over the wrist; (F) after gloves in place, fingers may be adjusted using gloved hands; (G) to remove first glove, grasp opposite glove in palm, pull down, and remove. To remove second glove, insert two fingers (ungloved) under the cuff of glove and peel down to remove; (H) peel second glove off hand over the balled-up first glove in hand without touching outside of contaminated gloves.

STERILE PACKETS

Sterile packets are prepared for use in minor surgery. Each one may contain either a single instrument or several items packaged together. These packets are then autoclaved with sterilization indicators and dated. Sterile packets may be purchased from medical supply companies or prepared in house by staff.

Prior to a procedure, all necessary equipment and supplies will be assembled and opened as they are needed to assist the physician. (Procedures 8-3 through 8-6 list the steps to open a sterile packet, drop sterile items on a sterile field, transfer sterile items onto sterile field using sterile transfer forceps, and pour sterile solutions onto a sterile field.)

PROCEDURE 8-3

OPENING A STERILE PACKET
ABHES VII.MA.A.1 9(o)(4)   CAAHEP III.P (5)

OBJECTIVE: To open a sterile packet and set up a sterile field without contamination.

STANDARD: This procedure takes 1 minute or less.

EQUIPMENT AND SUPPLIES: Sterile packet; Mayo stand; biohazard waste container; sterile forceps.

STEPS:

1. Perform hand hygiene.
2. Assemble equipment and adjust Mayo stand to correct height.
3. Place packet on Mayo stand with folded edge on top. Position packet on stand so that top flap will fold away from you so you will not have to reach over sterile field.

4. Remove tape or fastener. Check sterilization indicator and date. Pull corner of pack that is tucked under, and lay this flap away from you (Figures 8-4A and 8-4B).
5. With both hands pull next two flaps to each side (Figures 8-4C and 8-4D). (Packet will still be covered with last layer of outer wrap.)
6. Grasp corner of last flap without reaching over sterile field, and open flap toward your body without touching it. (Figure 8-4E). (Inside of this outer wrapper is now your sterile field.)
7. If you need to arrange items within sterile field, use sterile transfer forceps. If an inner packet on field needs to be opened, then someone wearing sterile gloves must open it.

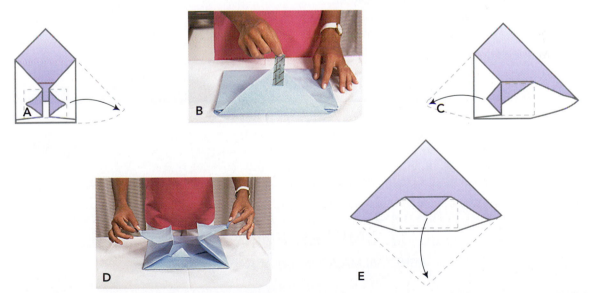

FIGURE 8.4 (A) Open the packet by removing tape; check the sterilization indicator and date; (B) pull the corner of the packet where tape is located, and open away from you; (C) open the next two flaps using both hands; (D) open the two side flaps using both hands; (E) open the last flap without touching or reaching over the field.

PROCEDURE 8-4

DROPPING A STERILE ITEM ONTO A STERILE FIELD

ABHES VII.MA.A.1 9(o)(4)   CAAHEP III.P (6)

OBJECTIVE: To drop a sterile item onto a sterile field or into a gloved hand without contaminating the packet or the field.

STANDARD: This task takes 1 minute or less.

EQUIPMENT AND SUPPLIES: Sterile pack containing prepackaged items such as specimen container or needle and syringe in a pull-apart packet.

1. Assemble equipment. Check expiration date and sealed condition of packet.
2. Locate edge of packet, and pull apart using thumb and forefinger of each hand. Do not let fingers touch inside of packet. Inside of packet is sterile, and outside is contaminated.
3. Pull apart packet by securely placing remaining three fingers of each hand against outside of packet on each side. Wrapper edges will be pulled back and away from sterile item.
4. Holding opened packet securely about 8 to 10 inches above sterile field, gently drop packet contents inside sterile field (Figure 8-5).

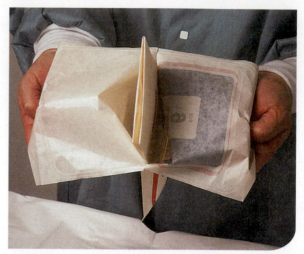

FIGURE 8-5   Dropping a sterile item onto a sterile field.

5. Physician may request you open sterile packet and hold it open so he or she may grasp item with gloved hand.
6. Discard paper wrapper in waste container.

WHY? Dropping packet from a height of 8 to 10 inches lessens the chances of contaminating the field. Remember that the outer 1-inch border around the field is considered contaminated.

PROCEDURE 8-5

TRANSFERRING STERILE ITEMS WITH STERILE TRANSFER FORCEPS

ABHES VII.MA.A.1 9(o)(4)   CAAHEP III.P (6)

OBJECTIVE: To move sterile items, such as instruments and supplies, within or onto a sterile field or into a gloved hand.

STANDARD: This task takes 1–2 minutes.

EQUIPMENT AND SUPPLIES: Sterile transfer forceps in forceps container with sterilant solution; Mayo stand with sterile field setup; sterile 4 × 4 gauze package.

STEPS:

1. Grasp forceps handle firmly without separating tips, and remove the instrument vertically from container. Removing vertically with closed tips helps prevent contaminating tips on sides of container and dripping on sterile field.

2. Hold forceps down. Gently tap tips together over a sterile dry gauze square, or touch tips to sterile dry gauze square to remove excess solution.

3. Pick up item to be transferred at its midsection, holding transfer forceps vertically with tips down. *Do not touch sterile field with tips.*

4. Place sterile item on sterile field inside 1-inch border that is considered contaminated (Figure 8-6).

5. Place forceps back into original container without touching sides of container.

6. Clean and sterilize forceps and container once a week or according to facility policy. Replace sterilant solution.

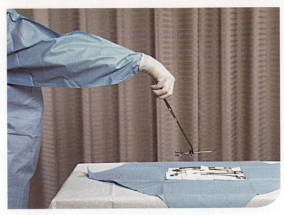

FIGURE 8-6 Proper technique to handle equipment with transfer forceps.

PROCEDURE 8-6

POURING FROM A STERILE CONTAINER ONTO A STERILE FIELD

ABHES VII.MA.A.1 9(o)(4)   CAAHEP III.P (6)

OBJECTIVE: To pour sterile solution onto a sterile field without spilling the solution or contaminating the field.

STANDARD: This task takes 5 minutes or less.

EQUIPMENT AND SUPPLIES: Sterile saline or other sterile solution; sterile basin or cup; Mayo stand; waste container.

STEPS:

1. Perform hand hygiene. Assemble equipment. Check expiration dates on solution and sterile basin pack.

2. Set up sterile basin on Mayo tray, using inside of wrapper to create a sterile field.

3. Remove cap of solution. Invert cap, and place it on a clean surface (inside facing up). Avoid touching inner surface of cap because it is considered sterile.

4. Recheck bottle label before pouring solution.

5. Pour a small amount of solution into waste container to clean lip of container.

6. Place label in palm of hand, and pour solution from height of about 6 inches above field. Pour slowly to avoid splashing (Figure 8-7).

7. Replace lid immediately after pouring.

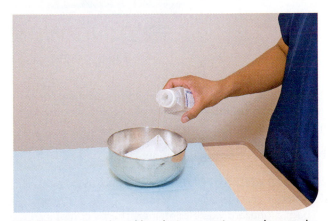

FIGURE 8-7 Pour liquid by placing container as close to the edge as possible while maintaining sterile 1-inch border. Then pour from 4 to 6 inches above field without spilling.

BOX 8-3 Minor Surgery Reminders

Prior to Procedure

- Review the patient's record and ascertain that the patient has a clear understanding of the procedure and postoperative care.
- Check to make certain the informed consent is signed and in the patient's record.
- Assemble all required equipment, including physician's preferences.
- Set up and cover the sterile field to maintain sterility.
- Position the patient.
- Prepare the patient's skin as required.

During the Procedure

- Adjust light.
- Remove cover from sterile field.
- Assist by adding to the sterile field (while maintaining sterility) supplies, instruments, and solutions as required.

- Use sterile gloves to hand instruments and supplies to the physician.
- Use sterile gloves to sponge the operative site, cut sutures, and retract tissue.
- Hold tissue container to obtain specimen for examination.

After the Procedure

- Clean the examination room.
- Label and prepare specimen for transport to the laboratory.
- Document the patient's record.
- Review the postcare information with patient or responsible adult, and verify understanding.
- Schedule a follow-up appointment.

Assisting with Minor Surgery

Minor surgery procedures may be carried out in an office or in an ambulatory care or clinic setting. A physician will perform the procedure, but the medical assistant or other health care assistant is responsible for assembling all necessary equipment and supplies and setting up a surgical field while maintaining sterility. Each physician has individual preferences for types of instruments and the manner in which the field is set up. It is helpful to keep an index card for each procedure, noting physician preferences. (Box 8-3 indicates some details to consider before, during, and after a minor surgical procedure. Procedure 8-7 lists the steps to set up and assist with a minor surgical procedure.)

PROCEDURE 8-7

ASSISTING WITH MINOR SURGERY

ABHES VII.MA.A.1 9(n) CAAHEP III.P (10)

OBJECTIVE: To prepare all material and equipment for use in a surgical procedure and assist physician, using sterile technique.

STANDARD: This task takes 15 minutes.

EQUIPMENT AND SUPPLIES: Mayo stand; side stand; transfer forceps and container with solution; waste container/plastic bag; biohazard waste container; sharps container; light; anesthetic; alcohol swab; sterile specimen container (depending on type of surgery); 2 or more pairs of sterile gloves (appropriate sizes); towel pack; 4 × 4 sponges; patient drape; needle pack; suture material; instrument packs, including towel clamp pack; syringe pack; 2 sterile basins; specimen container; patient's record; pen.

STEPS:

1. Perform hand hygiene.
2. Open sterile tray packs on Mayo stand and side stand, using sterile wrapper to create sterile field.
3. Use sterile transfer forceps to move instruments on tray or to place equipment from packets on tray.

4. Open sterile needle and syringe unit, and drop gently onto sterile field. Use care not to reach over sterile field.

5. Open sterile drape pack and towel clamp pack, if needed.

6. Open set of sterile gloves for physician.

7. After tray is ready with all equipment arranged, cover with sterile towel to protect from contamination. (Assistant should not leave room once tray is set up.)

8. After physician has donned sterile gloves, remove sterile towel covering sterile field setup. Remove towel by standing to one side and grasping two distal corners. Lift towel toward you so you do not reach over unprotected sterile field.

9. Cleanse top of anesthetic bottle with sterile alcohol swab and hold it upside down in palm of your hand with label facing toward physician. Hold it steady while physician draws up anesthetic.

10. Stand to one side and assist physician as requested. Provide additional supplies as needed. (If you assist by swabbing site or handing instruments, you must perform surgical scrub and wear sterile gloves and other PPE.)

11. Hold all containers for specimens, and provide container for disposal of contaminated sponges. Protect yourself by wearing nonsterile gloves.

12. Collect and place all soiled instruments in basin (out of patient's view, if possible).

13. Place all soiled items (4 × 4 gauze sponges) in plastic bag. Do not allow wet items to remain on sterile field.

14. Immediately label all specimens as they are obtained. Close each specimen container tightly.

15. Reassure patient periodically in a quiet voice.

16. When procedure is completed perform hand hygiene before touching patient.

17. Allow patient to rest and recover for time required. Periodically check vital signs according to facility policy.

18. Provide clear oral and written postoperative instructions for patient and caregiver. Make sure patient is stable before leaving facility.

19. Send specimens to laboratory with requisition slip.

20. Sanitize and sterilize instruments. Clean and disinfect room in preparation for next patient.

21. Dispose of soiled material in biohazard waste container.

22. Perform hand hygiene.

23. Document patient's record as needed.

NOTE: The physician charts the details of the procedure.

PREPARATION OF PATIENT'S SKIN

Although skin cannot be sterilized, it can be cleaned using medical aseptic technique. Careful cleansing of skin before performing a surgical procedure will reduce the number of microorganisms on it. This will decrease the chance of carrying infection-producing microorganisms through the skin during an invasive procedure. The physician may require that the surgical site be shaved prior to surgery; if so, care must be taken to avoid scraping or cutting the skin. Some physicians feel that the risks of shaving outweigh the benefits and prefer to have only skin cleansing prior to surgery. The Institute for Healthcare Improvement (IHI) states that using a razor for hair removal prior to surgery increases the incidence of wound infection when compared to close clipping of body hair or depilatory use. The ultimate decision rests with the physician. The shave may be wet or dry. (Procedure 8-8 lists the steps to follow to prepare a patient's skin for minor surgery.)

PROCEDURE 8-8

PREPARING A PATIENT'S SKIN FOR MINOR SURGERY

ABHES VII.MA.A.1 9(n)   CAAHEP III.P (10)

OBJECTIVE: To prepare a patient's skin for surgical procedure using sterile scrub and shave.

STANDARD: This task takes 10 minutes.

EQUIPMENT AND SUPPLIES: Antiseptic germicidal soap; sterile saline; antiseptic (e.g., povidone-iodine, Betadine); sterile applicators; Mayo tray; scissors; waste receptacle; hazardous waste container; plastic bag for soiled dressing;

sterile pack containing sterile gloves; 3 to 4 towel packs; sterile basin pack with 3 basins; patient drape; sterile gauze; 4 × 4 sponge pack with 12 to 24 sponges; shave preparation kit; patient's record; pen.

STEPS:

1. Check physician's orders, and check for patient allergies.
2. Perform hand hygiene.
3. Assemble equipment by placing pack on Mayo stand or side tray and opening outer wraps.
4. Identify patient, and explain procedure.
5. Have patient remove appropriate clothing and put on gown. Ask patient to void if necessary.
6. Position and drape patient to expose operative site.
7. Unwrap basin pack. Pour germicidal soap solution into one basin, sterile saline into second basin, antiseptic into third basin.

NOTE: Liquids are poured prior to donning sterile gloves.

8. Perform surgical scrub, and apply sterile gloves.
9. Drape skin with two towels placed 3 to 5 inches above and below surgical site.
10. With sterile gauze or a sponge, apply soapy solution to patient's skin. Using a circular motion, start at site of proposed incision and move outward (Figure 8-8). Pass over each skin area only once. Immediately place each used sponge into waste receptacle.
11. Use fresh gauze or a fresh sponge for each cleansing wipe. Repeat this process until area is completely washed. Last area cleansed will be outer edges.
12. Rinse using sterile saline on clean gauze or a clean sponge. Pat dry with dry gauze only on area that has been washed. Avoid touching any other skin area.

If shave is ordered, proceed as follows:

1. Apply soap solution to site area. Remove razor from shave preparation pack.
2. If hair is long, it may be cut with scissors prior to shaving.
3. Pull skin taut, and shave surgical site in same direction as hair is growing. Rinse with a saline solution using single-pass circular motion as before, and pat area dry.
4. Reapply soap solution to area, and repeat step 3, according to your office policy (about 5 minutes).
5. Pat entire area dry with third sterile towel.

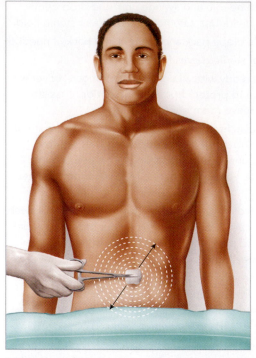

FIGURE 8-8   **Preparing the patient's skin at the surgical site.**

6. Apply antiseptic solution using two cotton applicators in same single pass in a circular motion. If povidone-iodine is used, be sure to ask patient about allergies to iodine or shellfish.
7. Cover prepared surgical site with remaining sterile towel.
8. Properly dispose of gloves and soiled materials in biohazard waste container.

To dispose of soiled dressings, use following steps:

1. Remove gloves.
2. Place one hand into empty plastic bag.
3. Using bag-covered hand, pick up all soiled materials. With other hand, pull outside of bag over soiled dressings. Dispose of bag in hazardous waste container.
4. Perform hand hygiene.
5. Document procedure in patient's record.

CHARTING EXAMPLE: 07/16/XX 9:00 A.M. Surgical prep on outer area of L forearm performed per physician's orders using povidone-iodine. No cuts or lesions noted in area. · · · · · · · · · · ·
· J. Keen, CMA (AAMA)

Cleansing Minor Wounds

A wound must be cleaned before suturing or sterile dressing can be applied. The physician determines the way wound cleansing is performed in a facility. Warm water and soap are used to remove surface dirt from around the wound area. To clean a wound, use sterile gauze square or a swab. Work from clean area near the wound outward to the less clean area. This is done to prevent dragging microorganisms over the wound. A linear wound is cleansed from top to bottom

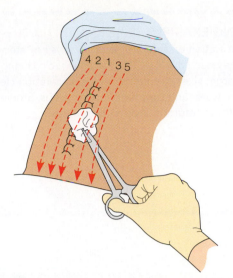

FIGURE 8-9 Cleanse a linear wound by using a new sterile gauze pad for each stroke. Begin next to the wound, and work from the top to the bottom of the wound area.

with one stroke per sterile gauze square or swab. Use a new sterile gauze square or swab for each stroke. (To cleanse an open wound, cleanse in circular manner as described in Procedure 8-8. Also see Figure 8-9 for cleaning a linear

wound.) Always clean at least 1 inch beyond the edges of the wound if a dressing is to be applied. If no dressing is to be applied, clean 2 inches beyond the edges of the wound.

Assisting with Sutures

Suturing is performed to close lacerations or incisions. Sterile scrub and materials are required. The size and depth of the wound or incision determine whether suturing will be performed. Suturing is also done to control bleeding. The type of suture materials used depends on the location of the wound. Some sutures are absorbable and do not need to be removed. Physicians usually suture a wound, but removing sutures may be done by medical assistants or other appropriately trained health care providers. Prior to suturing, the wound must be carefully cleaned as described in Procedure 8-9. The type and size of suture materials and needles are determined by the physician. After sutures are removed, the area may be redressed or left open, depending on the physician's orders. If the wound is deep and contains foreign material or excess **exudate** (discharge), wound irrigation may be requested. (Procedure 8-10 lists the steps for assisting with sutures. The steps for irrigating a wound are listed later in this chapter in Procedure 8-14.)

PROCEDURE 8-9

CLEANING A MINOR WOUND
ABHES VII.MA.A.1 9(n)   CAAHEP III.P (10)

OBJECTIVE: To clean a minor wound using aseptic technique

STANDARD: This task takes about 10 minutes, depending on the size of the wound area.

EQUIPMENT AND SUPPLIES: Sterile gauze; sterile gloves; sterile water or other cleaning solution ordered by the physician; sterile basin; sterile drapes; biohazard waste container.

STEPS:

1. Check physician's orders and patient allergies.
2. Perform hand hygiene.
3. Identify patient, and assess wound area to determine amount and size of supplies needed.
4. Only sterile solutions (water or other solutions per physician's orders) should be used to clean a wound.
5. Set up Mayo tray or side tray with sterile towel. Place sterile basin on field.
6. Pour sterile cleansing solution into sterile basin.
7. Place sterile gauze square of appropriate size in solution, or use commercially prepared swabs.
8. Drape wound as needed.
9. Open sterile dressing packs as needed.
10. Don sterile gloves.
11. Clean wound around site using one downward-motion swipe per gauze square or swab. If wound is rounded, start clean from area closest to center of wound, and work outward in circular motion. Do not go over same area with same gauze square or swab.
12. Clean gently. Repeat if wound still appears dirty.
13. Proceed as directed by physician to dress wound, or assist with suturing if necessary.
14. Anchor dressing according to facility policy.
15. Remove gloves. Dispose of soiled materials in biohazard waste container.

16. Perform hand hygiene.
17. Document patient's record, including size and appearance of wound and any treatment.

CHARTING EXAMPLE: 07/16/XX 10:00 A.M. Pt. presented with 2" laceration on sole of L foot. Pt. says he "stepped on a shell at the beach this A.M." Last tetanus rec'd during last visit. No discharge; sl. erythema on edges. Laceration cleansed with sterile water and povidone-iodine swabs. Sterile dressing applied. Pt. to return in 2 days for recheck. · P. Evans, CMA, (AAMA)

PROCEDURE 8-10

ASSISTING WITH SUTURING

ABHES VII.MA.A.1 9(n)   CAAHEP III.P (10)

OBJECTIVE: To assist with suture repair of an incision or laceration, using sterile technique.

STANDARD: This task takes 5–10 minutes, depending on size of incision or laceration.

EQUIPMENT AND SUPPLIES: Mayo stand; side stand; anesthetic; transfer forceps and container; sterile saline; waste container/plastic bag; biohazard waste container; sharps container; sterile gloves (2 pairs), sterile packs; (patient drape, towel pack with four towels); 4 × 4 gauze sponge pack; scalpel blades pack (Nos. 10 and 15); needle and syringe pack (syringe and needle pack per physician's orders); 2 sterile basins; suture pack (scalpel handle, needle holder, thumb forceps); 2 scissors; 3 hemostats; patient's record; pen.

NOTE: This procedure requires sterile scrub and gloving.

STEPS:

1. Check physician's orders, and check for patient allergies.
2. Perform hand hygiene.
3. Identify patient, and explain procedure.
4. Check that signed consent form is in patient's record.
5. Inquire about patient allergies and last tetanus injection.
6. Assemble and set up equipment and supplies on sterile field.
7. Perform surgical scrub, and don sterile gloves.
8. Clean and dry wound as in Procedure 8-9, using solutions per physician's orders.
9. Remove gloves, and dispose of them in biohazard waste container.
10. Perform hand hygiene, and assist physician either with sterile gloves or using transfer forceps to pass instruments and swab area with sterile gauze.
11. Pass instruments to physician, using a firm snap of handle into his or her hand.
12. Sponge wound area to keep free of drainage.
13. Mount needle into needle holder and pass as one unit to physician, using care to keep suture within sterile field. Pass needle holder with needle pointing outward. Hold suture with other hand, and do not let go of it until physician sees it.
14. Using suture scissors, cut suture as directed by physician (usually ⅛ to ¼ inch from knot).
15. Wipe closed wound once with a sponge and discard appropriately. Repeat as needed.
16. Dress wound per physician's orders.
17. When procedure is complete, remove gloves and perform hand hygiene before assisting patient.
18. Allow patient to rest and recover from procedure. Periodically check vital signs according to facility policy.
19. Provide clear oral and written postoperative instructions for patient and caregiver. Make sure patient is stable before discharging.

20. Don PPE.
21. Dispose of supplies per OSHA guidelines.
22. Clean, sanitize, and sterilize instruments. Clean and sanitize room in preparation for next patient.
23. Document procedure in patient's record.
24. Perform hand hygiene.

CHARTING EXAMPLE: 07/17/XX 1:00 P.M. Pt. presented with laceration to R forearm (1 × 2 cm). Wd cleaned and dried. Dr. Walsh used 8 nonabsorbable Ethicon sutures to close wound after injecting 1% lidocaine into site. Last tetanus 2 years ago. Postcare instructions given, verbal and written; understanding verified. Follow-up appointment scheduled for 7/22/XX. · B. Smith, RMA

DRESSING CHANGE AND REMOVING SUTURES AND STAPLES

When changing a dressing, it is important to note the type of drainage or exudate present. The following are the terms used:

- **Serous.** A watery clear exudate composed mainly of serum.
- **Purulent.** A thickish exudate composed of pus; may be greenish yellow, depending on causative agent.
- **Sanguineous.** A bright to dark red exudate that contains blood.
- **Serosanguineous.** A clear blood-tinged exudate that contains both blood and serum.

- **Purosanguineous.** An exudate containing blood and pus.

Both sutures and staples may be used to close an incision or laceration. Recently a topical glue (Dermabond) has been approved to close wounds. It is a noninvasive synthetic that acts like superglue on the wound, providing waterproofing and not requiring a dressing. It does not require removal and sloughs off after 7 to 10 days. Other types of skin closures, such as adhesive strips and butterfly bandages, are widely used for smaller wounds. Removing staples and sutures often requires removing a soiled dressing and applying a new sterile dressing and perhaps bandages. (Procedure 8-11 follows, as do the procedures listing the steps to remove sutures and staples and to apply and remove adhesive strips.)

PROCEDURE 8-11

CHANGING A STERILE DRESSING

ABHES VII.MA.A.1 9(n)   CAAHEP III.P (10)

OBJECTIVE: To change a sterile dressing maintaining sterile technique.

STANDARD: This task takes 5 minutes.

EQUIPMENT AND SUPPLIES: Mayo stand or side table; disposable gloves; antiseptic solution or swabs; solution container; prepackaged dressing pack containing antiseptic solution or swabs; sterile gloves; sterile thumb dressing forceps; sterile cotton balls; sterile gloves; sterile normal saline; tape; scissors; waste container for dressing; biohazard waste container; patient's record; pen.

STEPS:

1. Check physician's orders, and check for patient allergies.
2. Perform hand hygiene.

3. Identify patient, and explain procedure.
4. Assemble equipment on Mayo stand or side table.
5. Open sterile packs, preserving sterility.
6. Place bag for soiled dressing near incision. Arrange them so you avoid reaching across field.
7. Cut and place tape strips on table edge.
8. Don clean gloves.
9. Remove tape slowly, pulling tape toward wound on each side. If dressing is stuck to wound surface, moisten with sterile saline.
10. Remove soiled dressing, and dispose of it in bag provided.
11. Observe incision for signs of infection, swelling, or drainage. If discharge is excessive, obtain a wound culture according to facility policy.

12. Remove gloves and discard.

13. Perform hand hygiene.

14. Don sterile gloves.

15. Cleanse incision site according to facility policy with 4 × 4 gauze pads soaked in normal saline or with sterile antiseptic swabs. (Ask physician to view wound if infection is present.) Cleanse from top down with one swipe and discard, or cleanse outward from middle of incision in circular motion. Discard swab or gauze square after each swipe.

16. Place 4 × 4 gauze square over incision, taking care not to touch incision or patient with gloves to prevent contamination. If contamination occurs, reglove.

17. Secure dressing per physician's orders.

18. Remove gloves, and discard in hazardous waste container.

19. Perform hand hygiene.

20. Document patient's record.

CHARTING EXAMPLE: 07/17/XX 2:00 P.M. Dressing changed on R knee. Small amount of serosanguineous exudate present. Cleaned site and reapplied sterile dressing. Postcare instructions given, and understanding verified. Pt. to return in one wk. · L. Perez, CMA (AAMA)

PROCEDURE 8-12

REMOVING SUTURES AND STAPLES

ABHES VII.MA.A.1 9(n)   CAAHEP III.P (10)

OBJECTIVE: To remove sutures or staples per physician's orders using proper sterile technique.

STANDARD: This task takes 5 minutes.

EQUIPMENT AND SUPPLIES: Sterile suture removal pack (suture scissors, sterile gauze squares, thumb forceps); bag for dressing disposal; biohazard waste container; patient's record; pen; skin antiseptic; sterile gloves. For staple removal: sterile staple remover; clean gloves; dressing disposal bag; antiseptic solution; sterile dressings; adhesive strips or butterfly tape.

STEPS:

1. Review patient's record, and check for patient allergies.

2. Identify patient, and explain procedure.

3. Assemble equipment and supplies.

4. Perform hand hygiene.

5. Don gloves.

6. Remove soiled dressing as in Procedure 8-11.

7. Discard soiled dressing in bag.

8. Remove gloves.

9. Perform hand hygiene.

10. Open suture pack, and pour antiseptic solution into container.

11. Don sterile gloves.

12. Clean area around sutures to remove any exudate.

13. Using thumb forceps, gently lift one knot of suture away from skin and place curved tip of suture scissors under suture next to knot so contaminated portion of suture is not pulled through skin. (Figure 8-10A and 8-10B).

14. Cut suture, and with forceps pull suture up and out of incision, removing entire suture. Lay removed sutures on gauze square (to be counted when procedure completed).

15. Clean wound with antiseptic and allow to dry, wiping in one direction using new gauze square each time.

16. Redress wound. *If wound not entirely closed, apply sterile adhesive strips or butterfly strips per physician's orders.*

For staple removal:

1. Follow steps 1–11 above.

2. Clean and remove exudate with sterile 4 × 4 gauze square pad. Check to see if wound is **approximated** (edges brought together).

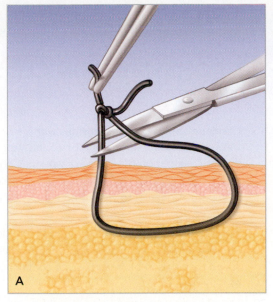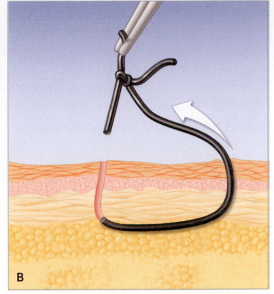

FIGURE 8-10 (A) Removal of sutures; (B) after cutting the suture, pull gently, taking care to pull so the suture material outside the wound is not pulled through the tissue.

3. Place lower tip of staple remover under staple (Figure 8-11A).

4. Press handles together to depress staple at center, and gently lift straight up (Figure 8-11B).

5. Lift staple remover device over disposal bag, and release handles to discard staple.

6. Continue until all staples are removed.

7. Cleanse wound area, and redress as above if ordered.

For both procedures:

1. Remove gloves.

2. Perform hand hygiene.

3. Document procedure in patient's record.

CHARTING EXAMPLE: 07/17/XX 3:00 P.M. Removed 5 sutures from well-healed incision. Steri-Strips applied. Postcare instructions, verbal and written, given to patient. Understanding verified. · · · · · · · · · · · · · · · · · · J. Sullivan, RMA

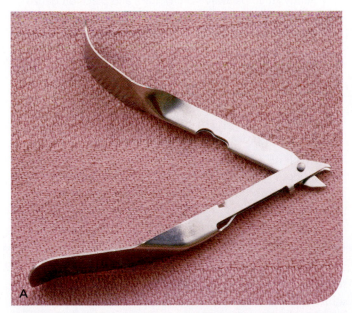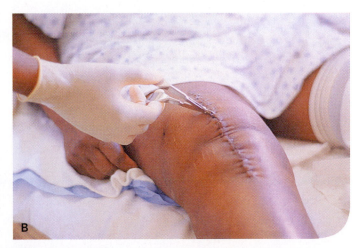

FIGURE 8-11 (A) Staple remover; (B) place lower tip of staple removal device under staple.

PROCEDURE 8-13

APPLYING AND REMOVING STERILE ADHESIVE SKIN CLOSURES

ABHES VII.MA.A.1 9(n)   CAAHEP III.P (10)

OBJECTIVE: Apply and remove sterile skin closure strips using sterile technique.

STANDARD: This task takes 5 minutes.

EQUIPMENT AND SUPPLIES: Clean gloves; sterile gloves; sterile adhesive skin closures; antiseptic solution; sterile 4×4 gauze pads; sterile dressing forceps; antiseptic swabs with povidone-iodine; tape; patient's record; pen; biohazard waste container.

STEPS:

1. Check physician's orders, and check for patient allergies.
2. Identify patient, and explain procedure.
3. Perform hand hygiene.
4. Assemble equipment and supplies.
5. Don gloves, remove dressing and bandages, and clean and dry wound per Procedure 8-11.
6. Remove gloves.
7. Perform hand hygiene.
8. Prepare a sterile field by opening packs on Mayo stand or side tray.
9. Open antiseptic solution (tincture of benzoin or as ordered by physician).
10. Apply antiseptic as ordered around wound.
11. Open sterile pack of adhesive strips and drop on sterile field.
12. Don sterile gloves.
13. Fold in half cardboard square on which adhesive strips are attached. Use sterile dressing forceps to peel off one strip at a time.
14. On dry skin surface, apply strip over center of wound, and press one end firmly to skin. Stretch strip over wound to approximate wound, and press firmly on other side of wound.
15. Continue applying adhesive strips with a strip midway between middle and one end of wound. Apply next strip in same manner on other side of wound. Continue to apply at ⅛-inch intervals until wound is closed.
16. Apply strips parallel to wound on either side once wound has been approximated.
17. Apply sterile dry dressing if ordered by physician.
18. Remove and discard gloves appropriately. Dispose of soiled materials in biohazard waste container.
19. Perform hand hygiene.
20. Provide postcare instruction and verify understanding.
21. Document procedure in patient's record.

To remove adhesive strips:

1. Follow steps 1–4 above.
2. Don gloves, and remove soiled dressing, checking for bleeding or drainage. Dispose of soiled dressing in bag provided.
3. Check incision for signs of infection and drainage.
4. Position a 4×4 gauze square next to wound area. Don gloves. Loosen skin closures toward incision line on both sides, leaving them intact on center of wound.
5. Gently lift strips away from wound, and place on gauze square.
6. Cleanse site with antiseptic swab, and apply a dry sterile dressing if ordered.
7. Dispose of all soiled materials in biohazard waste container, and perform hand hygiene.
8. Provide patient with postcare instructions, and verify understanding.
9. Document procedure in patient's record.

CHARTING EXAMPLE: 07/17/XX 4:00 P.M. Wound approximation good. No sign of infection. 3 strips removed from top of L foot. Cleansed area and provided postcare instructions, verified understanding. · · · · · · · · · · · · · · · Z. Armando, RMA

Wound Irrigation and Packing

A wound is a break in the skin, whatever the cause, and is prone to infection. Some wounds produce an excess of exudate that can delay healing. The physician may order irrigation of a wound with a specific type of sterile solution. Often sterile normal saline solution or **Ringer's solution** (an aqueous solution of the chlorides of sodium, potassium, and calcium) are used for irrigating. Strict observance of sterile technique is mandatory. To promote better drainage from certain types of wounds, the wound may be packed with sterile packing gauze or gauze squares. **Debridement** is a method of removing affected wound tissue that may be done surgically or using chemical, mechanical, or **autolytic** (self-dissolution or self-digestion of tissue) means.

Incision and drainage (I&D) is often performed as an outpatient procedure. (The steps for assisting with this procedure are a combination of Procedure 8-7 and Procedure 8-15 and are not listed separately in this text. Procedure 8-14 provides steps for irrigating a wound, and Procedure 8-15 lists steps for packing a wound.)

PROCEDURE 8-14

IRRIGATING A WOUND

ABHES VII.MA.A.1 9(n)   CAAHEP III.P (10)

OBJECTIVE: To irrigate a wound to remove excessive exudate using sterile technique.

STANDARD: This task takes 15 minutes.

EQUIPMENT AND SUPPLIES: Mayo tray/side table; sterile gloves; sterile irrigation kit (irrigating syringe, basin, container for solution); waterproof pad; nonsterile gloves; waterproof waste bag; equipment for dressing change; patient's record; pen.

STEPS:

1. Check physician's orders, and check for patient allergies.

NOTE: Administration of pain medication may be ordered for this procedure and should be given beforehand to allow time for its effects to begin (approximately 30 minutes).

2. Assemble equipment and supplies.
3. Identify patient, and explain procedure.
4. Perform hand hygiene.
5. Position patient for easy access to wound and patient comfort.
6. Place waterproof pad under area to be irrigated.
7. Don nonsterile gloves, and remove dressing noting discharge, color, and amount of drainage and odor.
8. Discard dressing into plastic bag.
9. Remove and discard gloves.
10. Perform hand hygiene.
11. Open sterile irrigation kit, and set up sterile field.
12. Pour room-temperature irrigating solution into sterile basin.
13. Don sterile gloves, and place sterile basin under wound area to collect irrigating solution.
14. Draw solution into irrigating syringe (35 mL) or bulb syringe and irrigate wound until all solution has been used and no further drainage noted (Figure 8-12).

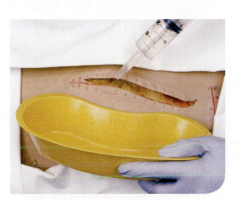

FIGURE 8-12   Irrigating a wound.

NOTE: The force with which the solution is introduced to the wound is important and is governed by the size of the syringe and tip and proximity to wound. Too much force may be damaging and painful. Too little pressure may not irrigate sufficiently.

15. Dry area around wound with sterile gauze square and examine wound again.
16. Apply sterile dressing as ordered.
17. Dispose of equipment and supplies properly.
18. Remove and dispose of gloves in biohazard waste container.
19. Perform hand hygiene.
20. Document procedure in patient's record.

CHARTING EXAMPLE: 07/19/XX 11:30 A.M. Wd. on L calf irrigated using 30 mL of sterile normal saline. Dressing showed mod. amt. of greenish yellowish exudate. Dr. Ames was notified about drainage. After irrigation wound appeared clean with some redness around edges. Pt. tolerated procedure well. Redressed wd. with sterile dry dressing. Pt. to return on 07/20/XX for wd. care. · K. Osaki, CMA (AAMA).

PROCEDURE 8-15

PACKING A WOUND

ABHES VII.MA.A.1 9(n)   CAAHEP III.P (10)

OBJECTIVE: To pack a wound per physician's orders using sterile technique.

STANDARD: This task takes 15 minutes, depending on condition of the patient.

EQUIPMENT AND SUPPLIES: Normal saline solution; dressing pack if available or sterile packing gauze or 4 × 4 gauze pads; sterile dressings; sterile forceps; sterile scissors; tape; plastic bag; clean gloves; sterile gloves; patient's record; pen.

STEPS:

1. Check physician's orders, and check for patient allergies. Follow orders for medication prior to procedure as needed.
2. Identify patient, and explain procedure.
3. Assemble equipment and supplies.
4. Perform hand hygiene, and don gloves.
5. Remove dressing (see Procedure 8-11) by pulling old tape toward wound from both sides and lifting off and discarding in plastic bag at site. (If dry, moisten dressing and old packing with sterile saline.)
6. Examine wound and surrounding skin area for size, shape, signs of infection, or exudate.
7. Check patient for level of pain, offer reassuring words to allay fears.
8. Remove and discard gloves properly, and perform hand hygiene.
9. Set up sterile field materials needed for dressing change, including packing materials.
10. Pour sterile saline solution into sterile container.
11. Don sterile gloves.
12. Clean area with sterile saline, and dry with sterile gauze.
13. Using sterile forceps, pack wound with appropriate sterile packing material.

NOTE: The type and size of packing material are dependent on size and type of wound and physician's orders. If gauze pads are used, they should be moistened with sterile saline before use.

14. When packing is complete, cut with sterile scissors and leave a small wick.
15. Redress wound with sterile dressing as ordered.
16. Dispose of used equipment and supplies appropriately. Remove gloves and dispose of them appropriately.
17. Perform hand hygiene.
18. Document procedure in patient's record.

CHARTING EXAMPLE: 07/19/XX 12:15 P.M. Dressing removed from Lg. abscess on R Thigh. Mod. amt. purulent discharge noted. Wd. culture obtained and sent to Memorial Lab for C&S. Wd. packed with ¼ inch iodoform gauze and redressed with dry sterile dressing. Written, verbal wound care provided. Understanding verified. Pt. tolerated procedure well. · H. Hansboro, CMA (AAMA)

Other Procedures

The number of minor surgery procedures performed in every specialty practice are too numerous to cover in this text; however, the three that follow are relatively common. Therefore Procedure 8-16: Assisting with Excision of a Sebaceous Cyst, Procedure 8-17: Assisting with Aspiration of Joint Fluid, and Procedure 8-18: Assisting with a Hemorrhoid Thrombectomy follow. Laser surgeries are frequently performed in a variety of specialty practices and facilities, thus Procedure 8-19: Preparing a Patient for Laser Surgery is also presented.

Biopsy Procedures

Biopsy is a diagnostic examination of tissue removed from a growth or organ. Biopsies are performed on many types of tissues, for example, liver, kidney, brain, breast, lymph nodes, lung, and bone marrow. A bone marrow biopsy specimen is removed from the iliac crest, sternum, anterior or posterior iliac spine in adults or from the tibia in children. Bone marrow biopsies are performed to detect diseases such as leukemia.

Several other procedures are performed to remove fluid from a body cavity or joint (Procedure 8-17). A **thoracentesis**

PROCEDURE 8-16

ASSISTING WITH EXCISION OF A SEBACEOUS CYST

ABHES VII.MA.A.1 9(n)   CAAHEP III.P (10)

OBJECTIVE: To assist with removal of a sebaceous cyst while observing sterile technique.

STANDARD: This task takes 15–20 minutes, depending on size and location of cyst.

EQUIPMENT AND SUPPLIES: Mayo stand/side table; iodoform gauze or sterile Penrose drains; gloves, sterile and nonsterile; PPE; skin prep supplies; sterile gauze squares; fenestrated drape; dressing; bandages; tape; alcohol pads; culture materials; antiseptic solution as ordered; sterile specimen container with preservative; minor surgery sterile pack containing curved scissors, curved hemostat, scalpel handle and blade, needle holder, suture material with needle, tissue forceps, and Mayo scissors; other items preferred by physician; biohazard waste container; sharps container; basin for soiled instruments; patient's record; pen.

STEPS:

1. Check patient's record for orders.
2. Check for signed consent form, allergies, date of last tetanus booster.
3. Assemble equipment and supplies.
4. Identify patient, and explain procedure.
5. Perform hand hygiene.
6. Place patient in comfortable position, lying down to avoid **vertigo** (dizziness).
7. Don PPE as needed, and perform skin preparation ordered by physician (Procedure 8-8).
8. Set up sterile field, and cover until physician is ready to perform procedure.
9. Clean top of vial of anesthetic, and hold vial for physician to aspirate required amount of medication.
10. Assist physician as in Procedure 8-7 either by donning sterile gloves or by assisting without sterile gloves using transfer forceps or dropping items onto sterile field.
11. Offer calming words to patient to relieve anxiety.
12. Hold specimen container as needed, and label immediately.

Postprocedure:

13. Don sterile gloves.
14. Clean area around wound with sterile 4 × 4 gauze squares.
15. Dress wound, and bandage as ordered. (Several layers of dressing may be necessary to absorb exudate.)
16. Dispose of soiled items appropriately. Discard items in sharps and biohazard waste containers as needed.
17. Clean examination room.
18. Check patient's vital signs per facility policy.
19. Provide postcare information in verbal and written form. Verify patient understanding.
20. Answer questions and schedule follow-up appointment.
21. Perform hand hygiene.
22. Document patient's record.
23. Phone or fax in medication orders as needed.

CHARTING EXAMPLE: 07/23/XX 10:15 A.M. Sebaceous cyst excised from R scapula by Dr. Rosen. Sm amt. of purulent exudate released. Specimen for C&S sent to Memorial Lab. Sterile Penrose drain inserted. Wd dressed. Pt. to return in A.M. for recheck. Written and verbal wound care instructions given. Verified patient understanding. BP 138/82, P 74. Pt. tolerated procedure well. · D. Patel, RMA

PROCEDURE 8-17

ASSISTING WITH ASPIRATION OF JOINT FLUID

ABHES VII.MA.A.1 9(n)   CAAHEP III.P (10)

OBJECTIVE: To assist physician with removal of excess synovial fluid from a joint while observing sterile technique.

STANDARD: This task takes 10–15 minutes.

EQUIPMENT AND SUPPLIES: Gloves sterile and nonsterile; PPE; skin preparation supplies; anesthetic as ordered; cortisone medication as ordered; sterile gauze pads; alcohol pads; dressing; bandages; tape; culture tube; specimen container; laboratory requisitions; minor surgery pack containing syringe and needles for anesthesia, sterile basin for aspirated fluid, fenestrated drape, syringe and needle for aspiration, hemostat, and sterile gauze pads; patient's record; pen; biohazard waste container; basin for soiled instruments.

STEPS:

1. Check patient's record for signed consent form and orders. Check for patient allergies.
2. Assemble equipment and supplies.
3. Identify patient, and explain procedure. Avoid false reassurance statements (e.g., "Everything will be fine"). Allay patient's fears as much as possible.
4. Perform hand hygiene.
5. Position patient in supine position.
6. Set up sterile field, and cover until physician is ready to perform procedure.
7. Don PPE as needed.
8. Perform skin preparation as in Procedure 8-8.
9. Assist physician by cleaning top of vial of anesthetic and holding it for physician to withdraw anesthetic.
10. Assist physician as needed while he or she inserts a sterile long needle into synovial sac to aspirate fluid. (A hemostat is used to stabilize needle hub, and syringe is removed from needle. Fluid is expelled into sterile basin. Syringe is reattached and aspiration by physician continues until all fluid removed.) Take care to observe sterile technique throughout procedure.

Postcare:

11. Apply sterile gloves.
12. Cleanse area around wound with sterile 4 × 4 gauze pads and antiseptic per physician's orders.
13. Dress and bandage wound as ordered.
14. Dispose of items in appropriate manner according to OSHA guidelines.
15. Remove gloves and dispose of them in biohazard waste container.
16. Provide written and verbal instruction on wound care to patient and caregiver. Verify patient and caregiver understanding.
17. Schedule follow-up appointment.
18. To send aspirated fluid to laboratory for testing, don PPE and gloves and put aspirated fluid into sterile container. Label immediately, and prepare for transport.
19. Remove gloves and PPE and dispose of appropriately.
20. Perform hand hygiene.
21. Document procedure in patient's record.

CHARTING EXAMPLE: 07/23/XX 1:00 P.M. 210 mL clear colorless fluid withdrawn from L knee by Dr. Ianucci after anesthesia given. Spec. sent to Memorial Lab for C&S, cell count. Written and verbal postcare instructions given. Verified patient understanding. Pt. to call to set up appointment for recheck next week. · S. English, RMA

PROCEDURE 8-18

ASSISTING WITH A HEMORRHOID THROMBECTOMY

ABHES VII.MA.A.1 9(n)   CAAHEP III.P (10)

OBJECTIVE: To assist physician with incising inflamed hemorrhoids and removal of thrombus and/or removal of hemorrhoids with laser, electrosurgery, cryosurgery, or banding while observing sterile technique.

STANDARD: This task takes 15–30 minutes.

EQUIPMENT AND SUPPLIES: *Mayo tray for sterile supplies;* syringe/needle for anesthesia; Mosquito hemostat (curved); sterile basin; sterile gauze sponges; fenestrated drapes; rubber bands if ordered by physician. *Off sterile field:* light; skin preparation supplies; sterile and nonsterile gloves; PPE; anesthesia as ordered; sterile gauze pads; perineal pad for postcare; bandage to hold pad in place; patient's record; pen; biohazard waste containers; basin for soiled instruments.

STEPS:

1. Check patient's record for signed consent form, date of last tetanus booster, and allergies.

2. Assemble equipment and supplies.

3. Identify patient, and explain procedure.

4. Allay patient's fears as much as possible.

5. Position patient in proctologic position or physician's preference.

NOTE: Hemorrhoids are internal or external varicose veins of the rectum. A thrombus can form and further inflame the vein. When this happens the vein is lanced and the thrombus is removed, observing sterile conditions, or a hemorrhoidectomy is performed. The anal sphincter is dilated, and the hemorrhoid is tied off and removed using laser surgery, cryosurgery, or electrosurgery. Elastic bands may be placed around the pedicle of the hemorrhoid to restrict the blood flow. The tissue will slough off after 7 to 10 days.

6. Drape patient, and make as comfortable as possible.

7. Set up sterile tray, and cover until physician is ready for procedure.

8. Apply PPE if necessary.

9. Perform skin preparation (as in Procedure 8-8).

10. Assist physician by cleaning top of vial of anesthetic, and hold vial while physician withdraws anesthesia.

11. Physician will continue with banding or excising of hemorrhoids. Provide comfort to patient as needed.

Postcare:

12. Assist physician with placing perineal pad on wound, and apply T-shaped bandage.

13. Dispose of used items as appropriate following OSHA guidelines. Clean area.

14. Remove gloves, and dispose of them in biohazard waste container. Perform hand hygiene.

15. Assist patient into a more comfortable position.

16. Explain postcare to patient and caregiver. A warm Sitz bath (bath taken in a sitting position) provides comfort if ordered by physician.

17. Provide written and verbal instructions, and verify understanding.

18. Schedule appointment for recheck.

19. Call or fax in medication order as needed.

20. Document procedure in patient's record.

CHARTING EXAMPLE: 07/23/XX 3:00 P.M. External hemorrhoids removed by electrosurgical procedure. Mod. amt of bleeding noted. Pt. tolerated procedure well. Verbal and written postcare instructions given with understanding verified. Rx given for Percodan 1 tab orally every 4–6 hrs as needed. Recheck scheduled for 1 week. · · · · · · · · · · · · N. Calvo, RMA

PROCEDURE 8-19

PREPARING A PATIENT FOR LASER SURGERY

ABHES VII.MA.A.1 9(l)   CAAHEP IV.P (6)

OBJECTIVE: To instruct patient about laser surgery and assist with laser surgery, observing safety precautions for patient and staff.

STANDARD: This task takes 5–10 minutes.

EQUIPMENT AND SUPPLIES: Equipment and supplies pertinent to the specific procedure, including a sterile basin with sterile saline to cool instrument quickly as needed; safety goggles for each staff member and patient; warning signs for door; patient's record; pen; gloves; biohazard waste container.

STEPS:

1. Check patient's record for signed consent form and allergies, date of last tetanus booster, and orders for type of procedure.

2. Assemble equipment and supplies.

3. Identify patient, and explain procedure.

4. Determine patient's willingness to accept instruction and level of understanding.

5. Reinforce explanation given by physician.

6. Describe operating room and equipment to be used.

7. Explain that all individuals in operating room, including patient, will wear goggles to protect eyes from damage.

8. Explain that wet drapes may be placed on patient's skin to prevent burns if needed.

9. Explain that laser surgery burns tissue and thus an odor and smoke may occur.

10. Describe machine and that physician may use a foot pedal that may be noisy.

11. Instruct patient to state if pain is felt. (Anesthetic is generally used.)

12. Explain that, depending on type of procedure, patient should not eat or drink (should be NPO) for 6 to 8 hours prior to the procedure.

13. Provide verbal and written postcare instructions, including that patient notify physician if fever over 100°F lasts for 24 hours or more postsurgery.

14. Answer questions as needed.

is performed to remove air or fluid from the pleural cavity to improve breathing. **Abdominal paracentesis** is done to remove fluid from the abdominal cavity. Excess fluid buildup in the abdominal cavity is known as **ascites** and may be found, for example, in cases of severe alcoholism. Any procedure involving penetration of a body cavity or organ requires surgical asepsis.

CRYOSURGERY

Cryosurgery involves the destruction of tissue by using extreme cold. A probe containing liquid nitrogen or carbon dioxide is used and applied directly on the involved area for a brief period. Tissue can be removed using surgical excision, cryosurgery, or cauterization. The physician determines which type of procedure will be utilized on individual patients.

9 Assisting with Medical Emergencies

PROCEDURES

Procedure 9-1 Placing a Victim in Recovery Position

Procedure 9-2 Administering Abdominal Thrusts (Heimlich Maneuver) for a Conscious Adult

Procedure 9-3 Performing Abdominal Thrusts for a Conscious Child

Procedure 9-4 Performing Back Blows and Chest Thrusts for a Conscious Choking Infant

Procedure 9-5 Performing Back Blows and Chest Thrusts for an Unconscious Infant

Procedure 9-6 Administering Abdominal Thrusts (Heimlich Maneuver) for an Unresponsive Adult or Child

Procedure 9-7 Performing Rescue Breathing for an Adult

Procedure 9-8 Performing Rescue Breathing for a Child

Procedure 9-9 Performing Rescue Breathing for an Infant

Procedure 9-10 Performing CPR for an Adult

Procedure 9-11 Performing CPR for a Child

Procedure 9-12 Performing CPR for an Infant

Procedure 9-13 Using an Automated External Defibrillator (AED)

Procedure 9-14 Maintaining the Emergency/Crash Cart

Procedure 9-15 Caring for a Fainting Patient

Procedure 9-16 Assisting a Patient During an Asthma Attack

Procedure 9-17 Assisting with an Anaphylactic Emergency

Procedure 9-18 Controlling Severe Bleeding

Procedure 9-19 Assisting with Burn Emergencies

Procedure 9-20 Assisting a Patient During a Seizure

Procedure 9-21 Applying a Tubular Gauze Bandage

Procedure 9-22 Applying an Arm Splint

TERMS TO LEARN

first responders

paramedics

intubate

logrolling

xiphoid process

umbilicus

hypovolemic shock

rule of nines

seizures

epilepsy

idiopathic

hyperthermia

hypothermia

An emergency can occur to anyone anywhere. Thus, obtaining cardiopulmonary resuscitation (CPR), automatic external defibrillator (AED), and first aid training is often a requirement of employment for all health care providers. Most medical assisting programs require students to have CPR/AED training before starting an externship. In fact it is important for everyone to have training for home and workplace emergencies.

Entire volumes are written about emergency care; however, this text addresses medical emergencies encountered in a medical office or walk-in medical facility, not in a hospital. In any medical emergency the physician on duty must be notified. In some cases emergency medical services (EMS) personnel must be notified by calling 911. EMS systems employ **first responders** who are trained to recognize medical conditions, initiate basic life support, and access other parts of the emergency medical system. The emergency crew may be staffed with **paramedics** who are licensed to provide more advanced emergency care; they may **intubate** a patient to open an airway and can start IVs and give emergency medications, provide oxygen, and perform other invasive procedures. Medical personnel must be prepared to provide EMS responders with pertinent patient information. In some cases they may be called upon to provide emergency care before the ambulance or rescue squad arrives, thereby increasing the patient's chances of survival.

Good Samaritan laws protect medical professionals and untrained bystanders who volunteer to provide aid in an emergency situation. Health care providers have the responsibility to provide care to victims according to the scope of practice in their field or, in other words, according to their license, certification, or other training. Each health care provider is required to stay with the victim until relieved by another health care provider with similar or higher level of training. All providers of care should be aware of the laws in their own state regarding emergency care. Caregivers should look for medical alert tags when assessing a patient during any emergency. It also is important to be aware of the triage policies of any facility to which the patient will be taken.

Emergency Action Planning

Each facility should have an action plan to deal with medical emergencies. The plan should include the following information:

- EMS local telephone number (if other than 911) displayed near all telephones
- Hospital emergency department's telephone number and address
- Regional poison control center telephone number
- Triage protocol for emergencies determined by physician(s) in charge
- Procedures for various emergencies determined by the physician(s) in charge
- List of personnel trained in CPR/AED
- Emergency medical cart containing items specified by physician(s) on duty

Remaining calm and being prepared are vital for providing the best emergency care to the patient. Box 9-1 lists the information to provide to EMS by telephone.

Documentation of a medical emergency should take place as soon as possible after the emergency is over. An incident report may be necessary, depending on facility policy. A copy of the incident report should be included in the patient's chart.

EMERGENCY EQUIPMENT

First aid kits should be available in all work areas and public buildings, including medical offices. A first aid kit contains supplies for dealing with minor injuries, such as gauze, tape, prepackaged antiseptic wipes, and chemical hot and cold packs. The location of first aid kits should be obvious, and kits should be easily accessible.

BOX 9-1 Information to Provide to EMS by Telephone

- Exact location of victim, including street name and number, room/apartment number if necessary
- Number of victims involved in emergency
- Conditions of victims including CC and symptoms
- Presence of Universal Emergency Medical Identification Symbol bracelet or card
- Caller's name
- Relationship of caller to victim
- Type of care already provided

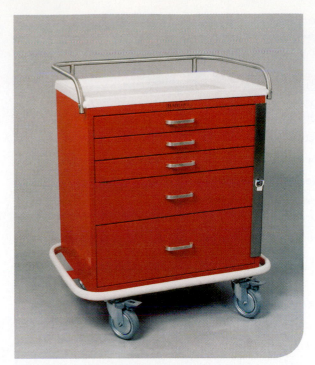

FIGURE 9-1 Emergency crash cart.

A medical emergency cart/crash cart (Figure 9-1) should contain all supplies that might be needed during an emergency and should be instantly accessible to anyone in the medical facility. A crash cart resembles a large roll-around toolbox with drawers used to store medications, intubation equipment, and other emergency supplies. (Box 9-2 lists general supplies needed in a crash cart. Table 9-1 lists emergency medications needed in each crash cart and their use.)

Crash cart supplies and equipment reflect the recommendations of the facility physician. Equipment and supplies should never be "borrowed" from a crash cart to supplement everyday supplies. The cart should be checked routinely for inventory and outdated medications and supplies. Battery-operated equipment must be recharged regularly with dates documented. In-house practice drills are helpful to prepare staff for real emergencies.

Primary Assessment

The first response to an emergency is to assess the situation and give assistance as quickly as possible without putting yourself at risk. Survey the scene to make sure it is safe to go to the victim, and don PPE if possible before providing assistance. Never move the victim of an accident or fall. The primary assessment should take not less than 5 seconds and no longer than 10 seconds. If the patient is unresponsive, check ABCs: airway, breathing, and circulation.

The airway must remain open. To establish an open airway, place one hand on the patient's forehead and the other under the patient's chin. If a neck injury *is not* a possibility, gently lift the jaw and push back; if a neck injury *is* a possibility, grasp both sides of the jaw and push forward. These positions help to keep the tongue from blocking the airway (Figure 9-2). Once the airway is open, do the following:

- Look at the chest for rise and fall of respiration.
- Listen for air moving into nose and mouth.
- Feel for pulse and movement of air from mouth.

BOX 9-2 General Supplies Needed in Crash Cart

- Adhesive tape (hypoallergenic tape)
- Airways of all sizes
- Alcohol wipes
- Bandage materials
- Bandage scissors
- Blood pressure cuff (standard, pediatric, large)
- Bulb syringe for suction
- Cardiac monitor/ECG machine
- Chemical hot and cold packs
- Defibrillator
- Elastic bandages of various sizes
- Sterile and nonsterile gloves of various sizes, including some latex free
- Intravenous tubing
- IV equipment, including poles and boards
- Laryngoscopes
- Manual resuscitator (e.g., Ambu bag)
- Needles and syringes for injection
- Otoscope/ophthalmoscope
- Oxygen mask
- Penlight
- PPE of all types
- Slings, triangle bandage
- Splints
- Sterile dressing materials
- Stethoscope
- Tongue depressors
- Tourniquet (constriction band)

TABLE 9-1 Emergency Medical Cart Medications and Medical Use

Product	Use
Activated charcoal	Binds with some poisons to prevent absorption
Adrenalin (epinephrine)	Constricts blood vessels and raises blood pressure; bronchodilator for asthma and anaphylaxis
Amobarbital sodium (Amytal)	Antianxiety, anticonvulsant
Apomorphine hydrochloride	Rapid-acting emetic
Aspirin	Heart attack; fever, except in children
Atropine	Slows heart rate, decreases body secretions, and relieves hypermotility of intestinal tract
Diazepam (Valium)*	Sedative and anticonvulsant
Digoxin (Lanoxin)	Strengthens heart muscle contractions
Dilantin	Anticonvulsant
Diphenhydramine hydrochloride (Benadryl)	Antihistamine, relieves allergic reactions
Dopamine	Increases blood pressure
Furosemide (Lasix)	Diuretic, to treat congestive heart failure (CHF)
Glucagon, sugar packets, dextrose 50%, orange juice	Hypoglycemic reactions, insulin reactions
Insulin	To reduce elevated blood sugar and hyperglycemia
Isoproterenol	Cardiac stimulant; antispasmodic for bronchospasm (injectable and inhalable forms)
IV dextrose in saline or Hater solution	Intravenous hydration
Lidocaine (Xylocaine) 0.5% or 1.0%	Local anesthetic, IV cardiac arrhythmia
Metaraminol (Aramine)	Shock
Nitroglycerin patches/tablets	Vasodilator for angina attacks
Phenobarbital*	Sedative
Prednisone	Corticosteroid for allergic reactions; respiratory symptoms
Ringer's solution	Intravenous hydration
Spirits of ammonia	Syncope
Sterile water, sterile saline	For injections
Syrup of Ipecac	Emetic

*Indicates controlled substance that must be kept in locked cabinet.

If the patient is not breathing, begin rescue breathing immediately once the airway is cleared. A face mask with a one-way valve or a bag-valve mask device, if available, is recommended when performing rescue breathing. Once the airway is open, (a) look, listen, and feel; (b) give 2 breaths; (c) check carotid/brachial pulse; and (d) perform compressions. To check for circulation, feel the carotid artery in an adult (Figure 9-3) and the brachial artery in an infant or small child. If no pulse is present, begin CPR at once. AEDs are available in many facilities, including schools and public buildings. Training in use of AEDs is included as part of most CPR classes.

Secondary Assessment

After breathing and circulation are reestablished, the patient may be evaluated for trauma or severe bleeding. If the victim is conscious, instruct him or her not to move, introduce yourself, and ask permission to treat. In an unconscious patient, immobilize the neck and spine if possible. This is done by **logrolling**, or moving the patient as a single unit to prevent spinal injury.

Questions are asked of the patient to discover further information about his or her condition and possibly to discover less obvious problems than those defined in the primary

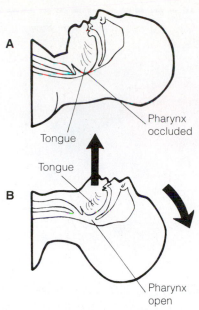

FIGURE 9-2   The position of an unconscious person's tongue: (A) airway occluded, (B) airway open.

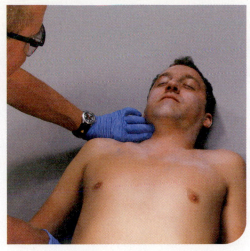

FIGURE 9-3   Checking the carotid pulse.

assessment. Evaluate the following during the secondary assessment evaluate the following:

- **General appearance.**   Facial expressions, motor activity, speech, medicine bottles in pocket/purse, medical bracelet or necklace, moisture, and color of skin.
- **Level of consciousness.**   Awake and Alert = A; responds to voice = V; responds only to pain = P; unresponsive = U.
- **Vital signs.**   Measure T, P, R, BP as soon as possible; monitor for changes while awaiting EMS.

- **Skin.**   Moist cool skin may indicate shock; note color of skin and extremities.
- **Location and level of pain.**

After the primary and secondary assessments are done, the patient is examined by a physician and a complete physical exam (PE) is done.

Recovery Position

The recovery position (Procedure 9-1) is used for an unresponsive patient who is breathing and has a pulse. It helps to maintain an open airway. Generally, no overt signs of trauma are present.

PROCEDURE 9-1

PLACING A VICTIM IN RECOVERY POSITION

ABHES VII.MA.A.1 9(o)(5)   CAAHEP XI.P (10)

OBJECTIVE: To place a victim in recovery position until EMS arrives.

STANDARD: The time this task takes depends on the condition of the patient.

EQUIPMENT AND SUPPLIES: Flat, firm surface.

STEPS:

1. Assess for potential trauma, especially to head and neck. If no trauma is obvious and breathing and pulse are present, place patient on a flat, firm surface if possible.
2. Kneel by victim's neck and straighten his or her legs.

3. Place victim's arm nearest to you at right angles to his or her body with elbow bent and palm upward.
4. Place victim's other arm across chest, and place hand near his or her cheek.
5. Grasp far side of victim's thigh above knee and pull thigh up toward his or her body.
6. Grasp victim's shoulder that is farthest away from you, and roll victim toward you onto his or her side.
7. Ensure upper leg, including knee and hip, are bent at right angles over lower leg.

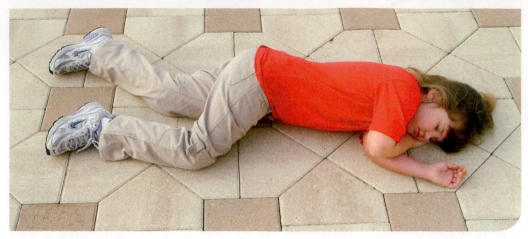

FIGURE 9-4 Patient in the recovery position.

8. Tilt head back to maintain open airway, and place victim's hand under his or her cheek to maintain head tilt (Figure 9-4).

9. Monitor victim closely for breathing and circulation until EMS arrives. If breathing or circulation stops, begin rescue breathing and CPR.

CHARTING EXAMPLE: 08/22/XX 9:10 A.M. Patient found unresponsive but with pulse and breathing. Found on floor of exam room 1A. No signs of trauma observed. Pt. placed in recovery position. EMS called at 9:13 A.M. · J. Lock, RMA

Blocked Airway, Rescue Breathing, Maintaining Circulation

Choking is a common cause of airway obstruction. If you think an individual is choking, ask if it is so. If the individual can speak, do not do anything except reassure and monitor the individual.

Barrier devices for performing rescue breathing and CPR offer protection for the rescuer. The two forms of barrier devices in use are the face shield and the face mask. The face shield is made of a clear plastic or silicon sheet and is placed over the victim's face to prevent direct contact with the victim during rescue breathing. Face shields are small, flexible, and portable. Face masks are hard-plastic devices that fit over the mouth and nose. They are more costly than face shields and not as easy for people to carry on their person. (See Figure 9-5A and Figure 9-5B for examples of a face mask and a face shield.)

If the situation deteriorates to a point where the person is unable to cough or speak, ask permission to assist; if possible, ask a co-worker to call 911 and proceed with the steps listed in Procedure 9-2.

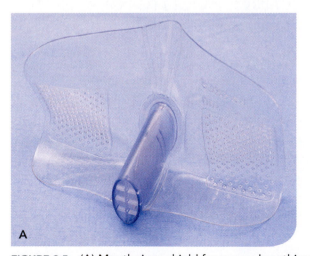

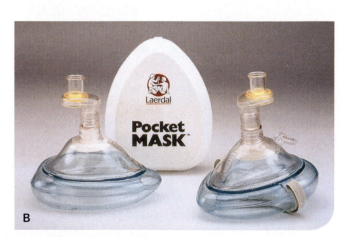

FIGURE 9-5 (A) Mouthpiece shield for rescue breathing; (B) pocket mask for rescue breathing.

ADMINISTERING ABDOMINAL THRUSTS (HEIMLICH MANEUVER) FOR A CONSCIOUS ADULT

ABHES VII.MA.A.1 9(o)(5)   CAAHEP XI.P (10)

OBJECTIVE: To be able to perform abdominal thrusts (Heimlich maneuver) on a conscious patient to expel a foreign object.

STANDARD: The time this task takes depends on the condition of the patient.

EQUIPMENT AND SUPPLIES: None.

STEPS:

1. Assess choking individual for pale color progressing to cyanosis.
2. Observe for familiar signs of choking.
   - Ask individual if he or she can speak?
   - Ask individual to hold hand on neck if choking (universal sign of choking). (See Figure 9-6A.)

> **HIPAA Alert!** Ask permission to assist patient if patient is conscious.

3. If unable to speak or coughing is ineffective, begin abdominal thrusts. (Hand and fist position for abdominal thrusts are illustrated in Figure 9-6C.)
4. Stand behind individual and place arms around individual's chest (Figure 9-6B).
5. Position hands halfway between **xiphoid process** (tip of the sternum) and **umbilicus** (belly button). Place thumb near xiphoid process and index finger on umbilicus.
6. Make a fist with one hand, and press thumb side of fist into individual's abdomen above umbilicus. Place other hand over fist.
7. Press fist into individual's abdomen.
8. Using a rotating motion of hands, forcefully thrust your hands in upward direction to assist in expelling foreign body. Individual may fall over your arms.

NOTE: Repeat until foreign body is expelled. If individual becomes unconscious, proceed with administering abdominal thrusts (Heimlich maneuver) on an unconscious patient (Procedure 9-6).

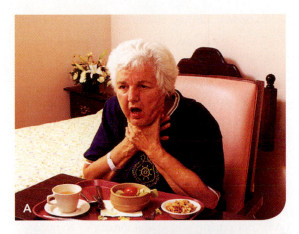

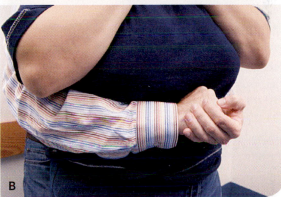

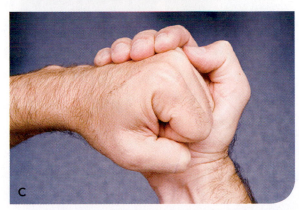

FIGURE 9-6 (A) Universal sign of choking; (B) position hands to perform abdominal thrusts (Heimlich maneuver); (C) make fist and place other hand on top to perform abdominal thrusts (Heimlich maneuver).

PROCEDURE 9-3

PERFORMING ABDOMINAL THRUSTS FOR A CONSCIOUS CHILD

ABHES VII.MA.A.1 9(o)(5) CAAHEP XI.P (10)

OBJECTIVE: To open a blocked airway for a conscious child.

STANDARD: The time this task takes depends on the condition of the patient.

EQUIPMENT AND SUPPLIES: None.

STEPS:

1. Place thumb side of fist of dominant hand just above umbilicus but below xiphoid process.
2. Place nondominant hand over fist and provide quick upward thrusts (Figure 9-7).
3. Repeat until object is expelled.
4. If child loses consciousness, proceed with steps in Procedure 9-6 for performing abdominal thrusts for an unconscious adult or child.
5. When emergency is over, perform hand hygiene.
6. Document procedure in patient's record.

CHARTING EXAMPLE: 8:35 A.M. Pt. choking on food. 4 abdominal thrusts performed with large piece of hot dog expelled. Breathing returned to normal, color good. Dr. Wing notified. · L. Cox, CMA (AAMA)

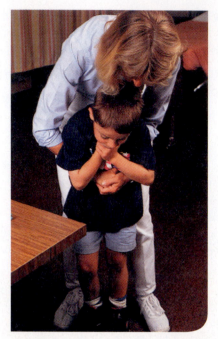

FIGURE 9-7 Conscious child being given abdominal thrusts.

PROCEDURE 9-4

PERFORMING BACK BLOWS AND CHEST THRUSTS FOR A CONSCIOUS CHOKING INFANT

ABHES VII.MA.A.1 9(o)(5) CAAHEP XI.P (10)

OBJECTIVE: To open a blocked airway for a conscious infant who is choking.

STANDARD: The time this task takes depends on condition of infant.

EQUIPMENT AND SUPPLIES: None.

STEPS:

1. Place infant face down on forearm, and give 5 back blows between scapula with heel of your hand (Figure 9-8A).
2. Turn infant over to face-up position on forearm.
3. Give 5 chest thrusts using two fingers on chest press ½ to 1 inch deep in center of sternum (Figure 9-8B).
4. Observe infant's mouth for foreign object.
5. Repeat alternating back blows and chest thrusts until object is expelled or infant resumes breathing on his or her own.

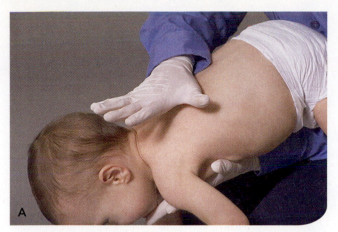

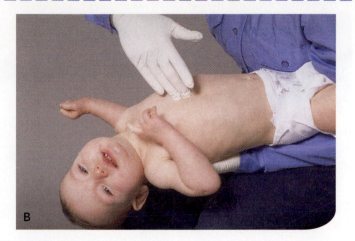

FIGURE 9-8 (A) Infant back slaps; (B) infant chest thrusts.

6. If infant becomes unconscious, notify EMS and use steps in Procedure 9-5 for using back blows and chest thrusts for an unconscious infant.

7. When emergency is over, perform hand hygiene.

8. Document procedure.

CHARTING EXAMPLE: 08/24/XX 8:05 A.M. Pt. choking. 3 cycles of back blows/chest thrust given. Round toy bead expelled. Pt. cried and pink color returned. Dr. Ames notified.
.... C. Kenney, CMA (AAMA)

PROCEDURE 9-5

PERFORMING BACK BLOWS AND CHEST THRUSTS FOR AN UNCONSCIOUS INFANT

ABHES VII.MA.A.1 9(o)(5)   CAAHEP XI.P (10)

OBJECTIVE: To open a blocked airway for an unconscious infant.

STANDARD: The time this task takes depends on condition of patient.

EQUIPMENT AND SUPPLIES: Rescue breathing mouth piece, gloves if available.

STEPS:

1. Notify EMS or call 911.

2. Don gloves. Check infant for consciousness/responsiveness.

3. Gently tilt back infant's head without hyperextending neck (Figure 9-9A).

4. Watch and listen for breathing.

5. If mouthpiece available, place it in position and give two breaths or cover mouth and nose of infant with your mouth and give two breaths (Figure 9-9B).

WHY? 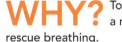 To protect against infection, use a mouthpiece whenever providing rescue breathing.

6. If airway is not open, retilt head and try to give two breaths again in same manner (Figure 9-9C).

7. If airway still blocked, use two fingers to give 5 chest compressions ½ to 1 inch deep.

8. Check mouth for foreign object by lifting jaw and tongue. If object visible, do a finger sweep.

9. Give 1 breath in same manner as before.

10. Repeat 2 breaths and 5 chest compressions, then check for object, until airway open and air goes in.

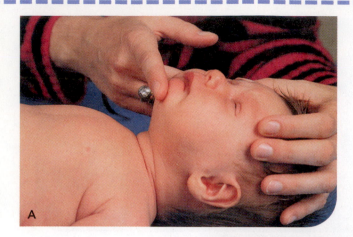

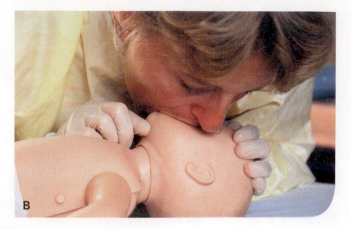

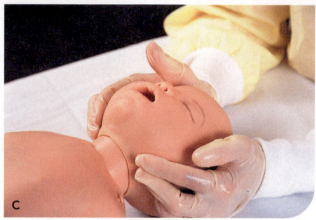

FIGURE 9-9 (A) Infant head tilt–chin lift maneuver; (B) infant mouth-to mouth rescue breathing; (C) infant jaw-thrust maneuver.

11. If infant does not breathe on own after airway open, perform CPR as in Procedure 9-12.

12. When emergency over, remove gloves.

13. Perform hand hygiene.

14. Document procedure in patient's record.

CHARTING EXAMPLE: 08/24/XX 10:10 A.M. Infant "turned blue while eating" according to mother. 911 called and Dr. Ames notified. No object seen in baby's mouth. 2 breaths given without success. Head retilted and 2 more breaths given. Airway open. Baby breathing on own, color pink. · · · · · · · · · ·
· C. L. Negri, CMA (AAMA)

PROCEDURE 9-6

ADMINISTERING ABDOMINAL THRUSTS (HEIMLICH MANEUVER) FOR AN UNRESPONSIVE ADULT OR CHILD

ABHES VII.MA.A.1 9(o)(5)   CAAHEP XI.P (10)

OBJECTIVE: To perform abdominal thrusts (Heimlich maneuver) for an unconscious adult or child to clear an obstructed airway.

STANDARD: The time this task takes depends on the condition of the adult or child.

EQUIPMENT AND SUPPLIES: None.

STEPS:

1. Place victim on back.
2. Establish unresponsiveness, shake, and shout.
3. Grasp jaw and tongue with one hand (Figure 9-10A).
4. Perform finger sweep with index finger of free hand only if object is visible (Figs. 9-10B and 9-10C).
5. Assess breathing.
   - Lean over victim and look at chest to determine if chest rises and falls.
   - Place ear and cheek near victim's mouth and nose to listen and feel for air movement.
6. Pinch nose and attempt to ventilate. Give 2 long ventilations of 2 seconds duration, and allow time for chest to rise.
7. Reposition head and attempt to ventilate a second time if chest does not rise and fall.
8. Kneel and straddle victim's thighs to prepare for abdominal thrusts (Heimlich maneuver).
9. Place hand just above umbilicus. Place second hand directly over first hand.
10. Press heel of hand toward head with 5 quick abdominal thrusts below the diaphragm (Figure 9-10D).
11. Repeat finger sweep.
12. Repeat abdominal thrusts until foreign object is cleared.
13. If pulse absent but airway open, begin CPR.
14. Following removal of foreign body, place victim in recovery position.

CHARTING EXAMPLE: 08/24/XX 5:15 P.M. Pt. began choking in waiting room. 4 abdominal thrusts performed. Large piece of hard candy expelled. Pt. breathing on own; appeared agitated. BP 138/82, P 98, R 18. Physician examined. After resting 10 min. Pt. felt fine. · C. Rodriguez, RMA

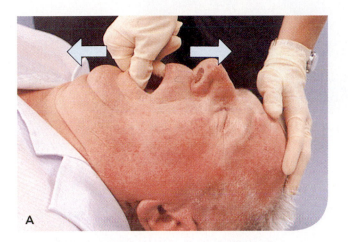
A

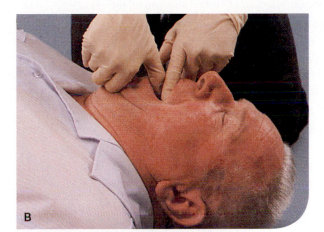
B

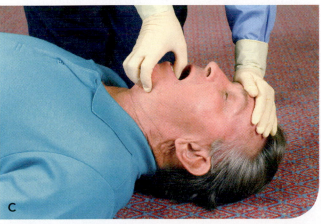
C

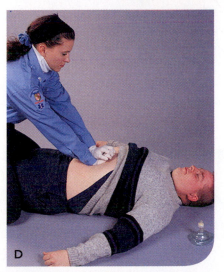
D

FIGURE 9-10 (A) Open the mouth with the crossed finger technique; (B) perform finger sweep to check for a foreign object; (C) tongue-jaw tilt; (D) deliver abdominal thrusts below the diaphragm.

PROCEDURE 9-7

PERFORMING RESCUE BREATHING FOR AN ADULT

ABHES VII.MA.A.1 9(o)(5)   CAAHEP XI.P (10)

OBJECTIVE: To perform rescue breathing for an adult in a breathing emergency.

STANDARD: The time this task takes depends on condition of patient.

EQUIPMENT AND SUPPLIES: Gloves; resuscitation mouthpiece; biohazard waste container; pen; patient's record.

STEPS:

1. Notify EMS by asking someone to call emergency services or 911.
2. Shout "Are you all right?! Are you all right?!"
3. Look, listen, and feel for breathing.
4. If no breathing detected, tilt head back, lift chin, place resuscitation mouthpiece in mouth, and pinch nose closed. If no mouthpiece is available, proceed with mouth-to-mouth rescue breathing (Figure 9-11).
5. Give patient 2 short breaths until chest rises.
6. Turn face to side, then look, listen, and feel for air to return.
7. Check carotid pulse.
8. If pulse present but victim not breathing, give 1 slow breath every 5 seconds for 1 minute.
9. Recheck breathing and pulse every minute.
10. Continue rescue breathing as long as pulse is present and victim unable to breath on his or her own or until someone relieves you.
11. If pulse ceases, begin CPR as explained in Procedure 9-10.
12. When emergency is over, dispose of waste in biohazard waste container.

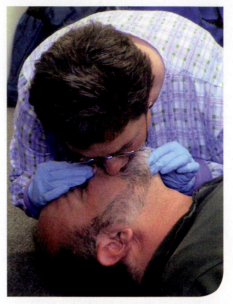

FIGURE 9-11   Mouth-to-mouth rescue breathing.

13. Perform hand hygiene.
14. Document patient's record.

CHARTING EXAMPLE: 08/24/XX 4:00 P.M. Began rescue breathing on Pt. after finding her unresponsive on floor in exam room 2. EMS activated at 4:03 P.M. Physician on duty notified. Pulse strong. Gave two breaths, no air returned. Continued until EMS arrived at 4:09 P.M. Pt. breathing on own with shallow respirations. Transported to Memorial Hosp. · N. Carroll, RMA

PROCEDURE 9-8

PERFORMING RESCUE BREATHING FOR A CHILD

ABHES VII.MA.A.1 9(o)(5)   CAAHEP XI.P (10)

OBJECTIVE: To perform rescue breathing for a child in response to a breathing emergency.

STANDARD: The time this task takes depends on condition of child.

EQUIPMENT AND SUPPLIES: Gloves; resuscitation mouthpiece; pen; patient's record; biohazard waste container.

STEPS:

1. Activate EMS procedure by having someone call EMS or 911.
2. Look, listen, and feel for breathing. If no breathing, proceed with following steps.
3. Don gloves.
4. Tilt head back, lift chin, place resuscitation mouthpiece in child's mouth, pinch nose closed, and give 2 short breaths.
5. If air does not go in, retilt head and breathe again.
6. Check carotid pulse.
7. If pulse present but child is not breathing, give 1 slow breath every 3 seconds for 1 minute.
8. Recheck pulse and breathing every minute.
9. Continue rescue breathing as long as pulse is present and child is not breathing on his or her own or until help arrives.
10. If pulse absent, begin CPR as in Procedure 9-11.
11. When emergency is over, remove gloves. Discard mask and gloves in biohazard waste container.
12. Perform hand hygiene.
13. Document patient's record.

CHARTING EXAMPLE: 08/24/XX 2:00 P.M. Pt. in clinic for PE; allergy injection. 15 min after injection she fell to floor and was unresponsive. EMS activated at 2:18 P.M. Physician notified at same time. Airway open two breaths given. Carotid pulse strong. One breath every 3 seconds for 2 minutes. Pt. began breathing on her own. Transported to ER at Memorial Hosp. · · · · · · · · · ·
· M. Woodhouse, CMA (AAMA)

PROCEDURE 9-9

PERFORMING RESCUE BREATHING FOR AN INFANT

ABHES VII.MA.A.1 9(o)(5)   CAAHEP XI.P (10)

OBJECTIVE: To perform rescue breathing for an infant in a breathing emergency.

STANDARD: The time this task takes depends on condition of infant.

EQUIPMENT AND SUPPLIES: Gloves; resuscitation mouthpiece; biohazard waste container; pen; patient's record.

STEPS:

1. Activate EMS procedure by having someone call EMS or 911.
2. Look, listen, and feel for breathing. If no breathing, proceed with following steps (Figure 9-12).
3. Don gloves.
4. Tilt infant's head back.
5. Place resuscitation mouthpiece in infant's mouth, or seal your lips tightly around infant's nose and mouth.
6. Give 2 slow breaths. Breathe into infant until chest rises.
7. Check brachial artery for pulse.
8. If pulse present but no air returned by infant, give 1 slow breath every 3 seconds for 1 minute.

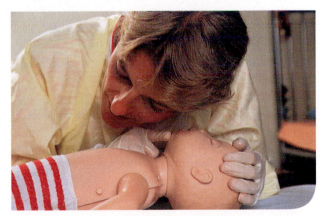

FIGURE 9-12 Assessing an infant's breathing.

9. Recheck for air return and pulse every minute.
10. Continue rescue breathing as long as pulse is present but infant not breathing or until help arrives to replace you.
11. If pulse not palpable, then proceed with CPR as indicated in Procedure 9-12.
12. When emergency is over, remove gloves and discard mask and gloves in biohazard waste container.

13. Perform hand hygiene.

14. Document patient's record.

CHARTING EXAMPLE: 08/24/XX 3:10 P.M. 8 mon. old female Pt. in Pedi Clinic for difficulty breathing. Pt. ceased breathing, was unresponsive, pulse present. Rescue breathing begun with 2 slow breaths. Breaths given every 3 seconds after 1.5 minutes. Pt. resumed breathing on own. Transported to Memorial Hosp. per Dr. Woo. · · · · · · · · · · · · · · R. Cohen, RMA

PROCEDURE 9-10

PERFORMING CPR FOR AN ADULT

ABHES VII.MA.A.1 9(o)(5)   CAAHEP XI.P (10)

OBJECTIVE: To perform CPR for an adult in a breathing and cardiac emergency.

STANDARD: The time this task takes depends on condition of patient.

EQUIPMENT AND SUPPLIES: Gloves; resuscitation mouthpiece; biohazard waste container; pen; patient's record.

STEPS:

1. Assess patient, and check for responsiveness by shouting "Are you okay?! Are you okay?!"

2. Call for help nearby or by phone. Get AED if nearby.

3. Move patient into position on a flat, firm surface. Position yourself on left side near patient's head.

4. Check airway. If obstructed, proceed to clear obstruction by pressing backward on forehead and lifting chin by placing 2 fingers on chin and lifting up and forward until teeth nearly closed.

5. Assess breathing by listening, looking, and feeling for air return for no more than 10 seconds. If airway open, evaluate respiratory function. If no respirations present, prepare to ventilate.

6. Leave dentures in place; pinch off nostrils.

7. Fully cover patient's mouth to form mouth-to-mouth seal, or place barrier device on patient's face and place your mouth on breathing piece or opening.

8. Continue to tilt head and lift chin before each ventilation.

9. Perform rescue breathing as in Procedure 9-7.

10. If no pulse and no air returned, begin CPR.

Single rescuer:

11. Position hands on lower half of sternum between nipples. See Figure 9-13A. (This location prevents damage to liver).

12. Place heel of one hand on sternum; superimpose other hand on top of first hand.

13. Interlace fingers, and extend fingers off rib cage.

14. Position your body directly over hands with shoulders above hands (Figure 9-13B).

15. Administer 30 compressions at a rate of 100 per minute. Compress chest 1½ to 2 inches each time.

16. Count compressions (compression time and release time should be equal). Count quickly to 30 as compressions are performed, and maintain rate of 100 compressions per minute.

17. Release pressure between compressions for cardiac refilling, but do not take heel of hand off chest.

18. Continue CPR at rate of 30 compressions and 2 rescue breaths for a single rescuer.

19. Pause 2 seconds for each ventilation.

20. Check carotid pulse for 5 seconds after 5 cycles of compression and ventilation.

Two professionals arrive together to do CPR:

1. Rescuer A assumes position at head of victim to perform ventilation.

2. Perform head tilt–chin lift maneuver for airway opening.

3. Assess breathing.

4. Ventilate with 2 slow breaths of 2 seconds each.

5. Observe for chest rise and fall.

NOTE: Longer ventilations allow time for chest to expand and reduce potential for abdominal distention.

6. Rescuer A checks for carotid pulse for 5 to 10 seconds.

7. Rescuer B assumes position of compressor at level of chest and locates site for compression.

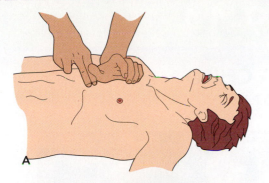

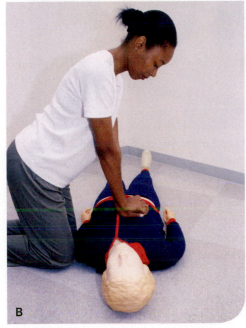

FIGURE 9-13 (A) Proper positioning of the hands during external cardiac compression; (B) arm and hand positions for external cardiac compressions.

8. If no pulse, Rescuer A states, "No pulse," and Rescuer B begins compressions.

9. Rescuer B completes 30 compressions (1½ to 2 inches) at rate of 100 per minute, then pauses after compressions.

10. Rescuer A gives 2 slow breaths.

11. Rescuer B maintains rhythm and counts out loud, "One, two, three," etc.

12. Rescuer B begins compressions again at ratio of 30 compressions to 2 ventilations.

13. Rescuer A checks carotid pulse after 2 minutes and then after every few minutes.

14. When Rescuer B becomes tired, he or she signals for a switch by saying "Change" or "Switch" before switching. Rescuer B signals and competes 30th compression, then both rescuers switch simultaneously. New Rescuer A at

head checks carotid pulse for 5 to 10 seconds. If no pulse, Rescuer A states, "No pulse," and gives 2 slow ventilations.

15. New Rescuer B begins cycle of compressions.

Continuing CPR:

1. Check carotid pulse and signs of circulation every few minutes during CPR.

2. Check pupils every 4 to 5 minutes unless third rescuer is present and can perform pupil check.

3. Observe for abdominal distention. If abdominal distention present, reposition airway and give longer ventilations.

4. Maintain enough air to elevate ribs.

5. Ventilators observe each breath for effectiveness.

6. If patient is in respiratory arrest, check only major pulse after 2 minutes for no longer then 10 seconds to ensure continuation of cardiac function.

7. If patient is breathing, place in recovery position unless cervical injury suspected.

8. Terminate CPR only if the following occurs:
   - Resuscitation is successful.
   - Vital functions return spontaneously.
   - Assisted support measures are initiated.
   - Patient is transferred to emergency vehicle or code team arrives.
   - Patient is pronounced dead by physician.
   - Rescuer is exhausted and cannot continue.

NOTE: Research shows chest compressions without ventilation provide significantly better outcomes than no CPR, so if rescuer does not or cannot perform rescue breathing, chest compressions still should be performed.

If AED is used:

1. Rescuer who handles AED is in charge of situation.

2. Rescuer B retrieves AED box, calls for help, and continues with the following:
   - Performs defibrillation after assessment
   - Places pocket face mask on patient in preparation for ventilations
   - Begins chest compressions
   - Maintains CPR protocol with Rescuer A

CHARTING EXAMPLE: 08/27/XX 11:00 A.M. 48 y old male Pt. complained of chest pain and stopped breathing. EMA activated. Two breaths given. No air returned, and no carotid pulse present. CPR started at 11:04 A.M. two breaths per 30 compressions given for 2 minutes. No breathing, no pulse. After next round of CPR, breathing and pulse returned. BP 94/60, R 10, P weak rapid 106. EMS stabilized patient and transported to Memorial ED. · · · · · · · · · · · · · · · · · J. Roberts, CMA (AAMA)

PERFORMING CPR FOR A CHILD

ABHES VII.MA.A.1 9(o)(5)   CAAHEP XI.P (10)

OBJECTIVE: To perform CPR on a child during a cardiac emergency.

STANDARD: The time required for this task depends on patient's needs.

EQUIPMENT AND SUPPLIES: Gloves and resuscitation device.

STEPS:

1. Put on gloves.
2. Tap child to check for consciousness. Notify EMS.
3. Tilt head. Look, listen, and feel for breathing.
4. If no breathing, give 2 breaths and check carotid artery.
5. If no pulse and no breathing, place one hand on breast-bone and one hand on forehead to open airway.
6. Place heel of hand above notch of xiphoid process. Position shoulders over child, and administer 5 chest compressions ⅓ to ½ depth of sternum (Figure 9-14).
7. Position resuscitation mouthpiece and give 1 slow breath while pinching nose closed.
8. Repeat cycles of 30 compressions and 2 breaths for a rate of 100 compressions per minute. Count "One, two, three," and up to 30, then breathe.
9. Check pulse and breathing for air return for 5 seconds.
10. If no pulse, continue sets of 30 compressions and 2 breaths at rate of 100 compressions per minute.
11. Recheck pulse and breathing every few minutes.

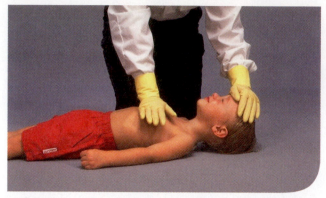

FIGURE 9-14   Chest compressions performed on a child.

12. Use AED only if child is age 8 years or older and weighs 55 pounds or more; or otherwise, follow protocol designated by facility.
13. Once emergency help arrives, remove gloves.
14. Perform hand hygiene.
15. Document procedure.

CHARTING EXAMPLE: 08/27/XX 2:00 P.M. 6 y old male child collapsed in waiting room of office. Child not breathing. 2 breaths given. No carotid pulse. EMS notified and CPR began at 2:03 P.M. CPR (30 compressions, 2 breaths) given for 2 minutes. Pt. began to move, and color and breathing returned. BP 74/56, P 114, R 10. EMS arrived and administered Adrenalin and O_2. Pt. transported to ED at Memorial Hosp. · C. Logan, RMA

PERFORMING CPR FOR AN INFANT

ABHES VII.MA.A.1 9(o)(5)   CAAHEP XI.P (10)

OBJECTIVE: To perform CPR for infant in cardiac emergency.

STANDARD: The time this task takes depends on condition of infant.

EQUIPMENT AND SUPPLIES: Gloves; resuscitation mouthpiece.

STEPS:

1. Don gloves.
2. Tap infant to determine consciousness level.
3. If no evidence of consciousness, notify EMS.
4. Tilt head. Look, listen, and feel for breathing.
5. If no breathing evident, position resuscitation mouthpiece and give 2 slow breaths while covering mouth and nose. If needed, give rescue breathing at rate of 40 to 60 breaths per minute.
6. Check brachial artery for 5 to 10 seconds. If heartbeat is lower than 60 beats per minute, it is not sufficient to support life and chest compressions must begin.
7. Place fingers on center of sternum just below nipples (Figure 9-15).
8. Compress chest ⅓ to ½ depth of chest 5 times.
9. Give 2 breaths.
10. Recheck brachial pulse and air return for 5 to 10 seconds.
11. If no pulse, continue CPR cycles (30 compressions to 2 breaths for a rate of 100 compressions per minute) and recheck pulse and breathing every few minutes.
12. Continue until EMS takes over or breathing and pulse return.
13. Remove gloves, and perform hand hygiene.
14. Document procedure in patient's record.

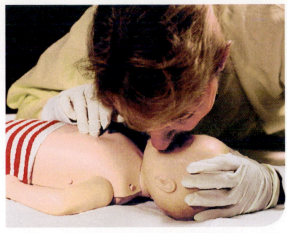

FIGURE 9-15 Performing CPR on an infant.

CHARTING EXAMPLE: 08/27/XX 7:15 P.M. 7-month-old infant brought in for exam with signs of croup. In exam room 1, infant ceased breathing, no pulse evident. EMS notified and CPR began at 7:20 P.M. 30 chest compressions per 2 breaths given for 2 minutes. No pulse or breathing after 1 minute. After 2 minutes no pulse, no breathing, no BP. CPR continued until EMS took over. Adrenaline and oxygen administered, and IV begun. Transported to ED at Memorial with mother at 7:30 P.M.
· I. Rodriquez, CMA (AAMA)

PROCEDURE 9-13

USING AN AUTOMATED EXTERNAL DEFIBRILLATOR (AED)

ABHES VII.MA.A.1 9(o)(5)   CAAHEP XI.P (10)

OBJECTIVE: To use an AED in a cardiac emergency.

STANDARD: This task takes 1–5 minutes, depending on condition of patient.

EQUIPMENT AND SUPPLIES: AED unit; face mask.

STEPS:

1. Open AED and turn on power. (In some devices, power turns on automatically once AED case is open. If power did not turn on automatically, press power button.)
2. Sound alerts, lights, and voice prompts will tell you that power is on and will instruct you on use of AED.
3. Place AED near head on left side (if possible, though that will vary with situation, space, etc.) of victim for easier use by rescuer.
4. Remove clothing from patient's torso.
5. Make certain chest is dry to provide better adhesion of electrode pads.
6. Open package of adhesive electrode pads. (Some electrode pads are preconnected to cables. If not preconnected, attach one end of each cable to AED and snap other end of each cable to an electrode pad.
7. Peel off protective plastic backing from pads to expose adhesive surface.
8. Place two adhesive pads on skin of chest as follows:
   - Right side of sternum with top edge of pad touching clavicle (Figure 9-16).
   - Pad marked with heart emblem (♥) outside of left nipple with top margin of pad at anterior axillary line.
   - Do not place pads over nitroglycerin patches or within 5 inches of implanted devices such as pacemakers.

9. A voice prompt or alarm may sound if electrode pads are not securely attached to chest or if cables are not fastened properly.

10. Stop CPR if it is being performed. Instruct everyone assisting with rescue not to touch patient to evaluate AED rhythm. (On some units, you may need to push ANALYZE button).

11. If analysis by AED indicates need for a shock, push SHOCK button on AED.

12. If necessary or if prompted by AED following each shock, press ANALYZE button for follow-up rhythm report.

NOTE: Follow AED voice or visual prompts. Shock sequence is usually completed three times if chest remains in fibrillation.

13. If patient is not in need of another shock, check at once for pulse and begin CPR. Provide 2 minutes of CPR. AED will perform another analysis.

14. After three shocks or NO SHOCK message on machine, check for signs of circulation. If signs are absent, begin CPR for 2 minutes. Press ANALYZE button on AED, and repeat until EMS arrives.

15. When patient is no longer in ventricular fibrillation or tachycardia, AED will signal "No Shock Indicated" or "No Shock Advised" or "Check Breathing and Pulse."

16. Leave AED electrodes attached to patient's chest, and leave AED on.

17. Follow protocol for rescue breathing or CPR as patient condition warrants.

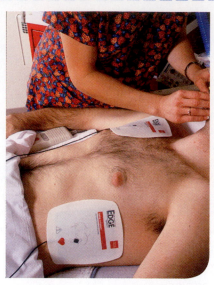

FIGURE 9-16 Placement of AED electrode pads.

CHARTING EXAMPLE: 08/28/XX 1:00 P.M. 56 y old female dropped to floor. No breathing or pulse detected. EMS notified. CPR started and two cycles of CPR completed while AED unit located. CPR ceased at 1:14 P.M. AED unit attached and activated. Three shocks given before breathing and pulse resumed. P 45, R 10, BP 86/48. EMS arrived at 1:19 P.M. Pt. stabilized and transported to ED of Memorial Hosp at 1:32 P.M. . . . . S. Patel, RMA

PROCEDURE 9-14

MAINTAINING THE EMERGENCY/CRASH CART
ABHES VII.MA.A.1 8(y); VII.MA.A.1 8(z)   CAAHEP V.P (9); V.P (10)

OBJECTIVE: To check the contents of an emergency cart for equipment and supplies and restock as needed and document correctly.

STANDARD: This task takes 10 minutes, depending on size of unit.

EQUIPMENT AND SUPPLIES: Emergency or crash cart; inventory control sheet; equipment and supplies designated by physician.

STEPS:

1. Check with physician regarding designated equipment and supplies to be included in emergency cart. (Refer to Box 9-2 for list of general supplies needed in emergency cart and Table 9-1 for list of medications required in most emergency carts.)

2. With inventory control sheet in hand, open each drawer to determine if each item listed is present and in correct location.

3. After checking each item, check each item's expiration date, and make a list of items to be replaced.

4. Gather replacement items, and restock cart. (Always check and resupply emergency carts after each use. Document each restocking.)

5. Check all batteries, and recharge or replace as needed.

6. Determine that all equipment is in working order.

7. Record information on inventory sheet. Date and initial when check of emergency cart is complete.

8. Secure crash cart with a device that is easily opened but discourages casual use of items in cart.

9. Keep cart in easy-to-access area.

Other Types of Medical Emergencies

In an emergency situation, check airway (A), breathing (B), and circulation (C), as described previously in this chapter. Once it is determined that the ABCs are functioning, check for bleeding; other signs and symptoms of injury, such as fainting, seizures, burns, shock, and poisoning; allergic reactions; and behavioral or psychiatric emergencies.

SYNCOPE

Syncope, or fainting, is the sudden loss of consciousness due to a sudden interruption of oxygen or blood supply to the brain. In and of itself, fainting is dangerous only if the patient sustains injury during the fall. The cause of the syncope is important, and further examination is warranted. The following are the warning signs of syncope:

- Dizziness
- Pallor
- Nausea
- Numbness in extremities

ASSISTING A PATIENT DURING AN ASTHMA ATTACK

Asthma is caused by exposure to an allergen that causes constriction of the bronchi. The symptoms of asthma include coughing, shortness of breath, wheezing, cyanosis, and choking. Severe asthma attacks require the use of epinephrine to dilate bronchioles and permit air flow into and out of the lungs. Asthma attacks are frightening for the patient, and every effort must be made to keep the patient as calm as possible.

PROCEDURE 9-15

CARING FOR A FAINTING PATIENT

ABHES VII.MA.A.1 9(o)(5)   CAAHEP XI.P (10)

OBJECTIVE: To care for patient experiencing syncope and protect him or her from injury.

STANDARD: This task takes 1–2 minutes.

EQUIPMENT AND SUPPLIES: None.

STEPS:

1. Determine level of responsiveness by shaking and shouting "Are you okay?!"

2. Call for assistance. Notify physician of patient's condition.

3. If there is no response, check ABCs and, if necessary, perform rescue breathing or CPR.

4. If patient is responsive and seated, ask him or her to lower head between knees to increase oxygen flow.

5. Elevate feet above head to increase blood flow.

6. Loosen tight clothing, and cover with drape or blanket.

7. Monitor vital signs.

8. Once fainting episode is over, assist patient to sitting position. Do not leave patient unattended until stable.

9. Perform hand hygiene.

10. Document episode in patient's record.

11. Schedule follow-up visits or tests ordered by physician to determine cause of syncope.

Safety Alert! A patient's safety is of prime importance. Protect the patient against injury and stay with the patient until he or she responds or other help arrives. If feasible, ask the patient to lie down to avoid injury due to falling.

CHARTING EXAMPLE: 08/29/XX 9:00 A.M. Pt. "felt dizzy" and was cold and clammy to touch after blood drawn. Assisted Pt. to lie down with feet raised and covered with blanket. BP 90/60, P 68, R 12. Dr. Welter ordered glucose stat. Gluc 58. OJ given. . . . . J. Lindsay, CMA (AAMA)

ANAPHYLAXIS

Today so many children and adults seem to have severe reactions to foods such as nuts, shellfish, and dairy products that the number of anaphylaxis cases is increasing. Anaphylaxis is an acute, life-threatening allergic reaction that can occur in minutes and results in airway obstruction, shock, coma, and death. Symptoms may include all symptoms associated with asthma attack, including swelling of airway tissue, tachycardia, hypotension, profuse sweating, and pallor. Each medical facility should have a protocol for treating anaphylaxis. Treatment usually includes close monitoring of breathing and vital signs and administration of epinephrine. Many medications cause allergic and sometimes anaphylactic reactions; thus, patients should be monitored closely after every medication dose is administered.

PROCEDURE 9-16

ASSISTING A PATIENT DURING AN ASTHMA ATTACK
ABHES VII.MA.A.1 9(o)(5)   CAAHEP XI.P (10)

OBJECTIVE: To assist patient during asthma attack and help restore normal breathing.

STANDARD: The time this task takes depends on condition of patient.

EQUIPMENT AND SUPPLIES: Gloves; patient's inhaler; nebulizer; epinephrine; oxygen.

STEPS:

1. Assess the patient's airway, breathing, and circulation. Proceed as indicated in previous procedures for opening airway, rescue breathing, and CPR.
2. Notify the physician that patient is having breathing problems.
3. Follow facility protocol for dealing with asthma attacks.
4. Try to calm patient as much as possible. Ask patient to assume a comfortable position (usually leaning forward with elbows on knees). Ask patient to inhale and blow out forcefully as if blowing out a candle.
5. If no protocol in place, locate patient's inhaler and assist patient to administer prescribed dose.
6. If inhaler is not effective, use nebulizer as defined by office protocol and physician's orders (Procedure 21-7).
7. Administer oxygen as ordered by physician (Procedure 21-8).
8. If breathing shows no improvement, notify physician and/or EMS.
9. Begin rescue breathing and CPR as needed.
10. When emergency is over, remove gloves.
11. Perform hand hygiene.
12. Document procedure in patient's record.

CHARTING EXAMPLE: 08/30/XX 12:15 P.M. Pt. waiting for PE began wheezing and coughing. Breathing labored and shallow, pulse rapid. Notified physician and Pt. given 2 doses from his inhaler. After 2 minutes breathing not improved. Physician ordered nebulizer treatment with Albuterol sulfate. Pt. breathing easier after 2 minutes. BP 138/88, R 26, P 90. Physician rechecked Pt. after 10-minute rest. Breathing normal.
· B. Macavoy, RMA

PROCEDURE 9-17

ASSISTING WITH AN ANAPHYLACTIC EMERGENCY
ABHES VII.MA.A.1 9(e); VII.MA.A.1 9(m)   CAAHEP I.P (10); XI.P (10)

OBJECTIVE: To assist patient during anaphylactic emergency to restore respiratory and circulatory function.

STANDARD: The time this task takes depends on condition of patient.

EQUIPMENT AND SUPPLIES: Gloves; emergency/crash cart; patient's record; pen; biohazard waste container.

STEPS:

1. Stay at patient's side.
2. Alert another staff person to notify physician and EMS. If a third person is present, ask him or her to bring emergency cart.
3. Assist patient into supine position. Drape as needed.
4. Try to calm patient.
5. Assess airway, breathing, and circulation, and proceed as indicated in procedures provided elsewhere in this chapter.
6. Monitor vital signs, skin color, and skin temperature.
7. Assist physician with starting an IV line as requested.
8. Administer oxygen or other medications as prescribed by physician.
9. Document all data, and communicate relevant information to EMS on arrival.
10. Once emergency is over, record all related information in patient's record.

CHARTING EXAMPLE: 08/30/XX 5:15 P.M. Co-worker began Tx of anaphylaxis after victim ingested candy provided by patient. Wheezing, SOB, swelling of tongue occurred 1 minute after ingesting candy. EMS and Dr. Ellison notified. Dr. administered epinephrine from EpiPen and started IV. O$_2$ started. EMS arrived at 5:26 P.M. Pt. stabilized in office. EMS transported Pt. to ED of Memorial for evaluation. ···········
··································· K. Oto, CMA (AAMA)

SEVERE BLEEDING

Severe bleeding or hemorrhage results when an artery or vein is punctured or torn inside or near the surface of the body. External bleeding originates in a wound in the skin or an opening in the body such as the mouth, nose, ear, anus, or vagina. Visible bleeding is controlled by direct pressure applied to the site, thereby compressing the blood vessels and facilitating formation of a clot and sealing off of the area. If direct pressure does not slow bleeding, then applying pressure to a nearby artery or pressure point may be necessary (Figure 9-17). Severe bleeding or hemorrhage can result in **hypovolemic shock** due to loss of blood volume. This results in low blood pressure and can be life threatening. The amount of blood loss needed to cause hypovolemic shock depends on the size, age, and general health of the individual. Internal bleeding is more difficult to discover and can result in hypovolemic shock.

BURN EMERGENCIES

Burns may be caused by heat, electricity, chemicals, or radiation. Burns are classified in two basic ways: by surface area affected and depth of burn. The **rule of nines** is useful for estimating the amount of body surface affected. Each of the areas indicated in Figure 9-19 represents 9% of body surface. For example 9% of skin covers the head. Each arm (front and back) is 9%. Each leg (front and back) is 18%. The genital area is 1% of total body surface. In infants and children, the rule of nines is modified because infant heads are much larger in relationship to the rest of the body. Thus the head is 18% and lower extremities are 13.5% each. Never break blisters as burns heal.

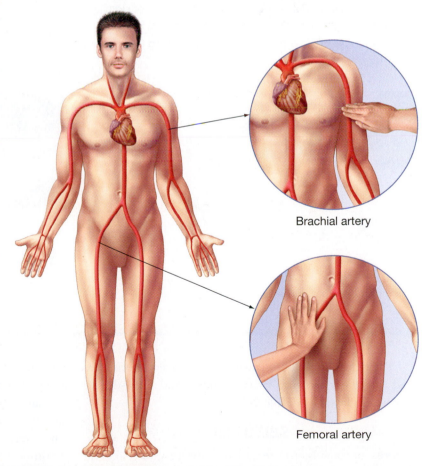

Brachial artery

Femoral artery

FIGURE 9-17 Arterial pressure points of the body.

PROCEDURE 9-18

CONTROLLING SEVERE BLEEDING

ABHES VII.MA.A.1 9(o)(5)   CAAHEP XI.P (10)

OBJECTIVE: To help control severe bleeding in a bleeding emergency.

STANDARD: The time this task takes depends on the condition of the patient.

EQUIPMENT AND SUPPLIES: Gloves; other PPE if available; sterile dressings; biohazard waste container; patient's record; pen.

STEPS:

1. Identify patient. Ask permission to treat.
2. If bleeding seems severe, contact EMS or 911. Notify physician on duty.
3. If time allows, perform hand hygiene and don PPE.
4. Remove or cut away clothing to expose wound (Figure 9-18A).
5. Apply sterile dressing over wound and press firmly. If sterile dressings unavailable use a clean towel, article of clothing, sanitary napkin, or other item on hand (Figure 9-18B).
6. If wound is on an extremity, elevate arm or leg to decrease blood flow.
7. Maintain pressure even if bleeding seeps through sterile dressing. Do not release pressure.
8. If bleeding pulsates and is bright red in color, apply and maintain pressure to nearest pressure point until help arrives. Use a tourniquet only as a measure of last resort.
9. When emergency is over, dispose of waste in biohazard waste container.
10. Clean area.
11. Remove PPE, and dispose of PPE in biohazard waste container.
12. Perform hand hygiene.
13. Document patient's record.

CHARTING EXAMPLE: 08/30/XX 8:50 A.M. Pt. presented in facility with a 4 cm puncture wound in L forearm. Sterile dressing applied. L arm elevated. Bleeding seeped through initial dressing, and another layer applied over first dressing. Physician notified. Bleeding stopped after 4 minutes. Dr. Elliot used 10 sutures to close WD. Pt. to return to office in 2 days for recheck. Verbal and written WD care information given. · · · · · ·
· S. Teta, RMA

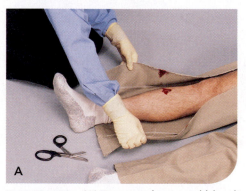 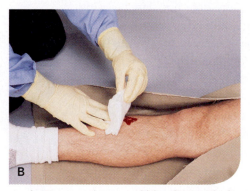

FIGURE 9-18   (A) To control external bleeding, first expose the wound; (B) control external bleeding with direct pressure or with direct pressure and elevation.

The depth of the burn and the tissue layers affected are used to classify burns as first-, second-, and third-degree burns, as indicated in Table 9-2.

SEIZURES

Seizures, or convulsions, are caused by disorganized electrical activity in the brain. They are characterized by involuntary muscle contractions and may be generalized over the entire body or localized and limited to a specific area. A seizure may be caused by many types of conditions or diseases that overstimulate neurons in the brain. **Epilepsy,** a chronic condition characterized by frequent seizures, may be due to injury to the brain or disease or may be **idiopathic** (no known cause). A generalized seizure is known as a grand mal or tonic-clonic

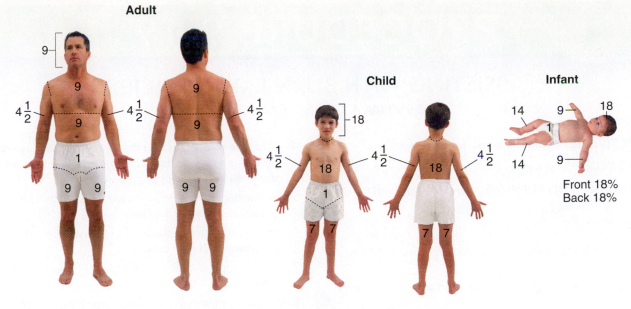

Note: Each arm totals 9% (front of arm $4\frac{1}{2}$%, back of arm $4\frac{1}{2}$%)

FIGURE 9-19 Rule of nines for burns.

seizure. The seizure itself lasts less than 30 seconds and is characterized by loss of consciousness; rigid muscle contractions; decreased respiration; cyanosis; and loss of control of the bladder, the bowel, or both. Once the seizure is over, the patient is disoriented for a period of 15 to 30 minutes. Emergency care of seizure patients focuses on preventing injury by removing furniture and other dangers as well as protecting the head from banging on the floor by placing articles of clothing or pillow under the head. Do not use restraint. Careful monitoring of the patient is vital, and once the seizure is over the patient should be placed in the recovery position (Procedure 9-1) to prevent choking on saliva or vomitus.

POISONING

Many poisoning incidents are accidental and occur in the home with children under age 5 years most often involved.

Poisons may be swallowed, absorbed through skin, inhaled, or injected. The poison control center number in your area should be located near each telephone in the facility. The American Association of Poison Control Centers (AAPCC) has established regional poison control centers and provides information about poisonous substances, antidotes if any are available, and immediate emergency treatment based on information provided. Follow-up telephone calls to monitor patient's progress also are provided by poison control centers. To respond to a telephone call about a possible poisoning incident, gather the following information:

- Who is calling and from where
- Age and weight of patient
- Nature of the poison (ingested, inhaled, or skin exposure)

TABLE 9-2 Burns Classified by Depth of Involvement

Depth	Cause	Skin Involvement	Symptoms	Wound Appearance
First degree (superficial)	Sunburn, low-intensity heat	Epidermis	Tingling, soothed by cooling	Reddened, turns white when pressure applied
Second degree	Flame, scalding	Epidermis and dermis	Pain, pain, sensitive to cold air	Blisters reddened, swelling and weeping surface.
Third degree	Longer exposure to flame, hot liquids, electric current	Epidermis, dermis, sub-cutaneous	Little pain, shock	Dry pale white or charred, edema

PROCEDURE 9-19

ASSISTING WITH BURN EMERGENCIES

ABHES VII.MA.A.1 9(o)(5)   CAAHEP XI.P (10)

OBJECTIVE: To perform burn care for a patient.

STANDARD: This task takes 2–5 minutes.

EQUIPMENT AND SUPPLIES: Water; cotton cloth (sterile if available); gloves.

STEPS:

1. Remove burn source, or move patient away from burn source.
2. Check patient's breathing status, and assess for severity of burns.
3. Call EMS or 911 for moderate or severe burns (extensive second-degree burns or third-degree on burns more than 2% of body area).
4. Flush chemical burns and thermal burns that have not penetrated to subcutaneous layer with large amount of sterile water if available or tap water if not.
5. If subcutaneous layer is affected, cover with cotton cloth or sterile dressing if available.
6. Monitor for signs of shock and for airway, breathing, and circulation until help arrives.
7. Do not apply ointment or antiseptics, unless ordered by physician.
8. When emergency is over, clean area and dispose of waste in biohazard waste container.
9. Perform hand hygiene.
10. Document patient's record.

PROCEDURE 9-20

ASSISTING A PATIENT DURING A SEIZURE

ABHES VII.MA.A.1 9(o)(5)   CAAHEP XI.P (10)

OBJECTIVE: To care for and protect from injury a patient having a seizure.

STANDARD: The time this task takes depends on condition of patient.

EQUIPMENT AND SUPPLIES: Firm surface.

STEPS:

1. Assist patient to floor.
2. Remove objects that may cause injury to seizing patient, such as chair, table, and other obstructions (Figure 9-20A).
3. Monitor airway, breathing, and circulation. Place towel or jacket under head to protect from injury on hard floor.
4. Do not restrain patient, and do not put anything in patient's mouth, in order to prevent patient from swallowing tongue.
5. Provide privacy, and protect patient as much as possible.
6. Do not attempt to give food or water to seizing patient.
7. Once seizure is over, place patient on side in recovery position to prevent aspiration of saliva or vomitus (Figure 9-20B).
8. Assess patient for injuries sustained during seizure, and provide care as needed.
9. Allow patient to rest for 30 minutes after seizure.
10. Obtain medical information about medications, past injuries, recent fever, and other signs of disease.
11. Once patient is stable and has been evaluated by physician, don gloves and clean area.
12. Remove gloves, and dispose of them in biohazard waste container. Perform hand hygiene.
13. Document patient's record.

CHARTING EXAMPLE: 09/02/XX 10:20 A.M. Patient began seizing in exam room 3. Assisted Pt. to floor. Notified physician. Seizure lasted 3 minutes with tonic-clonic movements. Pt. vomited during recovery period. No apparent injuries sustained. Dr. Elito requested CAT scan. Appointment scheduled for 09/07/XX at Memorial Hospital. · · · · · · · · · · · · F. Murray, RMA

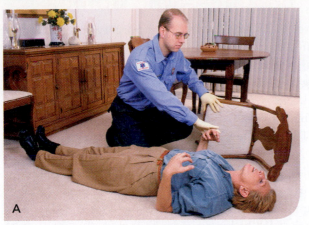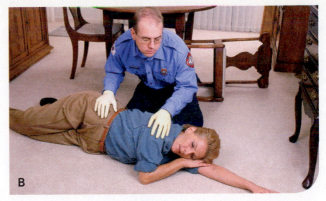

FIGURE 9-20A Move objects away from the seizure patient to help prevent injury; (B) when the seizure stops, position the patient to allow drainage of saliva and vomit.

- Name of substance, if known
- Amount of substance, if known
- When exposure happened
- Patient's signs and symptoms, including vomiting if it occurred
- Treatment given, if any

Be sure to keep the caller on the line while you gather the information and call the poison control center if the caller cannot. Relay all information regarding treatment from the poison control center to the patient.

Sometimes vomiting should be induced by using an emetic such as syrup of ipecac. If vomiting will cause further damage, as in the case of ingestion of a caustic substance such as lye or acid, milk or water may be administered to dilute the poison but only on the advice of the poison control center or physician. When poisons such as insecticides or fertilizers or parts of poisonous plants are absorbed through the skin, have the patient remove all clothing that came into contact with the poison and wash the affected skin area thoroughly with soap and water, then rinse skin thoroughly. In cases of inhaled poisons, move the individual into fresh air as soon as possible; monitor airway, breathing, and circulation; and notify EMS.

HEAT AND COLD EMERGENCIES

The human body normally controls its internal temperature effectively despite extreme variation in its surroundings. If the body is exposed to high or low temperatures for long enough, the result is **hyperthermia** (overheating) or **hypothermia** (lowering of body temperature).

The three main types of hyperthermia are heat cramps, heat exhaustion, and heat stroke. Heat cramps are muscle cramps following heavy exertion or sweating in a hot environment. Treatment depends on the severity of the cramps. In simple cases of muscle cramps, encourage the patient to drink water or electrolyte drinks such as Gatorade, cool down, and rest. If the patient is unable to drink liquids or is vomiting, intravenous infusion may be necessary.

Heat exhaustion results from exertion in a hot environment without fluid replacement. Heat cramps may or may not occur, but central nervous system symptoms such as headache, dizziness, syncope, moist skin, and high pulse rate are present. Treatment requires getting out of the heat immediately, lying down with feet raised, and hydrating with liquids such as water or Gatorade. If fever is greater than 102°F or confusion or seizures are present, notify EMS at once.

Heat stroke results when the body is no longer able to control the internal temperature, and it can result in brain damage or death. Symptoms of heat stroke are dry, hot skin with no sweating; confused, irritable, or unconscious state; and elevated vital signs that drop and may lead to cardiac arrest. Treatment includes moving the patient to a cooler area; removing clothing; and placing wet sheets or wet cloths on the head, neck, axilla, and groin; and notifying EMS.

Hypothermia results from exposure to very cold air or water. The symptoms are cool, pale skin, shallow and slow respiration, slow and faint pulse, and mental confusion. Treatment involves notifying EMS, removing wet clothing, and covering the patient to prevent further cooling.

Do not rub or massage the patient, and do not apply direct heat. Once the patient is alert and respirations are normal, administer warm fluids by mouth (avoid tea, coffee, and alcohol). Frostbite commonly occurs in the fingers, toes, ears, and nose after exposure to windy freezing weather. Superficial frostbite appears yellow or gray and waxy. Loss of sensation can lead to deep frostbite. Deep frostbite affects the hands and feet, and symptoms may appear after the initial loss of sensation. The skin becomes rigid and white. Deep frostbite can result in tissue necrosis. Treat superficial frostbite by warming the affected part of the patient's own body with part of your body. In severe cases notify EMS and rewarm affected tissue by immersing it in lukewarm water until it becomes flexible. Do not massage or apply dry heat.

Bandages and Splints

Chapter 8: Assisting with Minor Surgery covers cleaning and dressing wounds and applying dressings, figure-eight bandages, and slings. Applying a tubular bandage and applying a splint to immobilize a possible fracture are presented here.

Tubular gauze bandages are used to wrap around a body part. The bandage is a hollow tube that is stretchy and will mold itself to fingers, toes, and other hard-to-wrap areas. Tubular gauze is available in a variety of widths and is applied using a framelike applicator made of metal or plastic. The applicators are available in many sizes and should be larger than the body part to be bandaged. (Procedure 9-21 explains how to apply a tubular gauze bandage.)

PROCEDURE 9-21

APPLYING A TUBULAR GAUZE BANDAGE

ABHES VII.MA.A.1 9(o)(5)   CAAHEP XI.P (10)

OBJECTIVE: To apply a tubular gauze bandage to an extremity or digit.

STANDARD: This task takes about 10 minutes.

EQUIPMENT AND SUPPLIES: Tubular gauze and applicator of appropriate size; tape; scissors; patient's record; pen; gloves.

STEPS:

1. Perform hand hygiene.
2. Check patient's record for orders. Check for patient allergies.
3. Assemble equipment and supplies.
4. Identify patient, and explain procedure.
5. Select appropriate size applicator and gauze for area to be bandaged.
6. Cut tape in lengths to fasten gauze.
7. Place gauze bandage on applicator by placing applicator in upright position on a flat surface.
8. Pull some gauze from box, open end of gauze, and slide it over upper end of applicator.
9. Estimate amount of gauze needed to cover applicator, and cut when sufficient amount of gauze is on applicator.
10. Don gloves. Place applicator covered with gauze over distal end of area to be bandaged.
11. Apply bandage by pulling gauze over applicator onto skin.
12. Slide applicator to proximal end of affected part, hold gauze, and pull both applicator and gauze toward distal end.
13. While holding gauze in place at proximal end, pull applicator 1 to 2 inches past end of affected part if part is to be completely covered.
14. Turn applicator to anchor bandage.
15. Move applicator toward proximal body part about 1 inch past starting point, and anchor bandage by turning applicator.
16. Continue until affected area is sufficiently covered. End with final layer at proximal end of affected area.
17. Remove applicator, and cut extra gauze off applicator.
18. Secure bandage with tape.
19. Dispose of equipment and clean area.
20. Remove gloves, and perform hand hygiene.
21. Document procedure in patient's record.

CHARTING EXAMPLE: 09/02/XX 7:00 P.M. Sterile dressing applied to right thumb. Tubular bandage applied over dressing. Pt. received written and verbal wound care instructions. Pt. to return in 2 days for recheck. · · · · · · · · · · · · · · · · S. Greer, RMA

PROCEDURE 9-22

APPLYING AN ARM SPLINT

ABHES VII.MA.A.1 9(o)(5)   CAAHEP XI.P (10)

OBJECTIVE: To apply an arm splint to immobilize arm and reduce pain.

STANDARD: This task takes 10 minutes.

EQUIPMENT AND SUPPLIES: Splint, or piece of cardboard; gauze roller bandage; gloves; patient's record; pen.

STEPS:

1. Perform hand hygiene.
2. Assemble equipment and supplies.
3. Check physician's orders, and check for patient allergies. Identify patient, and explain procedure.
4. Place splint under injured area.
5. Holding splint in place, wrap roller gauze to secure arm to splint.
6. Provide extra padding at wrist between arm and board.
7. Check fingers for color and circulation. If splint too tight, reapply roller gauze.
8. Clean area.
9. Perform hand hygiene.
10. Document procedure in patient's record.

CHARTING EXAMPLE: 09/02/XX 5:00 P.M. Splint applied to L arm per physician's orders. Nail beds pink, and radial pulse palpated. Written and verbal follow-up information given patient. Sent to ED at Memorial for X-ray. · · · · · · · · · ·
· J. Hill, CMA (AAMA)

Emergency Preparedness

Emergency preparedness refers to the emergency plans developed to respond to a terrorist attack or natural disaster such as a hurricane, tornado, or flood. A brief discussion of emergency preparedness for situations such as earthquake, fire, flood, hurricane, terrorism, and environmental exposure follows.

The Federal Emergency Management Agency (FEMA) lists six steps involved in planning ahead for earthquakes:

1. Check for hazards around the facility. Make sure all shelves are secured to the walls; store heavy or breakable items on lower shelves; secure overhead lights; check wiring and gas connections and repair as needed; repair cracks in ceiling; store flammable materials on low shelves in locked closets.

2. Identify safe areas indoors and outdoors, such as an inside wall or under sturdy furniture that is away from glass and bookcases or other items that might fall over. Safe areas outside include places away from buildings, trees, wires, overpasses, or elevated roads.

3. Educate yourself and others by contacting the American Red Cross or civil preparedness centers for more information. Train all staff to turn off gas, electricity, and water in an emergency.

4. Have adequate supplies on hand, including flashlights, extra batteries an emergency first aid kit and manual, emergency food and water, sturdy shoes, and a manual can opener.

5. Develop an emergency communication plan, including a reuniting area in case of separation. Ensure that each staff member knows his or her responsibility, such as escorting patients out of the building.

6. Provide information at your facility to educate the public.

FIRE

Fire spreads rapidly and can engulf a building in 5 minutes.

1. All facilities must have working fire alarms, smoke detectors in each room that are tested monthly, and batteries replaced annually.

2. Escape routes must be clearly marked, and each staff member must be familiar with and practice these plans.

3. Flammable items should be stored in ventilated areas away from heat sources. Fire extinguishers should be located throughout the facility, and staff should be trained to use them.

4. Instruct person with clothing in flames to stop, drop, and roll.

5. Check closed doors for heat before opening. Feel the top of the door, doorknob and, crack around the door for heat. Do not open if it feels hot.

6. Stay low under smoke when escaping a fire. Close doors as you pass through them to prevent fire from spreading.

7. Do not reenter the premises unless the fire department has stated it is safe.

FLOODS

Floods are the most common disaster in the United States, according to FEMA. Be aware of the flood danger areas near your home and place of work. Water rises rapidly, so evacuate immediately when asked to do so. Move to a higher area if possible. Do not walk through moving water as only 6 inches of water can cause a person to fall. In a health care facility, be familiar with the emergency evacuation plan.

HURRICANES

Hurricanes can strike with little warning; however, today technology may warn us a week in advance that a hurricane is pending. It is important to prepare in advance of a hurricane in order to be able to respond quickly to an emergency or evacuation warning. Two examples of prehurricane preparation are trimming trees and shrubs in the immediate area and having hurricane shutters or plywood available to cover windows. Emergency supplies, such as those suggested in this chapter for earthquake preparedness, also should be readily accessible.

TERRORIST ATTACK

A terrorist attack may come in the form of explosions, biological agents, or a nuclear blast. Advance preparedness and emergency evacuation plans are essential. Follow the directions of civil preparedness units, listen to the radio or television, and follow the guidelines suggested in this chapter for earthquake or fire emergencies. Biological threats may come in several forms:

- **Aerosols.** Material spread through the air that may cover miles.

- **Animals.** Infected animals or insects.

- **Food or water contamination.** Agents placed in central water supplies or food production plants.

- **Person-to-person contact.** Agents spread by direct or droplet contact with infected persons.

NUCLEAR BLAST

In the event of a nuclear blast, take cover as quickly as possible below ground if there is a basement. Stay in the safe location and listen to instructions over the radio or television.

10 Clinical Laboratory Testing

PROCEDURES

Procedure 10-1 Completing a Laboratory Requisition and Preparing Specimen for Transport to Outside Laboratory

Procedure 10-2 Monitoring and Following Up on Patient Test Results

Procedure 10-3 Recording Quality Control Values on QC Control Record and Identifying Out-of-Control Values

Procedure 10-4 Using and Cleaning a Microscope

TERMS TO LEARN

qualitative test

analyte

quantitative test

turnaround time

outside laboratory

reference laboratory

precision

control samples

reagents

calibrate

accuracy

standard deviation

quantity not sufficient (QNS)

compound microscope

Clinical laboratory tests provide part of the framework upon which physicians base their diagnoses and monitor their patients' health. Clinical laboratory test results are an essential part of patient care and may be helpful to accomplish the following:

- Screen for disease
- Confirm a condition suspected by the physician
- Rule out a condition
- Monitor effectiveness of a treatment
- Assess the progress of disease
- Comply with employment, insurance, or legal requirements
- Contribute statistics for research and clinical trials

Laboratory data are used in conjunction with other clinical findings, patient history, and the expertise of the physician to provide quality care. However, relying on laboratory results alone is imprudent.

Clinical laboratories analyze specimens, report results, and provide reference ranges for comparison with patient results. Tests may be performed manually or automatically. The two common categories of laboratory tests are quantitative tests and qualitative tests. A **qualitative test** analyzes specimens for the presence or absence of a substance or analyte (the subject of an analysis). A **quantitative test** analyzes for the presence and amount of the analyte. Quantitative tests are reported using numerical values or units.

Laboratory results are reported using a universal system of metric units for weight, volume, and length. Table 10-1 lists the most common metric units used in reporting medical results. Centigrade units are used for recording temperatures. Refrigerators are generally kept at 4°C to 8°C, and room temperature is considered to be 15°C to 30°C. Storage of specimens, test kits, and analysis of specimens are often temperature sensitive. Temperature readings in all refrigerators, freezers, water baths, and incubators should be monitored daily and recorded on log sheets.

Clinical Laboratories

Three types of clinical laboratories perform tests of varying complexities: the physician's office laboratory (POL), the outside laboratory, and the reference or referral laboratory. The POL performs some of the tests ordered by the physician on site. The rapid **turnaround time** (time it takes to produce results) is an advantage of testing in a POL. However POL testing may also require more expensive equipment and more highly skilled employees to perform the tests. The **outside laboratory** is either a hospital-based or

TABLE 10-1 Metric Units of Measurements

Measurement	Metric Unit	Abbreviation	Comparison to Units in United States
Weight	gram	g or gm	1 g = approximately 1 raisin
	kilogram = 1,000 g	kg	1 kg = 2.2 lb
	decigram	dg	1/10 g (0.1)
	centigram	cg	1/100 g (0.01)
	milligram	mg	1/1,000 g (0.001)
	microgram	µg or mcg (use *mc* when writing by hand, not *µ*)	1/1,000,000 (0.000001) g
Volume	liter	L or l	1L = slightly more than 1 quart
	deciliter	dL or dl	1/10 liter
	milliliter	ml or mL	1/1,000 liter (same as cubic centimeter or cc)
	microliter	µl or µL	1/1,000,000 liter
Length	meter	M or m	1 meter = slightly longer than 1 mile
	kilometer	km	1,000 meters
	centimeter	cm	1/1,000 meter
	millimeter	Mm	1/1,000,000 of a meter
Temperature	Centigrade or Celsius	°C	0°C = freezing; 100° C = boiling = 212°F 37°C = body temperature = 98.6°F

Large clinical laboratories use cluster testing processes organized as follows:

Clinical chemistry	Routine and special chemistry testing
Cytogenetics	Genetic testing
Cytology	Review Pap tests and other cell detection testing
Hematology and coagulation	Blood counts (CBC) coagulation tests (PT, PTT)
Histology	Preparation of tissue samples, slides from biopsies, autopsies
Immunohematology	Transfusions, blood banking
Immunology, serology	Antibody detection testing for many illnesses
Microbiology	Detection and testing for bacteria, viruses, parasites, and fungus
Specimen collection/processing	Draw blood samples, process for testing, prepare for transportation to outside or reference lab
Urinalysis	Urine analysis (UA), special urine testing

independent laboratory capable of handling a large number of specimens and performing tests ranging from simple to complex. The referral or **reference laboratory** may be associated with a teaching or medical facility or be privately owned. Reference laboratories perform large numbers of complex tests that outside laboratories only occasionally receive requests to perform.

CLINICAL LABORATORY DEPARTMENTS

Clinical laboratories are divided into various departments that perform specific categories of tests. Box 10-1 lists sections of a clinical laboratory and a brief description of tests performed in each. For point-of-care, or near-patient, testing, the test procedure is performed where the patient is and the specimen is taken from there to the laboratory for analysis. This type of testing provides rapid results using small instruments that are accurate if used properly.

In 1988 the U.S. Congress enacted the Clinical Laboratory Improvement Amendments (CLIA) in response to widespread concern over the accuracy of laboratory tests results. CLIA was updated in 1992, and as a result tests are classified according to complexity and the level of training required to perform tests in each category. Tests are classified as Certificate of Waiver Tests (WTs), Level I Tests, and Level II Tests. The Health Care Financing Administration (HCFA), a division of the U.S. Department of Health and Human Services (DHHS) is responsible for monitoring compliance to CLIA regulations. Box 10-2 illustrates tests performed in each category under CLIA 1992. Laboratories performing moderate or high-complexity tests must adhere to CLIA regulations and are subject to unannounced inspections every 2 years by HCFA. CLIA regulations involve the following:

- **Patient Test Monitoring.** To ensure identification and integrity of patient specimens, results and reporting in every step of analysis process.

- **Quality Control (QC).** To ensure accurate, reliable, and precise results, QC procedures must be in place to monitor and evaluate each test process (laboratory procedure manual, two levels of controls daily, documenting problem identification and actions, QC documentation). (**Precision** of laboratory results refers to the reproducibility of results each time the test is performed.)

- **Proficiency Testing (PT).** External QC laboratory specimens prepared by a testing agency are sent and tested in a laboratory. The results are forwarded and graded by the testing agency and must meet certain requirements.

- **Personnel Requirements.** Education and training qualifications for laboratory directors, testing personnel, and consultants must be met before moderate- and high-complexity testing can take place.

QUALITY CONTROL

QC programs in the clinical laboratory monitor testing, analysis, and reporting of patient specimens and results to ensure reliable, valid, consistent results. Specimens or samples tested in clinical laboratories may be whole blood, serum, plasma, body fluids such as cerebrospinal fluid and urine, feces, tissue, and swabs of areas such as the vagina, the throat, and wounds. **Control samples** are samples that are similar to the testing specimen required and have been previously tested and have a known value. Controls are purchased from a manufacturer with an assigned lot number, value sheet, dilution instructions, storage instructions, and expiration date. **Reagents** are substances required for a chemical reaction or used to detect the presence of another substance, such as glucose. Many test kits contain positive and negative controls that must be run along with the test to ensure that the test is accurate and that the individual performing the test is performing it correctly. The results of the controls are posted on a QC sheet daily.

Some laboratory tests may require personnel to calibrate an instrument or machine prior to testing. To **calibrate** an instrument, a known standard is used to measure the accuracy of the equipment needed for testing procedures. Documentation of standardization must be done as part of QC. Maintenance of all laboratory equipment must be documented.

Manufacturers' recommendations should be followed, and a record of each piece of laboratory equipment with its model number, serial number, date of purchase, and manufacturer's insert must be maintained.

PROFICIENCY TESTING

Proficiency Testing is an external QC program that monitors the **accuracy** (correctness) of test systems by comparing an individual laboratory's results to results provided by a survey program. To be accurate, controls must consistently fall within two standard deviations of the mean. (**Standard deviation** is a statistical term describing the amount of variation from the mean in a set of data.) Any laboratory whose results for a specific analyte are unacceptable in two out of three testing surveys may lose its permission to perform that test. The laboratory may not perform that test for patients until appropriate action is taken and two subsequent proficiency tests are within acceptable limits.

LABORATORY SAFETY

Laboratory hazards include biohazards, chemical hazards, and physical hazards. Anyone working in a laboratory must be familiar with the following regulations:

- Hazard Communication Standards
- Standard Precautions and Bloodborne Pathogen Standards
- Hazardous Waste Operations
- Needlestick Safety and Prevention Act

Safety issues are discussed in Chapter 2: Infection Control, and further information may be found by checking Occupational Safety and Health Administration (OSHA) and Centers for Disease Control and Prevention (CDC) Web sites (osha.gov and cdc.gov).

LABORATORY REQUISITIONS

The laboratory testing process begins with the physician's request for a test. Careful completion of a laboratory requisition includes the information listed in Box 10-3. Reliable, accurate test results begin with the lab slip and patient data. Many facilities require specific requisition forms, and some other forms are not acceptable. (Figure 10-1 is an example of a laboratory requisition slip with procedure codes.)

Laboratory tests are often categorized into related groups or panels to provide information about a particular body organ, system, or part. For example, a cardiac panel would include tests associated with the heart. Medicare reimbursement requires that tests be ordered according to HCFA-approved organ- and disease-oriented panels, not as previously ordered with names such as CHEM 10 or SMAC 12. Each approved panel has its own CPT code.

BOX 10-3 Laboratory Requisition Information

- Physician's name, address, phone number, and account number
- Patient's full name, address, phone number
- Patient's age, sex, date of birth (DOB)
- Patient's complete insurance information
- Source of specimen
- Fasting or nonfasting specimen
- Date and collection time
- Specific tests requested per physician's orders, including five-digit procedure code
- Patient's present medications
- Diagnosis and diagnostic code, if possible
- Stat or regular request

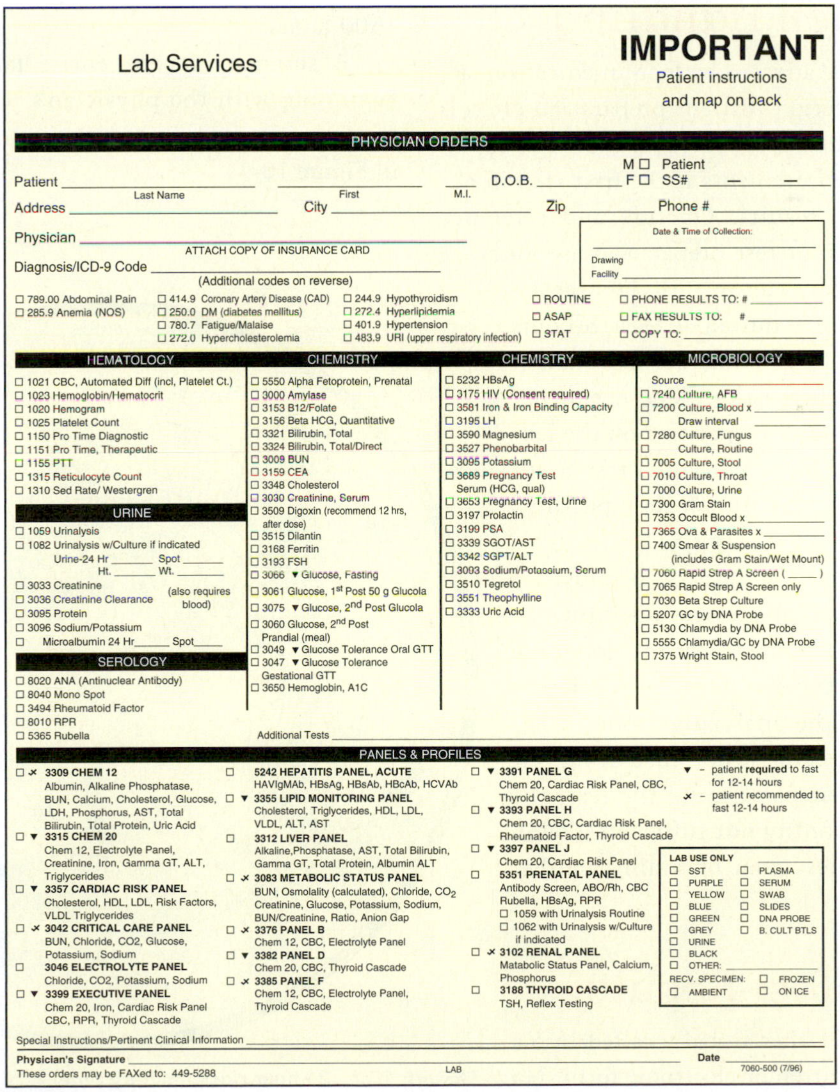

Lab Services

IMPORTANT
Patient instructions and map on back

PHYSICIAN ORDERS

Patient ____ (Last Name) ____ (First) ____ (M.I.) D.O.B. ____ M ☐ F ☐ Patient SS# ___ – ___ – ___
Address ____ City ____ Zip ____ Phone # ____
Physician ____
ATTACH COPY OF INSURANCE CARD
Diagnosis/ICD-9 Code ____
(Additional codes on reverse)

Date & Time of Collection: ____ ____
Drawing Facility ____

☐ 789.00 Abdominal Pain
☐ 285.9 Anemia (NOS)
☐ 414.9 Coronary Artery Disease (CAD)
☐ 250.0 DM (diabetes mellitus)
☐ 780.7 Fatigue/Malaise
☐ 272.0 Hypercholesterolemia
☐ 244.9 Hypothyroidism
☐ 272.4 Hyperlipidemia
☐ 401.9 Hypertension
☐ 483.9 URI (upper respiratory infection)

☐ ROUTINE
☐ ASAP
☐ STAT

☐ PHONE RESULTS TO: # ____
☐ FAX RESULTS TO: # ____
☐ COPY TO: ____

HEMATOLOGY
☐ 1021 CBC, Automated Diff (incl, Platelet Ct.)
☐ 1023 Hemoglobin/Hematocrit
☐ 1020 Hemogram
☐ 1025 Platelet Count
☐ 1150 Pro Time Diagnostic
☐ 1151 Pro Time, Therapeutic
☐ 1155 PTT
☐ 1315 Reticulocyte Count
☐ 1310 Sed Rate/ Westergren

URINE
☐ 1059 Urinalysis
☐ 1082 Urinalysis w/Culture if indicated
Urine-24 Hr ____ Spot ____
Ht. ____ Wt. ____
☐ 3033 Creatinine
☐ 3036 Creatinine Clearance (also requires blood)
☐ 3095 Protein
☐ 3096 Sodium/Potassium
☐ Microalbumin 24 Hr____ Spot____

SEROLOGY
☐ 8020 ANA (Antinuclear Antibody)
☐ 8040 Mono Spot
☐ 3494 Rheumatoid Factor
☐ 8010 RPR
☐ 5365 Rubella

CHEMISTRY
☐ 5550 Alpha Fetoprotein, Prenatal
☐ 3000 Amylase
☐ 3153 B12/Folate
☐ 3156 Beta HCG, Quantitative
☐ 3321 Bilirubin, Total
☐ 3324 Bilirubin, Total/Direct
☐ 3009 BUN
☐ 3159 CEA
☐ 3348 Cholesterol
☐ 3030 Creatinine, Serum
☐ 3509 Digoxin (recommend 12 hrs, after dose)
☐ 3515 Dilantin
☐ 3168 Ferritin
☐ 3193 FSH
☐ 3066 ▼ Glucose, Fasting
☐ 3061 Glucose, 1st Post 50 g Glucola
☐ 3075 ▼ Glucose, 2nd Post Glucola
☐ 3060 Glucose, 2nd Post Prandial (meal)
☐ 3049 ▼ Glucose Tolerance Oral GTT
☐ 3047 ▼ Glucose Tolerance Gestational GTT
☐ 3650 Hemoglobin, A1C

CHEMISTRY
☐ 5232 HBsAg
☐ 3175 HIV (Consent required)
☐ 3581 Iron & Iron Binding Capacity
☐ 3195 LH
☐ 3590 Magnesium
☐ 3527 Phenobarbital
☐ 3095 Potassium
☐ 3689 Pregnancy Test Serum (HCG, qual)
☐ 3653 Pregnancy Test, Urine
☐ 3197 Prolactin
☐ 3199 PSA
☐ 3339 SGOT/AST
☐ 3342 SGPT/ALT
☐ 3003 Sodium/Potassium, Serum
☐ 3510 Tegretol
☐ 3551 Theophylline
☐ 3333 Uric Acid

MICROBIOLOGY
Source ____
☐ 7240 Culture, AFB
☐ 7200 Culture, Blood x ____
☐ Draw interval ____
☐ 7280 Culture, Fungus
☐ Culture, Routine
☐ 7005 Culture, Stool
☐ 7010 Culture, Throat
☐ 7000 Culture, Urine
☐ 7300 Gram Stain
☐ 7353 Occult Blood x ____
☐ 7365 Ova & Parasites x ____
☐ 7400 Smear & Suspension (includes Gram Stain/Wet Mount)
☐ 7060 Rapid Strep A Screen (____)
☐ 7065 Rapid Strep A Screen only
☐ 7030 Beta Strep Culture
☐ 5207 GC by DNA Probe
☐ 5130 Chlamydia by DNA Probe
☐ 5555 Chlamydia/GC by DNA Probe
☐ 7375 Wright Stain, Stool

Additional Tests ____

PANELS & PROFILES
☐ ✗ **3309 CHEM 12** Albumin, Alkaline Phosphatase, BUN, Calcium, Cholesterol, Glucose, LDH, Phosphorus, AST, Total Bilirubin, Total Protein, Uric Acid
☐ ▼ **3315 CHEM 20** Chem 12, Electrolyte Panel, Creatinine, Iron, Gamma GT, ALT, Triglycerides
☐ ▼ **3357 CARDIAC RISK PANEL** Cholesterol, HDL, LDL, Risk Factors, VLDL Triglycerides
☐ ✗ **3042 CRITICAL CARE PANEL** BUN, Chloride, CO2, Glucose, Potassium, Sodium
☐ **3046 ELECTROLYTE PANEL** Chloride, CO2, Potassium, Sodium
☐ ▼ **3399 EXECUTIVE PANEL** Chem 20, Iron, Cardiac Risk Panel CBC, RPR, Thyroid Cascade
☐ **5242 HEPATITIS PANEL, ACUTE** HAVIgMAb, HBsAg, HBsAb, HBcAb, HCVAb
☐ ▼ **3355 LIPID MONITORING PANEL** Cholesterol, Triglycerides, HDL, LDL, VLDL, ALT, AST
☐ **3312 LIVER PANEL** Alkaline,Phosphatase, AST, Total Bilirubin, Gamma GT, Total Protein, Albumin ALT
☐ ✗ **3083 METABOLIC STATUS PANEL** BUN, Osmolality (calculated), Chloride, CO_2 Creatinine, Glucose, Potassium, Sodium, BUN/Creatinine, Ratio, Anion Gap
☐ ✗ **3376 PANEL B** Chem 12, CBC, Electrolyte Panel
☐ ▼ **3382 PANEL D** Chem 20, CBC, Thyroid Cascade
☐ ✗ **3385 PANEL F** Chem 12, CBC, Electrolyte Panel, Thyroid Cascade
☐ ▼ **3391 PANEL G** Chem 20, Cardiac Risk Panel, CBC, Thyroid Cascade
☐ ▼ **3393 PANEL H** Chem 20, CBC, Cardiac Risk Panel, Rheumatoid Factor, Thyroid Cascade
☐ ▼ **3397 PANEL J** Chem 20, Cardiac Risk Panel
☐ **5351 PRENATAL PANEL** Antibody Screen, ABO/Rh, CBC Rubella, HBsAg, RPR
☐ 1059 with Urinalysis Routine
☐ 1062 with Urinalysis w/Culture if indicated
☐ ✗ **3102 RENAL PANEL** Matabolic Status Panel, Calcium, Phosphorus
☐ **3188 THYROID CASCADE** TSH, Reflex Testing

▼ – patient **required** to fast for 12-14 hours
✗ – patient recommended to fast 12-14 hours

LAB USE ONLY ____
☐ SST ☐ PLASMA
☐ PURPLE ☐ SERUM
☐ YELLOW ☐ SWAB
☐ BLUE ☐ SLIDES
☐ GREEN ☐ DNA PROBE
☐ GREY ☐ B. CULT BTLS
☐ URINE
☐ BLACK
☐ OTHER: ____
RECV. SPECIMEN: ☐ FROZEN
☐ AMBIENT ☐ ON ICE

Special Instructions/Pertinent Clinical Information ____
Physician's Signature ____ **Date** ____
These orders may be FAXed to: 449-5288 LAB 7060-500 (7/96)

FIGURE 10-1 Laboratory requisition slip.

Chain of Custody

A patient must present picture identification at time of collection. Circumstances may arise which require that a specimen with medicolegal implications be obtained from a patient. Specimen collection in cases of rape, child, spousal, or elder abuse and drug or alcohol abuse could have important implications on the outcome of a legal case in a court of law. Proving chain of custody (COC) existed is vital for proving the integrity of the specimen. The term *chain of custody* refers to a specific set of procedures used to collect, process, test, and report results. A chain-of-custody form must be signed at each step of collection, processing, and reporting to prove that the chain of custody was unbroken. Proving a chain of custody existed is vital for the specimen to be considered valid.

Patient Preparation and Specimen Handling

Laboratory results can be affected by food, medication, activity, and time of collection. Patient preparation often is required before a specimen is collected. A thorough explanation of preparation requirements is the first step in obtaining valid accurate results. Outside and reference laboratory requirements for test preparation are found in the directory provided by the specific laboratory. For some tests, fasting is required at least 8 hours prior to testing, and 12 to 14 hours without food or drink are required in others cases. Whether or not the patient is fasting should be specified on the laboratory requisition slip. The quality of a test result is only as good as the quality of the specimen provided.

Once the specimen is obtained, it must be labeled immediately and processed according to the specific requirements of the laboratory doing the analyzing. Storage and transportation of specimens are done according to the analyzing laboratories' requirements. If the specimen obtained from the patient is insufficient for performing the test, the requisition is labeled **quantity not sufficient (QNS)**. Follow facility procedures about obtaining another specimen.

Patients' Test Results

Patients' test results are either verbally called into a facility or received in written or electronic form. No test results should be filed in a patient's record until the physician has reviewed them. It is the purview of the physician to explain test results to the patient. All laboratory results are confidential, and release of information must comply with HIPAA guidelines. Laboratory test results are compared to reference values provided by the testing laboratory. The reference values represent a range of results for the general population. If reference values vary due to gender, age, or race, these variations of values are included.

Laboratory Testing Cycle and Time

Time in most laboratories is based on International Military Time and must be used on all laboratory requisitions. Figure 10-2 is an illustration of a 24-hour clock with military and Greenwich Time. For example, 1:00 P.M. is 1300 hours.

A summary of the entire laboratory testing cycle, beginning with the physician's request and ending with transmission of results to the physician, is illustrated clearly in Figure 10-3.

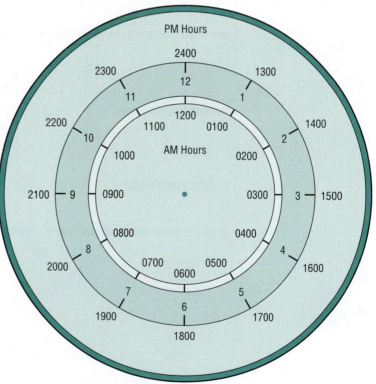

FIGURE 10-2 **24-hour clock (military time).**

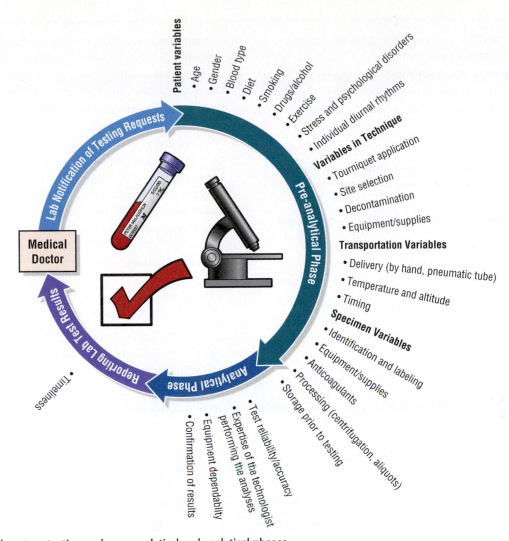

FIGURE 10-3 Laboratory testing cycle: preanalytical and analytical phases.

PROCEDURE 10-1

COMPLETING A LABORATORY REQUISITION AND PREPARING SPECIMEN FOR TRANSPORT TO OUTSIDE LABORATORY

ABHES VII.MA.A.1 10(d)   CAAHEP III.P (7)

OBJECTIVE: To accurately complete a laboratory requisition form for testing as ordered by the physician, obtain required specimen(s), and prepare specimen(s) for transport to outside laboratory.

STANDARD: This task takes 10 minutes to several hours, depending on type of specimen.

EQUIPMENT AND SUPPLIES: Physician's order for laboratory tests; patient's record; pen; laboratory requisition form;

gloves; specimen container; laboratory log book; biohazard waste container; pen.

STEPS:

1. Check patient's record for orders for specific lab tests.
2. Verify which lab will be doing testing, and locate required requisition form.
3. Complete patient demographic section.

4. Complete section requiring physician's name, address, phone number, and account number.

5. Complete patient's insurance and billing information.

6. Mark each box to indicate each test ordered by physician. If an ordered test is not listed on requisition, write in name of test on lines provided.

WHY? Recheck all tests ordered to avoid having to repeat blood draw and delaying results.

7. Indicate type and source of specimen to be tested.

8. Enter patient's diagnosis on requisition as needed. If no diagnosis has been made, then code patient's symptoms.

9. Complete patient authorization to release and assign benefits portion, as needed.

10. Assemble equipment and supplies needed to obtain specimen.

11. Perform hand hygiene, and don gloves.

12. Obtain specimen required after explaining procedure to patient.

13. Label specimen with patient's name, date, physician's name, time of collection, and other information required by facility.

14. Initial laboratory requisition, and complete date and time specimen was obtained.

15. Process specimens.

16. Attach laboratory requisition securely to specimen.

17. If specimens are not to be sent out right away, store sample according to laboratory requirements. Otherwise, follow laboratory requirements for sending sample to lab.

18. Remove gloves; dispose of them in biohazard waste container. Perform hand hygiene.

19. Document patient's record.

20. Record specimen in laboratory logbook, indicating date, time of collection, type and source of specimen, tests ordered, where samples were sent, and date sent.

CHARTING EXAMPLE: 08/04/XX 8:00 A.M. Venous blood sample for Stat CBC sent to Memorial Lab at 8:40 A.M. Lab will call back with results. · R. Patel, RMA

PROCEDURE 10-2

MONITORING AND FOLLOWING UP ON PATIENT TEST RESULTS

ABHES VII.MA.A.1 10(f)   CAAHEP I.P (16)

OBJECTIVE: Review incoming laboratory results and follow up with patient, per physician's orders.

STANDARD: This task takes 5 minutes.

EQUIPMENT AND SUPPLIES: Patient's record; laboratory test results; pen; log of patient's laboratory results.

STEPS:

NOTE: Follow facility policy on contacting patients with abnormal results. Results are not to be released to the patient unless authorized by the physician.

1. Review incoming lab results and compare with reference values provided by analyzing laboratory. Many laboratories highlight or indicate abnormal results on lab result sheets with "H" or "L."

2. Highlight any abnormal results per facility policy.

3. Obtain patient's medical record, attach new lab results, and submit to physician to review.

HIPAA Alert! Do not leave patient results anywhere they may be observed by others. Remember that results are governed by "need to know" as far as other employees are concerned. Patient confidentiality is mandatory.

4. Follow physician's orders regarding scheduling appointment or repeat testing.

5. Document patient's record accordingly.

CHARTING EXAMPLE: 08/04/XX 10:00 A.M.: Scheduled repeat lab test and follow-up appointment on 08/10/XX per physician's order. · · · · · · · · · · · · · · · · · C. Fisher, CMA (AAMA)

PROCEDURE 10-3

RECORDING QUALITY CONTROL VALUES ON QC CONTROL RECORD AND IDENTIFYING OUT-OF-CONTROL VALUES

ABHES VII.MA.A.1 10(a)   CAAHEP I.P (11)

OBJECTIVE: To record daily normal control values, recognize when control values are out of acceptable limits, and suggest possible reasons for out-of-control values.

STANDARD: This task takes 5 minutes.

EQUIPMENT AND SUPPLIES: QC record; three values for normal controls; pen.

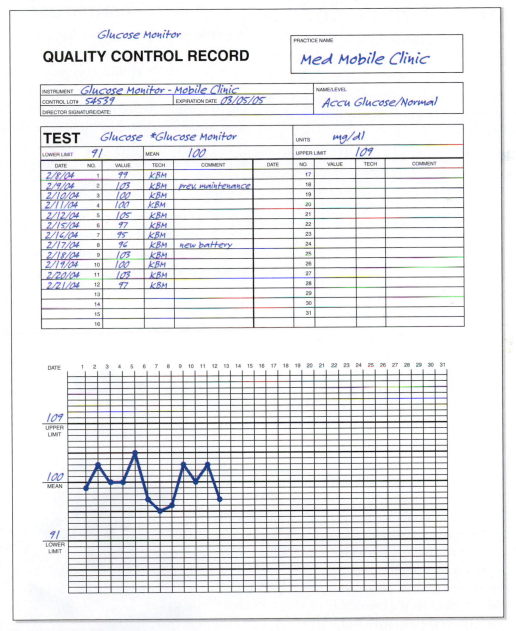

FIGURE 10-4   Quality Control Record.

STEPS:

1. Locate correct QC control sheet for a specific lot number and test protocol.

2. Given following values for dates provided, insert value for each of three controls, and place dot on correct line on QC Record (see Figure 10-4.)
   - 3/22/04   93 mg/dL
   - 3/23/04   112 mg/dL
   - 3/24/04   98 mg/dL

3. Connect dots. and write comment on sheet on action taken or reason for value beyond test control limits.

4. Follow up on reasons for out-of-control limits.

Safety Alert! If a control is outside of the expected limits, patient results are not reportable. Repeat the control with new control serum or another batch, and recheck results.

Laboratory Equipment

Clinical laboratories utilize a wide variety of equipment and supplies. A POL or point of care testing (POCT) site utilizes a smaller array of instruments; however, each one must be maintained well to ensure maximum performance. A few pieces of equipment are common to most small laboratories, including the following:

- Microscope
- Centrifuge
- Incubator
- Refrigerator and freezer
- Chemistry analyzer
- Automated cell counter
- Urine analyzer

MICROSCOPE

Microscopes are used to examine urine sediment, vaginal and bacteriological smears, and differential blood smears. The microscope magnifies structures unseen by the naked eye for the purpose of counting, naming, or differentiating. Figure 10-5 is an example of a **compound microscope** (one with two sets of lenses, oculars, and objectives) and its parts. The resolution of a microscope refers to the ability to distinguish clearly between two adjacent but distinct objects—the greater the resolution, the better the microscope. The components of a microscope are listed and briefly explained in Box 10-4.

The magnification of an object is calculated by multiplying the objective magnification by the eyepiece magnification. On low power, the magnification would be 100 times the size of the specimen under focus (10 for the objective times 10 for the eyepiece). (Procedure 10-4) lists the steps in using and cleaning a microscope.)

CENTRIFUGE

A centrifuge is an instrument that spins a specimen to separate it into component layers. A POL may use several centrifuges, each with a different purpose. One centrifuge is used to separate blood specimens into layers so the serum or plasma can be removed for testing without the red cells. Urines are spun in another centrifuge to separate the sediment (solids) from the liquid portion (supernatant) to perform a microscopic urine examination. Tiny capillary tubes are centrifuged in another centrifuge to measure a patient's hematocrit.

Balancing the tubes is the underlying concept when using any centrifuge. To maintain balance, a specimen container of the same type with the same amount of liquid should be placed in the position opposite the specimen container. Once the centrifuge is loaded correctly, it is closed, locked, and the amount of time is monitored. Different types of specimens are spun at different speeds and for different lengths of time. A centrifuge should not be opened before it comes to a complete stop.

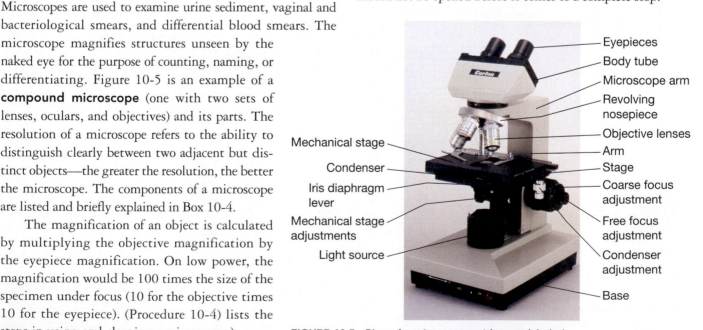

FIGURE 10-5 Binocular microscope with parts labeled.

BOX 10-4 Components of the Microscope

1. **Eyepiece(s).**   Monocular or binocular with magnification printed on each.
2. **Body tube.**   Directs light source.
3. **Arm.**   Used to carry the microscope along with the base.
4. **Revolving nosepiece.**   Holds objectives and rotates for selection.
5. **Objectives.**   Magnification is printed on each objective: 10 is low power; 40 is high dry setting; and 100 is for oil immersion setting.
6. **Stage.**   Holds the specimen.
7. **Mechanical stage.**   Device that holds the specimen or slide in place.
8. **Mechanical stage adjustment knobs.**   Two knobs, one small and one larger, that adjust stage up and down for focusing.
9. **Coarse and fine adjustment knobs.**   Small knob atop larger knob; adjust stage up and down for focusing.
10. **Condenser.**   Lens system used to increase light for sharper focus.
11. **Condenser adjustment knob.**   Adjusts the condenser.
12. **Light source or illuminator.**   Light usually set in the base of microscope.
13. **Iris diaphragm.**   Opens and shuts iris to increase and decrease light.
14. **Base.**   Holds the microscope upright, contains illuminator and rheostat, and is used together with arm to carry the microscope.

PROCEDURE 10-4

USING AND CLEANING A MICROSCOPE

ABHES VII.MA.A.1 8(y)   CAAHEP V.P (9)

OBJECTIVE: To observe a slide under 10×, 40×, and oil immersion properly and to clean and store microscope correctly.

STANDARD: This task takes 5 minutes.

EQUIPMENT AND SUPPLIES: Binocular compound microscope; specimen slide; lens paper; lens cleaner; dust cover for microscope.

STEPS:

1. Always carry microscope with one hand on arm and one hand under base.
2. Make sure stage is in down position before starting.
3. Clean objectives with lens paper starting with 10× and ending with oil immersion.
4. Place prepared slide on stage. Turn on light and rotate nosepiece until 10× objective is directly over slide.
5. Use coarse adjustment knob to raise stage until objective is close to slide on stage.
6. Look through eyepiece, and adjust coarse focus knob until microscope field is seen (a round circle of bright light).
7. Use fine adjustment knob for clearer image.
8. Open diaphragm, and adjust rheostat to focus if necessary.
9. Raise or lower condenser to alter light refraction. Condenser is usually lowered when using 10× power.
10. Observe slide.
11. Change objective to 40×, and readjust as needed. Move objective, and place a drop of oil on slide before completing turn in order to oil immersion lens.
12. When focusing and examination are complete, lower stage before removing slide.
13. Turn off light.
14. Clean eyepieces, and objectives with lens paper. Clean oil immersion lens with lens cleaner.
15. Unplug and wrap electrical cord around base.
16. Cover microscope with dust cover.
17. Clean slide and store.

INCUBATOR

An incubator is a piece of equipment that provides a stable temperature in which microorganisms can thrive and reproduce. Usually the internal temperature of an incubator is 98.6°F (37°C). Cultured media are placed in an incubator for 24 to 48 hours. A daily log of incubator temperature must be maintained.

REFRIGERATOR AND FREEZER

Refrigerators and freezers in a POL are used to store specimens, testing kits, and reagents at specific temperatures. Many tests are temperature sensitive, and test kits and reagents must be stored at the manufacturers' designated temperatures. A refrigerator should maintain a temperature of 39.2F° (4°C to 8°C), and a daily log of temperature variations must be kept.

CHEMISTRY ANALYZER

Chemistry analyzers vary from a simple instrument that performs one or two tests to complex computerized analyzers that perform multiple tests on each specimen rapidly and prints out results. In a POL a number of benchtop chemistry analyzers may be found. These instruments test for a few analytes and use dry reagent technology in the form of a special card or strip to which a drop of specimen (whole blood, serum, or plasma) is applied. An automated pipette is used to deliver the precise amount of specimen required. Hand-held devices for bedside testing of glucose are another type of analyzer. Whatever the type of analyzer, the manufacturer's instructions must be followed exactly for testing, use, and care.

AUTOMATED CELL COUNTER

A cell counter is an automated analyzer used to count the size and number of blood cells. The simpler ones count red and white cells and measure hemoglobin and hematocrits. The specimen sample is inserted manually, and results are reported on a digital screen or printed out. Complex cell counters handle hundreds of specimens and perform many tests and calculations on each specimen. Cell counters are operated by medical assistants who have received documented training from a CLIA-qualified individual.

URINE ANALYZER

Special urine analyzers are used in some POLs. A urine specimen is placed on a reagent strip and inserted into the analyzer, and a printout of results is produced shortly. Manufacturers' directions must be followed exactly, and QC performed to ensure accurate results.

11 Urinalysis

PROCEDURES

Procedure 11-1 Instructing a Patient How to Collect a 24-Hour Urine Specimen

Procedure 11-2 Instructing a Male Patient How to Collect a Clean-Catch Midstream Urine Specimen

Procedure 11-3 Instructing a Female Patient How to Collect a Clean-Catch Midstream Urine Specimen

Procedure 11-4 Collecting a Urine Specimen for Drug Screening

Procedure 11-5 Evaluating the Color, Clarity, and Volume of Urine

Procedure 11-6 Measuring Specific Gravity of Urine with Refractometer

Procedure 11-7 Testing Urine with Chemical Reagent Strips

Procedure 11-8 Performing a Complete Urinalysis

Procedure 11-9 Performing Clinitest Tablet Test for Glucose and Other Reducing Substances in Urine

Procedure 11-10 Testing for Ketones in Urine Using Acetest (Nitroprusside Reaction)

Procedure 11-11 Testing for Protein in Urine Using Sulfosalicylic Acid (SSA)

Procedure 11-12 Testing Urine Using Ictotest (Diazo Tablet) for Bilirubin

Procedure 11-13 Performing a Urine Pregnancy Test Using the Enzyme Immunoassay Method

TERMS TO LEARN

aliquot

sediment

turbid

fetid

polyuria

oliguria

anuria

supernatant

casts

hematuria

pyuria

parasites

Urinalysis refers to testing of urine for the presence of infection or disease. A routine urinalysis consists of examining the physical, chemical, and microscopic characteristics of urine. It is one of the most frequently performed laboratory tests. Urine is readily available, easily collected, and often provides the first clues to illness. The patient needs to receive clear instructions about methods of collection in simple terms.

Collecting a Urine Specimen

The method of collection and storage for urine specimens is governed by the type of test requested. All types of urine collections have the following general guidelines:

- Correctly label the specimen container with patient's name, date, type of specimen collected (random, first morning, 24 hour, clean catch, or catheterized).

- 10 to 30 mL is usually needed for most procedures.

- After collection, clean the outside of the specimen container with disinfectant to avoid spreading disease. (See Figures 11-1A, 11-1B, and 11-1C for examples of urine containers.)

- Obtain the right specimen in the correct type of container (sterile, disposable, 24 hour).

- Avoid collecting urine samples during menses; if menses present, note it on the laboratory requisition slip.

- Test urine as soon as possible after collection, refrigerate it, or add preservative if it is to sit more than 1 hour, depending on the facility's recommendations.

RANDOM URINE SAMPLE

A random sample of urine is the most commonly collected type of urine specimen. This specimen is collected in a nonsterile container and can be collected at any time, even though the composition of urine changes during the day. Urine containers should be provided by the facility to the patient, who may bring a sample from home in certain cases.

Guidelines for collecting a routine, random sample of urine in the office are as follows:

- Provide patient with nonsterile container labeled with patient's name and date.

- Ask patient to use the lavatory and void initial small amount of urine into the toilet before filling the container about two-thirds with urine.

- Explain where you want the patient to leave the container of urine.

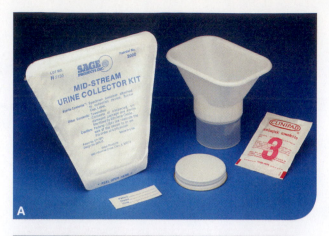

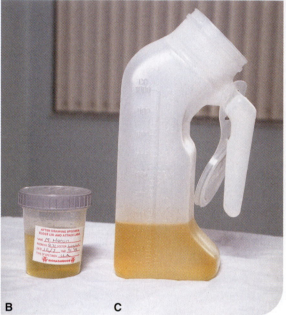

FIGURE 11-1   Various urine containers: (A) a midstream clean-catch container; (B) urine collection cup; (C) 24-hour urine container.

- Provide a paper towel on which to place and with which to carry the container to prevent contamination.

- Wear nonsterile gloves to test the specimen.

- Test the sample as soon as possible after collection, or store it in the refrigerator if more than 1 hour will pass prior to testing.

First Voided Morning Specimen

A first voided morning specimen is the most concentrated specimen of the day and therefore is the specimen of choice because it has the greatest amount of dissolved substances. It is easier to detect abnormalities in a more concentrated sample of urine. The collection process is the same as for a random specimen. The patient is asked to obtain a first morning specimen on arising and store it in the refrigerator in the container provided until able to drop it off at the facility for testing.

Timed Urine Specimen

Timed specimens are necessary for quantitative analysis of substances such as protein, creatinine, or glucose. Timed specimens also are necessary for certain types of urine testing, such as a 24-hour urine sample or a 2-hour postprandial sample. To obtain an adequate 24-hour specimen, patient directions must be thorough, clear, and in writing when the container is presented to the patient.

To collect a 24-hour specimen the patient is given a large, clean, and properly labeled container to take home. Collection begins after voiding the first morning specimen into the toilet and collecting every drop of urine voided during the next 24-hour period, including the first morning specimen on the following day. Refrigeration of the specimen during the 24-hour period may slow growth of microorganisms but not prevent it all together. Depending on the test to be performed, a preservative may be added before providing the patient with the container. The preservative should be noted clearly on the label because certain preservatives may be caustic. The patient must use caution when pouring sample into the container and avoid splashing the preservative. (Procedure 11-1 addresses how to collect a 24-hour urine specimen follows.)

PROCEDURE 11-1

INSTRUCTING A PATIENT HOW TO COLLECT A 24-HOUR URINE SPECIMEN

ABHES VII.MA.A.1 10(e)   CAAHEP IV.P (5); III.A (2)

OBJECTIVE: To instruct a patient how to properly collect a 24-hour urine specimen.

STANDARD: This task takes about 5 minutes, depending on patient's ability to understand directions.

EQUIPMENT AND SUPPLIES: 24-hour urine containers (2 may be necessary for some patients); toilet insert for collection; funnel for pouring; label; chemical hazard label, as needed; preservatives as required by specific test; graduated cylinder; 10 mL pipette; gloves; written instruction sheet for specific test; requisition slip; patient's record; pen.

STEPS:

1. Check patient's record for orders for specific test. Check for patient allergies.
2. Assemble equipment and supplies needed.
3. Consult laboratory directory for special instructions regarding dietary restrictions and preservative for test ordered.
4. Perform hand hygiene.
5. Label container with patient's name and dates and times to start and stop collection of specimen.
6. If required, add exact amount of preservative using a pipette. If preservative is caustic, add chemical hazard label.
7. Identify patient, and thoroughly explain directions for collection as follows:
   - Void into toilet and flush.

- Note exact time and date as beginning of 24-hour collection.
- Collect all voided urine after start time for next 24-hour period ending exactly 24 hours after start time on following day.
- Note times and dates on label.
- Instruct patient not to urinate directly into container or place anything other than urine in container. Ask patient to use a toilet or urinal insert for collection of specimen and then pour urine into 24-hour container. Explain specimen may need refrigeration, depending on test, in which case it should be refrigerated for entire 24-hour period.
- Patient is to return container(s) as soon as possible after ending collection to ensure accurate results.

8. Provide written copy of instructions to patient with prepared container(s).
9. Record supplies and instructions given to patient and name of test requested.
10. Verify collection dates and times when specimen is returned to facility.
11. When sample returned and before sending to testing laboratory, check in the outside laboratory's procedures manual to see if other additives are to be included.
12. Don gloves.

13. Mix urine sample by swirling carefully. Measure volume of urine collected exactly by pouring into a large graduated cylinder that holds 1 L.

14. Pour an **aliquot** (a small sample representative of the entire specimen) of urine into appropriate container for delivery to testing facility. Record total volume of urine collected and preservative added. Dispose of remainder of urine according to laboratory directions.

15. Record date, time, and volume of urine and where specimen was sent.

16. Clean cylinder as appropriate. Dispose of container in biohazard waste container.

17. Clean area.

18. Remove gloves, and perform hand hygiene.

CHARTING EXAMPLE: 08/06/XX 7:00 A.M. Pt. given 2 24-hour urine containers and instructions for collection of specimen for protein. Timing to begin at 7:00 A.M. 08/07/XX after voiding and discarding first A.M. specimen. Pt. to return containers in 24 hours. · C. Cox, RMA

2-HOUR POSTPRANDIAL SPECIMEN

A 2-hour postprandial specimen is collected 2 hours after a meal is eaten. This test is done to screen for glucose that may be spilled into the urine once the blood levels of glucose exceed the renal threshold. Renal threshold is the concentration at which a substance is excreted by the kidneys. For example, a normal blood glucose level is 70 to 110 mg/dL. If a patient is diabetic, once the blood glucose level exceeds 168–180 mg/dL the kidneys will remove the excess glucose, and it will be detectable in the urine.

CLEAN-CATCH MIDSTREAM SPECIMEN

Catheterization is used to collect a sterile sample of urine. The procedures for female (Procedure 5-19) and male (Procedure 5-21) catheterization are presented in Chapter 5. Collection of a pediatric urine sample is found in Procedure 6-8 in Chapter 6. A clean-catch midstream specimen (CCMS) is a satisfactory alternative since it is not always practical to collect a catheterized specimen. A clean-catch midstream specimen is used to detect urinary tract infections and other urinary dysfunctions.

To properly collect a clean-catch midstream specimen, male and female patients need separate sets of clear instructions to ensure that specimens will be free of contamination. If clean-catch midstream sample is to be used for drug testing, alcohol-free antiseptic wipes should be used. Use terms appropriate to the patient's level of understanding when giving instructions. Medical terms such as *void* may not be understood. Everyday words for urinating may be necessary to get the point across. (Procedure 11-2: Instructing a Male How to Collect a Clean-Catch Midstream Urine Specimen and Procedure 11-3: Instructing a Female Patient How to Collect a Clean-Catch Midstream Urine Specimen follow.)

PROCEDURE 11-2

INSTRUCTING A MALE PATIENT HOW TO COLLECT A CLEAN-CATCH MIDSTREAM URINE SPECIMEN

ABHES VII.MA.A.1 10(e)   CAAHEP IV.P (5); III.A (2)

OBJECTIVE: To instruct a male patient to correctly obtain a contaminant-free clean-catch midstream urine specimen or assist patient if necessary following facility protocol.

STANDARD: This task takes 5–10 minutes, depending on patient's level of understanding.

EQUIPMENT AND SUPPLIES: Sterile midstream urine container; label; gloves; antiseptic towelettes; soap; water; written patient instructions; patient's record; pen.

STEPS:

1. Perform hand hygiene.

2. Check patient's record for physician's orders. Check for patient allergies.

3. Assemble equipment and supplies.

4. Identify patient, and explain procedure. Determine patient's level of understanding. If patient does not comprehend

directions, you will have to don gloves and perform procedure for him following facility protocol.

5. Label container. Explain procedure to male patient using diagrams and written instructions for him to take into lavatory. Instruct patient to do the following:
   a. Wash and dry hands.
   b. Loosen top of urine container.
   c. Expose head of penis. If foreskin is present, retract it and hold back until collection complete.
   d. Cleanse head of penis around urethral opening from top to bottom, using a separate antiseptic wipe for each side and wiping in one direction only.
   e. Cleanse across top of urethral opening with a third antiseptic wipe. Wipe only in one direction and discard (Figure 11-2).
   f. Void a small amount of urine into toilet.
   g. While voiding, pass sterile container under stream of urine to collect sample until container is two-thirds full. Continue voiding into toilet.
   h. Recap container immediately, taking care not to touch inside of lid at any time. Wipe outside of container as needed.
   i. Deliver specimen as instructed.

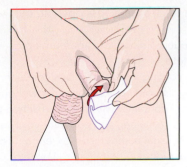

FIGURE 11-2 Cleansing the male urinary meatus.

   j. Discard wipes and rest of packaging.
   k. Wash hands with soap and water.

6. Don gloves to receive specimen from patient. Make sure specimen is labeled, attach a laboratory requisition to it immediately, and process it per facility policy.

7. Provide patient with further instruction.

8. Remove gloves, and perform hand hygiene.

9. Document patient's record.

CHARTING EXAMPLE: 08/06/XX CC 9:00 A.M. CCMS urine collected for C&S. Sent to Memorial Lab 10:00 A.M. · · · · · · · · ·
· L. O'Connell, CMA (AAMA)

PROCEDURE 11-3

INSTRUCTING A FEMALE PATIENT HOW TO COLLECT A CLEAN-CATCH MIDSTREAM URINE SPECIMEN

ABHES VII.MA.A.1 10(e)   CAAHEP IV.P (5); III.A (2)

OBJECTIVE: To instruct a female patient to correctly obtain a contaminant-free clean-catch midstream urine specimen or perform or assist patient if necessary following facility protocol.

STANDARD: This task takes about 5–10 minutes, depending on patient's level of understanding.

EQUIPMENT AND SUPPLIES: Sterile midstream urine container; label; gloves; antiseptic towelettes; soap; water; written patient instructions; patient's record; pen.

STEPS:

1. Perform hand hygiene.
2. Check patient's record for physician's orders. Check for patient allergies.
3. Assemble equipment and supplies.

4. Identify patient, and explain procedure. Determine patient's level of understanding. If patient does not comprehend directions, you will have to don gloves and perform procedure for her following facility protocol.

5. Label container. Explain procedure to patient using diagrams and written instructions for her to take into lavatory. Instruct patient to do the following:
   • Wash and dry hands.
   • Remove underwear and sit on toilet.
   • Expose urinary opening by pulling back labia with nondominant hand.
   • Use dominant hand to cleanse around one side of urinary meatus from front to back with one antiseptic wipe.
   • Use second wipe to cleanse other side in same manner.

Use third wipe to cleanse across opening of meatus (Figure 11-3).

- Continue holding labia apart until procedure is complete.
- Begin voiding into toilet. Place container into position, and begin voiding into container without touching inside of container with fingers. Fill two-thirds full.
- Remove container, and continue voiding into toilet.
- Wipe in usual manner, and cover container with lid while avoiding contaminating inside of lid. Wipe outside of container.
- Wash and dry hands.
- Deliver container as instructed.

6. Don gloves to receive specimen from patient. Make sure container is labeled appropriately, attach requisition slip immediately, and process per facility policy.
7. Provide patient with further instruction.
8. Remove gloves, and perform hand hygiene.
9. Document patient's record.

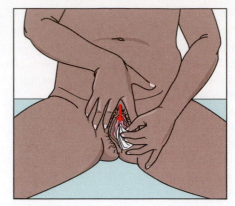

FIGURE 11-3 Cleansing the female urinary meatus.

CHARTING EXAMPLE: 08/08/XX CC 11:00 A.M. CCMS urine collected for C&S. Sent to Memorial Lab 11:30 A.M. · · · · · ·
· L. Tebow, CMA (AAMA)

URINE SPECIMEN FOR A DRUG SCREEN

Employees, athletes, and others may be required to undergo a urine drug screen test to qualify for sports teams or employment opportunities. A signed consent form is necessary for any drug screening test to be performed. A copy of a photo identification from the urine donor may also be required as part of chain-of-custody requirements and should accompany the signed consent form. Drug collection kits vary and require amounts from 1 to 40 mL of urine. Some kits require a bluing agent to be placed in the toilet prior to the sample collection to prevent fraudulent substitutions of water from the toilet. If the drug screen is part of a crime investigation, then the patient must be observed during the collection of the sample. Otherwise the assistant should stand outside the door of the lavatory and receive the sample directly from the donor. Chain-of-custody procedures for the facility must be followed exactly. (See Procedure 11-4 for the steps involved in collecting a drug sample for drug screening.)

PROCEDURE 11-4

COLLECTING A URINE SPECIMEN FOR DRUG SCREENING

ABHES VII.MA.A.1 10(b)(1)   CAAHEP I.P (14)

OBJECTIVE: To obtain a urine specimen from a patient for detection of drugs following explicitly all instructions and complying with chain-of-custody protocol.

STANDARD: This task takes 5–10 minutes, depending on patient's level of understanding.

EQUIPMENT AND SUPPLIES: Urine drug kits (at least two choices); gloves; biohazard waste container; patient's record; pen.

STEPS:

1. Have patient sign consent form and show photo identification. Copy and retain photo identification with signed consent form.
2. Perform hand hygiene.
3. Assemble equipment, and explain procedure to patient.
4. Ask patient to choose urine collection kit to be used, thus avoiding a patient claiming wrong urine sample was tested.

5. Ask patient to remove outer garments and empty pockets, wash and dry hands. This eliminates chances of substituting another specimen.

6. Instruct patient to collect at least 40 mL of urine in collection container.

7. Put on gloves, and measure temperature of urine sample provided. (Fresh urine will be at least 98.6°F/37°C.)

8. Label container, and have patient sign and initial lid.

9. Place specimen in bag, seal bag, and have patient initial it.

10. Sample must be kept in a locked container until it is picked up in compliance with chain-of-custody protocol.

11. The collector and donor must sign off on collection process to make sure all steps were followed.

12. Remove gloves, and perform hand hygiene.

13. Document procedure in patient's record.

CHARTING EXAMPLE: 08/06/XX 5:00 P.M. Urine for drug screen collected. T of spec. 98.2° F. Pt. initialed lid. Spec delivered to lab and handed to technician in charge. · · · · · · · ·
· A. Martin, RMA

Routine Urinalysis

A routine urinalysis consists of describing color and appearance of urine and performing tests for pH and specific gravity and chemical analyses for glucose, bacteria, protein, and other chemical elements. Lastly, the **sediment** (solid material remaining at bottom of test tube after centrifugation) is examined. Table 11-1 lists the categories of tests performed during a routine urinalysis.

PHYSICAL CHARACTERISTICS

Urinalysis begins with an examination of the physical characteristics of a well-mixed urine sample: appearance, color, odor, quantity, and specific gravity.

Appearance

When observing a urine specimen, first notice if the specimen is clear or cloudy. If it is cloudy, more specific terms are needed to describe the appearance, such as slightly cloudy or **turbid** (opaque). Turbidity is caused by a number of factors, including

bacterial infection, white or red cells, epithelial cells, yeast, or vaginal contaminants. Always report exactly what is seen in the sample. Urine should be evaluated when fresh or within 2 hours of collection. Urine may be stored in the refrigerator and should be brought to room temperature before testing.

Color

The normal color of urine is straw or pale yellow. However, concentrated urine and other variables including medications, vitamins, and some foods can cause urine colors to range from pale yellow to amber. Occasionally, urine will appear brown or black, indicating serious illness. Reddish-brown urine may indicate bleeding. Orange urine may be a result of phenazopyridine HCl (Pyridium), a medication used to treat bladder spasms. Large amounts of B vitamins can cause the urine to appear bright yellow. Figure 11-4 shows the color range of urine and the terms used to describe the colors.

Odor

Odor is not usually recorded, but any abnormal aroma should be documented. Individuals testing positive for ketones may

TABLE 11-1 Routine Urinalysis Categories of Characteristics

Physical	Chemical	Microscopic
Appearance (clarity/turbidity)	Reaction	Cells
Color	Protein	Blood (RBCs, WBCs)
Specific Gravity	Glucose	Epithelial cells (squamous, transitional, renal)
Odor	Blood	Casts (hyaline, cellular, granular, waxy)
Quantity (24-hour specimen only)	Ketones	Crystals (acid/alkaline)
	Bilirubin	Other: bacteria, spermatozoa, parasites, yeast
	Urobilinogen	Artifacts
	Nitrite	
	Leukocytes	

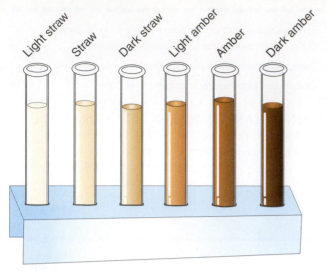

FIGURE 11-4   Color range of urine specimens.

Light straw   Straw   Dark straw   Light amber   Amber   Dark amber

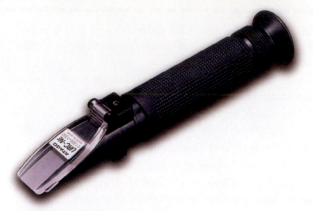

FIGURE 11-5   Portable digital refractometer.

have a fruity odor to their urine. This may indicate uncontrolled diabetes. **Fetid** (foul) odors might indicate infection. Ammonia odors, similar to the odor of a diaper that needs to be changed, usually result from urine breaking down over time.

Quantity (Volume)

Quantity is measured when timed urine specimens are collected but is not usually noted for routine samples. A 24-hour urine specimen should yield between 700 and 2,000 mL with the average being 1,500 mL. The volume of urine produced in 24 hours varies depends on the amount of fluid ingested by the patient. **Polyuria** (excessive amount of urine) may indicate disorders such as diabetes or kidney disease. **Oliguria** (decreased amounts of urine production) can be indicative of dehydration, bleeding, decreased fluid intake, or kidney disease. If renal failure or an obstruction is present, then **anuria** (absence of urine) may result.

Specific Gravity

Specific gravity (SG) is the weight of a substance in relation to the weight of the same amount of distilled water. The concentration of urine changes during the day, depending on the amount of fluid intake. Specific gravity is a rough estimate of the amount of substances dissolved in urine. These measurements indicate how well the kidneys can concentrate or dilute urine. Normal specific gravity ranges between 1.010 and 1.030. Readings outside this range may be the first indication that the kidneys are not working properly. The presence of protein, glucose, or X-ray dyes may increase the specific gravity of urine.

Several methods are used to test a urine specimen's specific gravity: the dipstick or reagent strip method, the refractometer method, and the infrequently used urinometer. The latter method requires a larger sample of urine and is more prone to error.

The dipstick method is the most commonly used method of measuring the specific gravity of urine. It is done by dipping a chemically treated piece of plastic into the sample of urine and reading the chemical reaction that takes place on the dipstick. Reading the test strip is performed by chemical analyzer or visual comparison with the results provided on the side of the strip container.

A refractometer uses light, a prism, and a calibrated scale to measure the concentration level of the specimen. (Figure 11-5 is an example of a portable refractometer.)

PROCEDURE 11-5

EVALUATING THE COLOR, CLARITY, AND VOLUME OF URINE
ABHES VII.MA.A.1 10(b)(1)   CAAHEP I.P (14)

OBJECTIVE: To evaluate the physical characteristics of urine.

STANDARD: This task takes 5 minutes.

EQUIPMENT AND SUPPLIES: Gloves; labeled urine specimen; centrifuge tube; laboratory requisition; PPE, as needed; patient's record; pen.

STEPS:

1. Perform hand hygiene.
2. Don gloves.
3. Check label for patient's name and identifying information. Reject unlabeled samples.
4. Evaluate approximate volume of urine in sample, according to facility policy. If specimen is for 24-hour urine, volume must be measured exactly.
5. Mix urine carefully by swirling with top fastened securely.
6. Label centrifuge tube with patient's name.
7. Assess color of specimen, and record using appropriate terms.
8. Assess clarity, and record using appropriate terms (clear, slightly cloudy, cloudy, turbid).
9. If microscopic examination is to follow, pour an aliquot of urine into centrifuge tube.
10. Clean area.
11. Remove gloves, and perform hand hygiene unless proceeding with complete urinalysis.

CHARTING EXAMPLE: 08/08/XX 2:00 P.M. Random Ur. spec collected. Clear, pale yellow. · · · · · · · · · · · · · · · · · · ·
· M. Donohue, CMA (AAMA)

PROCEDURE 11-6

MEASURING SPECIFIC GRAVITY OF URINE WITH REFRACTOMETER

ABHES VII.MA.A.1 10(b)(1)   CAAHEP I.P (14)

OBJECTIVE: To measure the specific gravity of urine with a refractometer.

STANDARD: This task takes 1 minute.

EQUIPMENT AND SUPPLIES: Antiseptic cleaner; biohazard waste container; PPE; nonsterile gloves; distilled water; medicine dropper/pipette; pen; paper; paper towels; refractometer; urine specimen patient's laboratory requisition.

STEPS:

1. Perform hand hygiene.
2. Don gloves and PPE as needed.
3. Assemble equipment and supplies.
4. Perform QC check on refractometer by using a drop of distilled water first. Distilled water value: 1.000.
   a. Clean prism and refractometer cover with distilled water and wipe dry.
   b. Close cover. Using a dropper or pipette, place a drop of distilled water on notched area of cover. If refractometer does not have an attached cover, place water directly onto prism, then place cover plate on top of prism.
   c. Tilt refractometer to allow light to enter. Read specific gravity by noting division line between light and dark area. This reading should be 1.000. If it is not, retest with fresh distilled water.
5. To test urine sample, swirl urine specimen gently with lid on to avoid splashing. Using medicine dropper, remove a small sample and place one to two drops onto notched area of cover.
6. Follow instructions in step 4c to read specific gravity.
7. Record reading on a piece of paper.
8. Discard urine appropriately if testing is complete, or proceed with testing if ordered.
9. Clean work area and equipment.
10. If testing is completed, remove gloves disposing of them in biohazard waste container. Perform hand hygiene.
11. Document findings in patient's record or on laboratory requisition.

CHARTING EXAMPLE: 08/08/XX 1:00 P.M. SG 1.012. · · · · · ·
· L. Clark, RMA

TABLE 11-2 Chemical Characteristics Associated with Urinalysis and Their Significance

Chemical Characteristic	Significance	Urine Normal Values
Bilirubin	By-product of hemoglobin breakdown, liver disease, obstructive biliary disease, infectious mononucleosis, jaundice	Negative
Blood	Urinary tract infection, kidney stones, trauma, some medications, menses	Negative
Glucose	Diabetes mellitus, extreme stress, Cushing's syndrome, infection	Negative
Ketones	Acidosis, diabetes mellitus, dehydration, starvation	Negative
Leukocytes	Leukocytes release esterase when lysed; correlate with nitrite test and C&S and microscopic examination	Negative; false positive possible from sample sitting too long at room temperature
Nitrites	Used to detect bacteria; some bacteria convert nitrates to nitrites; may indicate UTI if correlated with positive leukocyte test and C&S	Negative
pH/reaction	Ability of urine to concentrate and dilute urine; helps maintain pH of blood	4.6–7.9
Protein	Renal dysfunction, preeclampsia in pregnancy, congestive heart failure	Negative
Urobilinogen	Results from RBC breakdown; same conditions as bilirubin	Small amount

CHEMICAL CHARACTERISTICS

Chemical analysis using a dipstick is the most common method of measuring the chemical characteristics of urine. The dipstick has small chemically treated pads that react with specific chemicals in the urine to allow for measurement of specific elements. The color changes caused by the chemical reactions are then compared to charts on the outside of the reagent strip container with the normal and abnormal value of each provided. In many facilities the color changes on the dipstick are evaluated by chemical urine analyzer. Dipstick tests are available for pH, protein, glucose, ketones, blood, specific gravity, bilirubin, urobilinogen, nitrite, and leukocytes. Facilities select which combination of chemical tests to perform and then purchase the appropriate strips. Dipstick tests are time sensitive, and the time needed for reading each test is provided on the reagent strip container. (Table 11-2 presents the chemical characteristics and normal values associated with urine and the significance of the findings. Procedure 11-7 lists the steps for performing manual chemical reagent tests on urine.)

Automated analyzers are available for evaluating chemical tests strips with 1 to 10 individual chemical tests per strip. Automated analyzers use light photometry to test the strips, which reduces human error associated with color recognition. Whichever method is used, quality control must be performed.

Performing a Complete Urinalysis

The third component of a complete urinalysis is the microscopic examination of urine sediment. Examination of urine sediment is *not* considered a CLIA Waived test. The facility performing urine microscopics must be granted a provider-performed microscopic procedure (PPMP) certificate, in which case the physician in charge is responsible for performing it, or a medical technologist on staff may do it. Otherwise, urine microscopic examinations must be sent to an outside facility certified to perform the examination. Medical assistants and other health care workers must be able to properly prepare a urine specimen for examination and understand the significance of the results of urine microscopy. (See Procedures 11-5, 11-6, and 11-7 for preliminary steps for performing a complete urinalysis. Procedure 11-8 lists all the final steps, including those needed to prepare urine sediment for microscopic examination.)

Understanding and reporting urine microscopic examinations is important to ensure quality care for the patient. Several urine atlases provide excellent diagrams or photos with explanations of all urine microscopic elements.

Cells and other elements of various types may be found during a microscopic examination:

- The presence of red blood cells in urine is known as **hematuria** and is an abnormal finding or may indicate

TESTING URINE WITH CHEMICAL REAGENT STRIPS

ABHES VII.MA.A.1 10(b)(1)   CAAHEP I.P (14)

OBJECTIVE: To perform manual chemical testing on urine using chemical reagent strips to determine any abnormal components.

STANDARD: This task takes 2–5 minutes.

EQUIPMENT AND SUPPLIES: Urine specimen; reagent test strips; timer; paper towel; laboratory requisition; pen; PPE; biohazard waste container; disinfectant.

STEPS:

1. Perform hand hygiene and don personal protective gear.
2. Check specimen for patient identity date and time of collection.
3. Check expiration date on chemical reagent strips.
4. Follow manufacturer's suggested directions to perform quality control using reagent strips. Observe facility policies for frequency of QC. As with all QC, record and log results.

WHY? To provide valid, reliable results, the equipment and supplies used in testing procedures should be tested routinely and results documented. Each manufacturer provides information about QC.

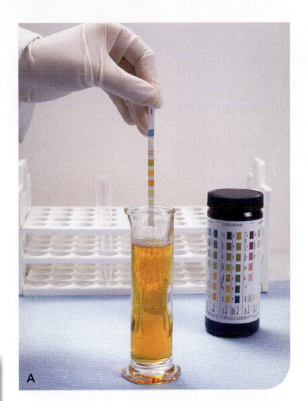

A

5. Bring specimen to room temperature, and swirl gently to mix, taking care not to spill.
6. Remove reagent strip from container, and close container immediately to prevent deterioration of strips.
7. Dip chemical reagent strip in urine, making sure all pads on strip are moistened (Figure 11-6A). Tap strip on paper towel to remove excess urine.
8. Read each pad by comparing to chart on side of bottle, appropriately timing each test (Figure 11-6B). Do not hold test strip against bottle as contamination will result. Ignore color changes after prescribed time has elapsed.
9. Record results on patient's laboratory requisition. Clean work area. Dispose of used supplies in biohazard waste container.

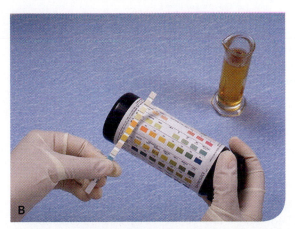

B

FIGURE 11-6 **(A)** Dip reagent strip into urine and withdraw; **(B)** compare color changes on reagent strip to chart on side of container without touching strip to side of container.

10. Remove gloves, dispose of them properly, and perform hand hygiene.

PERFORMING A COMPLETE URINALYSIS

ABHES VII.MA.A.1 10(b)(1)   CAAHEP I.P (14)

OBJECTIVE: To perform complete urine examination, including physical, chemical, and microscopic examination within 30 minutes of obtaining the specimen

STANDARD: This task takes 10 minutes.

EQUIPMENT AND SUPPLIES: Gloves; microscope; centrifuge; centrifuge tubes and rack for tubes; coverslips; disposable pipettes; Sedi-Stain (optional); biohazard waste container; other PPE as needed; pen; laboratory requisition.

NOTE: Medical assistants are not expected to perform a microscopic examination but should be able to prepare the specimen for examination.

STEPS:

1. Perform hand hygiene.
2. Don gloves and other PPE as required.
3. Assemble equipment and supplies.
4. Examine specimen for proper label.
5. Swirl specimen with cap on to mix. Pour 10 mL of well-mixed urine into a labeled centrifuge tube, and cap tube.
6. Place tube in centrifuge, and balance with another tube containing same amount of urine or water. Spin tube in centrifuge at 1,500 rpm for 5 minutes.
7. While sample is centrifuging, assess and record color and clarity.
8. Perform specific gravity using a refractometer if it is not part of chemical reagent testing procedure. Record results.
9. Perform chemical examination of urine and record results. When centrifugation is complete, remove tube and pour off **supernatant** (clear fluid above sediment or precipitate), leaving a small amount of liquid in bottom of tube.

NOTE: The Kova system, a standardized method for measuring and resuspending urinary sediment, may be used. Follow the manufacturer's directions.

10. Resuspend sediment by flicking bottom of tube to mix. Add Sedi-Stain if desired. Remix by tapping tube bottom gently with fingertip.

11. Place a drop of well-mixed sediment onto a clean slide with coverslip (avoiding forming bubbles under coverslip).
12. Place slide onto microscope stage, and notify physician or medical technologist that slide is ready for examination.

HIPAA Alert! Understanding the significance of test results to provide more informed health care while guarding patients' health care rights is of prime importance.

NOTE: The following steps are presented to further familiarize anyone preparing sediment with how calculation of microscopic elements is obtained. Explanation of the elements and their significance is covered in the text following the procedure:

*   Focus under low power (10×) with low light, and scan the slide for casts, especially near the edges of the coverslip.
*   Change to high power by rotating the high-power objective into place. Focus with fine adjustment knob, and increase light. Identify the **casts**, which are protein structures formed in kidney tubules. (Casts are reported by averaging each type of cast found in 10 to 15 fields under low power.)
*   Evaluate other formed cellular elements, such as epithelial cells, RBCs, and WBCs, on high power by scanning 10 to 15 fields and averaging each type of formed element.
*   Observe for crystals and identify. Observe for bacteria, sperm, yeast, and parasites. Report using terms *rare*, *few*, *mod*, *many*, or *1+*, *2+*, *3+*, *4+*, and *TNTC* (too numerous to count).
*   Record results.

13. Do not discard the sediment until the slide has been evaluated in case a repeat slide is necessary.
14. Dispose of specimen. Dispose of urine in designated sink. Discard all tubes and slides in biohazard waste and sharps containers.
15. Remove gloves, and perform hand hygiene.

menses in a female patient. RBCs are small, pale, and round with no nucleus. They are difficult to see in un-stained urine. They may be mistaken for yeast or other structures. RBCs are counted per high power field. The normal range is 0 to 3 RBCs per high-power field.

*   The presence of white blood cells in urine is known as **pyuria** and may indicate infection in the urinary system. WBCs contain a nucleus, are larger than RBCs, and have a granular appearance. The normal range is 0 to 5 WBCs per high-power field.

- Several types of epithelial cells are found in urine. All have a nucleus and are larger than WBCs. Squamous epithelial cells are most frequently seen and are the least significant type of epithelial cell found in urine; they are found lining the urinary tract from the external meatus to the bladder and are considered contaminants in the vaginal tract. A few (0 to 5) squamous epithelial cells per high-power field are considered normal. Finding bladder or renal epithelial cells in urine is considered an abnormal finding and may indicate bladder or kidney disease.

- Casts result from protein formation in the kidney tubules as a result of decreased urine flow, increased acidity, increased solute concentration, and increased protein formation. Different types of casts are classified according to the substances that form them. Casts are classified as hyaline, granular (coarse or fine), cellular (WBC or RBC or epithelial or mixed), waxy, or fatty. Casts dissolve in alkaline urine, thus fresh urine is needed for valid evaluation.

- Crystals are formed by precipitation of urine salts when pH or temperature changes. Urine crystals are found in either acid or alkaline urine, not in both. Most crystals are normal, with a few indicating liver disease, metabolic disorder, or renal damage. Certain radiographic dyes may cause the formation of crystals. Crystals should be identified and counted under high power.

- Bacteria are normally not found in fresh urine and would indicate a UTI. Bacteria are tiny, rod or round shaped, and sometimes motile.

- Yeast are small oval organisms that may be budding in appearance. Difficult to differentiate from RBCs, yeasts may be found in women with candidiasis or in males and females with diabetes.

- Spermatozoa can be found in either male or female urine after sexual intercourse. Sperm are oval, have long whiplike tails or flagella, and are reported as 1+ to 4+ (0 = none visible; 4+ = many).

- **Parasites** are organisms that live in other organisms. One of the most common urinary parasites is *Trichomonas vaginalis,* a pear-shaped organism with four terminal flagella that provide a characteristic rapid darting movement. Parasites are reported in the same manner as bacteria.

- Mucus is a protein substance that appears thread like under the microscope. Mucus is not significant and is viewed with low light.

- Artifacts are contaminants of urine—such as fecal matter, clothing fibers, hair, talc, air bubbles, and starch granules from gloves—and are insignificant except for the fact that they may be misidentified.

Confirmation of Chemical Reagent Stick Testing

Prudent laboratory practice requires that further testing be performed to confirm a positive result obtained with a urine dipstick. A backup test should be performed prior to releasing any positive test results. Facility policies dictate which procedures are to be used to confirm a positive test result. Some of the tests performed as backup tests are the Clinitest tablet test for sugars in addition to glucose, the Acetest for ketones, and the Ictotest for bilirubin. (Procedures 11-9, 11-10, 11-11, and 11-12 for the above mentioned tests follow.

PROCEDURE 11-9

PERFORMING CLINITEST TABLET TEST FOR GLUCOSE AND OTHER REDUCING SUBSTANCES IN URINE

ABHES VII.MA.A.1 10(b)(1)   CAAHEP I.P (14)

OBJECTIVE: To perform Clinitest Tablet 5 Drop test method for glucose.

STANDARD: This task takes 1 minute.

EQUIPMENT AND SUPPLIES: Clinitest Tablet bottle; clean empty test tube; test tube of water with pipette; urine sample with pipette; Clinitest Reference Chart; patient's record; pen; gloves; antiseptic cleaner; biohazard waste container.

STEPS:

1. Perform hand hygiene.
2. Assemble equipment and supplies. Check expiration of Clinitest Tablets.
3. Check specimen label and date and time of collection.
4. Don gloves and other PPE as needed. Do not touch bottom of test tube as it is hot from chemical reaction.
5. Add 10 drops of water to test tube.
6. Add 5 drops of urine.
7. Place tube in rack.
8. Drop in one Clinitest Tablet by shaking one tablet into cap of reagent bottle and inverting cap so tablet falls into prepared tube. Do not touch bottom of tube.
9. Observe boiling reaction in tube carefully for color change. Occasionally, in samples with very high amounts of sugars, a "pass-through effect" occurs: color change may quickly pass through positive color changes and go to negative. To report this finding, record greater than 2% for 5 drop method or greater than 5% if using 2 drop method. Do not use color chart for final color if you notice the pass-through effect.
10. For samples not exhibiting a pass-through effect, mix tube for 15 seconds after boiling ends, compare to color chart for 5 drop method, and record results.
11. Discard equipment in appropriate biohazard waste container. Discard urine in designated sink and wash down with water.
12. Clean work area.
13. Remove gloves, and perform hand hygiene.
14. Document results in patient's record.

CHARTING EXAMPLE: 1:15 P.M. Clinitest 5 Drop Test ¾%.
·· S. Gupta, RMA

PROCEDURE 11-10

TESTING FOR KETONES IN URINE USING ACETEST (NITROPRUSSIDE REACTION)

ABHES VII.MA.A.1 10(b)(1)   CAAHEP I.P (14)

OBJECTIVE: To determine the ketone level in labeled sample of urine using Acetest tablets.

STANDARD: This task takes 1 minute.

EQUIPMENT AND SUPPLIES: Urine sample with label; white filter paper; plastic transfer pipette; Acetest tablet; manufacturer's color comparison chart; gloves; other PPE as needed; antiseptic solution; patient's record; pen.

STEPS:

1. Perform hand hygiene.
2. Assemble equipment and supplies.
3. Don gloves and other PPE.
4. Check sample to see if it is properly labeled.
5. Place Acetest tablet in cap of container without handling it with fingers.
6. Swirl urine specimen with lid on to mix. Use transfer pipette, and place 1 drop of well-mixed urine on top of tablet.
7. Wait 30 seconds for reaction to complete.
8. Compare color of tablet to color chart, and record results as negative, trace, small, moderate, or large amount.
9. Dispose of equipment and supplies appropriately.
10. Clean area with antiseptic.
11. Remove gloves, and perform hand hygiene.

CHARTING EXAMPLE: 08/11/XX 8:00 A.M.: Urine spec. for ketones with Acetest tab showed large amount of ketones present. Physician notified. ··········· L. Tracy, CMA (AAMA)

PROCEDURE 11-11

TESTING FOR PROTEIN IN URINE USING SULFOSALICYLIC ACID (SSA)

ABHES VII.MA.A.1 10(b)(1)   CAAHEP I.P (14)

OBJECTIVE: To determine level of protein in urine using 3% sulfosalicylic acid (SSA) solution.

STANDARD: This task takes 10 minutes.

EQUIPMENT AND SUPPLIES: Urine sample with label; test tube rack; clear test tube; transfer pipettes; control (positive & negative) timer; 3% SSA solution; laboratory requisition; gloves and other PPE as needed; pen; log sheet.

STEPS:

1. Perform hand hygiene.
2. Assemble equipment and supplies.
3. Don gloves and other PPE as needed.
4. Check sample for label and requisition for test ordered.
5. Record on log sheet if required.
6. Label three clean test tubes: one with "N" for *normal* or negative (control), one with "P" for *positive* (control), and one with patient's name or ID number.
7. After balancing centrifuge, run a sample at 1,500 rpm for 5 minutes.
8. Add 1 to 3 mL of urine supernatant to labeled tube.
9. Add correct controls to corresponding labeled tubes in same amount as patient sample.
10. Add equal amount of 3% SSA to each tube.
11. Mix tubes. Using a timer, let stand for minimum of 2 minutes and maximum of 10 minutes.
12. Mix tube contents again, and observe degree of turbidity. Record results as follows:
    - Neg: clear
    - Trace: slightly cloudy or turbid
    - 1+: turbid with no precipitation
    - 2+: heavy turbidity with fine granulation
    - 3+: heavy turbidity with granulation and flakes
    - 4+: clumps of precipitated protein
13. Clean area and dispose properly of waste and equipment.
14. Remove PPE, and perform hand hygiene. Record results.

CHARTING EXAMPLE: 08/11/XX Dipstick urine positive for protein. 3% SSA test used to confirm results 2+. · H. McDonald, CMA (AAMA)

PROCEDURE 11-12

TESTING URINE USING ICTOTEST (DIAZO TABLET) FOR BILIRUBIN

ABHES VII.MA.A.1 10(b)(1)   CAAHEP I.P (14)

OBJECTIVE: To determine presence of bilirubin in urine using Ictotest.

STANDARD: This test takes 2–4 minutes.

EQUIPMENT AND SUPPLIES: Urine sample with label; paper towel; transfer pipette; Ictotest tablets (Diazo tablets); timer; Ictotest white mats; gloves and other PPE; antiseptic solution; patient's record; pen.

STEPS:

1. Perform hand hygiene.
2. Assemble equipment and supplies.
3. Don gloves and other PPE as needed.
4. Check label on sample and requisition for agreement.
5. Place Ictotest mat on dry paper towel.

6. Using a transfer pipette, add 10 drops of urine to center of mat. (If sample is red in color, centrifuge for 5 minutes and use supernatant for testing.)

7. Shake tablet into bottle cap and put in center of mat. Recap container immediately. Do not touch tablet or mat with hands.

8. Using clean transfer pipette, place 1 drop of water on tablet and wait for 5 seconds.

9. Add another drop of water to top of tablet and *within* 60 seconds observe mat around tablet for positive reaction of color change of either blue or purple. Pink or red color is considered negative.

NOTE: QC must be performed daily and recorded following facility policy.

10. Clean area with antiseptic, and dispose of waste properly.

11. Remove gloves and other PPE, and perform hand hygiene.

12. Record results.

CHARTING EXAMPLE: 08/11/XX 10:10 A.M. Urine spec tested Pos with Dipstick. Confirmed with Ictotest. Results: positive. · P. Russo, RMA

Urine Pregnancy Testing

Pregnancy testing is based on the detection of human chorionic gonadotropin (hCG), which is produced by the placenta and is present in the blood and urine of pregnant women. Levels of hCG may be detectable as early as 1 to 5 days after fertilization has taken place. Levels increase and peak between the fiftieth and eightieth days of pregnancy, then decline and remain low and disappear a few days after birth. A first morning specimen is preferred for this test because the concentration of the hormone is greater at that time of day. If a first morning sample is unavailable, a urine sample with a specific gravity of at least 1.010 is acceptable.

A variety of commercial over-the-counter pregnancy tests are available, easy to use, and accurate. Any home test should be confirmed by laboratory testing using quality control and CLIA trained personnel.

CLIA Waived status is granted to all pregnancy tests that use visual color comparison. Two testing methods are used: slide or tube agglutination inhibition tests and enzyme immunoassay tests. A positive pregnancy test result alone does not always indicate pregnancy. Pregnancy is confirmed after a positive test result and a pelvic examination by a physician. Abnormal conditions—such as ectopic pregnancy, choriocarcinoma, and hydatidiform mole—may cause a positive pregnancy test reaction.

Test kits must be stored and used at temperatures according to manufacturers' instructions. Most kits contain built-in quality control. Positive and negative urine controls must be used with patient sample. (Box 11-1 lists guidelines for urine pregnancy testing. Procedure 11-13 lists the steps for performing a urine pregnancy test using an enzyme immunoassay method.)

BOX 11-1 Guidelines for Urine Pregnancy Testing

- Use clean disposable container for collection of specimen.
- First A.M. urine is recommended.
- Test urine specimen specific gravity. If less than 1.010, sample may be too dilute and cause a false-negative result.
- Test fresh urine, or refrigerate up to 24 hours.
- Allow sample to come to room temperature before testing.
- Follow manufacturer's directions exactly.
- Always check expiration date of kits before beginning test. Do not use expired test kits.
- Do not use reagents or tubes from one kit in another test kit of a different lot number or from a different manufacturer.
- Always chart as positive for pregnancy or negative *for pregnancy*, not just "pos." or "neg."

PROCEDURE 11-13

PERFORMING A URINE PREGNANCY TEST USING THE ENZYME IMMUNOASSAY METHOD

ABHES VII.MA.A.1 10(b)(1)   CAAHEP I.P (14)

OBJECTIVE: To perform and interpret an enzyme immunoassay (EIA) urine pregnancy test for hCG.

STANDARD: This task takes 5 minutes.

EQUIPMENT AND SUPPLIES: Patient's first A.M. urine specimen; EIA test kit for hCG; timer; gloves; laboratory report; pen.

STEPS:

1. Perform hand hygiene, and don gloves.
2. Gather equipment and supplies. Check expiration date on test kit.
3. Allow testing materials and specimen to come to room temperature.
4. Verify that name on specimen and requisition match.
5. Label one test pack with patient name or ID number.
6. Label one test pack positive and one test pack negative for controls. (See Figure 11-7.)
7. Place patient's urine on test chamber following manufacturer's directions. Use dropper or pipettes provided in test kit.
8. Place positive and negative controls in correct areas following manufacturer's directions.
9. Time test according to manufacturer's directions.
10. Interpret results correctly.
11. Record results on patient's laboratory requisition.
12. Record positive and negative controls in quality control logbook, according to office policy.
13. Dispose of equipment, and perform hand hygiene.

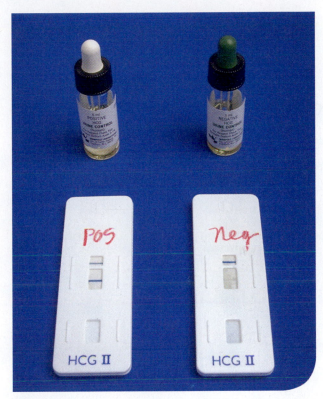

FIGURE 11-7   Urine pregnancy control test: positive and negative.

CHARTING EXAMPLE: 08/17/XX 4:00 P.M. Preg test positive. · M. King, CMA (AAMA)

12 Microbiology

PROCEDURES

Procedure 12-1 Preparing a Direct Smear

Procedure 12-2 Performing a Gram Stain

Procedure 12-3 Streaking a Blood Agar Plate for Colony Isolation

Procedure 12-4 Performing a Urine Culture for Colony Count

Procedure 12-5 Obtaining a Stool Specimen for Ova and Parasites

Procedure 12-6 Obtaining and Examining a Specimen for Pinworms

TERMS TO LEARN

ubiquitous

orifices

normal flora

transudate

colony

morphology

Petri dish

aerobes

facultative anaerobes

anaerobes

The field of microbiology involves the study of living organisms too small to be seen with the naked eye (microorganisms). This fascinating field includes the study of bacteria, fungi, viruses, parasites, and algae. Microorganisms are divided into two categories based on their ability to cause disease. Disease-producing microorganisms are known as pathogens, and those that do not cause disease are known as nonpathogens. Microorganisms are **ubiquitous** (widespread) in our environment and are found on the skin and in body **orifices** (openings). The term **normal flora** refers to microorganisms that are normally present in or on the body and are usually nonpathogenic.

One of the main tasks for all health care providers is to protect patients and themselves from nosocomial infections. (infections acquired in a medical setting). Proper use of PPE and especially proper hand washing are important in the battle against nosocomial infections.

Naming Microorganisms

Scientists use a binomial system to name all living organisms: animals, plants, bacteria, fungi, and protozoa. Each organism has two names: genus (always capitalized) and species (lowercase). For example, the organism that causes strep throat is known as *Streptococcus pyogenes.*

Health care providers are often charged with the task of obtaining specimens from the patient that will allow the laboratory to identify the causative agent of an illness so that the prescribed medication will, hopefully, kill the organism effectively.

Specimen Collection

The term *culture* refers to the process of taking a small sample of a specimen (aliquot) and transferring it to a culture medium that contains nourishing ingredients for microorganisms. The task of specimen collection when obtaining cultures is critical. If the material to be cultured is not obtained correctly (free of contamination) and handled, stored, and tested according to specific guidelines, the test results are worthless, and treatment of the patient is delayed. The requirements for collection of microbiological specimens must be performed based on protocols and guidelines established by the laboratory performing the testing. Proper patient instruction and closely following the collection guidelines are necessary for proper specimen collection. Some examples of collection devices for microbiology samples are sterile swabs and culture tubes

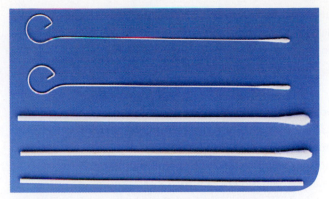

FIGURE 12-1 Examples of sterile swabs (removed from protective wrappers).

(Figures 12-1 and 12-2). Once the specimen is obtained from the patient, the material collected may be tested by placing a small amount of the specimen on a special culture media to enhance the growth of suspected microorganisms and permit easier identification. Special equipment known as an inoculating loop may be used to transfer an aliquot of the specimen to culture media. Another aliquot of specimen may be placed on a glass slide to make a direct smear. The smears are then stained with special dyes to enhance the structural characteristics of the microorganisms (Gram stain). The Gram-stained smears are examined under a microscope by physicians, medical technologists, or laboratory specialists who then report their findings to the attending physician.

Specimens can be collected from eyes, nose, mouth, throat (Procedure 5-33), ears, anus, vagina, wounds (Procedure 5-3), blood, cerebral spinal fluid (Procedure 5-11), exudates, **transudates** (substances that pass through membranes) such as urine (Procedure 11-1), feces (Procedure 5-7), and sputum (Procedure 21-9). The collection process for stool for ova and parasites and obtaining a pinworm specimen are covered in this chapter, as are procedures for preparing a direct smear, performing a Gram stain, streaking a culture

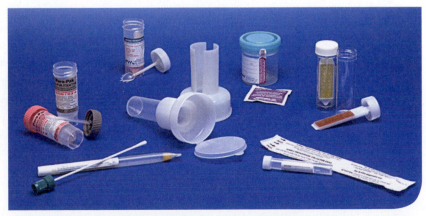

FIGURE 12-2 Examples of specimen collection containers.

plate, and performing a urine culture for colony count. Chapter 10 provides more details for the collection, preparation, and transportation of specimens to an outside laboratory.

Preparing a Direct Smear

Two methods are used to prepare a specimen for direct examination under the microscope: the direct smear and the wet mount preparation (Procedure 5-14). A direct smear preparation is prepared from a swab of the specimen or from a **colony** (a macroscopic growth of a microorganism on a culture plate composed of one type of microbe) on a culture plate. Each microbe produces a specific type of colony on culture media. A direct smear from the specimen swab is made after the culture media has been inoculated to prevent contamination of the specimen from the surface of the glass slide. Once the culture is prepared, the swab is rolled carefully across the slide so all areas of the swab touch the slide. The slide is labeled with the patient's name and type of specimen (throat, wound, etc.) and allowed to air-dry. Do not fan or wave or blow-dry a smear to hasten drying as this may cause the spread of pathogens. After drying, the slide must be fixed to ensure the specimen material adheres to the slide when it is stained. Fixing may be done by passing the underneath part of the slide through an open flame three or four times or flooding the slide with methanol and letting it dry. If a direct smear is to be made from a colony on a culture, place a drop of sterile distilled water or sterile saline on a slide and use a sterilized inoculating loop or needle to pick up a small amount of the colony in question, transfer it to the slide, mix it with the sterile water, and spread it evenly over the slide. Sterilize the loop again when finished making the slide, then allow the slide to dry and fix it before staining. (Be sure to use PPE when handling biological specimens)

PROCEDURE 12-1

PREPARING A DIRECT SMEAR

ABHES VII.MA.A.1 10(b)(5)   CAAHEP III.P (7)

OBJECTIVE: To prepare a smear for microscopic examination

STANDARD: This task takes 30 minutes.

EQUIPMENT AND SUPPLIES: Frosted glass slides; gloves; sterile distilled water; inoculating loop or specimen swab; forceps; Bunsen burner or incinerator; biohazard waste container; patient's record; pen.

STEPS:

1. Perform hand hygiene, and don gloves.
2. Assemble equipment and supplies.
3. Verify that name on laboratory requisition and specimen are same.
4. Label a clean slide with patient's name, date, and type of specimen.
5. Inoculate slide from specimen swab by rolling swab across slide or from a colony on a culture as follows:
   - Sterilize inoculating loop in open flame.
   - Place a loop full of sterile distilled water on slide.
   - Sterilize inoculating loop again.
   - Pick up a small amount of colony in question with loop, and transfer it to slide; mix it with sterile water, and spread thinly.
   - Sterilize loop again, and return it to storage rack.

To prepare a slide from a liquid culture medium:

   - Sterilize inoculating loop.
   - Dip loop in liquid culture medium, and remove a loop full of material.
   - Spread loop full of specimen on a prepared glass slide.

6. Allow prepared slide to air-dry completely (15–20 minutes).
7. Fix slide by picking it up with forceps and passing underside of slide through an open flame three to four times. Let slide cool before proceeding with staining process, or flood dry slide with methanol and let it dry to fix slide before staining.
8. Clean area, and dispose of biohazard waste in designated containers.
9. Remove gloves, and dispose of them properly.
10. Perform hand hygiene.
11. Document procedure in specimen log.

CHARTING EXAMPLE: 09/18/XX 8:00 A.M. Direct smear prepared from swab of abscess on R thigh. · · · · · · · · · · · · · · · ·
· M. Klee, CMA (AAMA)

Staining a Direct Smear

Many types of stains are used in microbiology to help distinguish the **morphology** (form and structure) and staining properties of microbes. Some staining procedures are tedious and beyond the scope of this text. The Gram stain, however, is widely used to differentiate bacteria into two groups: Gram positive or Gram negative.

The compounds that make up the cell walls in bacteria pick up and retain specific stains and release other stains. Gram-positive microorganisms pick up and retain crystal-violet stain and appear purple under the microscope. Gram-negative microorganisms retain only safranin stain and appear pink. The Gram stain procedure must be timed carefully, and manufacturer's directions must be carefully followed. If the slide is decolorized too long, the color differences are difficult to distinguish.

Acid-fast stains are used to stain slides made from specimens suspected of containing *Mycobacterium* genus. (*Mycobacterium tuberculosis* is the causative agent of tuberculosis.) This category of organisms resists decolorization with acid-alcohol solution.

PROCEDURE 12-2

PERFORMING A GRAM STAIN

ABHES VII.MA.A.1 10(b)(5)   CAAHEP III.P (8)

OBJECTIVE: To perform the Gram stain process on a direct smear and allow microscopic examination of Gram-positive and Gram-negative bacteria.

STANDARD: This task takes 10 minutes.

EQUIPMENT AND SUPPLIES: Gram stain kit, including crystal violet, Gram's iodine, decolorizer (alcohol/acetone mixture), safranin dye; direct smear prepared as in Procedure 12-1; wash bottle of distilled water; sink; watch; rack and tray for staining; forceps; paper towel; biohazard waste container; slide stand; gloves.

STEPS:

1. Perform hand, hygiene and don gloves.
2. Assemble equipment and supplies.
3. Verify that name on laboratory requisition and specimen are identical.
4. Make and fix smear according to steps in Procedure 12-1.
5. Place fixed dry slide on staining rack.
6. Cover slide with crystal violet, and let stand for 1 minute. (See Figure 12-3A.)
7. Tilt slide, and rinse with water (Figure 12-3B).
8. Pour Gram's iodine all over slide, and let stand 1 minute.
9. Tilt slide, drain excess iodine solution, and rinse with water.
10. Tilt slide, and gently pour decolorizer all over slide for 15 seconds or until blue color stops running.

WHY? Timing is critical in performing a Gram stain. If slide is decolorized too much, it will be difficult to determine Gram-staining properties of organisms.

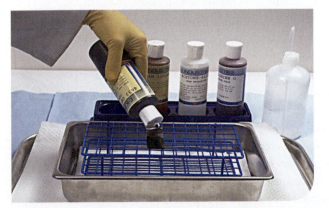
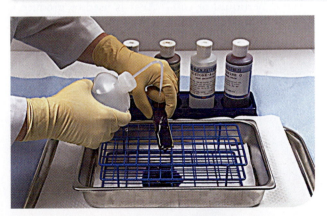

FIGURE 12-3 (A) Pour crystal violet all over fixed slide and time for one minute; (B) rinse crystal violet off slide with water before applying Gram's iodine.

11. Rinse with water immediately.

12. Pour safranin stain all over slide, and let stand 30 seconds.

13. Tilt slide to drain excess stain, and rinse with water. Wipe back of slide.

14. Stand slide on end on paper towel or in slide drying rack, and let air-dry.

15. Mount slide on microscope for examination.

NOTE: Examination of a Gram-stained slide is beyond the scope of medical assistants and should be performed by a physician, medical technologist, or laboratory specialist.

16. Clean area. Dispose of biohazard waste and gloves in designated containers.

17. Perform hand hygiene.

18. Document procedure.

CHARTING EXAMPLE: 09/18/XX 8:45 A.M. Gram-stained spec from Rt thigh to be examined by physician. · · · · · · · · · · ·
· C. Lasso, RMA

In addition to the Gram-staining properties of bacteria, it is possible to distinguish the shape and size of organisms from a Gram-stained slide. This information is helpful to distinguish pathogenic from nonpathogenic bacteria.

Bacteria are divided into three basic shapes: round (coccus), rod shaped (bacillus), and spiral (spirilla). Cocci found in grapelike clusters are grouped as staphylococci; those in chains are called streptococci (Figure 12-4), and those grouped in pairs are diplococci. Members of each of these groups include both pathogens and nonpathogens. Table 12-1 illustrates examples of classes of microorganisms with a brief description of each and examples of several diseases they cause.

Culture and Sensitivity Testing

After preparing a specimen for culture, the preparation is incubated to optimize growth of the microorganisms to permit identification of pathogenic microorganisms. Culture medium may be liquid or solid. Agar is used to produce a gelatinlike texture that is poured into a **Petri dish** (a glass or plastic dish with a loose cover that is used in culturing bacteria) to solidify. A slant media is prepared by pouring the liquid agar medium into a tube and placing the tube on an angle so it solidifies and forms a slanted surface. Liquid media is also used with nutrients added but without agar so no gel forms. Special commercially prepared media contain a variety of substances either to enhance or inhibit the growth of certain categories of microorganisms.

Microorganisms require nourishment and moisture, and each organism has individual temperature and oxygen requirements. Most organisms require body temperature to grow; however, some fungi grow better at room temperature. Organisms that require oxygen are known as **aerobes**. Those that require a reduced amount of oxygen are called **facultative anaerobes**. Those that grow best in the absence of oxygen are known as **anaerobes**.

Outside testing laboratories specify what type of media specimens should be placed on and with what oxygen requirements and at what temperature the specimens should be stored and transported. Dryness kills most types of microbes, and thus microbiological samples should not be allowed to dry out during transportation to outside testing facilities. Table 12-2 lists several types of culture media and the organisms each media aids in isolating.

Inoculating culture media is performed to separate the colonies and thereby more easily identify the causative agents involved in the patient's illness. Streaking for isolation requires applying the specimen material to one section of the agar plate and then using an inoculating loop to spread the material to thin out the growth in the remaining sections of the plate.

A sensitivity test is ordered when the physician would like to know which antibiotic is most effective in killing the causative agent of a patient's illness. A Petri dish containing Mueller-Hinton agar is streaked heavily with the specimen over the entire surface of the plate. A special type of dispenser is placed over the media plate, and after a lever is pushed, a series of small discs impregnated with an assortment

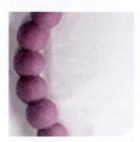

FIGURE 12-4 Streptococci: round bacteria in chains.

TABLE 12-1 Classes of Microorganisms

Microorganism	Description	Example
Bacteria	Most numerous of all microorganisms Identified by shape and appearance Many pathogenic to humans	*See* cocci, bacilli, and spirilla
• Cocci	Round or spherical bacteria	
1. Staphylococci	Grapelike clusters of pus-producing organisms	Boils, acne, osteomyelitis
2. Streptococci	Form chains of cell	Rheumatic fever, scarlet fever, strep throat
3. Diplococci	Form pairs of cells	Pneumonia, gonorrhea, and meningitis
• Bacilli	Rod-shaped bacteria	Gram-positive bacilli: tetanus, diphtheria, gas gangrene; Gram-negative bacilli: *E. coli* (urinary tract infection), *Bordetella pertussis* (whooping cough)
• Spirilla	Spiral-shaped organisms	Syphilis, cholera
• Rickettsia	Tiny Gram-negative type of bacteria transmitted by ticks	Rocky Mountain spotted fever
• Chlamydia	Tiny bacteria; require host cell to live; once thought to be viruses	Sexually transmitted disease, trachoma (eye infection)
• Mycoplasmas	Tiny, unusual, bacterialike with no cell wall	Pneumonia
Fungi	Parasitic and some nonparasitic plants and molds; depend on other life forms for nutrition; reproduce by budding (e.g., yeast)	Candidiasis (yeast infection), histoplasmosis, athlete's foot, ringworm
Viruses	Smallest of microorganisms; can only be seen with electron microscope; can only live in living cell; difficult to kill; many varieties	Herpes virus I and II, HIV, ARC, AIDS, common cold, influenza, smallpox, chicken pox, hepatitis A, hepatitis B, hepatitis C, shingles, mumps
Protozoa	Parasitic; one-celled organisms; can move with cilia or pseudopods	Amoebic dysentery, malaria, *Trichomonas vaginalis* (vaginal infection)

of antibiotics falls to the surface of the plate. The Petri dish is inverted and incubated for 24 hours. After 24 hours the organism will have grown over the whole plate except in a zone around the disc or discs containing antibiotics effective in killing the organism (Figure 12-5). These zones are measured in millimeters and compared to known values provided by the manufacturer. If an antibiotic inhibits growth of the microorganism, then it is reported as "S" (sensitive); if moderate inhibition is noted, it is reported as "I" (intermediate); and if no inhibition of the growth of the organisms occurs, then it is reported as "R" (resistant). The physician then selects the antibiotic most suited for his or her patient based on patient history and sensitivity to certain medications.

Streptococci organisms are Gram-positive cocci in chains. They can produce toxins that hemolyze (break down blood cells) red blood cells on blood agar plates. It is possible to classify *Streptococcus* organisms according to their hemolytic properties:

- Alpha hemolysis is the partial breakdown of red blood cells; it causes a greenish area around some types of strep colonies.

- Beta hemolysis is the complete breakdown of red blood cells; it is indicated by a clear zone around certain types of strep colonies.

- Gamma hemolysis refers to no breakdown of red blood cells; no change occurs in the media around certain colonies.

TABLE 12-2 Culture Media and Isolates

Common Culture Media	Isolates
Blood agar	Most bacteria
Chocolate agar	*Neisseria, Haemophilus*
EMB	Gram-negative bacteria
MacConkey agar	Gram-negative bacteria
Thioglycollate broth	Anaerobic microorganisms
GN broth	Fecal microorganisms

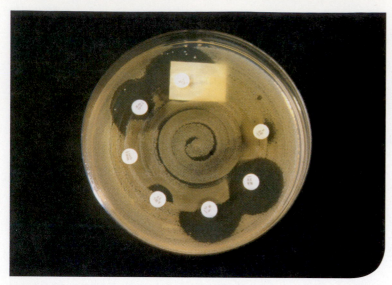

FIGURE 12-5 Culture plate showing antibiotic discs on sensitivity plate.

This differentiation aids in the identification of *Streptococci pyogenes*, the causative agent of strep throat. This bacteria's susceptibility to bacitracin further differentiates the normal flora type of strep from *S. pyogenes*. Strep organisms are divided into sub Groups A through O, with Group A being the virulent type that causes strep throats. A blood agar plate should be streaked for isolation as indicated in Procedure 12-3, and then a disc of bacitracin is placed on the surface of the agar before the plate is inverted and incubated. Group A beta-hemolytic strep causes an area of no growth around the small disc of bacitracin antibiotic placed on a blood agar plate (Figure 12-6). This bacitracin method is sometimes used as a backup to a rapid strep test.

PROCEDURE 12-3

STREAKING A BLOOD AGAR PLATE FOR COLONY ISOLATION

ABHES VII.MA.A.1 10(b)(5)   CAAHEP III.P (8)

OBJECTIVE: To inoculate a blood agar plate to isolate colonies for easier identification of pathogens.

STANDARD: This task takes 5 minutes.

EQUIPMENT AND SUPPLIES: Blood agar plate; inoculating loop; heat source (incinerator or Bunsen burner); permanent marker; forceps; patient's swab specimen; patient's record; pen; gloves; face mask; biohazard waste container.

STEPS:

1. Perform hand hygiene, and don gloves. Don PPE as needed.
2. Verify that name on laboratory requisition and specimen are identical.
3. Remove swab from culture tube, remove cover from Petri dish, and place cover on table with inside facing up.
4. Roll swab over upper quadrant of agar plate.
5. Replace swab in tube. Sterilize loop in heat source, and touch to side of agar in dish to cool loop. Streak over a small area of section already streaked with swab to pick up some of specimen, turn plate a quarter turn, and streak unmarked area.
6. Sterilize and cool loop again. Pick up small amount of specimen from last section streaked. Turn plate again to

unmarked quadrant, and streak again. (This process allows for further separation of colonies and, thereby, easier differentiation of pathogens from normal flora.) Continue until all four quadrants of plate have been streaked with successively lesser amounts of specimen.

7. To decrease possibility of contamination, replace Petri dish cover as soon as possible after inoculating.
8. Invert plate, and incubate blood agar plate at 98.6°F (37°C) for 24 to 48 hours.
9. After inoculating to allow for growth, prepare a secondary culture by picking an isolated colony. Using a sterilized loop, inoculate a new second plate (as above). if done correctly, this process will yield a pure culture (a culture containing only one type of microorganism).
10. Dispose of biohazard waste correctly.
11. Clean area, and remove and dispose of gloves in designated container.
12. Perform hand hygiene.

CHARTING EXAMPLE: 09/21/XX 4:00 P.M. Inoculated blood agar plate with WD spec R calf and incubated/physician's orders. · J. Scotti, RMA

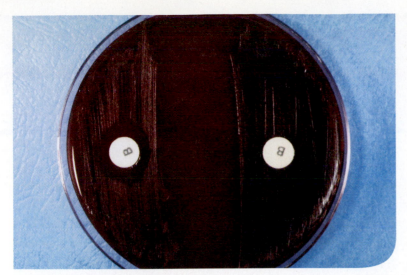

FIGURE 12-6 Bacitracin Group A test.

RAPID STREP TESTING

There are many CLIA-Waived Group A strep kits available that test for the extracted Group A beta-hemolytic *Streptococcus* antigen. These are self-contained tests that can be done while the patient waits. These tests are particularly useful in pediatric offices and clinics. Each manufacturer provides instructions, which must be followed exactly. Directions for storage of the test kits and strict adherence to expiration dates also are critical. Controls must be run with each test based on the manufacturer's directions.

URINE CULTURES

Specimens for urine culture are obtained from clean catch midstream (CCMS), voided midstream, or catheterized urine and placed in a sterile container. The collection methods for these types of specimens are covered in Chapters 5 and 11. A urine culture involves performing a colony count to determine if enough organisms are present to cause a UTI and thus warrant treatment. The colony count technique requires that the whole agar plate be streaked (lawn technique) using a loop calibrated to contain 0.001 mL of urine. The plate is then incubated overnight. The colonies that grow on the medium are counted, and the number is multiplied by 1,000. Fewer than 10 colonies are normal. Considered suspicious are 10 to 100 colonies, and more than 100 colonies are indicative of an infection. (Procedure 12-4: Performing a Urine Culture for colony count follows.)

PROCEDURE 12-4

PERFORMING A URINE CULTURE FOR COLONY COUNT

ABHES VII.MA.A.1 10(b)(5)   CAAHEP III.P (8)

OBJECTIVE: To perform a urine culture for colony count without contamination.

STANDARD: This task takes 5 minutes.

EQUIPMENT AND SUPPLIES: Gloves; mask; incinerator or Bunsen burner; calibrated loop; urine specimen midstream clean catch, catheterized at room temp; pen; biohazard waste container.

STEPS:

1. Assemble equipment and supplies.
2. Perform hand hygiene, and don gloves. Don mask if needed.
3. Verify that name on laboratory requisition and specimen are identical.
4. Swirl urine specimen to mix with lid on to prevent spills.
5. Sterilize calibrated urine culture loop (0.001 mL), and allow it to cool briefly.
6. Dip sterilized loop in urine, and remove a loop full of urine. Streak blood agar plate using "lawn technique" and cover entire plate.
7. Repeat procedure, and inoculate MacConkey agar plate.

NOTE: This is a selective medium that only permits Gram-negative bacteria to grow. UTIs are most often caused by Gram-negative organisms.

8. Replace lids and label bottom of both agar plates with patient's name, date, and type of specimen (urine). Do not write all over plate bottom but confine labeling to edges of plate to permit easier examination of growth.
9. Place inoculated plates in incubator inverted with bottom side up to avoid condensation on surface of plate.
10. After 24 hours, remove plates and notify physician, medical technologist, or clinical laboratory scientist, who may interpret results.
11. Discard waste in appropriate biohazard waste containers.

12. Clean area.
13. Remove and discard gloves properly.
14. Perform hand hygiene.
15. Document procedure.

Collecting Specimens for Ova and Parasites

Parasites cause illnesses varying from mild to fatal. They vary in size from very tiny to many feet long. They can be detected in blood, urine, feces, and vaginal specimens. Traveling to and from countries is easier than ever before, and as a result more parasitic infections are being seen in areas not previously affected.

Procedure 5-8 covers collecting a stool specimen for occult blood and culture. Collection of a fecal specimen for ova and parasites (O&P) utilizes a commercial transport system of two containers. One container holds formalin and the other polyvinyl alcohol. Each container must be filled to the designated line with fecal specimen. These solutions help to preserve ova and parasites if any are present. The container is then returned or mailed to the testing facility in a container with a biohazard waste label attached. Detection of ova and parasites is usually done by direct wet mount slide but requires expertise usually available only in outside or reference laboratories.

Three separate collections of samples may be requested to enhance the possibility of detecting either ova or parasites or both. Clear instructions for the patient are important.

PROCEDURE 12-5

OBTAINING A STOOL SPECIMEN FOR OVA AND PARASITES

ABHES VII.MA.A.1 10(d)   CAAHEP III.P (7)

OBJECTIVE: To properly instruct a patient to collect fecal specimens for ova and parasites and process correctly.

STANDARD: This task takes 10 minutes.

EQUIPMENT AND SUPPLIES: Collection kit for ova and parasites with one vial of formalin and one of polyvinyl alcohol; specimen pan or bed pan; tongue depressors; sterile applicator sticks; mailing container with biohazard label; patient labels; laboratory requisition; gloves; biohazard waste container; patient's record; pen.

STEPS:

1. Check patient's record for orders. Check for patient allergies.
2. Assemble equipment and supplies.
3. Identify patient, and explain procedure. Provide verbal and written instructions for patient to take home if multiple samples are required.
4. Instruct patient to defecate into container provided. Remind patient not to urinate into container or put toilet tissue into it. Remind patient not to take a laxative or enema before collecting samples to avoid destroying any ova or parasites.
5. Remind patient to use tongue depressors provided to take stool samples from different parts of fecal material and place samples in appropriate containers. Remind patient to fill containers to designated lines if so requested.
6. Instruct patient to return specimens to office or designated testing facility immediately after collection.
7. Fill out and label correctly all necessary paperwork.
8. Place specimens in transport envelope with biohazard label affixed, and deliver or mail to testing laboratory.
9. Dispose properly of waste materials. Clean area, and remove and dispose of gloves in biohazard waste container.
10. Perform hand hygiene.
11. Document patient's record.

CHARTING EXAMPLE: 09/19/XX 10:00 A.M. Stool for O&P returned to office by patient and sent to Memorial Lab for testing. · K. Lito, RMA

Collecting Pinworm Specimens

A tiny round worm known as *Enterobius vermicularis*, more commonly known as pinworm, causes nighttime anal itching in humans. Scratching the area infects the hands and fingernails and can spread the parasite to others. This common parasite inhabits the lower gastrointestinal tract. Mature female pinworms migrate out of the anus at night to lay eggs.

Collection of a specimen for pinworms is performed using cellulose tape attached to a tongue depressor. The tongue depressor is then pressed around the anal opening to pick up ova, mature worms, or both. The tape is placed sticky side down on a glass slide and examined for the presence of ova; this examination must be done by a physician or medical technologist. (See Procedure 12-6 for examples of the steps involved in collecting a specimen for pinworms.)

Testing for Influenza

Influenza is an upper respiratory illness caused by a virus. Symptoms include chills fever, cough, sore throat, runny nose, headache, and muscle aches. The elderly and patients who are immunocompromised are at greater risk. Certain individuals may develop complications, such as pneumonia. The three types of flu are A, B, and C. Types A and B are usually the organisms that cause epidemics each year. Several CLIA-Waived quick influenza tests are available commercially; most are based on immunoassay, which detects influenza A and B, and some differentiate between the two. As with any commercial kit, manufacturer's directions must be followed closely.

PROCEDURE 12-6

OBTAINING AND EXAMINING A SPECIMEN FOR PINWORMS

ABHES VII.MA.A.1 10(b)(5)   CAAHEP III.P (7); III.P (8)

OBJECTIVE: To collect an anal specimen using cellulose tape for examination for pinworms.

STANDARD: This task takes 10 minutes.

EQUIPMENT AND SUPPLIES: Glass slide; tongue depressor; cellulose tape; gloves; patient's record; pen.

STEPS:

1. Check patient's record for orders. Check for patient allergies.
2. Assemble equipment and supplies.
3. Identify patient, and explain procedure to patient/caregiver.
4. Perform hand hygiene, and don gloves.
5. Prepare slide by attaching sticky side of a piece of cellulose tape to a glass slide, and leave one end available to make it easy to remove when performing procedure. Leave room on slide for labeling at other end of slide.
6. Before leaving room, provide a gown and ask patient to remove clothing from waist down. Give patient privacy to disrobe or, for a child, assist caregiver as needed.
7. Position patient on examination table with anus exposed, and drape patient for privacy.
8. Peel tape off slide by labeled end and wrap around tongue depressor or swab with sticky side out.
9. Press taped tongue depressor firmly around anus on both sides.
10. Remove tape from tongue depressor, and place on slide with sticky side down.
11. Label slide with patient's name and date. Fill out laboratory requisition form.
12. Physician or medical technologist will examine slide for presence of pinworms or their ova.
13. Dispose of all waste in biohazard waste container.
14. Clean area, and remove and dispose of gloves properly.
15. Perform hand hygiene.
16. Document patient's record.

CHARTING EXAMPLE: 09/19/XX 11:00 A.M. Specimen obtained for pinworm examination. Slide prepared for physician to examine. · · · · · · · · · · · · · · · · · H. Herboldt, CMA (AAMA)

13 Phlebotomy

PROCEDURES

Procedure 13-1 Performing a Skin Puncture for an Adult or Child

Procedure 13-2 Performing a Heelstick for an Infant

Procedure 13-3 Collecting a Heelstick Blood Specimen for PKU Screening

Procedure 13-4 Obtaining a Skin Puncture Specimen in a Microtainer Unit

Procedure 13-5 Identifying the Patient Correctly Prior to a Phlebotomy Procedure

Procedure 13-6 Performing a Venipuncture Using the Evacuated Tube Collection Method

Procedure 13-7 Performing a Venipuncture Using the Syringe Method

Procedure 13-8 Performing a Butterfly/Winged Infusion Blood Draw from a Patient's Hand

Procedure 13-9 Collecting a Specimen for Blood Culture

Procedure 13-10 Performing a Bleeding Time Test with a Surgicutt Device

TERMS TO LEARN

interstitial fluid

phenylketonuria (PKU)

hypothyroidism

hematoma

lumen

septicemia

bacteremia

Phlebotomy, the collection of blood specimens, is performed by a number of different health care providers: phlebotomists, laboratory technicians, medical assistants, respiratory therapists, and nurses. In this text, we use the term *phlebotomist* to mean anyone who obtains blood specimens as ordered by the physician. The blood samples are then analyzed by the clinical laboratory to help pinpoint a diagnosis, develop effective treatment, and monitor a patient's illness.

To provide accurate reliable results, a quality specimen must be obtained in the right container, be identified properly, and stored and transported correctly. Chapter 10 covers the importance of correctly identifying the patient and labeling the specimen.

The chief methods for collecting blood are skin puncture and venipuncture. In addition, arterial blood samples may be obtained by a respiratory therapist or physician for analysis of blood gases.

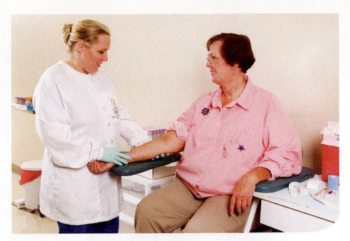

FIGURE 13-1 **Blood drawing chair.**

Basic Procedural Steps

Regardless of the method used for collecting a specimen, the initial steps are the same:

- Correctly complete the requisitions for testing
- Properly identify the patient
- Properly position the patient
- Correctly label the sample
- Use the correct type of blood sample device
- Correctly transport the sample to the testing facility

In addition, infection control precautions must be observed, including the following:

- Frequent hand washing
- Barrier precautions (PPE)
- Needlestick protection devices
- Proper disposal of biohazard waste in appropriate containers (sharps, etc.)
- Employing sterile technique when necessary

Basic Blood Drawing Equipment

Blood drawing by skin puncture or venipuncture may be done at the patient's bedside, at a blood drawing station, in a physician's office, or at a clinic. The basic necessary equipment includes the following:

- Chair with armrest, which prevents the patient from falling if syncope occurs (Figure 13-1).

- Examination table for anxious, acutely ill patients
- Table at the same height as chair to hold equipment
- PPE, including gloves of various sizes
- Antiseptic and gauze
- Bandages to cover puncture site
- Sharps container for soiled needles and other sharp objects
- Tourniquets
- Biohazard waste container

Specimen collection trays are made of a plastic material and must be sterilizable. The tray may be carried to the patient's bedside or any other area to obtain blood samples. The tray should contain all the collection equipment necessary to obtain blood samples, depending on the patient population.

Skin Puncture

To perform a skin puncture, the skin is pierced with a lancet. The composition of blood obtained is not the same as from a vein. Skin puncture blood contains blood from arterioles, venules, capillaries, and **interstitial fluid** (fluid among the cells or tissue fluid). Generally, laboratory results are more accurate on larger samples of blood; however, improvements in testing procedures have been achieved for microsamples of blood.

Skin punctures are performed on the elderly, small children and infants, patients with difficult veins, patients with scarring or damage at venipuncture sites; to preserve veins for dialysis or chemotherapy; at point of care testing (POC); and per physician's orders. A fleshy,

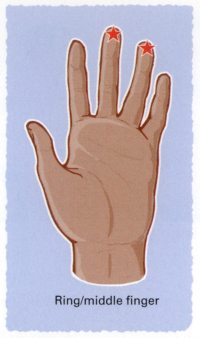

Ring/middle finger

FIGURE 13-2 Preferred finger puncture sites in adults and children are the distal portions of the third and fourth fingers. Note the circled fleshy areas.

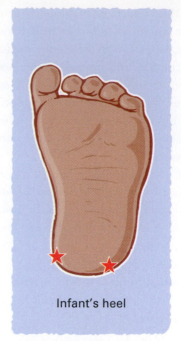

Infant's heel

FIGURE 13-3 Heel sites for skin puncture on infants. Note the areas on the lateral portions of the heel.

vascular site free of calluses and scars is preferred. In adults and children, the sites generally used are the middle or ring finger (Figure 13-2). The pinkie finger is too slender, and the index finger and thumb are generally more callused and sensitive. In an infant or child who is not walking, the sides of the heel are used for skin puncture (Figure 13-3). To avoid bone injury, the puncture must not be more than 2 mm deep in a child and 2 to 3 mm deep in an adult.

If the site is too cold or cyanotic, it will be difficult to obtain a sufficient amount of sample. Warming the area to be punctured improves the supply of blood. Warming may be done by massaging the area or applying a warmed towel or commercially available warming device. The temperature of the warming device should not be higher than 107.6°F (42C°). The site should be cleaned with 70% isopropyl alcohol and allowed to dry to avoid contaminating or hemolyzing the sample. The first drop of blood obtained by skin puncture should be wiped away with gauze because it may contain tissue fluid and could dilute the sample.

SKIN PUNCTURE DEVICES

Lancets are capillary puncture devices available in various lengths to puncture at different depths, depending on the patient's age and medical status. The safest lancets are retractable and nonreusable. They are color coded according to the puncture depth each one accomplishes. Figure 13-4 provides an example of various microcollection lancet devices. Many home use devices achieve a specific depth and protect against puncturing too deeply. Home monitoring devices are used to test glucose, cholesterol, and hematocrit levels. Lasers are now

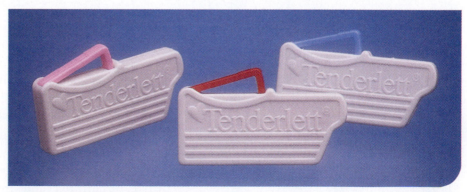

FIGURE 13-4 Single use fully automated disposable lancet devices of varying penetration depths for adult, children, and infants.
Courtesy of ITC, Edison, NJ.

sometimes used to puncture skin and provide a small opening 1 to 2 mm deep.

Collection tubes for skin puncture samples are available in a variety of sizes. They are made of glass or plastic, with plastic preferred for safety reasons. Blood is pulled into capillary tubes by capillary action. Some capillary tubes contain anticoagulants such as heparin (red-marked tubes) to keep the sample from clotting. It is essential to mix these tubes to prevent coagulation. Blue-marked capillary tubes do not contain anticoagulants. BD Microtainer capillary blood collection tubes are available with color-coded caps to indicate what additive is present in the tube. Each has a small capillary tube leading into the collection tube. Each collection tube is marked at 250 µL and 500 µL (microliters).

The following guidelines should be observed when performing a skin puncture collection:

1. Hold capillary collection tube horizontal to the site to avoid air bubbles.

2. After collection, seal the tube end with clay or the color-coded lid provided.

3. Place the sealed capillary tube in an unfilled vacuum tube, and label with patient's information.

Unopette collection devices (Figure 13-5) are used to collect specimens for white blood cell count, red blood cell count, platelet count, and red blood cell fragility test. Arterial blood gas samples should be placed immediately in ice water until delivered to the testing site. The order of draw for skin puncture samples is different than for

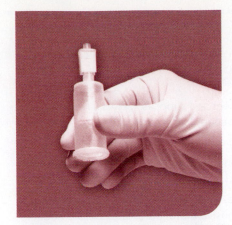

FIGURE 13-5 A microcollection device that is a dilution unit for blood for WBC count, RBC count, platelet count, and RBC fragility tests.
Courtesy and © Becton, Dickinson and Company.

venous samples. The Clinical and Laboratory Standards Institute (CLSI), formerly the National Committee for Clinical Laboratory Standards (NCCLS), recommends the following order of draw:

1. Lavender tubes with ethylenediaminetetraacetic acid (EDTA) for hematology testing

2. Additive tubes with anticoagulant heparin and serum separating tubes with separating gel

3. Nonadditive tubes (red-topped tubes with no anticoagulants, clot accelerators or gel

Differential smears often are made at the time of collection. Two smears must be made for each patient, and care must be taken to label each of the two smears correctly. The

PROCEDURE 13-1

PERFORMING A SKIN PUNCTURE FOR AN ADULT OR CHILD

ABHES VII.MA.A.1 10(d)(2)   CAAHEP I.P (3)

OBJECTIVE: To perform a successful skin puncture for an adult or child and obtain the required specimen.

STANDARD: This task takes 10 minutes or less.

EQUIPMENT AND SUPPLIES: Automated skin puncture device or sterile disposable lancet; 70% alcohol wipes; 2 × 2 sterile gauze pads; microcollection tubes based on tests ordered; sealant; sharps container; gloves; towel or washcloth to warm site; marking pen; laboratory requisition; labels; glass slides if needed for differential smear; biohazard waste container; patient's record; pen.

STEPS:

1. Check requisition slip for tests ordered, or check patient's record and complete a requisition slip for ordered tests.

2. Assemble equipment and supplies. (Select a lancet appropriate for age of patient.)

3. Perform hand hygiene.

4. Identify patient, and recheck requisition slip for patient's name and ordered tests.

5. Explain procedure. Always check to make sure patient is not allergic to adhesive materials or latex before beginning. If patient is a child, take extra time to explain what you are going to do. Request assistance to hold child steady if necessary.

6. Don gloves.

7. Select site for puncture (palmar surface of middle or ring finger).

8. Warm surface by rubbing or using a warmed cloth.

9. Clean site with 70% alcohol pad, and allow to air-dry. Do not blow on it or fan it dry as this spreads microorganisms.

10. Check that you have appropriate lancet device for age of patient.

11. Remove puncture device, lancet, or both from packaging, and keep sterile.

12. Holding patient's finger firmly, state that a stick will be felt. Puncture site, then discard lancet into sharps container.

13. Wipe away first drop of blood with sterile gauze because it contains tissue fluid and will dilute sample.

14. Massage gently from base of finger to allow a free-flowing drop of blood to form.

15. Fill appropriate container for tests ordered using correct order of draw.

16. Hold capillary tubes horizontal to site to avoid air bubbles. Mix tubes with additives gently to avoid coagulation. Cap or seal collection tubes after filling.

17. Place sterile gauze on site. Ask patient to apply pressure if able, or apply pressure for patient.

18. Recheck site to determine bleeding has stopped. Bandage per facility guidelines. Label tubes with patient's name, any identification number, date, time drawn, and your name or initials as indicated by facility guidelines.

19. Dispose of soiled materials in biohazard waste container, and remove gloves and dispose of them properly.

20. Perform hand hygiene.

21. Document patient's record.

CHARTING EXAMPLE: 10/18/XX 11:00 A.M. Fingerstick for in-house Hct performed. Hct 38%. · · · · · V. Vecchito, CMA (AAMA)

---

procedure for making a differential smear is covered in Chapter 14: Hematology.

HEELSTICK PROCEDURE

Skin puncture on the heel of an infant is performed after warming the heel. The medial and plantar surfaces of the heel are used, and the first drop of blood is wiped away as in fingerstick procedures. Swaddling the infant helps to calm and restrain. Recommendations for relieving neonatal pain also include applying EMLA (a topical anesthetic applied by nurse or physician, oral sucrose (12%–24% solution) if ordered by the physician, a pacifier, or both. Facility protocols should be observed. There are guidelines for the amount of microcapillary blood samples that can be safely collected based on weight and blood volume of the infant.

Neonatal screening for **phenylketonuria (PKU)** and **hypothyroidism** is mandated in the United States for all newborns. Babies born with low thyroid function suffer arrested physical and mental development, a condition formerly known as cretinism. Newborns with PKU lack enzymes for breaking down specific proteins, and that can result in severe mental retardation. Some states require screening for other abnormalities such as sickle cell anemia, cystic fibrosis, and HIV. PKU testing is performed between 24 to 72 hours after birth. A drop of blood is applied to each circle on the specimen collection card. Each circle is filled completely and the card allowed to dry before it is mailed to the testing facility in envelopes provided by state health departments.

Newborns who show signs of jaundice are screened for elevated bilirubin levels due to liver dysfunction. Failure to treat newborns with direct light to break down excess bilirubin may result in brain damage and other problems. When transporting bilirubin samples it is important to keep them from excessive exposure to light as this will result in lower values. The procedure for performing a heelstick follows.

PROCEDURE 13-2

PERFORMING A HEELSTICK FOR AN INFANT
ABHES VII.MA.A.1 10(d)(2)   CAAHEP I.P (3)

OBJECTIVE: To obtain sufficient blood sample from heel of an infant to perform tests ordered by physician.

STANDARD: This task takes 10 minutes or less.

EQUIPMENT AND SUPPLIES: Sterile automated heelstick safety device in different incision depths (0.65–0.85 mm for premature neonates, 1.0 mm for larger infants); 70% alcohol wipes; sterile 2 × 2 gauze sponges; collection tubes appropriate for tests ordered; sharps container; washcloth to warm heel; marking pen; laboratory requisition; labels; gloves; other PPE as needed.

STEPS:

1. Check laboratory requisition or patient's record for tests ordered. Check for patient allergies.
2. Assemble equipment and supplies.
3. Identify infant by identification bracelet, or ask floor nurse to identify infant by name, address, identification number, and birth date. Compare name with laboratory requisition.
4. Perform hand hygiene.
5. Don gloves and PPE as required.
6. Place infant in supine position, and swaddle. If possible, allow infant's foot to hang lower than torso.
7. Select a site, and warm with moist washcloth. Dry after warming.
8. Clean site with alcohol wipe, and allow to air-dry without allowing foot to touch any nonsterile surface.
9. Remove appropriate automated lancet device from its package, and remove safety clip.
10. Raise foot, and place blade opening flush against heel with middle at center point of intended incision site (medial or lateral plantar surface of heel).
11. Make sure both ends of device come in contact with skin, then push trigger. Immediately remove device after triggering (Figure 13-6).

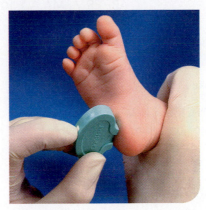

FIGURE 13-6   Performing a heelstick on an infant.
Courtesy and © Becton, Dickinson and Company.

12. Gently dry area with a sterile dry gauze sponge.
13. Fill collection tube by placing it close to but not touching wound. Fill to correct level. Gently milk foot to produce additional drops of blood.
14. When collection is complete, place a dry sterile gauze pad on wound using gentle pressure until bleeding stops. This step helps to prevent a **hematoma** (mass of clotted blood) from forming.
15. Label a specimen container properly, and record time and date of collection.
16. Dispose of lancet device in sharps container. Remove and dispose of gloves and PPE in biohazard waste container.
17. Perform hand hygiene.
18. Document procedure in patient's record.

CHARTING EXAMPLE: 10/12/XX 10:00 A.M. Heelstick for blood glucose level performed. Gluc. 92 mg/dL. · · · · · · · · · · ·
· S. Curley, RMA

VENIPUNCTURE EQUIPMENT

Venipuncture is defined as the collection of blood from a vein. A venipuncture can be accomplished using evacuated tubes, a sterile syringe, or a sterile butterfly setup. Vacuum tubes are tubes from which air has been removed. They come in sizes ranging from 2 mL to 15 mL. The larger tubes are used for adult blood collection, and the smaller ones (2 mL, 3 mL, 4 mL) are used for collection of blood from children. Tubes are made of glass or plastic, with plastic preferred to prevent breakage and spills. Each tube has an expiration date printed on it and should not be used after that date. Tubes may be purchased with conventional stoppers or BD (Becton,

PROCEDURE 13-3

COLLECTING A HEELSTICK BLOOD SPECIMEN FOR PKU SCREENING

ABHES VII.MA.A.1 10(d)(2)   CAAHEP I.P (3)

OBJECTIVE: To collect sufficient blood from a heelstick for PKU screening.

STANDARD: This task takes 10 minutes.

EQUIPMENT AND SUPPLIES: Sterile automated heelstick safety device in different incision depths (0.65–0.85 mm for premature neonates, 1.0 mm for larger infants); 70% alcohol wipes; sterile 2 × 2 gauze sponges; PKU collection cards from state health department; sharps container; washcloth to warm heel; marking pen; laboratory requisition; labels; gloves; other PPE as needed.

NOTE: To prevent contamination do not touch any part of the filter paper circle with hands or gloves at any time before during or after collection.

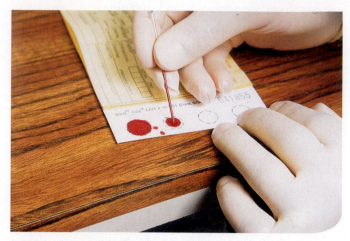

FIGURE 13-7   Collecting a blood sample for neonatal screening test.

STEPS:

1. Check patient's record for physician's orders. Check for patient allergies.
2. Assemble equipment and supplies.
3. Perform hand hygiene.
4. Identify infant correctly. If caregiver is present, explain procedure.
5. Don gloves.
6. Position infant, and warm heel as for a heelstick (Procedure 13-2).
7. Cleanse infant's heel with 70% alcohol pad.
8. Wipe puncture site dry with sterile gauze.
9. Puncture site.
10. Allow large drop of blood to form, gently squeezing heel if necessary.
11. Lightly touch printed side of filter paper collection card to blood and completely fill each circle (usually 4 or 5). Allow blood to soak through card. Label card.
12. If unable to fill all circles with original drop, wipe heel and express another drop. Fill remaining circles as before.

NOTE: Do not add second drop of blood to a circle that is incompletely filled. At no time should filter paper collection card touch skin at puncture site of patient.

13. Use only one side of filter paper collection card.

14. Allow blood-sampled circles to dry flat on nonabsorbent surface for 4 hours.

NOTE: Directly applied heelstick blood is preferred; however, blood from a heparinized capillary tube may be used. Care must be taken not to scratch or dent filter paper collection card. (See Figure 13-7.)

15. Following blood collection, gently press a dry sterile gauze pad to incision site until bleeding has stopped. (This helps prevent a hematoma.)
16. When filter paper collection cards are dry, place them in state-provided envelope, and mail within 24 hours.
17. Rewrap infant, and place safely in bassinett or caregiver's care.
18. Dispose of sharps in sharps container. Remove and dispose of PPE and gloves in biohazard waste container.
19. Perform hand hygiene.
20. Complete information on screening card to allow for follow-up care if results are abnormal.
21. Record procedure in patient's record.

CHARTING EXAMPLE: 10/13/XX 6:00 P.M. Heelstick sample for PKU obtained from L heel and sent to state laboratory on 10/14/XX 9:00 A.M. · · · · · · · · · · · · · S. Hadijian, CMA (AAMA)

OBTAINING A SKIN PUNCTURE SPECIMEN IN A MICROTAINER UNIT

ABHES VII.MA.A.1 10(d)(2)   CAAHEP I.P (3)

OBJECTIVE: To successfully obtain a skin puncture specimen of blood in the correct Microtainer unit, based on tests ordered.

STANDARD: This task takes 10 minutes.

EQUIPMENT AND SUPPLIES: Gloves; alcohol wipes; sterile 2 × 2 gauze; safety lancet; correct microcollection tube units based on the tests ordered; sharps container; biohazard waste container; pen; patient's record; laboratory requisition; specimen transport container.

STEPS:

1. Check requisition slip for tests ordered, or check patient's record and make out a requisition slip for ordered tests.
2. Check for patient allergies.
3. Assemble equipment and supplies.
4. Perform hand hygiene.
5. Identify patient, and recheck requisition slip for correct patient's name and ordered tests.
6. Explain procedure. If patient is a child, take extra time to explain what you are going to do. Request assistance to hold child steady if necessary,
7. Don gloves.
8. Select site for puncture (palmar surface of middle or ring finger).
9. Warm surface by rubbing or using a warmed cloth.
10. Clean site with 70% alcohol, and allow it to air-dry. Do not blow on it or fan it dry.
11. Determine appropriate lancet device for age of patient.
12. Remove puncture device, lancet, or both from packaging, and keep sterile.
13. Holding patient's finger firmly, state that a stick will be felt. Puncture site, and discard lancet into biohazard sharps container.
14. Wipe away first drop of blood with sterile gauze because it contains tissue fluid and will dilute sample.
15. Massaging gently from base of finger, allow a free-flowing drop of blood to form.
16. Using correct microcollection device based on tests ordered, scoop specimen into container with scoop-shaped projection. Tip microcontainer to allow drop to slide into tube so it can mix with any additive present.
17. Gently mix container, and then proceed to collect another drop in same manner. Fill microcontainer to designated

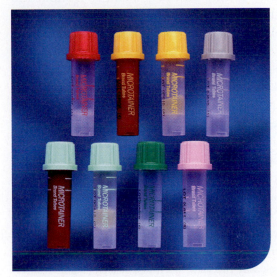

FIGURE 13-8   BD Microtainer tubes with different additives for collection of skin puncture sample. Each tube has 250 mL and 500 mL markings.
Courtesy and © Becton, Dickinson and Company.

line to ensure correct blood-to-additive ratio. Mix as needed based on manufacturer's directions.

18. Place a gauze sponge on site, and ask patient to hold it on puncture site; if patient is a child, hold site until bleeding stops.
19. Remove end with collection device (scoop), and discard in sharps container.
20. Place cap provided with container onto end to seal it (Figure 13-8). Label with patient's name, date, and time of collection and your initials.
21. Place microcollection container in a specimen container such as a urine specimen cup. Place lid on it, and label container.
22. Fill out laboratory requisition with all information needed. Place specimen in labeled container in biohazard transport bag, and attach laboratory requisition.
23. Remove and dispose of gloves in biohazard waste container. Perform hand hygiene.
24. Document procedure in patient's record.

CHARTING EXAMPLE: 10/13/XX 5:00 P.M. R middle finger stick sample for electrolytes collected and sent to Memorial Lab for stat testing at 5:25 P.M. · · · · · · · · G. Koll, CMA (AAMA)

Dickinson and Company) Hemogard closures that help reduce blood splatter when tubes are opened.

The tubes are produced with a variety of different color tops, each indicating what additive if any is in the tube. The additives may be anticoagulants to prevent blood from clotting, preservatives, or serum separator substances; some tubes contain no additive. Some additives, such as silicone and glass beads, can accelerate clotting so specimens are ready for testing more quickly than they would be if allowed to clot undisturbed.

Blood collected into a tube with no additives will coagulate after 30 to 45 minutes. The blood separates into serum (the straw-colored liquid portion of blood that remains after clotting) and the clot itself (made of white blood cells, red blood cells, and platelets). Spinning the blood in a centrifuge for 15 minutes increases the amount of serum recovered. Some tubes have serum separator substances that act as a barrier between the clot and the serum to facilitate pouring off serum free of blood cells. Blood collected in tubes with an anticoagulant will separate into blood cells and plasma; the clotting factors in such tubes remain present in the plasma, and the plasma can be resuspended with the cells to form whole blood.

Laboratory tests require serum, plasma, or whole blood. Some additives may interfere with test reactions and results. Before performing a venipuncture it is important to know the following:

- The test(s) to be performed
- The type of specimen(s) required by the testing facility
- The color tube to be used
- How much specimen is needed
- How the specimen should be stored and transported

Figure 13-9 illustrates a variety of Vacutainer evacuated specimen tubes with Hemogard closures. Table 13-1 lists stopper colors, what type of specimen each yields, laboratory use, and number of times a specimen should be inverted at the time of collection.

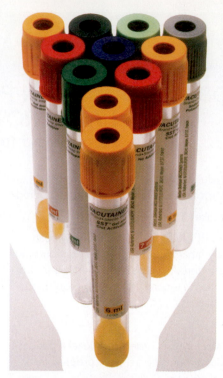

FIGURE 13-9 Vacuum tubes with Hemogard caps to prevent splatters when opening tube.

1. **Yellow.**   Blood for blood cultures; always drawn first to protect sterility of specimen

2. **Light blue.**   Drawn next for coagulation studies to prevent anticoagulants from other tubes interfering with some studies

3. **Red or gold.**   Either with or without clot activators and serum separators to yield serum

4. **Green.**   Either with or without gel separators, drawn before EDTA (lavender) tubes

5. **Lavender.**   Containing EDTA

6. **Gray.**   Always drawn after EDTA (lavender) tubes because potassium levels and RBC morphology may be affected

WHY?
Do not shake specimens; only invert gently. Each tube should be filled completely to prevent incorrect blood/anticoagulant ratio, which could affect test results.

Order of Draw

When drawing a blood specimen using evacuated tubes, it is important to fill the tubes in the order recommended by the CLSI.

Needles, Holders, and Syringes

Needles used for blood drawing are usually 20–21 gauge. The smaller the gauge number of the needle, the larger the bore or diameter of the needle. For children, a 21–23 gauge needle is used. Blood donor centers generally use an 18 gauge needle to collect a pint of blood. The needles vary between 1 to 1½ inches in length. Several types of safety shield needles are available to help prevent needlesticks

TABLE 13-1 Vacutainer Tubes and Their Uses

Stopper Color	Additive	Specimen Yield	Laboratory Use	Inversions at Time of Collection
Gray and Red	Polymer barrier	Clotted blood/serum	Chemistry tests	5
Gold	Polymer barrier	Clotted blood/serum	Chemistry tests	5
Red	None (glass)	Clotted blood/serum	Chemistry, serology, blood bank	0
Orange	Thrombin	Clotted blood/serum	Stat serum chemistry	8
Yellow/Gray	Thrombin	Clotted blood/serum	Stat serum chemistry	8
Royal Blue	No additive; sterile tube	Clotted blood/serum	Trace elements, toxicology screen, nutritional-chemistry studies	0
Green/Gray	Lithium, heparin, and polymer barrier	Whole blood/plasma	Plasma chemistry tests	8
Green	Sodium or lithium, heparin	Whole blood/plasma	Plasma chemistry tests	8
Light Green	Lithium, heparin with polymer barrier	Whole blood/plasma	Plasma chemistry tests	8
Gray	Sodium fluoride, potassium oxalate	Whole blood/plasma	Glucose determinations	8
Royal Blue	Sodium, heparin, or EDTA–Na$_2$	Whole blood/plasma	Trace elements, toxicology screen, nutritional studies	8
Pink	Dried K$_2$ EDTA	Whole blood/plasma	Blood bank, whole blood hematology	8
Tan	K$_2$ EDTA	Whole blood/plasma	Lead determinations	8
Yellow	Acid citrate, dextrose/SPS	Whole blood	SPS tubes for blood culture, ACD for blood bank, HLA studies, paternity testing	8
Lavender (purple)	EDTA with Na$_2$ or K$_2$ or K$_3$	Whole blood	Whole blood hematology determinations, blood bank ABO/Rh	8
Light Blue	Sodium citrate and CTAD	Whole blood/plasma	Coagulation studies, platelet function studies (may require chilling)	3–4

(Figures 13-10A and 13-10B). A double-ended needle attaches to an adapter or holder and is used to collect blood into evacuated tubes; the long end of the needle is inserted into the vein, and the protected short end punctures the top of the stopper on the tube once the tube is placed into the holder (Figure 13-11) Once the stopper is pierced, the vacuum is released and blood will flow into the tube. Syringes are also used to obtain blood from veins too fragile for collection with the evacuated tube system. Safety syringes generally are used to decrease the risk of accidental needlesticks. Syringes are also used for collection of arterial blood samples. Syringes for blood specimen collection vary from 5 mL to 20 mL, with needles of the same length and gauge used for evacuated tube samples. To transfer blood from a syringe to evacuated tubes, a safety transfer device (Figure 13-12) is used; the syringe needle is safely removed and discarded into a sharps container, a blood transfer device is attached to the syringe, and a vacuum tube is inserted into the transfer device.

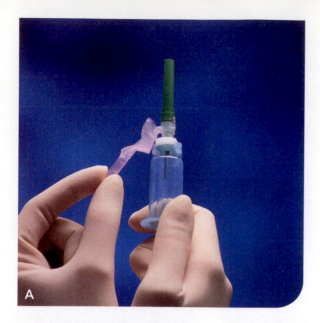

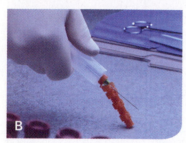

FIGURE 13-10   (A) Blood collection attached to holder with needle shield attachment. *Courtesy and © Becton, Dickinson and Company;* (B) Venipuncture Needle-Pro Protection Device to be activated after withdrawing the needle from the patient and pressing hard on a surface. *Courtesy of Protex, Inc., Keene, NH.*

BUTTERFLY/WINGED INFUSION SETS

Butterfly or winged infusion sets consist of a specially designed short, small bore needle with plastic wings (to grasp while inserting the needle), tubing, and devices to attach either to a syringe or Vacutainer collection system (Figure 13-13). These sets are designed for use on children or individuals with tiny, fragile veins. Winged infusion sets are commonly used intravenous devices. Some have safety features that automatically resheath the needle when it is withdrawn.

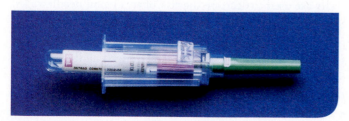

FIGURE 13-11   Assembled evacuated tube system.

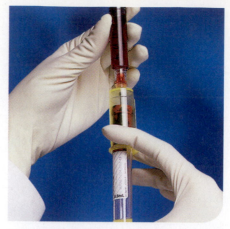

FIGURE 13-12   An example of a syringe attached to a safety syringe shielded transfer device.

TOURNIQUETS

Tourniquets are used to make veins more prominent. The variety of types available includes latex and nonlatex bands 1 to 1½ inches wide and about 15 inches long. All are easily cleaned or may be discarded after use. Velcro tourniquets allow for easy adjustment during venipuncture. A blood pressure cuff may be used with the pressure kept below the patient's diastolic pressure.

Patient Identification and Laboratory Test Orders

Laboratory testing requests are computer generated or handwritten on a laboratory requisition form. The patient information section is filled out completely along with the complete list of tests requested. This information can be handwritten on the specimen container once it is obtained. Clerical errors may result. Many facilities also generate

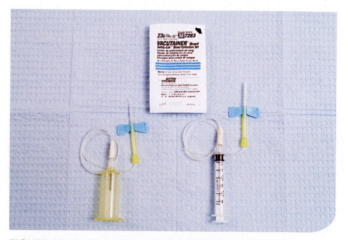

FIGURE 13-13   Examples of butterfly/winged infusion sets.

PROCEDURE 13-5

IDENTIFYING THE PATIENT CORRECTLY PRIOR TO A PHLEBOTOMY PROCEDURE

ABHES VII.MA.A.1 8(ff)   CAAHEP I.P (6)

OBJECTIVE: To correctly identify a patient before performing a phlebotomy procedure.

STANDARD: This task takes 2 minutes.

EQUIPMENT AND SUPPLIES: Patient's record; laboratory requisition; pen; identification bracelet.

STEPS:

1. Review patient's record for physician's orders for blood tests, or check patient's name, date of birth, address on form, if laboratory requisition has been filled out identifying tests to be performed by physician.

2. Check for patient allergies.

> **HIPAA Alert!** If calling patient in from a waiting room, call patient by name or use a sign-in sheet and numbering system to avoid revealing any confidential information.

3. After reaching patient's side, greet and ask conscious patient to state his or her full name, address, and date of birth (DOB).

4. Compare information provided by patient with laboratory requisition information, making sure name, address, and DOB agree.

5. Confirm information provided by patient and laboratory requisition form with a third source such as an identification bracelet, printed identification number, driver's license, nurse, caregiver, or parent.

6. If a patient is an unconscious inpatient, first check laboratory requisition patient identification information, then check wrist bracelet identification information. A third identification may be obtained from a nurse, close relative, or friend.

---

barcode labels for specimens along with the requisition to reduce error and speed up specimen processing. Once the specimen is obtained the barcode label is then attached to the specimen; when the specimen reaches the laboratory, both requisition and barcode label are rechecked. Radio frequency identification (RFID) tags are becoming more widely used. These tiny silicon chips are attached to specimen, and data are then sent to a wireless receiver. No line-of-sight reading is necessary, thus human errors are reduced. It is possible to track many specimens simultaneously. Cost, standardization, and privacy measures are being studied and addressed.

Proper patient identification is crucial. Use at least two patient identifiers when drawing blood. Identification of a patient varies whether the patient is an inpatient or outpatient or in the attending physician's office. The patient's condition, age, and ability to understand English are factors to take into consideration. In-house patients wear identification bracelets with their first name, last name, date of birth, and hospital number. A match should be made with the test requisition, the patient's identification bracelet and by patient saying his or her name and DOB. If patients are unconscious, mentally unable to answer correctly, or non–English speaking, a nurse or relative may identify the patient. The bracelet and test requisition should be checked as well. The same process is used for infants and young children as for unconscious patients.

Venipuncture Sites

The veins of the antecubital space just below the elbow are most commonly used for venipuncture. (See Figure 13-14 for a drawing of a human arm with veins labeled.) The median cubital is the most commonly used vein. Next choice would be the cephalic vein on the outer edge of the arm, and lastly the basilic vein on the inner edge of the arm. Veins on the dorsal side of the hands and wrists may be used

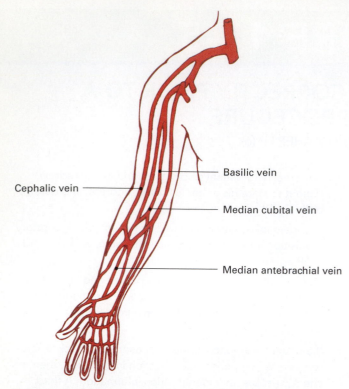

FIGURE 13-14 Drawing of a human arm with the main veins labeled.

Cephalic vein

Basilic vein

Median cubital vein

Median antebrachial vein

as venipuncture sites if the antecubital veins are not available. Veins in the foot and ankle may be used only with permission of the physician. Venipuncture sites that must be avoided are as follows:

- On the side on which mastectomy was performed
- Above an IV (specimen will be diluted)
- Close to hematomas, burns, or scar tissue
- Near chemotherapy or dialysis sites
- In areas with edema (specimen may be diluted with tissue fluid)

Proper positioning of the patient and the phlebotomist is important to perform a successful phlebotomy procedure. If the patient is ambulatory, ask him or her to sit in a phlebotomy chair with adjustable arm supports at a height comfortable for the phlebotomist. Syncope is not uncommon; therefore, a chair that has a device to pull across in front of the patient and lock is helpful to prevent dangerous falls. If the patient is in bed or on a stretcher, a pillow or arm rest device that is wedge shaped is helpful to provide extension of the arm. Blood collecting equipment should be kept accessible but not where it could be overturned if the patient moved suddenly.

PROCEDURE 13-6

PERFORMING A VENIPUNCTURE USING THE EVACUATED TUBE COLLECTION METHOD

ABHES VII.MA.A.1 10(d)(1)   CAAHEP I.P (2)

OBJECTIVE: To perform a venipuncture by correctly assembling equipment and locating, entering, and withdrawing a blood sample from the vein using the evacuated tube collection method.

STANDARD: This task takes 10 minutes.

EQUIPMENT AND SUPPLIES: Gloves; tourniquet; 70% alcohol wipes; nonalcohol cleansers for collection of blood alcohol levels; Band-Aids or comparable bandages; sterile 2 × 2 gauze squares; iodine solution for blood culture; needles of varying gauges; tube holders; evacuated blood collection tubes with a variety of colored stoppers; test tube rack; marking pen; sharps container; laboratory labels; patient laboratory requisition; pen.

STEPS:

1. Review patient's record or laboratory requisition.
2. Perform hand hygiene.
3. Greet and identify patient.
4. Ask patient if he or she is allergic to latex or adhesive materials. Use equipment and supplies appropriate for patient.
5. Assemble evacuated tubes and equipment needed for tests requested.
6. Prepare equipment by attaching needle to tube holder. Select evacuated tubes required for tests ordered. Check expiration date on each, and gently tap tubes with additive to dislodge additives from stopper or wall. Prepare gauze and 70% alcohol wipe (if drawing blood for blood culture, take out iodine solution wipes or swabs).
7. Position patient's arm comfortably with arm extended slightly downward and elbow slightly bent.
8. Apply tourniquet by passing it under patient's arm about 2 inches above antecubital area; cross ends of tourniquet, and pull them taut against skin; hold them in place with nondominant hand. With dominant hand, tuck top

piece of tourniquet under bottom part, leaving one end of tourniquet projecting upward for easy release.

9. Palpate across antecubital area in search of a vein, which will feel spongy to touch of index finger. If no suitable vein is palpated, reapply tourniquet to other arm and palpate in same manner. Select vein that feels fullest. Tourniquet should not be left on more than 1 minute.

10. Don gloves.

11. Disinfect area, and let it air-dry without fanning or blowing on it. Make sure that all equipment and supplies are prepared and available. Tubes should be in order of draw with first tube in tube holder pushed on as far as thin line on holder but no farther because vacuum will be released and tube would be useless.

12. Reapply tourniquet, and ask patient to close his or her fist without pumping it.

13. If you need to repalpate, apply alcohol to your finger and recheck vein.

14. Explain that patient will feel a stick and that it is important for him or her to hold very still.

15. Remove needle cover, anchor vein with thumb of nondominant hand, line up needle with vein, and insert needle at a 15- to 30-degree angle to skin.

16. Push tube into place with nondominant hand while steadying needle and holder with dominant hand. Switch tubes after first tube is full by gently twisting and pulling tube off and replacing it. Gently invert tubes collected with additives to mix them with blood. If tubes are filling well, carefully release tourniquet. If blood is slow, leave tourniquet in place.

NOTE: Some phlebotomists switch hands after inserting needle to use their dominant hand to switch tubes. This is permissible as long as it is easiest way for phlebotomist to achieve a "good draw."

17. After filling last tube, remove it from holder. Then withdraw needle and place a gauze pad over puncture site until bleeding stops (or ask patient to apply pressure if able to do so for 3 to 5 minutes). Tell patient not to bend the arm because this may cause a hematoma.

18. Activate needle safety device according to manufacturer's directions. Dispose of needle and holder in sharps container.

19. Invert tubes with additives again, per manufacturer's guidelines. Do not shake.

20. Label tubes with preprinted labels if available or print patient's first and last names, identification number if assigned, date of collection, and your name or initials as facility policy dictates. Place labeled tubes safely in rack until ready to be transported to testing laboratory.

21. Check puncture site for bleeding and bandage. Instruct patient to remove bandage after 15 minutes. If bleeding has not stopped after 5 minutes, notify physician.

22. Clean area. Remove and dispose of gloves in biohazard waste container. Perform hand hygiene.

23. Document patient's record if applicable.

CHARTING EXAMPLE: 10/16/XX 4:00 P.M. Venous blood for CBC obtained from Rt arm and sent to Memorial Laboratory at 5:00 P.M. · C. Popke, CMA (AAMA)

PROCEDURE 13-7

PERFORMING A VENIPUNCTURE USING THE SYRINGE METHOD

ABHES VII.MA.A.1 10(d)(1)   CAAHEP I.P (2)

OBJECTIVE: To perform a venipuncture using the syringe method and correctly dispense blood samples into specified tubes.

STANDARD: This task takes 5–7 minutes.

EQUIPMENT AND SUPPLIES: Gloves; tourniquet; 70% alcohol wipes; nonalcohol cleansers for collection of blood alcohol levels; Band-Aids or comparable bandages; sterile 2 × 2 gauze squares; iodine solution wipes or swabs for blood culture; needles of varying gauges; syringes of several sizes; evacuated blood collection tubes with a variety of colored stoppers; safety transfer device; test tube rack; marking pen; sharps container; laboratory labels; patient laboratory requisition.

STEPS:

1. Review laboratory requisition, and check supplies.

2. Perform hand hygiene.

3. Greet and identify patient.

4. Ask patient if he or she is allergic to latex or adhesive materials. Use equipment and supplies appropriate for patient.

5. Assemble evacuated tubes and equipment needed for tests requested.

6. Prepare syringe and needle by removing them from sterile packaging while preserving sterility. Move syringe plunger back and forth several times to break seal on syringe. Select evacuated tubes required for tests ordered, and place them in a rack in correct order of draw. Check expiration date on each, and gently tap tubes with additive to dislodge additives from stopper or wall. Prepare gauze and 70% alcohol wipe (if drawing blood for blood culture, take out iodine solution wipes or swabs).

7. Position patient's arm comfortably with arm extended slightly downward and elbow slightly bent.

8. Apply tourniquet by passing it under patient's arm about 2 inches above antecubital area; cross ends of tourniquet and pull them taut against skin; hold in place with nondominant hand. With dominant hand, tuck top piece of tourniquet under bottom part, leaving end pointed toward shoulder long enough to pull for easy release.

9. Palpate across antecubital area in search of a vein, which will feel spongy to touch of index finger. If no suitable vein is palpated, reapply tourniquet to other arm and palpate in same manner. Select vein that feels fullest. Tourniquet should not be left on more than 1 minute.

10. Don gloves.

11. Disinfect area, and let it air-dry without fanning or blowing on it. Make sure that all equipment and supplies are prepared and within easy reach.

12. Reapply tourniquet, and ask patient to close fist without pumping it.

13. If you need to repalpate vein, apply alcohol to your finger and recheck vein.

14. Explain that patient will feel a stick and that it is important to hold very still.

15. Before inserting needle, move plunger back and forth to expel any air. Insert needle at a 15- to 30-degree angle to skin (Figure 13-15). When needle is in vein, blood is visible in hub of syringe.

16. Gently pull back on plunger while holding needle steady, taking care not to pull needle out when pulling plunger back. (Pulling too vigorously may cause hemolysis of blood cells or collapse of vein.)

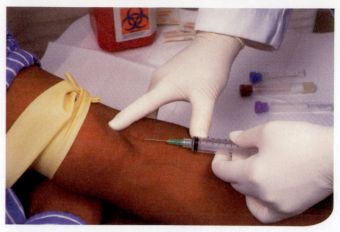

FIGURE 13-15 **An example of drawing blood with a syringe using two-finger anchor.**

17. When required amount of blood is withdrawn, release tourniquet and have patient release fist. Place sterile gauze over puncture site, and apply pressure. To avoid causing pain to patient, do not apply pressure on gauze until needle is out.

18. Activate safety device according to manufacturer's directions; detach and discard immediately in sharps container.

19. Ask patient to apply pressure to gauze with arm straight for 3 to 5 minutes.

20. Using a syringe transfer device, fill evacuated tubes in order of draw. (This must be done as quickly as possible to avoid blood coagulating in syringe. Vacuum in tubes draws blood from syringe automatically.) Never push plunger to expel blood (this action will cause hemolysis of red blood cells).

21. Mix tubes containing additives 5 to 8 times, following manufacturer's directions, and immediately label them at patient's side.

22. Dispose of entire syringe safety device setup in sharps container. Dispose of all biohazard waste in appropriately marked container.

23. Check puncture site for bleeding, and apply bandage using materials appropriate for that patient. If bleeding has not stopped after 5 minutes, notify physician.

24. Remove and dispose of gloves in proper manner.

25. Perform hand hygiene.

26. Document procedure in patient's record.

CHARTING EXAMPLE: 10/17/XX 10:00 A.M. VP with syringe on Rt. Arm for CBC, FBS & lytes. Spec sent to Memorial Lab at 12:00 P.M. · E. Zandri, CMA (AAMA)

PROCEDURE 13-8

PERFORMING A BUTTERFLY/WINGED INFUSION BLOOD DRAW FROM A PATIENT'S HAND

ABHES VII.MA.A.1 10(d)(1)   CAAHEP I.P (2)

OBJECTIVE: To successfully obtain required venous blood samples from a patient's hand using the butterfly/winged infusion method.

STANDARD: This task takes 10 minutes.

EQUIPMENT AND SUPPLIES: Gloves; tourniquet; 70% alcohol wipes; nonalcohol cleansers for collection of blood alcohol levels; Band-Aids or comparable bandages; sterile 2 × 2 gauze squares; iodine solution wipes or swabs for blood culture; sterile winged infusion set with adapter to connect to tube holder; evacuated blood collection tubes with a variety of colored stoppers, or syringe and safety transfer device; test tube rack; marking pen; sharps container; laboratory labels; patient laboratory requisition.

STEPS:

1. Review laboratory requisition and check supplies.
2. Perform hand hygiene.
3. Greet and identify patient.
4. Ask patient if he or she is allergic to latex or adhesive materials. Use equipment and supplies appropriate for patient.
5. Assemble evacuated tubes and equipment needed for tests requested.
6. Open sterile butterfly package, and uncoil tubing. When using hand, use a syringe with butterfly setup. (Evacuated tubes may cause vein to collapse.) Prepare syringe by removing it from sterile packaging while preserving sterility. Move plunger back and forth several times to break seal on syringe. Attach syringe to end of butterfly setup by screwing infusion set end into hub of syringe. (Use a Luer adapter at end of tubing if you are using a Vacutainer holder and evacuated tubes).
7. Select evacuated tubes required for tests ordered and place them in a rack in correct order of draw. Check expiration date on each, and gently tap tubes with additive to dislodge additives from stopper or wall.
8. Prepare gauze and 70% alcohol wipe (if drawing blood for blood culture, take out iodine solution wipes or swabs).
9. Position patient's arm comfortably and extended slightly downward with elbow slightly bent.
10. Apply tourniquet near wrist bone about 3 inches above appropriate hand site (a butterfly setup may be used to draw blood from antecubital area also), cross ends of tourniquet, and pull them taut against skin; hold in place with nondominant hand. With dominant hand, tuck top piece of tourniquet under bottom part leaving end pointed upward and long enough to pull for easy release. Have patient make a fist or hold a roll of gauze or stress ball to slightly elevate hand.
11. Palpate across hand/wrist area in search of a vein, which will feel spongy to touch of index finger. If no suitable vein is palpated, reapply tourniquet above other wrist and palpate in same manner. Select vein that feels fullest. Tourniquet should not be left on more than 1 minute.
12. Don gloves.
13. Disinfect area, and let it air-dry without fanning or blowing on it. Make sure that all equipment and supplies are prepared and within easy reach.
14. Reapply tourniquet and ask patient to close his or her fist without pumping it.
15. If you need to repalpate vein, apply alcohol to your finger and recheck vein.
16. Explain that patient will feel a stick and that it is important to hold very still. Remove needle sheath from butterfly needle, and anchor vein with a single- or double-finger anchor to keep vein taut.
17. Holding plastic wing part of needle, insert needle ¼ to ½ inch at a 15-degree angle (if successful you will see blood come immediately come into tubing). Thread needle slightly into **lumen** (cavity) of vein to secure it. If using a syringe, gently pull back on plunger to extract correct amount of blood. If using a Vacutainer adapter and tube holder, push tube into holder until it fills, then remove it and gently mix. Insert remaining tubes in order of draw.
18. First tube drawn with a butterfly setup should be red stopper tube without additive. Tubing contains air, thus first tube is underfilled by approximately 0.5 mL. Then order of draw is same as for Vacutainer or syringe method of venipuncture. Tubes must be held horizontally or slightly downward to avoid additives transferring from one tube to next.
19. After obtaining required amount of blood, release tourniquet and ask patient to release fist. Place sterile gauze

20. Activate needle safety device. Discard butterfly needle and tubing.

21. Ask patient to apply pressure to gauze with arm straight and elevated for 3 to 5 minutes.

22. In order of draw and using syringe transfer device, fill evacuated tubes as quickly as possible to avoid blood coagulating in syringe (See Figure 13-12). (Vacuum in tubes draws blood from syringe automatically. Never push plunger to expel blood as this action will cause hemolysis of red blood cells.)

23. Mix tubes containing additives 5 to 8 times, following manufacturer's directions, and immediately label them at patient's side.

over puncture site, and avoid pushing down on gauze until after needle is extracted from vein.

24. Dispose of entire syringe safety device setup in sharps container. Dispose of all biohazard waste in appropriately marked container.

25. Check puncture site for bleeding, and apply bandage using materials appropriate for that patient. If bleeding has not stopped after 5 minutes, notify physician.

26. Remove and dispose of gloves in proper manner.

27. Perform hand hygiene.

28. Document procedure in patient's record.

CHARTING EXAMPLE: 10/17/XX 3:00 P.M. Butterfly setup used to draw blood for lipid profile, CBC from back of Lt hand. Spec. sent to Memorial Lab at 5:00 P.M. · · · · E. Sokoloski, RMA

Phlebotomy Problems

Problems or complications are always a possibility when performing a phlebotomy procedure. The problems may be as simple as repositioning the needle in the vein to increase blood flow or as difficult as a combative patient or one who has a seizure.

SYNCOPE

Syncope or fainting is covered in Chapter 9 (Procedure 9-15). Question the patient about problems with blood drawing in the past before beginning the procedure. If the patient feels "uneasy" at all, ask him or her to lie down to prevent injury. Always be sure that the arm of the phlebotomy chair is in place to prevent falls. If syncope should occur during a blood drawing, withdraw the needle, apply pressure to the site, and ask the patient to lower his or her head between the knees. If possible, ask for help before assisting the patient into a lying position.

HEMATOMAS

A hematoma is a collection of blood at the puncture site that occurs when some of the blood escapes the vein and enters the surrounding tissue. Hematomas occur when any of the following occurs:

- The needle goes through the vein.
- The needle is only partially in the vein.
- The vein is very fragile.
- The needle is removed with tourniquet still on.
- Not enough pressure is applied to the puncture site when the procedure is over.

Hematomas may cause bruising at the site area and may be painful or painless. A cold compress over the area may reduce discomfort and swelling.

FAILURE TO OBTAIN BLOOD

The many reasons for "missing the vein" include the following:

- Failure to insert the needle deep enough
- Needle penetrating through the vein
- Bevel of the needle hitting against the wall of the vein
- No vacuum in tube
- Veins rolling when the needle is inserted

Patient-associated problems may cause a failure to obtain blood, including situations and conditions such as the following:

- Obesity
- Edema from intravenous infusion (if unavoidable, draw blood from below the IV)
- Seizure (remove needle and tourniquet, apply pressure, and protect patient from harm)
- Refusing to have blood drawn (follow facility protocol and document)
- Excessive bleeding
- Excessive pain in arm due to hitting a nerve (remove needle and tourniquet, apply pressure)
- Collapsed veins (use smaller needle, smaller tubes, butterfly setup)

SPECIMEN PROBLEMS

Many problems are associated with specimen collection and processing. Among them are the following:

- Wrong tubes drawn on correct patient
- Correct tubes drawn on wrong patient
- Incorrect labeling of specimen
- Illegible writing on specimen label
- Incomplete labeling (not enough patient information to differentiate patients with the same name)
- Improper timing of collection of specimens
- Hemolyzed sample (too small a needle, vigorous shaking, drawing sample before alcohol dry, excessive hand pumping, physiological conditions)
- Improper transporting conditions
- Delayed processing or testing

Special Collection Procedures

Most special collection procedures are performed on inpatients by professionals specifically trained to perform the procedures. However, any discussion of phlebotomy would be incomplete without mentioning the procedures and providing a general overview.

ARTERIAL BLOOD GASES

Arterial blood gases (ABG) are obtained to provide information about the patient's respiratory condition. The radial artery is used most frequently as long as the blood flow in the artery is adequate. The brachial artery or femoral artery may be used. Blood is drawn in specially designed syringes. Arterial blood gas analysis should take place within 10 minutes of being drawn. If longer time than 10 minutes will elapse, the specimen should be transported in a container with a "slurry" (a mixture of water and ice).

CAPILLARY BLOOD GASES

Capillary blood gas analysis is often performed on small children or infants for whom arterial sticks would be dangerous. These samples are collected from the same sites as other capillary samples (heel, finger). Special blood collection capillary tubes are used, and both ends of the tubes are sealed after the collection is complete. The sample should be analyzed as soon as possible or transported in a container with a "slurry" of water and ice.

BLOOD CULTURES

Blood cultures are ordered when **septicemia** (pathogenic organisms in the bloodstream) or **bacteremia** (bacteria in the blood) is suspected or when patients have a fever of unknown origin (FUO). The procedure for drawing blood cultures involves a more detailed venipuncture site preparation. Designated Vacutainer tubes, butterfly setups, or syringes may be used for these collections, depending on the preferences of the testing laboratory and your facility. Check the laboratory testing facility manual for detailed information.

PROCEDURE 13-9

COLLECTING A SPECIMEN FOR BLOOD CULTURE
ABHES VII.MA.A.1 10(d)(1)   CAAHEP I.P (2)

OBJECTIVE: To collect a specimen for blood culture without contamination.

STANDARD: This task takes 10 minutes.

EQUIPMENT AND SUPPLIES: Blood culture collection supplies or prepared kit; 2 blood culture vials (one aerobic, one anaerobic); gloves; iodine solution swabs; 2 additional antimicrobial swabs; additional needles; 2 × 2 sterile gauze; tape; tourniquet; labels; sharps container; safety syringe or evacuated tube holder.

NOTE: Blood cultures can be collected with Vacutainer tube, syringe, or butterfly setup. Essentially, cleansing of the skin and tops of the collection tubes are the major differences between these three methods and standard collection.

STEPS:

1. Review laboratory requisition, and check supplies.
2. Perform hand hygiene.
3. Greet and identify patient.

4. Ask patient if he or she is allergic to latex or adhesive materials. Use equipment and supplies appropriate for patient.

5. Assemble evacuated blood culture tubes and equipment needed for tests requested.

6. Check expiration date on each tube. Don gloves, apply tourniquet as previously described, locate vein, loosen tourniquet, and begin site preparation with 70% alcohol wipe for 1 minute, then scrub for at least 30 seconds with iodine tincture or chlorhexidine gluconate for patients sensitive to iodine or for infants. Swab in circles about 4 inches in diameter without overlapping from center of puncture site outward. (Facility protocols may differ on preparation for blood culture. Check with procedure manual on site).

NOTE: Some blood culture kits have an antiseptic mixture provided that is used for a total of 30 seconds.

7. Allow area to dry 1 minute to permit antiseptic to work against microorganisms on skin. Do *not* repalpate site before puncturing skin.

8. While waiting for skin to dry, cleanse tops of blood culture tubes with a new iodine tincture swab, then wipe with a new alcohol pad. This cleansing should take place immediately before collecting specimen.

9. Using a Vacutainer tube holder and needle assembly and a cleansed blood culture bottle that fits into holder, puncture vein as previously explained, then push blood culture tube into place. Collect designated amount of blood first in anaerobic, then in aerobic, containers.

NOTE: Yellow-top tubes are also used to collect blood cultures.

10. Withdraw last culture bottle before withdrawing needle. Apply gauze as explained for 3 to 5 minutes. Follow manufacturer's directions for inversion of blood culture bottles. Label with patient's name, time, date of collection, and your initials. Timing is important since multiple blood cultures are often ordered times three at intervals of 15, 30, or 60 minutes.

For syringe collection, proceed as in Procedure 13-7 with the following changes:

- Use a safety syringe for an adult (follow facility protocol for collection of blood culture from pediatric patients), and transfer first 10 mL into anaerobic vial and second 10 mL into aerobic vial for a total of 20 mL.
- After withdrawing sample with syringe, activate safety needle cover and dispose of it in sharps container.
- Place a special blunt connector on syringe, and attach it to direct draw holder/adapter.
- Place anaerobic vial in an upright position, put direct draw adapter over blood culture vial, and allow desired amount (10 mL) to enter vial.
- Remove vial, and repeat with aerobic vial. Do not push plunger on syringe to dispense blood. Vacuum in vial will pull blood.

For butterfly collection, proceed as in Procedure 13-8 with following changes:

- Use a butterfly safety collection device to puncture vein after appropriate skin cleansing.
- Use a direct draw adapter that fits over blood culture vial to transfer blood into vials. Fill aerobic vial first since tubing contains some air, then collect anaerobic sample. See manufacturer's directions for vial inversion.
- Label vials with patient's name, date, time of draw, and your initials.

11. Remove iodine from patient's skin with alcohol pad after collection of samples with any of methods described.

12. Check puncture site for bleeding and bandage. Instruct patient to remove bandage after 15 minutes. If puncture site is still bleeding after 5 minutes, notify physician.

13. Clean area. Remove and dispose of gloves in biohazard waste container. Perform hand hygiene.

14. Document patient's record if applicable.

CHARTING EXAMPLE: 10/18/XX 8:15 A.M. Bld culture ×3 drawn from Lt arm every 30 minutes at 8:15, 8:45, 9:15. · A. Byron, CMA (AAMA)

Bleeding Times

A bleeding time test is used to determine how rapidly a small wound will cease to bleed. The procedure is performed to test for platelet plug formation in the capillaries and is often performed as a screening test prior to surgery. The normal bleeding times range from 2 to 8 minutes. Abnormal bleeding times may result when platelets are low in number or when they are not functioning normally. A variety of devices are available.

An incision 5 mm long and 1 mm deep is made in the patient's forearm, and after 30 seconds white filter paper is used to blot the incision without directly touching the skin. This wicking is continued every 30 seconds until blood no longer stains the filter paper. Patients should be made aware that slight scarring may result from the test. In the case of prolonged bleeding, butterfly bandages or a pressure bandage should be applied after the test. If bleeding continues for more than 15 minutes, the physician should be notified. Ingestion of aspirin within 2 weeks of the test may interfere with results. Patients should be asked about aspirin and response noted prior to testing. (Procedure 13-10 lists the steps for using the disposable Surgicutt device with a retractable blade.)

PERFORMING A BLEEDING TIME TEST WITH A SURGICUTT DEVICE

ABHES VII.MA.A.1 10(b)(2)   CAAHEP I.P (12)

OBJECTIVE: To successfully perform a bleeding time test using a Surgicutt device.

STANDARD: This tasks 15–20 minutes.

EQUIPMENT AND SUPPLIES: Surgicutt device; gloves; blood pressure cuff; 70% alcohol pad; bleeding time blotting paper; butterfly bandage; sterile 2 × 2 gauze; tape; patient's record; watch with a second hand; pen; biohazard waste container; sharps container.

STEPS:

1. Check patient's record or laboratory requisition for test orders. Check for patient allergies.
2. Identify patient, and explain procedure, including fact that slight scarring may result.
3. Inquire whether or not patient has taken aspirin within 2 weeks and how much was ingested.
4. Place patient's arm in a well-supported, comfortable position. Expose forearm, and examine area about 5 cm below antecubital crease on lateral surface of forearm. Avoid areas with scars, abscesses, bruises, or surface veins.
5. Put blood pressure cuff on upper arm and inflate to 40 mm Hg pressure (adults).
6. Clean area with alcohol pad, and allow to air-dry.
7. Remove safety clip, and hold instrument between thumb and index finger. Rest it gently on cleansed area so both ends of device are touching surface of skin.
8. Push trigger on device, and make an incision parallel to antecubital crease (5 mm long ×1 mm deep). Start timing immediately.
9. After 30 seconds touch blotter paper to flow of blood without touching incision. (Touching incision may disturb clot and change results.)
10. Blot in same manner every 30 seconds until no blood stains are present on blotter paper, and then stop timer immediately. Results are reported to nearest 30 seconds.
11. Deflate and remove blood pressure cuff, and cleanse site again with antiseptic swab. Apply butterfly bandage. Ask patient to leave bandage in place for 24 hours. If site bleeds longer than 15 minutes, apply a pressure bandage and notify physician.
12. Clean area, and dispose of Surgicutt device in sharps container. Dispose of other materials, including gloves, in biohazard waste container.
13. Perform hand hygiene.
14. Document patient's record.

CHARTING EXAMPLE: 10/18/XX 9:20 A.M. BT performed on RT forearm. BT 4 min 30 seconds. Butterfly bandage applied. · R. Roberts, RMA

14 Hematology

PROCEDURES

Procedure 14-1 Performing a Manual Microhematocrit

Procedure 14-2 Performing a Hematocrit Using the HemataSTAT II Instrument

Procedure 14-3 Performing a Hemoglobin Determination Using HemoCue Method

Procedure 14-4 Preparing a Dilution of Whole Blood Using a WBC Unopette System

Procedure 14-5 Performing a CBC Using QBC STAR Centrifugal Hematology

Procedure 14-6 Preparing a Peripheral Blood Smear

Procedure 14-7 Staining a Peripheral Blood Smear

Advanced Procedure 14-8 Performing a Differential Blood Smear Evaluation

Procedure 14-9 Performing an Erythrocyte Sedimentation Rate Using the Wintrobe Method

Procedure 14-10 Performing an Erythrocyte Sedimentation Rate Using the Westergren Method

TERMS TO LEARN

hematopoiesis

erythrocytes

leukocytes

thrombocytes

serum

anemia

polycythemia

leukocytosis

leukopenia

indices

corpuscular

Hematology is the study of blood and the tissues that produce it. Blood and its components are analyzed to detect pathological conditions and to determine appropriate courses of treatment. Complete blood counts (CBC) are one of the most frequently ordered diagnostic tests. A complete blood count includes hemoglobin, hematocrit, WBC count, red blood cell count, red blood cell indices, and differential smear evaluation. Each of these tests is discussed in more detail in this chapter.

Blood Components

The formation of blood is known as **hematopoiesis** and begins with stem cell formation in the bone marrow. Blood is composed of plasma (liquid portion) and the formed elements: **erythrocytes** (red blood cells), **leukocytes** (white blood cells), and **thrombocytes** (platelets).

Blood

White blood cells (WBCs) are formed in the bone marrow and provide the main line of defense against infection. There are five types of leukocytes. They are divided into granulocytic and nongranulocytic categories. Granulocytic WBCs have lobed nuclei and granules in their cytoplasm. Nongranulocytic cells generally have nuclei without lobes and no granules in the cytoplasm.

1. Granulocytes: the three types of granulocytes each have lobed nucleus and granules in the cytoplasm.
   - Neutrophils
   - Eosinophils
   - Basophils
2. Nongranulocytic cells
   - Lymphocytes: formed in bone marrow and lymph nodes
   - Monocytes: formed in bone marrow and able to migrate into the tissues as macrophages to engulf invading microorganisms.

Red blood cells (RBCs) are formed in the bone marrow. Their main function is to carry oxygen to the cells and remove carbon dioxide from the cells as waste.

Platelets are formed in the bone marrow and are cell fragments whose main function is to assist in the coagulation of blood.

Plasma, the liquid portion of blood, comprises about 55% of blood, and the formed elements make up the remaining 45% of blood. Plasma is made of 90% water and 10% dissolved solids. Plasma contains all the clotting factors. The dissolved solids in plasma include the following:

- Plasma proteins (albumin, globulin, fibrinogen, prothrombin); plasma without fibrinogen = **serum**
- Electrolytes (sodium, potassium, chloride)
- Glucose
- Amino acids
- Lipids
- Cholesterol
- Carbohydrates
- Waste products (urea, lactic acid, uric acid), creatinine
- Respiratory gases (oxygen and carbon dioxide)
- Miscellaneous substances (hormones, enzymes, vitamins)

Blood samples for most hematology tests require an anticoagulant to prevent clotting. When performing a venipuncture, a lavender top tube (EDTA) is required for a CBC, and a blue top tube (sodium citrate) is required for prothrombin. For skin puncture, heparinized capillary tubes are required.

Safety Alert! When opening evacuated blood tubes, protect yourself from fine drops of blood (aerosols of blood) by wearing PPE and by using either safety-capped tubes or cap shields when opening standard tops or, if neither is available, a folded paper towel over the top.

Microhematocrit

Hematocrit is a measurement of the percentage of packed red blood cells in a blood sample and reflects the ratio of red blood cells to plasma in the body. The normal values for hematocrits vary depending on the sex of the individual. As with all laboratory values, the results should be compared to the reference ranges of the testing laboratory. The following are the average hematocrit levels:

Adult males	41%–53%
Adult females	36%–46%

Performing a hematocrit is a quick, easy, useful test for screening for anemia and polycythemia. **Anemia** is a decrease in the number of red blood cells or amount of hemoglobin in the red blood cells indicated in a decreased hematocrit and hemoglobin. **Polycythemia** is an overproduction of blood cells as indicated by elevated hematocrit level. Children have slightly lower hematocrits than adults. Generally, measuring a hematocrit involves placing a sample of antico-agulated blood into a capillary tube and the capillary tube in a centrifuge at 10,000 to 15,000 rpm for 5 minutes (or according to manufacturer's guidelines). After the tubes are spun, they will separate into the plasma layer, the buffy coat (a small layer of white cells between the plasma and the RBCs), and the red blood cells. The volume of packed RBCs is compared to the total blood volume in the tube.

The hematocrit tubes are read on a built-in scale in the centrifuge or on a separate variable volume scale. The HemataSTAT II by Separation Technology, Inc., is a small and lightweight centrifuge system for performing rapid and accurate microhematocrits. It contains a built-in reader that instructs the tester through each step of the procedure. It is a CLIA Waived procedure. (Procedures 14-1 and 14-2 describe how to perform a manual microhematocrit and use a HemataSTAT II.)

PROCEDURE 14-1

PERFORMING A MANUAL MICROHEMATOCRIT

ABHES VII.MA.A.1 10(b)(2)   CAAHEP I.P (12)

OBJECTIVE: To perform a microhematocrit from a skin puncture or EDTA venous sample, using aseptic technique and obtaining correct values within ± 2.

STANDARD: This task takes less than 15 minutes.

EQUIPMENT AND SUPPLIES: Microcollection tubes, heparinized and plain; sealant clay; a microhematocrit centrifuge and reading device; sharps container; gloves; pen; laboratory requisition; gauze squares; patient's record; biohazard waste container.

NOTE: Blood for a microhematocrit may be obtained from a skin puncture using a heparinized capillary tube (Procedure 13-1) or from a lavender top tube collected by venipuncture using a plain capillary tube (Procedure 13-6). These steps are not repeated in this chapter.

STEPS:

1. Check laboratory requisition or patient's record for tests ordered. Check for patient allergies.
2. Assemble equipment and supplies.
3. Verify that name on laboratory requisition and EDTA tube agree.
4. Identify patient, and explain procedure.
5. Perform hand hygiene, and don gloves.
6. Perform either a skin puncture or venipuncture.

    From a skin puncture:
    - Fill 2 heparinized capillary tubes three-quarters full.
    - Place a gloved finger over one end to prevent blood from running out, and seal other end in clay sealant. Use caution; do not push so hard that tube breaks.

- If more than one patient is to be tested, place first 2 tubes in clay and write patient's name and numbers above slots in clay corresponding to patient's capillary tubes.

From a well-mixed EDTA (lavender) tube:
- Fill 2 plain capillary tubes three-quarters full of EDTA well-mixed anticoagulated blood by carefully removing top using a paper towel over top unless a safety cap is present.
- Holding tube at an angle, touch tip of capillary tube to blood and fill tube; place your finger over end, wipe excess blood off exterior of tube, and place gently in clay sealant. Repeat with second tube.
- If more than one patient is to be tested, place first 2 tubes in clay and write patient's name and numbers corresponding to patient's capillary tubes locations in sealant.

7. Place tubes with clay end touching outside rim of centrifuge in grooves opposite one another.
8. Attach lid, and tighten. Close lid on centrifuge, and set for 10,000 to 15,000 rpm for 2 to 5 minutes (or whatever manufacturer's guidelines specify).
9. Either read tubes on built-in scale in centrifuge, *or* remove capillary tubes carefully after centrifuge has stopped spinning and place first tube in groove on microhematocrit reader with clay end down; follow directions on reader to determine hematocrit values. Read second tube in same way as first.
10. Record results.

11. Dispose of capillary tubes in sharps container and other waste in biohazard waste container.

12. Remove and dispose of gloves properly.

13. Perform hand hygiene.

14. Document results in laboratory log and patient's requisition or patient's record.

CHARTING EXAMPLE: 10/23/XX 3:00 P.M. Capillary puncture for HCT = 41%. · L. Lee, RMA

PROCEDURE 14-2

PERFORMING A HEMATOCRIT USING HEMATASTAT II INSTRUMENT

ABHES VII.MA.A.1 10(b)(2)   CAAHEP I.P (12)

OBJECTIVE: To perform a microhematocrit test using the HemataSTAT II Instrument.

STANDARD: This task takes 5 minutes or less after the specimen is obtained.

EQUIPMENT AND SUPPLIES: Skin puncture or venous EDTA specimen in appropriate capillary tubes; HemataCHEK controls; HemataSTAT II instrument; gauze; clay sealant; gloves; laboratory requisition; pen; sharps container; biohazard waste container.

STEPS:

1. Check laboratory requisition or patient's record for tests ordered. Check for patient allergies.

2. Assemble equipment and supplies.

3. Check expiration date and storage requirements on all supplies and control specimens.

4. Verify agreement of name on laboratory requisition and patient's sample.

5. Identify patient, and explain procedure.

6. Perform hand hygiene, and don gloves.

7. Perform either a skin puncture or venipuncture.

   From a skin puncture:
   - Fill 2 heparinized capillary tubes one-half to three-quarters full.
   - Place gloved finger over one end to prevent blood from running out, and seal other end in clay sealant. Use caution not to push so hard that tube breaks.
   - If more than one patient is to be tested, place first 2 tubes in clay and write patient's name and numbers corresponding to patient's capillary tubes location in sealant.

From a well-mixed EDTA (lavender) tube:
- Fill 2 capillary tubes one-half to three-quarters full of anticoagulated blood by carefully removing top, using a paper towel over top unless a safety cap is present.
- Holding tube at an angle, touch tip of capillary tube to blood and fill tube; place your finger over end, and wipe excess blood off exterior of capillary tube; place gently in clay sealant. Repeat with second tube.
- If more than one patient is to be tested, place first 2 tubes in clay and write patient's name and numbers corresponding to patient's capillary tubes location in sealant.

WHY? Two tubes are always tested in a hematocrit test done for quality control purposes. The tube readings should be ± 2, or the test must be repeated. Normal and abnormal controls should be run following the protocol of the testing facility. The N, A controls readings should be recorded on the daily QC log.

8. Fill 2 normal control capillary tubes and 2 abnormal control capillary tubes in same manner as above. All readings on each pair of specimens should be within ±2, or tests must be repeated.

9. Place all six capillary tubes into HemataSTAT centrifuge rotor tube holder (Figure 14-1).

10. Close centrifuge lid, and lock it.

11. Press RUN button to spin tests for 60 seconds.

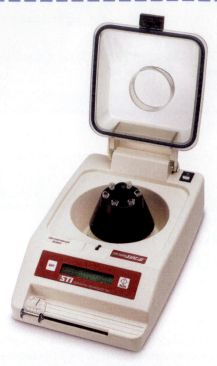

FIGURE 14-1 HemataSTAT II hematocrit machine.
Courtesy of Thermo Fisher Scientific.

12. After instrument beeps, open lid.

13. Move sealed end of tube and slider all the way to left side on reader tray. Follow directions on instrument display. Move slider to interface of red cells/sealant; then red cells/plasma; and then plasma and air interface. Press ENTER button at each interface to mark each one of the three.

14. Hematocrit percentage reading will be displayed automatically.

15. Repeat with all remaining tubes.

16. Record results of each reading. Log results of normal and abnormal controls in QC log.

17. Dispose of capillary tubes in sharps container and remaining waste in biohazard waste container.

18. Remove and dispose of gloves properly.

19. Perform hand hygiene.

20. Document results in laboratory log and patient's requisition or patient's record.

CHARTING EXAMPLE: 10/24/XX 9:00 A.M. HemataSTAT HCT 46% using EDTA venous spec. ⋯⋯⋯⋯⋯⋯
⋯⋯⋯⋯⋯⋯⋯⋯⋯⋯⋯⋯ B. Peters, CMA (AAMA)

Hemoglobin

Hemoglobin is the molecule in red blood cells that transports oxygen to the cells and carbon dioxide from the cells in the body. Each hemoglobin molecule is composed of heme and globin, with iron the main component in the heme molecules. Oxygenated (arterial) blood is bright red, and deoxygenated (venous) blood is dark red. Several disease conditions are caused by abnormal forms of hemoglobin. Sickle cell anemia is one example. Iron deficiency anemia is, as the name implies, a decrease in the amount of iron in red blood cells. Thus measurement of hemoglobin levels is another important source of diagnostic information for the physician. Many methods of measuring hemoglobin are available, with the most accurate involving automated analyzers of various types. One older method uses a hemoglobinometer, which requires hemolyzing the red cells and matching the color on a small lighted device. Newer point of care (POC) testing devices have replaced the hemoglobinometer. Instruments such as the HemoCue system (Figure 14-2A), HGB Meter (Figure 14-2B), and I-STAT Point-of-Care analyzer are easy to use, and results are less subject to error than those of the hemoglobinometer. Normal values for hemoglobin differ in males and females. They are as follows:

Adult male	13.5–17.5 g/dL
Adult female	12–16 g/dL

As a rule of thumb, three times the hemoglobin value should equal the hematocrit value plus or minus two. If these values do not check out using this basic formula, both tests must be repeated. If they still do not agree after repeating them, the report should be repeated and verified. Some facilities have protocols governing results that are out of the norm. These policies should be followed. However, it is possible in certain types of anemias that these values will not agree; however, human or machine error must be ruled out first.

White and Red Blood Cell Counts

White and red blood cell counts are performed manually or by automated analyzers. Neither testing option is CLIA Waived and cannot be performed without proper certification from the Centers for Medicare and Medicaid Services

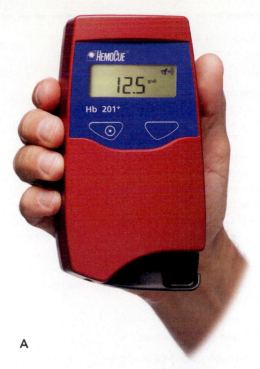
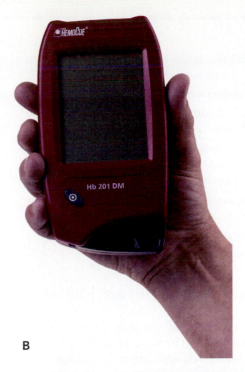

A

B

FIGURE 14-2 (A) HemoCue Instrument for measuring hemoglobin; (B) an example of CLIA Waived POC hemoglobin testing equipment. *Courtesy of HemoCue® AB.*

(CMS). Individuals performing these tests must obtain further training. Running daily quality control and having proficiency testing done by an outside proficiency testing laboratory twice a year are required as well. However, the collection of samples for manual method of WBC, RBC, and platelet counts may be required in many facilities. The methods for collection of samples are all similar but use different diluting solutions, depending on the test. The procedure for obtaining a WBC count sample is covered here. The procedure for cell counting using a hemocytometer with Neubauer ruling is an advanced procedure and is not covered. The automated hematology system QBC STAR Centrifugal Hematology System by Becton, Dickinson and Company is rated by CLIA as moderately complex and is covered in this chapter but does not require the use of a microscope.

PROCEDURE 14-3

PERFORMING A HEMOGLOBIN DETERMINATION USING HEMOCUE METHOD

ABHES VII.MA.A.1 10(b)(2)   CAAHEP I.P (12)

OBJECTIVE: To perform a hemoglobin test using the HemoCue method following manufacturer's directions using either capillary or EDTA venous sample.

STANDARD: This task takes 10 minutes or less.

EQUIPMENT AND SUPPLIES: Laboratory requisition; gloves; capillary puncture equipment or EDTA venous blood sample; HemoCue system with supplies and daily controls for the analyzer; biohazard waste container; sharps container; pen; gauze pads.

STEPS:

1. Check laboratory requisition or patient's record for tests ordered. Check for patient allergies.
2. Assemble equipment and supplies.
3. Verify agreement of name on laboratory requisition and name on EDTA tube.
4. Turn on HemoCue machine to warm up.
5. Check expiration date and storage requirements for all supplies and control specimens.
6. Identify patient, and explain procedure.
7. Perform hand hygiene, and don gloves.
8. Perform either a skin puncture or venipuncture using previously explained procedures.

   Skin puncture:
   - Perform capillary puncture, and wipe away first drop.
   - Fill HemoCue cuvette without stopping and without topping off (to prevent formation of bubbles).
   - Wipe off outside of cuvette with gauze, taking care not to touch gauze to point and cause blood to be withdrawn.
   - Inspect for air bubbles. If air bubbles are found, fill a new cuvette.
   - Insert filled cuvette within 10 minutes of filling into black cuvette holder, and push into HemoCue instrument.
   - Read hemoglobin level from display, and record.
   - Run controls daily and log QC results to ensure that both machine and reagents are working correctly.

   Venous EDTA specimen:
   - Using previously obtained EDTA venous specimen, fill HemoCue cuvette without topping off and without bubbles by holding point of a cuvette into well-mixed sample of EDTA blood.
   - Wipe off exterior of cuvette without touching point and reducing amount of blood in cuvette.
   - Inspect for air bubbles. If air bubbles are present, fill a new cuvette.
   - Insert filled cuvette into black cuvette holder, and push into HemoCue instrument within 10 minutes of filling.
   - Read hemoglobin level from display, and record.
   - Run controls daily and log QC results to ensure machine is working correctly.

9. Dispose of cuvettes in sharps container and remaining waste in biohazard waste container.
10. Remove and dispose of gloves properly.
11. Perform hand hygiene.
12. Document results in laboratory log and laboratory requisition or patient's record.

CHARTING EXAMPLE: 10/24/XX 10:00 A.M. Hgb. HemoCue 12.4 g/dL (skin puncture). ················· J. Fleming, RMA

Coulter Counters by Beckman Coulter are more complex systems seen in larger testing facilities. These automated systems use electrolyte solution diluents capable of conducting electricity. The blood is diluted, and the sample is aspirated into the machine through an opening. The cells cause an interruption of electrical impulse, each of which is counted. The pulses are counted, analyzed, and calculated by the instrument, and a readout is produced. The readout provides values for WBC, RBC, Hgb, Hct, RBC indices, platelets, and types and percentages of the WBC, plus evaluation of RBC morphology.

WHITE BLOOD CELL COUNT

WBC counts provide the patient's total WBC count. The normal reference value for a total WBC is 4,000–11,000 WBC/mm^2 of blood. There is some variation in children and among different races. An elevated WBC count, **leukocytosis**, indicates an increase in the number of WBCs, and **leukopenia**, a decrease in WBCs. Leukocytosis occurs in infections or certain types of leukemia. Leukopenia is seen in cases of bone marrow suppression, overwhelming infection, and some types of leukemia. The procedures for using a Unopette to dilute blood for WBC count and the procedure for QBC STAR semi-automated method for CBC follow.

Unopette

The Unopette System for counting blood cells is not widely used at this time; however, a familiarity with the workings of Unopette devices is helpful when automated equipment is malfunctioning. Blood for a manual WBC using a Unopette System may be obtained by skin puncture or from an EDTA venous specimen. Figure 14-3 illustrates a complete WBC Unopette System for one patient. The reservoir contains diluent (3% acetic acid), which hemolyzes RBCs and leaves WBCs intact for easier counting. Once the sample is obtained and mixed in the Unopette, the Neubauer hemocytometer is

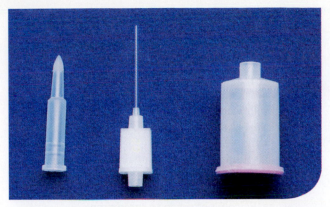

FIGURE 14-3 Unopette System, left to right: pipette shield, pipette, and reservoir.

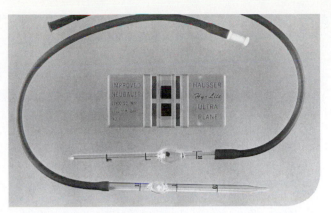

FIGURE 14-4 Hemocytometer.

"charged," or filled carefully, using the Unopette pipette as a capillary tube to facilitate filling both chambers (sides) of the hemocytometer (Figure 14-4). The hemocytometer is then placed under the microscope using low light and low power, and the four corner squares are counted on each side of the chamber. The count is calculated by averaging the total number of cells counted on both sides of the chamber and using the following formula:

$$\text{Average of cells counted} \times 50 = \text{Total WBC/mm}^2$$

The Unopette for RBC contains 0.85% normal saline as a diluent, which preserves the RBCs. The blood is diluted the same way. Unopettes for RBC counts have a red bottom. The chambers are filled in the same way; however, $40\times$ power and low light are used. The five squares in the center area of the small squares are counted.

The Unopette for platelet count uses 1% ammonium oxalate solution. The platelets are counted in the entire center square using $40\times$ with lowered light. Platelets are tiny fragments of cells much smaller than RBCs, and they are more difficult to see and count. Automated equipment offers more accurate, valid, reliable results if used properly and monitored by routine maintenance, daily quality control, and proficiency testing.

PROCEDURE 14-4

PREPARING A DILUTION OF WHOLE BLOOD USING A WBC UNOPETTE SYSTEM

ABHES VII.MA.A.1 10(b)(2)   CAAHEP I.P (12)

OBJECTIVE: To prepare a WBC Unopette dilution with whole blood.

STANDARD: This task takes 5 minutes or less.

EQUIPMENT AND SUPPLIES: WBC Unopette reservoir; pipette and pipette shield; gloves; sharps container; biohazard waste container; marking pen; laboratory requisition; patient's record; gauze; blood sample from skin puncture or EDTA venous specimen.

STEPS:

1. Check laboratory requisition or patient's record for tests ordered. Check for patient allergies.
2. Assemble equipment and supplies.
3. Verify that name on laboratory requisition and EDTA tube match.
4. Check expiration date and storage requirements for all supplies and control specimens.

5. Identify patient, and explain procedure.

6. Perform hand hygiene, and don gloves.

7. Using pipette shield, puncture an opening in top of Unopette reservoir.

8. Perform either a skin puncture or venipuncture.

For skin puncture:

- Remove Unopette capillary tube from shield. While holding capillary tube horizontal to blood flow to prevent bubbles, fill capillary tube completely. (It will automatically stop when filled.)
- Wipe off exterior of Unopette capillary tube with a gauze square without removing any blood from tip.
- Squeeze reservoir slightly to expel some air before inserting Unopette pipette.
- With an index finger, cover end of pipette not used to obtain blood, and insert pipette into reservoir. Remove index finger, and blood from pipette will be drawn into reservoir diluent.
- Gently squeeze sides of reservoir to rinse pipette with diluent. Be careful not to do it so forcefully that you expel some of blood/diluent mixture, which would lower results. Rinse pipette two to three times.
- Swirl reservoir gently to mix blood, and allow to stand for 10 minutes to hemolyze RBCs. Swirl sample again to remix cells before charging counting chamber.

Venous EDTA sample:

- Remove Unopette capillary tube from shield. Hold EDTA tube at an angle, and touch tip of capillary tube to blood, taking care not to cause bubbles; fill capillary tube. It will automatically stop when filled.

- Wipe off exterior of Unopette capillary tube with gauze square without removing any blood from tip.
- Squeeze reservoir slightly to expel some air before inserting Unopette pipette.
- With index finger, cover end of pipette not used to obtain blood, and insert pipette into reservoir. Remove index finger, and blood from pipette will be drawn into reservoir diluent.
- Gently squeeze sides of reservoir to rinse pipette with diluent. Be careful not to do it so forcefully that you lose some of blood/diluent mixture, which will lower results. Rinse pipette two to three times.
- Swirl reservoir gently to mix blood and allow to stand for 10 minutes to hemolyze RBCs. Swirl sample again to remix cells before charging counting chamber.

9. Label Unopette reservoir with patient's name, date, and ID number if applicable. Notify laboratory specialist that in 10 minutes Unopette will be ready to be counted on hemocytometer.

10. Dispose of sharps in container. Clean area, and dispose of other biohazard waste and gloves in biohazard waste container.

11. Perform hand hygiene.

12. Document procedure in laboratory log, on laboratory requisition, and in patient's record.

CHARTING EXAMPLE: 10/29/XX 1:00 P.M. Fingerstick for Unopette CBC performed. Technologist notified at 1:25 P.M.
· A. Newlon, CMA (AAMA)

PROCEDURE 14-5

PERFORMING A CBC USING QBC STAR CENTRIFUGAL HEMATOLOGY

ABHES VII.MA.A.1 10(b)(2)   CAAHEP I.P (12)

OBJECTIVE: To perform a QBC STAR moderately complex test following manufacturer's directions and quality control procedures.

STANDARD: This task takes 10 minutes.

EQUIPMENT AND SUPPLIES: QBC STAR Instrument; QBC STAR tubes; controls; capillary or EDTA venous blood sample; gauze; gloves; laboratory requisition; patient's record; pen; sharps container; biohazard waste container.

STEPS:

1. Check laboratory requisition or patient's record for tests ordered. Check for patient allergies.

2. Verify that name on laboratory requisition and EDTA specimen tube agree.

3. Assemble equipment and supplies.

4. Check expiration date and storage requirements for all supplies and control specimens.

5. Perform hand hygiene, and don gloves.

6. Turn on machine, perform quality control and follow steps 7 and 8. Perform patient's test by following steps 9 through 15 below (Figure 14-5). Figure 14-6 shows an enlargement of a QBC STAR tube.

7. Record quality control results as facility protocol demands. If controls are not within acceptable limits, repeat as protocol requires.

8. Identify patient, and explain procedure.

9. Place collection tip of QBC STAR tube in contact with blood as shown. Using either skin puncture or EDTA venous blood, fill a QBC STAR tube. So tube will fill, do

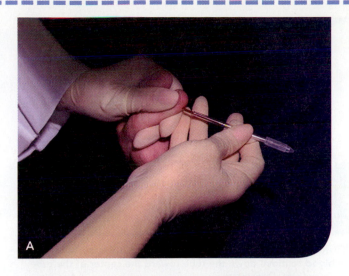

A

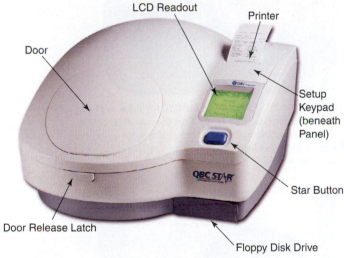

FIGURE 14-5 QBC STAR Hematology System provides ambulatory settings with Hct, Hgb, WBC, and platelet counts and distribution of granulocytes and nongranulocytes.
Courtesy of QBC Diagnostics.

Labels: Door, LCD Readout, Printer, Setup Keypad (beneath Panel), Star Button, Floppy Disk Drive, Door Release Latch

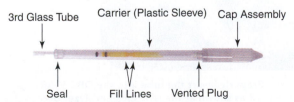

Labels: 3rd Glass Tube, Carrier (Plastic Sleeve), Cap Assembly, Seal, Fill Lines, Vented Plug

FIGURE 14-6 QBC STAR tube.
Courtesy of QBC Diagnostics.

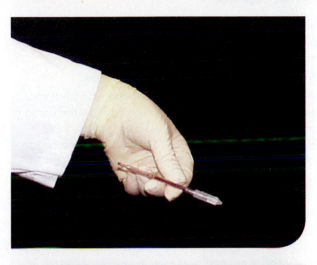

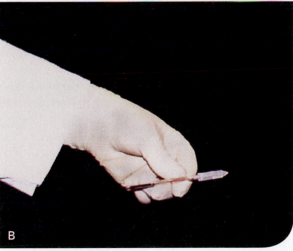

B

FIGURE 14-7 (A) Place the collection tip of the QBC STAR tube in contact with blood. Fill tube beyond the first black line and up to the second black line; (B) rock the QBC STAR tube back and forth at least four times to mix the blood with the orange coating.
Courtesy of QBC Diagnostics.

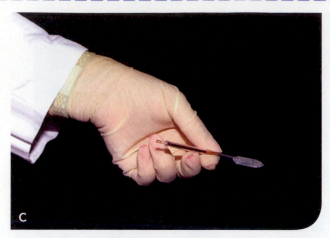

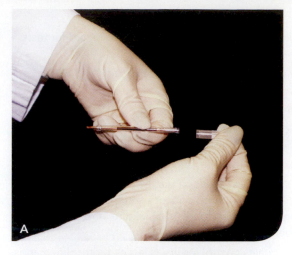

C

FIGURE 14-7 (Continued) (C) Tilt the QBC STAR tube, allowing the blood to move down the tube toward the center of the tube. *Courtesy of QBC Diagnostics.*

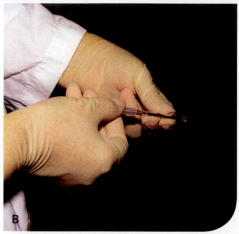

A

B

not allow plastic sleeve of QBC STAR tube to contact blood. Fill tube by capillary action to second black line. Hold tube so no bubbles form. (See Figure 14-7A.)

10. Wipe off excess blood from outside of tube.

11. Mix blood by carefully tilting or rocking tube back and forth four times then tilting the tube to allow the blood to move down the tube toward the center of the tube (Figure 14-7B and Figure 14-7C). Do not allow blood to touch white plug at end of tube.

12. Remove cap from end of tube by holding tube in a horizontal position and pulling it straight off as shown in Figure 14-8A. Do not allow blood to touch white plug at end of tube.

13. Place cap on collection end of tube (opposite white cap), push it on, and twist to seal tube as shown in Figure 14-8B.

14. Place QBC STAR tube in QBC STAR analyzer and close and lock door (Figure 14-9).

15. Press STAR button to start.

16. During spinning, cells are packed into distinct bands layered in tube. Results will be displayed automatically and printed.

17. Label printout results with patient's name and your initials.

18. Dispose of sharps in sharps container. Dispose of all other medical waste in biohazard waste container.

19. Clean area. Remove and dispose of gloves properly.

20. Perform hand hygiene.

21. Document QC log, patient's record, and patient's requisition.

22. Identify abnormal values, and notify physician.

FIGURE 14-8 (A) Hold the QBC STAR tube as shown. Remove the cap from the tube by pulling the cap straight off; (B) place the cap over the collection end of the tube by guiding the glass end of the tube into the center of the cap. *Courtesy of QBC Diagnostics.*

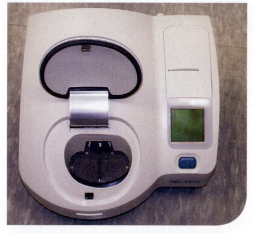

FIGURE 14-9 Properly insert the tube into the QBC STAR analyzer, oriented as shown at the left. Close analyzer door, and press STAR button. *Courtesy of QBC Diagnostics.*

CHARTING EXAMPLE: 10/24/XX 11:00 A.M. QBC STAR done on EDTA sample. Printout attached. · · · · · · · · · · J. Watts, RMA

Test	Result	Reference Range
HCT % (men)	44%	41–53
HCT % (women)	—	36–46
HGB (men) (g/dL)	14.2 g/dL	13.5–17.5 g/dL
MCHC (g/dL)	35 g/dL	31–37 g/dL
PLT ($\times 10^9$)/L	355 ($\times 10^9$)	150–450 ($\times 10^9$)/L
WBC ($\times 10^9$)/L	5.7 ($\times 10^9$)/L	4.3–11.0 ($\times 10^9$)/L
Granulocytes ($\times 10^9$)/L	5.0 ($\times 10^9$)/L	1.8–7.2 ($\times 10^9$)/L
Lymphocytes/Monocytes ($\times 10^9$)/L	2.9 ($\times 10^9$)/L	1.7–4.9 ($\times 10^9$)/L

Peripheral Blood Smears

A differential smear count indicates the percentages of each type of WBC, describes the RBC morphology, and estimates the number of platelets. For this procedure, a drop of blood is applied to a slide and spread out thinly using a special technique. The prepared slide is then stained with Wright's or Wright-Giemsa stain to help differentiate the cells by color. The stained slide is then observed under the microscope using the 100× oil immersion lens, and a total of 100 WBCs are counted, differentiating one from another. The appearance, size, shape, and color of RBCs are described. The number of platelets is estimated based on the number of thrombocytes seen per field. This test may be performed manually by professionally trained medical technicians, technologists, or hematologists. Wright's or Wright-Giemsa stain is a polychromatic stain that contains methylene blue and eosin. On a slide with these stains, RBCs stain a light pink color. WBCs pick up the stains differently, depending on their affinity for either the methylene blue basic stain or eosin acidic stain. The appearance of the cells is discussed more completely later in this chapter.

The slide(s) are then stained with Wright's or Wright-Giemsa stain (Procedure 14-7) and viewed and counted by a laboratory specialist using 100× oil immersion (Procedure 14-8). Wright's staining procedures differ from one

PROCEDURE 14-6

PREPARING A PERIPHERAL BLOOD SMEAR

ABHES VII.MA.A.1 10(b)(2)   CAAHEP I.P (12)

OBJECTIVE: To prepare two peripheral blood smears from a skin puncture or EDTA venous sample so there is a thick end, a thin end, and a feathered edge on each one.

STANDARD: This task takes 5 minutes or less.

EQUIPMENT AND SUPPLIES: Clean glass slide; EDTA venous whole blood sample or skin puncture blood sample; gloves; biohazard waste container; dropper or Diff safety device (Becton Dickinson); laboratory requisition; patient's record; pen.

STEPS:

1. Check laboratory requisition or patient's record for the tests ordered. Check for patient allergies.
2. Assemble equipment and supplies.
3. Identify patient, and explain procedure.

4. Perform hand hygiene.

5. Don gloves.

6. Obtain a drop of blood by skin puncture or well-mixed EDTA venous sample.

For a skin puncture:

- Puncture skin using skin puncture method covered previously. Wipe away first drop. Touch next drop of blood to slide close to end of slide (Figure 14-10A). Two slides should always be prepared when obtaining blood from skin puncture in case one slide is destroyed.

For EDTA venous sample:

- Verify that name on laboratory requisition and patient sample are identical. Mix venous tube well by inverting eight to ten times. Do not shake tube. Remove top using a paper towel to cover tube's stopper if safety stoppers are not present. Fill a capillary tube in manner described previously, and place a drop of blood near end of slide. Or use a Quick Diff (Becton, Dickinson and Company) safety device to obtain a

drop of blood from an EDTA tube without removing top of tube. Push small device into top of EDTA tube, and invert and press tube against slide to produce a drop of blood.

7. With end of a second clean "spreader" slide held at a 30° angle, allow drop of blood to spread evenly along edge of "spreader" slide (Figure 14-10B).

8. Using smooth even motion, quickly move "spreader" slide forward (Figure 14-10C) until drop of blood is spread out. A thick end (near drop of blood), a thin area, and a feathered edge should be apparent (as in Figure 14-10D).

9. Label slide with patient's name and date.

10. Allow slide to air-dry.

WHY? Slides should be allowed to air-dry to avoid distortion of the cells.

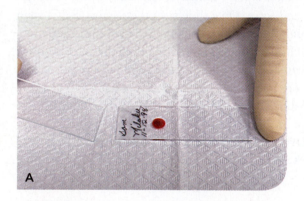
A

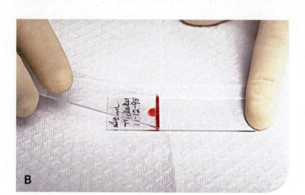
B

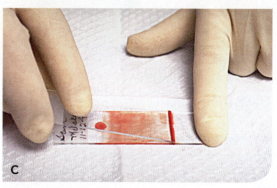
C

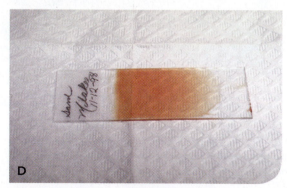
D

FIGURE 14-10 (A) Place a drop of blood close to one end of the clean glass slide; (B) using a clean glass "spreader" slide, allow the drop to spread out evenly along the edge; (C) using gentle continuous pressure, spread drop out along slide in a gliding motion; (D) a correctly made smear should have a thick end, a thin end, and a feathered edge.

PROCEDURE 14-7

STAINING A PERIPHERAL BLOOD SMEAR

ABHES VII.MA.A.1 10(b)(2)   CAAHEP I.P (12)

OBJECTIVE: To stain a peripheral blood smear with Wright's stain following manufacturer's timing and directions.

STANDARD: This task takes 10 minutes or less.

EQUIPMENT AND SUPPLIES: Dry peripheral blood smears; staining rack or jar; Wright's stain kit (methylene blue methanol fixative, eosin, buffer solution); thumb forceps; drying rack; timer; paper towel; pen; laboratory requisition; gloves; sharps container; biohazard waste container.

STEPS:

1. Make sure that slides are labeled correctly and legibly.
2. Verify that name on laboratory requisition and patient's slide are identical.
3. Place peripheral blood slides on a staining rack or in a staining jar containing Wright's stain. (Some procedures call for fixing slide with methanol as a separate step; in other procedures methanol, methylene blue, and eosin are all in one solution.)
4. Following manufacturer's directions, place stain on slide or place slide in staining jar for required time.
5. After correct amount of time has elapsed, flood slide on staining rack with buffer solution for required time, or remove slide from staining jar and place it in second jar with buffer for required time.
6. After correct amount of time has elapsed, gently wash slide with water and wipe off back of slide with paper towel to remove excess stain; or when time has elapsed, remove slide from last staining jar and proceed to wash and dry as described.
7. After slide is dry, it is ready for laboratory specialist to count and differentiate WBCs under 100× oil immersion lens.

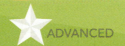 ADVANCED

PROCEDURE 14-8

PERFORMING A DIFFERENTIAL BLOOD SMEAR EVALUATION

OBJECTIVE: To perform a differential blood smear evaluation and report the results.

STANDARD: This task takes 20 minutes or less.

EQUIPMENT AND SUPPLIES: Stained peripheral blood smear; microscope; immersion oil; a differential calculator; pen; laboratory requisition; patient's record.

STEPS:

NOTE: This procedure should only be performed by trained laboratory specialists or physicians.

1. Perform hand hygiene.
2. Assemble equipment and supplies. Verify that patient's name on slide and name on requisition match.
3. Place stained peripheral blood smear on microscope focus with low power near feathered edge of smear.
4. Focus on low power, then high power, and switch objective. Before clicking it into position, place a drop of immersion oil over lighted area on slide.
5. Then click oil immersion lens into place.
6. Increase amount of light somewhat.
7. Focus on slide in an area where RBCs are touching but not overlapping. Begin at top of slide and move downward in snakelike pattern shown in Figure 14-11.
8. In each field, count and identify each WBC encountered using a differential tabulator (a hand tabulator) with a button for each type of WBC, neutrophil, lymphocyte,

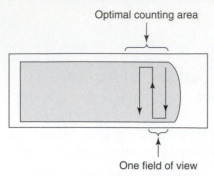

Optimal counting area

One field of view

FIGURE 14-11 A differential is counted in the thinner area where RBCs are touching but not overlapping, in a pattern similar to the one illustrated in this diagram.

monocyte, eosinophil, and basophil. Stop when bell rings at 100 cells.

9. Record number of each type of WBC as shown on differential tabulator. These numbers reflect percentage of each type of WBC and make up 100 cell differential count.

10. In optimal viewing area on slide, examine size, shape, and color of RBCs. If they appear normal in size, shape, and color, report it as follows: RBCs appear normal. If a significant number of RBCs are too small, large, pale, or odd shaped, use terms from Table 14-1 to describe RBCs and, if possible, quantify them as sl, 1+, 2+, 3+, 4+, with 4+ being most abnormal in appearance.

11. Next, in optimal viewing area on slide, observe five fields and count number of platelets in each field (a normal estimate is 5 to 20 per field), or calculate platelets using formula established in your facility. Record an estimate of platelets.

12. Complete laboratory requisition.

13. If any findings are abnormal, repeat entire count. If findings are still abnormal, ask a supervisor or physician to review slide and your abnormal findings before reporting results.

CHARTING EXAMPLE: 11/01/XX 4:00 P.M. Segs 55%, lymphs 35%, monos 5%, eos 4%, basos 1%; RBCs appear normal, platelets adequate. · · · · · · · · · · M. Roberti, MT (ASCP)

manufacturer to another. Basically the slide is fixed with methanol to ensure the cells do not wash off the slide. Next the slide is flooded with Wright's stain or Wright-Giemsa stain. A buffer is added to the slide, and then the slide is washed off gently. The back side of the slide is wiped to remove excess stain for better viewing, then tilted upright to air-dry.

Automated machines are available that prepare, stain, and evaluate peripheral blood smears and produce a printout that highlights abnormal values. The slides are then reviewed manually under the microscope by a hematologist or other laboratory specialist for a final evaluation and report. Examination of a well-prepared, well-stained peripheral blood smear is valuable as a screening tool to identify an illness, for definitive diagnosis of a suspected illness, and/or to monitor a patient's progress in response to treatment.

A peripheral blood smear count includes the following:

- Counting a 100 cell leukocyte differential
- Estimating the number of platelets
- Evaluating the RBC and platelet morphology
- Detecting and identifying abnormal WBCs and RBCs

After staining a slide, the appearance percentage of WBCs in a normal smear is as follows:

Neutrophils	50% to 70%	dark purple–lobed nucleus; pale pink cytoplasm with light purple to pink fine granules in the cytoplasm
Eosinophils	0% to 5%	dark purple–lobed nucleus, pink cytoplasm with reddish-orange large granules in cytoplasm
Basophils	0% to 2%	dark purple–lobed nucleus; light purple cytoplasm with deep blue-purple large granules in cytoplasm
Monocytes	2% to 10%	dark purple–lobed nucleus; pale blue-gray cytoplasm; largest white cell
Lymphocytes	25% to 35%	dark purple round to oval nucleus; in small amount of blue cytoplasm

RBCs appear pale pink with no nucleus in the mature form. Platelets appear as small noncellular fragments, sometimes in clumps that stain purple.

The differential smear is focused under a 100× immersion oil lens. The area best for counting cells is a short distance from the feathered edge where the RBCs appear to be touching but not overlapping. A definite pattern should be followed to prevent recounting the same area or missing a section in the optimal counting area. Once the slide is in focus, the area in view is known as a field. Using the pattern, every WBC encountered is identified and counted until 100 WBCs have been tallied in each field. The percentage of each type of WBC is reported. The result is the differential count. RBCs are reviewed in the optimal area of the slide, and a description of their morphology is reported. Red cells are normally biconcave discs similar in size, shape, and color. (Descriptive terms and definitions are listed in Table 14-1.) The number of platelets in each of five fields is counted, with 5 to 20 platelets estimated per field considered normal. This value should correlate with the total platelet count if it was performed. Abnormal or immature cells, either white or red, are identified as well.

TABLE 14-1 Red Blood Cell Descriptive Terms and Definitions

Macrocyte	large cell
Microcyte	small cell
Polychromatic	multicolored cells
Dacryocyte	tear-shaped cell
Elliptocyte	oval-shaped cell
Spherocyte	ball-shaped round cell
Sickle cell	C-shaped cell
Anisocytosis	when RBCs vary in size
Poikilocytosis	when RBCs vary in shape
Hypochromia	when RBCs are deficient in color or pale
Hyperchromia	when RBCs are darker in color

Red Blood Cell Indices

Red blood cell **indices** are hematology screening tests that are calculated from hematocrit, hemoglobin, and RBC count values. RBC indices define the size of RBC (mean **corpuscular** volume, or MCV), the hemoglobin content of RBCs (mean corpuscular hemoglobin concentration, or MCHC), and the weight of hemoglobin (mean corpuscular hemoglobin, or MCH). The reference values for RBC indices for adult males and females are as follows:

MCV	80–100 fL	(femtoliters; fL is a unit of volume 10^{-15}, formerly reported in cubic microns)
MCH	26–34 pg	(picograms) (pg = a micro microgram or 1×10^{-12})
MCHC	31–37 g/dL	(grams per deciliter)

RBC indices are important in classifying and treating different types of anemias. Since the use of automated hematology instruments is more common today and more reliable values for RBC counts are available, RBC indices are included in a CBC report. The values for RBC count, Hgb, and Hct are parameters that are determined with most automated instruments, and indices are calculated using these results.

MCH and MCV are decreased in anemias in which the RBCs are small and pale in color, as in iron deficiency anemia. The MCH and MCV are increased in anemias in which the RBCs are larger in size, as in pernicious anemia. MCHC is decreased in iron deficiency anemia.

The formulas for calculating RBC indices are as follows:

$$MVC = Hematocrit \div RBC \text{ in millions} \times 10$$

$$MCH = Hemoglobin \text{ in grams} \div RBCs \text{ in millions} \times 10$$

$$MCHC = Hemoglobin \text{ in grams} \div Hematocrit \times 10$$

Although only experienced laboratory specialists perform differential smears, most assistive personnel will encounter CBC results and are responsible for receiving CBC results over the phone from testing facilities. It is then important to be familiar with these terms since they may be part of any CBC report.

Erythrocyte Sedimentation Rate (ESR)

The erythrocyte sedimentation rate (ESR) is a measurement of how far the RBCs in an EDTA sample of whole blood will settle out or fall in 1 hour. This value is reported in millimeters per hour. Expected ESR values are as follows:

Adult males	0–10 mm/hour
Adult females	0–20 mm/hour

The rate at which the cells fall depends on the size of the RBCs, the shape of the RBCs, the number of RBCs, and the concentration of proteins in the plasma. For example, RBCs such as sickle cells fall at a slower rate because of the pointed ends. An individual with an elevated hemoglobin and hematocrit will have a slower rate of falling cells than an individual with anemia because with fewer cells the RBCs will settle out of the plasma more quickly.

The ESR, or sed rate test, is used to detect the presence of inflammation in the body. It is a nonspecific test that does not pinpoint the location of infection or inflammation.

Conditions such as arthritis, carcinomas, and autoimmune diseases have increased ESR values. The sed rate test is also used to monitor the progress or change in conditions. Two methods are used to measure ESR: the Wintrobe method and the Westergren method. The Westergren method differs from the Wintrobe in that the blood sample is mixed with a solution of sodium citrate or normal saline first. In both methods the filled tubes are placed in a rack, held in vertical position on level counter, free of bubbles and from movement or drafts, undisturbed for 1 hour. Exactly at the end of 1 hour the value is read as the number of millimeters the RBCs have fallen in millimeters, and it is reported as the sedimentation rate. EDTA blood not more than 2 hours old, or 6 hours old if the sample was refrigerated, is required. The Westergren Method is a closed system available now from several manufacturers. It offers a safer procedure with less exposure to bloodborne pathogens. (Procedure 14-9 and Procedure 14-10 present both methods.)

PROCEDURE 14-9

PERFORMING AN ERYTHROCYTE SEDIMENTATION RATE USING THE WINTROBE METHOD

ABHES VII.MA.A.1 10(b)(2)   CAAHEP I.P (12)

OBJECTIVE: To properly perform an ESR using the Wintrobe method.

STANDARD: This task takes 65 to 70 minutes.

EQUIPMENT AND SUPPLIES: EDTA whole blood specimen; Wintrobe tubes; clock; Pasteur pipette; Wintrobe pipette rack; laboratory requisition; patient's record; gloves; biohazard waste container; sharps container; pen.

STEPS:

1. Check laboratory requisition or patient's record for tests ordered. Check for patient allergies.
2. Assemble equipment and supplies.
3. Perform hand hygiene.
4. Don gloves.
5. Verify that name on laboratory requisition and name on patient's tube match.
6. If EDTA is not available, draw a tube using venipuncture method previously described. Be sure to invert tube 8 times to mix anticoagulant and blood immediately before setting up test.

7. Remove stopper of EDTA tube using paper towel method to cover top if tubes do not have safety stoppers.
8. Insert transfer pipette into specimen, and squeeze bulb to withdraw blood.
9. Insert transfer pipette into bottom of Wintrobe tube, and slowly raise it while keeping tip of pipette below level of blood to prevent bubbles from forming. Dispense blood while withdrawing transfer pipette slowly until blood is at 0 line of Wintrobe tube.
10. Place Wintrobe pipette rack in an area free of drafts and where it will be unmoved or disturbed and on a level surface. Then place filled Wintrobe tube in Wintrobe pipette rack. Set timer for 60 minutes exactly.
11. Dispose of all used sharps and biohazard waste in appropriate containers.
12. Remove and dispose of gloves properly.
13. After timer goes off to signal 60 minutes have elapsed, record number of millimeters RBCs have fallen as ESR result.
14. Document patient's record and laboratory requisition.

CHARTING EXAMPLE: 10/28/XX 4:15 P.M. ESR Wintrobe method = 15 mm/hr. · V. Zachs, RMA

PROCEDURE 14-10

PERFORMING AN ERYTHROCYTE SEDIMENTATION RATE USING THE WESTERGREN METHOD

ABHES VII.MA.A.1 10(b)(2)   CAAHEP I.P (12)

OBJECTIVE: To perform an ESR using the Westergren method for erythrocyte sedimentation rate determination.

STANDARD: This task takes 65–70 minutes.

EQUIPMENT AND SUPPLIES: EDTA whole blood sample less than 2 hours old, 6 hours if refrigerated; Westergren Dispette system with auto-zeroing pipette; vial prefilled with 0.2 mL of 3.8% sodium citrate; Westergren sed rate rack; disposable transfer pipette; sharps container; biohazard waste container; laboratory requisition; patient's record; pen; clock; gloves.

STEPS:

1. Check laboratory requisition or patient's record for tests ordered. Check for patient allergies

2. Assemble equipment and supplies.

3. Perform hand hygiene, and don gloves

4. Use EDTA whole blood sample well mixed at room temp if sample was refrigerated. Or perform venipuncture to obtain specimen following venipuncture steps previously explained in Procedure 13-6.
   Verify that name on laboratory requisition and name on patient's tube match.

5. Immediately before testing, invert vial eight times (do not shake) to thoroughly mix specimen. Remove stopper on EDTA tube using paper towel safety precautions if safety stopper not on tube.

6. Remove top from prefilled vial containing diluent. Using a transfer pipette, fill vial to fill line with 0.8 mL of blood to make required 4:1 dilution of blood to diluent.

7. Replace stopper, and invert several times to mix.

8. Place vial of diluted blood in Westergren rack on a level surface away from draft and danger of movement. Insert auto zeroing pipette through stopper of vial of blood/diluent, rotating it downward until pipette reaches bottom of vial.

9. Diluent blood mixture will fill automatically to zero line, and any excess will go into reservoir area.

10. Let filled Westergren pipette stand undisturbed for exactly 1 hour.

11. Read results at end of hour.

12. Record level of how far RBCs have fallen in millimeters per hour (mm/hr).

13. Document patient's record or laboratory requisition.

14. Discard tubes in sharps container. Discard other equipment and gloves in biohazard waste container.

15. Perform hand hygiene.

CHARTING EXAMPLE: 10/29/XX 8:20 A.M. Westergren ESR = 32 mm/hour. Physician notified of elevated results. · · · ·
· C. Olsen, CMA (AAMA)

Coagulation Studies

In human plasma, 13 coagulation factors are involved in the two pathways that are activated to cause the formation of a clot. These two pathways, extrinsic and intrinsic, are involved in coagulation. The factors in the extrinsic system are dependent on vitamin K, and the intrinsic factors are not. Prothrombin time (PT) measures extrinsic pathway factors, and partial thromboplastin time (PTT) measures intrinsic pathway factors. Vitamin K is produced in the large intestines. Green leafy vegetables and liver are two good sources of this important vitamin.

Clot formation is also dependent on an adequate number of platelets and normal blood calcium levels. Table 14-2 presents the stages of coagulation. If any one of the factors or ions is deficient, then a normal clot will not form. For example, the hereditary condition hemophilia is due to a deficiency in Factor 8.

TABLE 14-2 Stages of Coagulation

Stage	Factors Necessary	Reaction
Stage 1	• Platelet factors • Substances released by damaged tissue (tissue thromboplastin) • Factors 5, 7, 8, 9, 10, 11, 12 • Calcium ions	Platelet factors + tissue thromboplastin + other clotting factors + calcium ions form prothrombin activator
Stage 2	• Prothrombin activator from Stage 1 • Prothrombin • Calcium ions	Prothrombin activator converts prothrombin to thrombin
Stage 3	• Thrombin from Stage 2 • Fibrinogen (plasma protein) • Calcium ions • Factor 13 (fibrin stabilizing factor)	Thrombin converts fibrinogen to fibrin, which becomes the clot

Coagulation Testing

Prothrombin time (PT) is a CLIA Waived test that measures the time it takes for a sample of a patient's blood to form a fibrin clot. This is used to screen or monitor patients who may be lacking clotting factors, have liver disease or a deficiency in vitamin K, or are on anticoagulant therapy. Patients who have a tendency to produce clots—such as stroke, heart attack, or heart surgery patients—are given anticoagulant drugs such as warfarin (Coumadin) to lengthen the time it takes them to clot. However, these patients must be monitored closely to prevent too much medication from causing excessive bleeding. (The bleeding time procedure was discussed in Chapter 13.)

Prothrombin times are measured on fresh whole blood collected in sodium citrate tubes (blue top). Capillary blood instruments that measure prothrombin time are available now and are being used in some physicians' offices. The ProTime Microcoagulation time device manufactured by International Technidyne Corporation and the HemoSense INR meter by HemoSense Inc. are devices mentioned in recent literature.

The sodium citrate tubes should be centrifuged as soon as possible. If testing is delayed, the plasma should be separated from the cells. The plasma may need to be refrigerated or placed on ice, depending on the requirements of the testing facility. Some automated procedures, such as the Hemochron Microcoagulation System (International Technidyne Corporation), are available and use a skin puncture sample of whole blood with the POC testing instrument. Normal reference range for patients not on anticoagulant therapy is 11 to 14 seconds. Sometimes results are reported in terms of the international normalized ratio (INR), which is the PT of the patient divided by the normal control. This INR value can then be easily compared, using different testing methods, to other results performed and can help to standardize results.

PTT is used to assess individuals on heparin therapy. This is a two-stage test. Testing protocol depends on the manufacturers of the testing reagents and equipment. Patients on anticoagulant therapy are usually kept at a PTT of 16 to 18 seconds, or 2.0 to 2.5 INR.

15 Serology/Immunology

PROCEDURES

Procedure 15-1 Performing a Test for Infectious Mononucleosis Using the BioStar Acceava Mono II Test

Procedure 15-2 Performing BioStar Acceava Strep A Test

Procedure 15-3 Performing a QuickVue Test for *Helicobacter pylori*

Advanced Procedure 15-4 Performing Agglutination Slide Testing for ABO Blood Grouping

Advanced Procedure 15-5 Performing Rh Typing by Slide Method

TERMS TO LEARN

antigen
antibodies
specificity
sensitivity

in vivo
in vitro
ELISA
external controls

internal controls
lipemic
in utero
antisera

The immune system is the defense system of the body, and it protects against toxic agents, pathogens, and other foreign substances. An **antigen** is a substance that appears foreign to the body and causes production of a specific antibody. **Antibodies** are protein in nature and are usually found in serum, the liquid portion of blood after the blood has coagulated and fibrinogen has been removed. Substances such as bee sting toxins, bacteria or viruses, cancer cells, and allergens are antigenic. The **specificity** of antigen/antibody reactions is the basic framework of the testing system. For example, if a patient had chicken pox, then he or she has an antibody that is specific against the chicken pox virus. This antibody will not protect against other diseases, such as measles or mumps. This property is referred to as specificity.

The laboratory department responsible for performing antigen/antibody testing is known as the serology department. The immunology or immunohematology department is the laboratory section devoted to blood banking. Testing prior to transfusing patients is performed in the immunology department. Each specimen is tested for blood group and Rh type and cross-matched to evaluate compatibility between the patient's and donor's blood before a transfusion. An antibody is named using the prefix anti before the name of the specific antigen: for example, Rh (D) antigen and anti-Rh or anti-D antibody.

Antibodies usually have a fairly strong affinity for specific antigens, and this property makes testing possible. This is known as **sensitivity**. Antigen/antibody test reactions are both specific and sensitive.

Serology Tests

To be effective, a serology test must induce a visual reaction between an antigen and its specific antibody. Tests maybe done **in vivo** (in the living body) like allergy testing, with an antigen injected to produce a wheal, or **in vitro** (outside the body) in the laboratory. Many CLIA Waived test kits are available to detect the present of an antigen (direct test), while others detect the presence of an antibody (indirect test) associated with specific diseases. These tests exhibit their results by agglutination or clumping or by color formation with enzyme-linked immunosorbent assay (**ELISA**) tests for antibody–antigen reactions. Procedure 11-13 in Chapter 11 is an example of an ELISA test. Table 15-1 lists common serology tests and their clinical significance.

Agglutination is the clumping together of particles caused by the binding of antigens/antibodies. In most agglutination tests, the reagent (antibody) is combined with the patient's specimen and mixed by rocking gently for a short time, and then the reaction is observed for clumping together of cells or particles. In any case the procedure must be followed exactly to produce reliable results.

Enzyme-linked immunosorbent assays involve more reagents, but the end reaction results in a color change, which makes it easier to read the final outcome.

Quality Control

Serology tests are produced in kits containing all the equipment, supplies, reagents, and directions needed to perform the test. Tests must be stored exactly according to manufacturer's specifications. This information is found on the package or on the package insert. Each kit also has an expiration date and a lot number. Test kits should never be used after their expiration date. Reagents from one test kit may not be used in another test kit with a different lot number. Equipment and supplies such as droppers, cards, and tubes included in the test kit are the only ones to be used with that specific test kit. Exchanging equipment between test kits is not acceptable laboratory procedure.

Each time a test kit is opened, the date it was opened should be written on the outside of the package. Sometimes the expiration date changes once the kit is opened. Quality control should be performed upon opening a new test kit to ensure the reagents are functioning properly.

External controls are tested exactly the way the patient's sample is tested and have known results. If the result is not as expected according to the manufacturer, the patient's results may not be reported. Many test kits include **internal controls**, also called built-in controls or technique controls, which indicate what positive and negative reactions look like. Separate positive and negative zones are built into the test. This information indicates to the tester that the test kit is functioning as it was meant to function. Controls should be used each time a test is performed and when the test is initially opened.

False-negative and false-positive reactions sometimes occur even when the control results are as expected. False-negative reactions mean that the patient tests negative but does indeed have the condition as confirmed by other tests or physical examination. False-positive reactions occur when the patient tests positive but does not have the condition or disease. False-positive and false-negative reactions may occur because of medications or a patient's biological conditions, out-of-date tests, or improperly performed procedures. Technical difficulties with the sample such as hemolysis or **lipemic** serum (high fat content) may impact results in certain tests.

TABLE 15-1 Common Serology Tests

Bacterial Tests	Significance
Group A *Streptococcus*	Strep throat and secondary infections such as endocarditis, rheumatic fever; CLIA Waived rapid screening tests for strep antigens
Helicobacter pylori	Stomach ulcers; CLIA Waived screening tests for *H. pylori* antibodies
Syphilis (*Treponema pallidum*)	Potentially fatal sexually transmitted disease (STD) caused by *Treponema pallidum*; Venereal Disease Research Laboratory (VDRL), rapid plasma reagin (RPR), and fluorescent treponemal antibody tests
Chlamydia (*Chlamydia trachomatis*)	Common STD; immunoassay tests that direct detection from endocervical swabs
Gardnerella vaginalis	Vaginal infection; enzyme test on vaginal secretions
Borrelia burgdorferi	Lyme disease; ELISA, fluorescent antibody test, or Western immunoblot
Respiratory syncytial virus (RSV)	Acute respiratory illness
Viral Infections	**Significance**
Epstein-Barr virus (EBV)	Infectious mononucleosis; CLIA Waived test to detect heterophile antibody
Types A and B influenza	FLU; CLIA Waived test for antigens for influenza A and B from nasal specimens
HIV/AIDS	Human Immunodeficiency Virus/Acquired Immune Deficiency Syndrome; CLIA Waived tests for antibodies in blood or mouth specific for HIV-1
Rubella	German measles; serum of pregnant women tested for presence of antibody; Rubella during pregnancy results in fetal defects.
Hepatitis C	Liver infection from bloodborne pathogen; at-home tests available
Varicella zoster	Chicken pox/shingles; immunofluorescent tests on secretions from blisters
Other Tests	**Significance**
Human chorionic gonadotropin (HCG)	Pregnancy tests: CLIA Waived immunoassay detection of HCG hormone
CA 125	Ovarian cancer; tests for antigen for ovarian cancer
Prostate-specific antigen (PSA)	Prostate cancer
Bladder tumor-associated antigen (BTA)	CLIA Waived tumor marker test detects antigen in urine
Rheumatoid factor (RF)	Rheumatoid arthritis; antibody detected in blood
Antinuclear antibody (ANA)	Systemic lupus erythematosus

CLIA Waived Serology Tests

Procedures for several CLIA Waived serology tests are presented in this chapter. However, these tests refer to specific tests by manufacturer's name, and if different manufacturer's tests are used only the directions from that kit must be followed.

MONONUCLEOSIS TESTS

The Epstein-Barr virus (EBV) is the causative agent of mononucleosis. It is transmitted by direct contact through saliva and thus is often called the "kissing disease." Signs and symptoms are low-grade fever, fatigue, sore throat, swollen lymph glands, and enlarged liver. On a differential smear, atypical or reactive lymphocytes may be present. The antibody produced by the EBV infection is a heterophile antibody that is produced between the fifth and eighth day of infection. The majority of patients produce heterophile antibodies. Some patients test negative although their clinical examination and hematology results confirm the presence of the disease. Slide tests for infectious mononucleosis are available. These tests are based on agglutination reaction

BOX 15-1 Agglutination Testing Guidelines

- Read directions thoroughly before beginning.
- If glass slides are used, make sure they are clean and free of lint.
- Follow timing directions exactly.
- If a slide is not labeled with positive and negative areas for controls for the patient sample, use a marking crayon to mark +, −, Pt. to distinguish the readings at the conclusion of the test.

- Mix reagents before using.
- Mix samples before using.
- Do not touch droppers to the test area to avoid cross contamination.
- Use a separate applicator stick to mix each sample.
- View the test results under direct light.
- Do not rock too forcefully or to lightly.

---

and involve mixing together, on an area of glass or paper card, the patient sample and a reagent containing an antibody. The slide is gently rocked for a specified time and then observed for clumping or agglutination. These tests are inexpensive and easy to perform; however, they are more subject to error in reading results than those tests that have color change as an end point. (The guidelines in Box 15-1 should be observed when performing any agglutination test.)

The widely used QuickVue+ Mononucleosis Test (Quidel) has been discontinued by the manufacturer. BioStar Acceava Mono II test is a sensitive CLIA Waived test using whole blood only and a non-Waived test using serum, plasma, or whole blood. This test is stored either at room temperature or refrigerated. The test is based on the patient sample reacting with bovine erythrocyte extracted antigen on the test strip. If heterophile antibodies are present, a positive reaction will result.

PROCEDURE 15-1

PERFORMING A TEST FOR INFECTIOUS MONONUCLEOSIS USING THE BIOSTAR ACCEAVA MONO II TEST

ABHES VII.MA.A.1 10(b)(4) CAAHEP I.P (15)

OBJECTIVE: To perform a CLIA Waived BioStar Acceava Mono II Test for infectious mononucleosis using quality control.

STANDARD: This task takes 10 minutes.

EQUIPMENT AND SUPPLIES: BioStar Acceava Mono II test kit containing supplies: test strips, disposable sample tubes, disposable droppers, heparinized capillary tubes and dispensing bulb, positive and negative controls, sample buffer, package insert workstation (Figure 15-1A); timer; gloves; venous blood collection equipment; lancet; pen; laboratory requisition; patient's record.

STEPS:

1. Check laboratory requisition or patient's chart for tests ordered. Check for patient allergies.
2. Assemble equipment and supplies.

3. Check expiration date of test kit. Confirm that storage conditions were observed. If test kit was refrigerated, allow test strips, buffer, and controls to come to room temperature.

4. Before beginning, read package directions through completely. When opening a new kit, perform positive and negative external controls and record results in quality control log. To perform external controls, use positive and negative control serum in place of patient sample:
   - Add 1 drop of positive serum to a tube and 1 drop of negative serum to another tube. Label each tube. Add 1 drop of buffer to each. Set timer, place test strip in tube, and after 5 minutes read results. Positive control = two red lines, negative control = one red line in "C" region (Figure 15-1B).

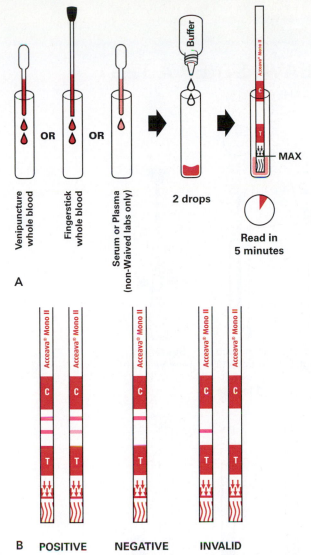

B POSITIVE   NEGATIVE   INVALID

FIGURE 15-1 (A) Add sample to tube using either drops of whole blood from venipuncture or full capillary tube for fingerstick (1 drop serum or plasma for CLIA non-Waived procedure); (B) read results in 5 minutes.
Courtesy of Inverness Medical.

5. Identify patient, and explain procedure.
6. Perform hand hygiene, and don gloves.
7. If blood sample is not available, perform a finger puncture and, with a heparinized capillary tube from test

kit, fill tube; or if other tests are ordered. perform a venipuncture and obtain an anticoagulated whole blood sample. Use pipette in kit to withdraw whole blood from tube.

8. For whole blood, fill dropper provided with whole blood and dispense 2 drops into bottom of tube. Avoid getting blood on sides of tube.

9. If capillary blood is used, insert capillary tube nearly to bottom of tube and dispense full capillary tube of blood into tube.

10. For either type of sample, add 2 drops of buffer solution to bottom of tube and tap tube to mix.

11. Remove test strip from container, and recap immediately. To avoid contamination, keep test strips in closed container until just before using. Place test strip into tube containing sample and buffer mixture.

12. Set timer for 5 minutes. Wait for red line(s) to appear at end of 5 minutes. Background should be clear before reading results. (Results will be inaccurate if you do not read results before a total of 10 minutes elapse.)

13. Interpret results as follows:
    - *Positive:* two distinct red lines with one line in "C" control region and one in "T" region. Shade of red depends on amount of heterophile antibody in sample. Any shade of red is considered positive.
    - *Negative:* one red line in "C" control region and no red line in "T" test region.
    - *Invalid result:* no line appears in control region.

14. Dispose of used equipment in appropriate biohazard waste containers. Clean area.

15. Remove and dispose of gloves in biohazard waste container.

16. Perform hand hygiene.

17. Document results in patient's record and on laboratory requisition. Post external control results in QC log.

CHARTING EXAMPLE: 11/04/XX 10:15 A.M. BioStar Acceava Mono II test for infectious mono is neg. · · · · · · · G. Patel, RMA

STREP TESTS

Serologic tests for Group A beta hemolytic *Streptococcus pyogenes* are frequently performed as rapid screening tests. If the results are negative, a throat culture on blood agar using a bacitracin disk (Chapter 12) may be required. Many CLIA Waived

ELISA serology tests are available for strep testing. The ELISA kits test for antigen extracted from a throat culture swab using solutions provided in the kit. Complications from strep throat include glomerulonephritis, scarlet fever, and rheumatic fever. The procedure for CLIA Waived Acceava Strep A Test follows.

PERFORMING BIOSTAR ACCEAVA STREP A TEST

ABHES VII.MA.A.1 10(b)(4)   CAAHEP I.P (15)

OBJECTIVE: To perform a BioStar Acceava Strep A Test following manufacturer's directions and using quality control.

STANDARD: This task takes 10 minutes.

EQUIPMENT AND SUPPLIES: BioStar Acceava Strep A test kit including reagent 1 and 2, positive and negative controls, test tubes, test stick container, rayon swab; sterile tongue depressor; gloves; mask; patient's record; pen; timer; biohazard waste containers.

STEPS:

1. Check patient's record or laboratory requisition for tests ordered. Check for patient allergies.

2. Assemble equipment and supplies.

3. Check expiration date of test kit and storage requirements.

4. Read directions completely before beginning test.

5. Perform hand hygiene, and don PPE.

6. Run external positive and negative controls when test kit is opened. (Running controls ensures that test reagents are working properly and that operator knows how to perform procedure.) Log QC results. (External control procedures differ from positive controls in that no patient swab is used.)

   - Add 1 drop of positive control to one tube and negative control to another tube. Place a separate sterile swab in each. Label both tubes. Add 3 drops of reagent 1 and 3 drops of reagent 2 into tubes. Mix well by rotating swab against side of tube 10 times and let stand 1 minute. Then squeeze swabs against side of tube, and discard in biohazard waste container. Place test stick in each tube, and set timer for 5 minutes. After 5 minutes read results. Positive control = blue line in "T" area and pink line in "C" area. Log control results.

7. Identify patient, and explain procedure.

8. Immediately before testing place 3 drops of reagent 1 and 3 drops of reagent 2 into test tube provided in test kit. Mixture should turn yellow.

9. Obtain throat swab (Procedure 5-33), and immediately put throat swab into solution to prevent drying and contamination (Figure 15-2A).

10. Mix well by rotating swab against side of tube 10 times and let stand 1 minute.

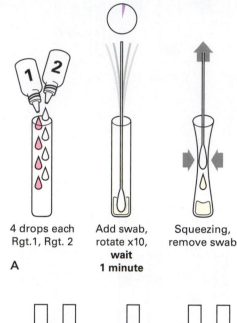

4 drops each
Rgt.1, Rgt. 2

Add swab,
rotate x10,
**wait
1 minute**

Squeezing,
remove swab

A

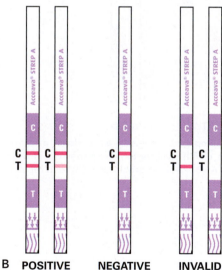

B   POSITIVE   NEGATIVE   INVALID

FIGURE 15-2 (A) Add reagents to tube. Insert patient swab. Mix well. Wait 1 minute. Remove sample swab; (B) place test strip into sample tube. Read result in 5 minutes.
Courtesy of Inverness Medical.

11. Squeeze swab by rolling against side of tube as it is withdrawn.

12. Discard swab in biohazard waste container.

13. Remove a test stick from container, and recap container immediately.

14. Place absorbent end of stick into tube with extracted sample.
15. Set timer for 5 minutes and then read.
16. Interpret results as follows (Figure 15-2B):
    - Positive = a blue line in "T" test area and pink line in "C" control area and indicates presence of *Streptococcus pyogenes* antigen.
    - Negative = no blue line in "T" test area and a pink line in "C" control area.

17. Discard all test material in biohazard waste container. Clean area. Remove and dispose of gloves in same manner.
18. Perform hand hygiene.
19. Document procedure in patient's record or on laboratory requisition.

CHARTING EXAMPLE: 11/04/XX Acceava Strep A test = Pos. · T. Russo, CMA (AAMA)

TESTING FOR *HELICOBACTER PYLORI*

Several immunoassay tests are available for testing for *Helicobacter pylori*, the bacteria associated with gastric ulcers. It is believed that this spiral-shaped bacteria causes the majority of gastric and duodenal ulcers. Quidel's QuickVue *Helicobacter pylori* gII test is a qualitative CLIA Waived immunoassay test for the rapid detection of antibodies specific to *H. pylori* in whole blood samples. The test requires 50 microliters (50 µL) of anticoagulated blood from green top tube (heparin tube) or EDTA lavender tube. Blood may be stored for up to 4 hours at room temperature or refrigerated for up to 72 hours prior to testing. Capillary blood may also be used.

PROCEDURE 15-3

PERFORMING A QUICKVUE TEST FOR *HELICOBACTER PYLORI*

ABHES VII.MA.A.1 10(b)(4)   CAAHEP I.P (15)

OBJECTIVE: Perform a CLIA Waived *H. pylori* test using quality control and following manufacturer's directions.

STANDARD: This task takes 10 minutes.

EQUIPMENT AND SUPPLIES: QuickVue *H. pylori* gII test kit including foil-wrapped test cassette, plastic capillary tubes for skin puncture sample, disposable droppers for venous sample, positive and negative controls, package insert directions, and procedure card; capillary and venous puncture supplies; timer; gloves; biohazard waste containers; sharps container; pen; patient's record.

STEPS:

1. Check patient's record or laboratory requisition for tests ordered. Check for patient allergies.
2. Assemble equipment and supplies.
3. Check expiration date of test kit and storage requirements.
4. Read all directions prior to starting test.
5. Identify patient, and explain procedure.
6. Don gloves.
7. Obtain specimen from patient by fingerstick or from venous blood in green or lavender top tube.
    - Fill capillary tube to black line from a fingerstick.
    - Or using dropper provided in kit, obtain anticoagulated blood from EDTA or heparin tube (room temperature, well mixed).
8. Add 1 capillary tube of whole blood to sample well on test cassette (Figure 15-3A); or add 2 hanging drops from fingerstick directly to well (Figure 15-3B); or add 1 large drop of venous anticoagulated blood to sample well with disposable dropper (Figure 15-3C).
9. Do not move test cassette until test is complete.
10. Set timer for 5 minutes.
11. Read immediately.
12. Interpret results as follows:
    - Positive = Any shade of pink to red line near letter "T" and a blue procedural control line near letter "C" visible within 5 minutes or less indicates presence of *H. pylori* specified IgG antibodies.

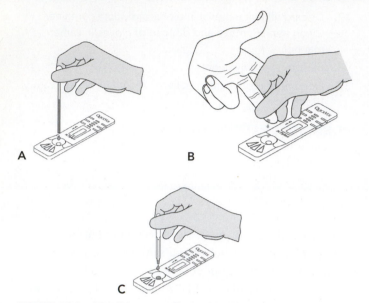

FIGURE 15-3 (A) Add one capillary tube of blood to sample well on test cassette; (B) add two hanging drops from fingerstick directly to sample well; (C) add one drop of venous anticoagulated blood to the sample well with disposable dropper.
Courtesy of QUIDEL® Corporation, San Diego, CA. Used with permission.

- Negative = Only a blue procedural control line near letter "C" at 5 minutes.
- Invalid = If blue procedural control line is not visible at 5 minutes after sample application even if test line is visible. Retest with a new cassette.

13. External positive and negative controls should be performed with opening of a new kit. Procedure is identical except that in place of whole blood 2 drops of positive control are added to 1 test cassette, and 2 drops of negative control are added to a second test cassette. Each is read in the same manner after 5 minutes. QC results should be logged and dated.

14. Dispose of all testing materials in biohazard waste container as appropriate.

15. Remove and dispose of gloves in biohazard waste container.

16. Perform hand hygiene.

17. Document results in patient's record or on laboratory requisition.

CHARTING EXAMPLE: 11/04/XX 2:00 P.M. QuickVue gII for *H. pylori* neg. · A. Ralph, RMA

Other Serology Tests

There are many other serology tests on the market for a variety of illnesses and conditions. Some are very complex and are beyond the scope of this text. The following are examples of more frequently performed tests:

- Influenza tests using nasal swabs are available to test for presence of influenza A and B. The principles are similar to the tests already described.

- Antistreptolysin O Test (ASO) detects ASO antibodies in a patient's serum. It is used to test for secondary infections associated with *Streptococcus pyogenes* infections.

- C-Reactive protein (CRP) appears in the blood during inflammation and tissue destruction. It is also useful in monitoring the progress of conditions such as rheumatoid arthritis, malignancy, and bacterial infections.

- Cold Agglutinins tests detect the presence of antibodies known as cold agglutinins. The patient's serum is incubated at cold temperatures, and a positive reaction indicates cold agglutinins are present and cause agglutination of RBCs. These antibodies are found in patients with mononucleosis, lymphoma, and mycoplasmal pneumonia.

Blood Antigens

An individual's blood type is determined by the presence or absence of two antigens (A antigen and B antigen) on the surface of his or her RBCs. The presence or absence of these two antigens determines which of the four blood groups a person inherits: A, B, AB, or O. To provide safe transfusions a patient's blood group antigen must be determined. In addition to the inherited antigen, each individual has a naturally occurring antibody that fights against any antigen missing from the surface of his or her red blood cells. For example, a person with an A antigen on his or her RBCs has anti-B antibodies naturally occurring in his or her plasma. Table 15-2 illustrates the ABO blood groups and the naturally occurring antibodies in the plasma of each individual. Figure 15-4A illustrates the content of Table 15-2. In addition to the A and B antigens, about 85% of the population has Rh (D) antigen on their red cells and are considered Rh positive, whereas 15% do not have the gene and are considered

TABLE 15-2 ABO Blood Groups

Blood Group	Antigen on RBCs	Antibodies in Plasma
A	A antigens	Anti-B antibodies
B	B antigens	Anti-A antibodies
AB	Both A and B antigens	Neither anti-A nor anti-B antibodies
O	Neither A nor B antigens	Both anti-A and anti-B antibodies

Rh negative. No anti-Rh (D) antibodies occur naturally. Rh antibodies develop when an Rh negative patient is transfused with Rh positive blood or if an Rh negative mother is exposed to the Rh positive blood cells of a fetus before or during childbirth. In some Rh negative mothers the anti-D antibody develops and then crosses the placenta into the fetus, causing destruction of red blood cells and a condition known as erythroblastosis fetalis. In some cases this may be fatal to the fetus or newborn. Exchange transfusions may be performed in utero (in the uterus) to alleviate the symptoms. If an Rh negative mother has never built up anti-D antibodies, she may receive an injection of RhoGAM within 72 hours after birth. This prevents the mother from building up antibodies resulting from the delivery and prevents erythroblastosis fetalis in the next pregnancy. RhoGAM should be administered after each pregnancy during which no anti-Rh antibodies are formed.

Other important antigens and antibodies can impact transfusion compatibility. Immunology departments in testing facilities handle these types of evaluations.

The properties of blood cell antigens and antibodies are useful in testing procedures designed to determine the patient's blood group and Rh type. **Antisera** (anti-A, anti-B, and anti-D) are used to test the ABO blood group and Rh type of patients and donors. If the same blood group antigen and antibody are present together in the body, in a tube or on a slide, agglutination or clumping together of the cells results (Figure 15-4B). In the body this clumping could result in death of the patient because the blood clumps would not pass through the capillaries and small vessels of the kidneys and other organs.

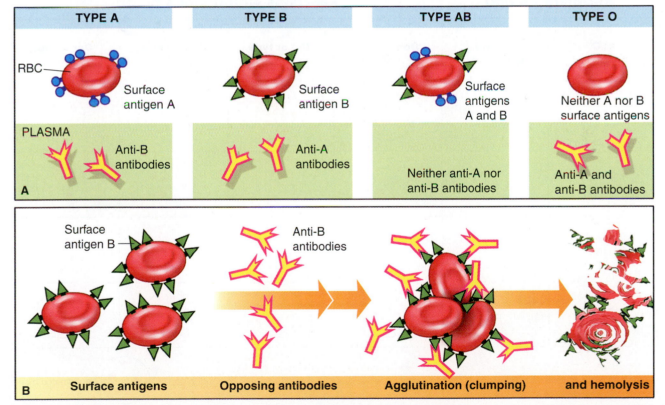

FIGURE 15-4 (A) Naturally occurring RBC antigens and plasma antibodies that make up the four blood groups; (B) antigens on RBCs that encounter their specific antibodies lead to agglutination and hemolysis of the affected RBCs.

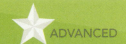
PROCEDURE 15-4

PERFORMING AGGLUTINATION SLIDE TESTING FOR ABO BLOOD GROUPING

OBJECTIVE: To perform agglutination slide testing to determine the ABO blood group of a patient from a blood sample.

STANDARD: This task takes 10 minutes.

EQUIPMENT AND SUPPLIES: Anti-A antisera (blue solution); anti-A antisera (yellow solution); clean glass slide;

	TYPE A	TYPE B	TYPE AB	TYPE O
RBC	Surface antigen A	Surface antigen B	Surface antigens A and B	Neither A nor B surface antigens
PLASMA	Anti-B antibodies	Anti-A antibodies	Neither anti-A nor anti-B antibodies	Anti-A and anti-B antibodies

Recipient's blood		Reactions with donor's blood			
RBC antigens	**Plasma antibodies**	**Donor type O**	**Donor type A**	**Donor type B**	**Donor type AB**
None (Type O)	Anti-A Anti-B				
A (Type A)	Anti-B				
B (Type B)	Anti-A				
AB (Type AB)	(None)				

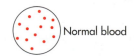 Normal blood   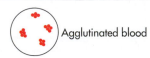 Agglutinated blood

FIGURE 15-5 Typing and cross-matching.

wooden applicator sticks; disposable droppers; capillary and venous blood supplies; gloves; biohazard waste container; glass marker; patient's record.

NOTE: The procedures to determine blood group and type are usually performed in an outside clinical laboratory or hospital immunology department and are not CLIA Waived tests.

STEPS:

1. Check patient's record for tests ordered.
2. Assemble equipment and supplies.
3. With a glass marker, divide slide in two. Label left side A and right side B.
4. Identify patient or verify that name on patient's sample and on patient's test order are identical.
5. Explain procedure.
6. Perform hand hygiene, and don gloves.
7. Perform a skin puncture, or obtain an anticoagulated venous sample of patient's blood following previously cited procedural steps.
8. With a disposable dropper or capillary tube of patient's blood, place 1 drop of patient's blood in center of A side of slide and 1 drop in center of area marked B.
9. Place 1 drop of anti-A antisera next to drop of blood on side A and 1 drop of anti-B antisera next to drop of blood on side B. Do not allow dropper of antisera to touch blood or be contaminated by splashes of patient's blood.

10. Stir mixture on A side with an applicator until well mixed, and spread out slightly on slide. Use a new applicator, mix solutions on side B together, and spread out slightly.
11. At room temperature, tilt slide gently to enhance mixing and examine for agglutination. Read results as follows (Figure 15-5):
    - Agglutination on side A means patient is blood group A.
    - Agglutination on side B means patient is blood group B.
    - Agglutination on both sides means patient is blood group AB.
    - No agglutination on either side means patient is blood group O.
12. Dispose of glass slides in sharps container and other equipment in biohazard waste container.
13. Clean area. Remove and dispose of gloves in biohazard waste container.
14. Perform hand hygiene.
15. Document in patient's record if approved to perform this non–CLIA Waived procedure.

CHARTING EXAMPLE: 11/07/XX 2:00 P.M. Blood grouping performed per orders of Dr. Zhao. Pt. tested as blood group A. · C. Sanchez, RMA

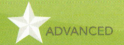 ADVANCED

PROCEDURE 15-5

PERFORMING Rh TYPING BY SLIDE METHOD

OBJECTIVE: To perform Rh typing procedure by slide method on a sample of patient's blood.

STANDARD: This task takes 10 minutes.

EQUIPMENT AND SUPPLIES: Anti-Rh (D) antisera; negative control serum or saline; clean glass slide; wooden applicator sticks; disposable droppers; capillary and venous blood supplies; gloves; heated slide warmer; biohazard waste container; glass marker; patient's record.

STEPS:

1. Check patient's record for tests ordered.
2. Assemble equipment and supplies.

3. With a glass marker, divide slide in two. Label left side as Rh (D) and right side as negative control.
4. With a disposable dropper or capillary tube of patient's blood, place 1 drop of patient's blood in center of Rh (D) side of slide and 1 drop in center of area marked negative control.
5. Place 1 drop anti-Rh (D) antiserum next to drop of blood on Rh side and 1 drop of negative control serum next to drop of blood on negative control side. Do not allow dropper of antiserum or control serum to touch or be splashed with blood of patient and cause contamination.
6. Stir mixture on RH side with an applicator until well mixed, and spread out slightly on slide. Use a new

applicator, mix together solutions on negative control side, and spread out slightly.

7. Place slide on a lighted slide warmer, and tilt and rock gently for 2 minutes to enhance mixing. Then examine for agglutination. Anti-Rh (D) antibodies react better with warming.

8. Read results as follows:
   - Agglutination on left side with anti-Rh (D) antiserum means patient is Rh positive.

NOTE: This reaction may take full 2 minutes and not be a strong clumping reaction. Do not read test after 2 minutes have elapsed. If in doubt, ask supervisor to observe or repeat test.

   - Agglutination on right side with negative control serum (where there should be no agglutination)

means control serum might be in question and test must be repeated.

9. Dispose of glass slide in sharps container and other waste in appropriate containers.

10. Clean area. Remove and dispose of gloves in biohazard waste container.

11. Perform hand hygiene.

12. Document procedure in patient's record if approved to perform this non–CLIA Waived procedure.

CHARTING EXAMPLE: 11/07/XX 9:00 A.M. Rh typing performed per Dr. Zhao, Pt. tested Rh pos. · L. Tracy, CMA (AAMA)

16 Blood Chemistry

PROCEDURES

Procedure 16-1 Calibrating a Blood Glucose Meter (One Touch Ultra)

Procedure 16-2 Performing a Blood Glucose Test Using One Touch Ultra Device

Procedure 16-3 Performing Quality Control for Blood Glucose Testing Using SureStep Flexx Glucose Monitor

Procedure 16-4 Monitoring Blood Glucose with a SureStep Flexx Monitor

Procedure 16-5 Performing a Glycosylated Hemoglobin Test Using a Bayer DCA 2000+ Analyzer

Procedure 16-6 Performing a Cholesterol Test Using a ProAct Testing Device

Procedure 16-7 Performing Lipid Profile and Glucose Testing Using a Cholestech LDX Analyzer

TERMS TO LEARN

analytes

hyperglycemia

hypoglycemia

metabolic syndrome

impaired glucose tolerance (IGT)

lipidemia

atherosclerosis

lipoproteins

Blood chemistry tests reflect the manner in which the body and its organs control the chemicals or **analytes** in the bloodstream. For example, the blood level of glucose, which is determined in one of the most commonly performed chemistry tests, is elevated if the pancreas is not producing enough insulin or if glucose cannot be transported into the cells for energy. Chemistry tests are available for the many naturally occurring chemicals found in the blood and body fluids. They are performed on various types of body fluids, including urine, spinal fluid, pleural fluid, and pericardial fluid as well as whole blood, plasma, and serum. Physicians use the results from chemistry tests to detect or confirm existing conditions in a body system or specific organ.

Chemistry tests often are grouped together in panels, a series of tests related to a system or organ. For example, a lipid panel includes tests for cholesterol, high-density lipids, low-density lipids, very low-density lipids, and triglycerides.

Elaborate chemistry analyzers used in reference and hospital laboratories produce a large number of test results from a small amount of specimen in a short time with great accuracy. These sophisticated analyzers require calibration, daily quality control, and careful maintenance by trained technicians. Reference and hospital laboratory chemistry analyzers generally require serum specimens and sometimes plasma samples. Smaller analyzers (benchtop analyzers) are used in ambulatory care facilities, physicians' offices, and clinics. Some benchtop analyzers perform CLIA Waived tests. They test for fewer analytes and frequently utilize whole blood samples. Other CLIA Waived single-test analyzers are used by patients or for point of care testing. Dozens of glucose analyzers are available commercially for home and POC use.

Chemistry analyzers measure the color change produced by the patient's sample and the chemical reagents used in the procedure. A spectrum of light passes through the resulting colored substances, and a photometer measures the amount of light that passed through the specimen or is reflected off the specimen. The intensity of the color change is proportional to the concentration of the analyte in the specimen. For example, the deeper the color produced during a glucose analysis, the higher the glucose level in the patient. This is known as the Beer-Lambert law and is the basis for many chemical analyzer instruments.

Before discussing the actual tests, we need to review the reference values and types of vacuum tubes needed to perform chemistry tests. Processing blood samples correctly after they are drawn is important to ensure the reliability and accuracy of test results. The type of vacuum tube used to obtain a blood sample is determined by the testing laboratory. Check the reference laboratory's manual for the type of tube, amount of sample, and how it should be processed and transported.

For serum samples, the gold serum separator tube (SST) with gel and clot activator is widely used. This tube must be allowed to sit 30 minutes after drawing before being centrifuged for 15 minutes. Centrifuging pushes the cells to the bottom of the tube, and the gel moves over the cells to separate them from the clot. Some chemical analytes are affected by the gel or clot activator and must be drawn in plain red top tubes. These tubes must be allowed to sit 30 minutes before being centrifuged for 15 minutes. When pouring off serum from a plain red top tube, care must be taken that red cells are not poured off with the serum. Red cells in serum may affect certain tests and lead to erroneous results. Pouring off serum from a gold stopper tube is easier because the gel acts as a barrier.

Labeling mistakes are often the cause of errors in laboratories. The original vacuum tube must be labeled clearly with the patient's name, date, time of draw, and phlebotomist's initials. The tube into which the serum is poured during processing must also be clearly labeled. Any tube unlabeled should be rejected for testing.

Reference values vary from laboratory to laboratory because methods, instrumentation, or both for testing differ. Reference or "normal values" are given in this chapter with the caveat that the reference manual of the testing laboratory must be checked for their values. Usually, to make it easier to compare values, each testing laboratory lists its reference values on the laboratory requisition next to the space for the patient's test results.

Blood Glucose

Glucose is a simple sugar required by all body cells to produce energy. The liver and muscles store glucose as glycogen. The pancreas secretes insulin and glucagon, the two hormones responsible for maintaining glucose levels at a normal range. Insulin helps lower blood sugar, and glucagon increases the blood sugar level by converting glycogen to glucose. When this intricate balancing system between these two hormones is working effectively, blood glucose levels stay in the normal range of 70 to 110 mg/dL of blood. Elevated blood glucose is known as **hyperglycemia**, and decreased level of blood glucose is known as **hypoglycemia**. Box 16-1 provides guidelines for working with controls. Table 16-1 illustrates how blood glucose levels are controlled by the secretions of the alpha and beta cells of the islets of Langerhans in the pancreas.

One of the most common hormonal imbalances encountered today, diabetes mellitus (DM), occurs when glucose levels are consistently out of normal range. There are two types of diabetes mellitus: type 1 or insulin dependent

BOX 16-1   Guidelines for Working with Controls

Repeat controls if they do not check out the first time. Then check for the following:

- Technique for possible errors
- Expiration dates on controls
- Expiration dates on reagents
- Temperature requirements for all substances
- Optics scan and maintenance requirements

If these check out, repeat controls with a new set of controls

If these do not check out, call the manufacturer for troubleshooting advice.

diabetes mellitus (IDDM) was previously known as juvenile diabetes, and type 2 or noninsulin dependent diabetes mellitus (NIDDM). Table 16-2 compares the onset, symptoms, and treatment of type 1 and type 2 diabetes mellitus.

Blood Glucose Testing

Two tests are recommended by the American Diabetes Association to identify diabetes and a condition known as prediabetes: fasting blood glucose (FBS or FBG) and glucose tolerance test (GTT). Many screening tests for FBG are CLIA Waived and can be performed in ambulatory care centers or at home. If the FBG is elevated, the physician will order the GTT. For either test, the patient must fast for 10 to 14 hours and may drink only water during that time. Facility protocols for fasting may differ, however, and should be checked and observed. If a fasting blood glucose is over between 100 and 130 mg/dL on two separate occasions, the patient is considered prediabetic by most physicians, and if the FBG is over 130 mg/dL most physicians would consider the patient diabetic. CLIA Waived glucose screening tests should be followed up with fasting plasma glucose levels using a specimen from a gray top tube.

POSTPRANDIAL BLOOD GLUCOSE TEST

The postprandial blood glucose test is another glucose screening test. A fasting blood glucose specimen is obtained, and the patient is given a glucose drink or meal with a designated amount of carbohydrates. The blood glucose level is measured exactly 2 hours after the drink or meal ended. This is known as 2-hour postprandial glucose (2hPP). Normally an individual's glucose level falls to less than 140 mg/dL 2 hours after eating or drinking the glucose-laden offerings. A glucose level of over 200 mg/dL after 2 hours is considered diabetic range. With levels between 140 and 200 mg/dL, a patient would be considered prediabetic.

GLUCOSE TOLERANCE TESTS

The GTT is a more informative test performed on plasma. A fasting blood glucose is drawn in a gray top tube after fasting 10 to 14 hours. A drink containing a 100 gram dose of glucose is given to the patient to drink. Additional specimens are drawn in gray top tubes at ½, 1, 2, 3, and up to 6 hours after consuming the glucose drink. Careful labeling of each specimen with the time of draw is important. Physicians may have individual preferences for the timing of GTT specimens.

Urine samples are collected each time a blood sample is obtained, and each must be carefully labeled. Urine is tested to see if the renal threshold (160–180 mg/dL) of glucose is exceeded. The values obtained after all the GTT specimens are tested indicate a normal pattern (glucose back to normal range after 2 hours), a hypoglycemic pattern (glucose levels peak but drop rapidly to below normal range), or a hyperglycemic pattern (glucose levels are elevated and never return to normal level).

TABLE 16-1 Control of Blood Glucose Level

Elevated Blood Glucose	Low Blood Glucose
↓	↓
Beta Cells in Pancreas	Alpha Cells in Pancreas
↓	↓
Insulin	Glucagon
↓	↓
Glucose enters cells	Liver releases glucose from stored glycogen
↓	↓
Blood glucose level lowered	Blood glucose level raised

TABLE 16-2 Characteristics of Type 1 and Type 2 Diabetes Mellitus

Characteristics/Symptoms/Treatment	Type 1	Type 2
Features	• Onset usually before age 30 years • Autoimmune condition destroys beta cells • Rapid onset • Little or no insulin produced • Weight thin to normal • Acidosis/ketosis	• Onset usually after age 30 years • Slow onset • Few symptoms • Insulin present • Overweight • Ketosis/acidosis rare
Symptoms	• Excessive thirst and urination • Urine positive for glucose • Often hungry	• Excessive urination possible • Excessive thirst in some cases • Occasional complaints of hunger
Treatment	• Insulin • Dietary changes	• Dietary changes • Oral medication or insulin

GLYCOSYLATED HEMOGLOBIN (HgbA1c)

If a patient has persistently high levels of glucose, the hemoglobin A molecule inside the red blood cells may be permanently changed or glycosylated and becomes hemoglobin A1c (HgbA1c). RBCs live 90 to 120 days, thus the percentage of HgbA1C molecules in a specimen reflects the overall concentration of blood glucose during that time. Normal HgbA1c range in an adult using whole blood specimen is 2.2%–4.8%. Thus this test gives a long-term view of a patient's average blood glucose during the previous 90 to 120 days, and it does not fluctuate the way blood glucose levels do. An HgbA1c test result between 6% and 8% means the patient is prediabetic and at risk for developing cardiovascular and small blood vessel complications. In type 1 diabetes, complications from long-term elevated blood glucose include the following:

- Cardiovascular problems due to plaque formation in arteries leading to heart disease, stroke, and hypertension.

- Elevated ketone levels and/or acidosis due to cells burning fat instead of glucose, which is unavailable to the cells. The by-products of fat metabolism are ketones, three types of fatty acids. If ketone levels are high enough, the pH of the blood lowers and is followed by acidosis resulting in a diabetic coma.

- Microvascular problems due to excessive amounts of glucose blocking small blood vessels leading to kidney failure, retinopathy, blindness, poor circulation in the extremities, and gangrene.

Thus the type 1 diabetes patient must monitor glucose levels several times a day and administer insulin, follow a low-carbohydrate diet, and exercise moderately to reduce blood glucose levels.

Type 2 diabetes is epidemic in the United States, including in many more children than ever before. A sedentary lifestyle and ingestion of huge amounts of carbohydrate-rich foods are mainly to blame. In type 2 diabetics or prediabetics also known as **metabolic syndrome**, the following are observed:

- Insulin resistance occurs. Insulin is produced but is ineffective in taking glucose into the cells where it can be used for energy. This lead to impaired glucose tolerance.

- In **impaired glucose tolerance (IGT)**, beta cells in the pancreas become sluggish; that decreases insulin production and leads to periods of high and low blood sugar.

- IGT leads to elevated insulin levels, which causes elevated fat levels in blood and leads to lipidemia and atherosclerosis.

- **Lipidemia, atherosclerosis** (plaque buildup in blood vessels), and the same problems experienced by type 1 diabetics (acidosis, cardiovascular and microvascular problems) occur.

Gestational diabetes may occur during pregnancy, and it usually disappears after delivery. Women with gestational diabetes often give birth to large babies (over 9 pounds) and are more prone to type 2 diabetes later in life.

CLIA WAIVED GLUCOSE TESTS

Many glucose screening devices have been approved by CLIA for home and POC use. In general, modern devices use less blood and provide faster results, and some can even collect blood from sites other than the finger. Infrared absorption technology makes it possible to measure blood glucose without drawing blood at all. Newer glucose devices are technologically more advanced and can store multiple results, provide daily graphs of results, and generate printouts of values. (One Touch and SureStep Flexx BG meter procedures are presented in Procedures 16-1 through 16-4.)

PROCEDURE 16-1

CALIBRATING A BLOOD GLUCOSE METER (ONE TOUCH ULTRA)

ABHES VII.MA.A.1 10(b)(3)   CAAHEP I.P (13)

OBJECTIVE: To calibrate a One Touch blood glucose meter correctly.

STANDARD: This task takes 5 minutes or less.

EQUIPMENT AND SUPPLIES: One Touch blood glucose meter; glucose test strips and calibration strip; cotton ball; gloves; QC log; pen.

STEPS:

1. Obtain a new container of glucose test strips required by manufacturer for model device used, and remove calibration strip.
2. Compare lot numbers on calibration strip to lot number on side of strip container. (These numbers must be identical to proceed with test procedure. If they are not identical, open a new container and repeat procedure.)
3. If numbers match, place calibration strip in meter by opening door and inserting top of strip into slot on right side of meter.
4. Insert strip until a click is heard.
5. Close door.
6. Push ON/OFF button. Numbers "888" should appear on screen.
7. Open door of monitor.
8. Push black button on left side of door, and slide test strip under strip guide with test pads facing up.
9. Quickly close door. Numbers "000" should be displayed on screen indicator. If not, open and close door again.
10. Open door, remove strip, and leave door open.
11. Log QC and prepare to perform procedure on patient.

PROCEDURE 16-2

PERFORMING A BLOOD GLUCOSE TEST USING ONE TOUCH ULTRA DEVICE

ABHES VII.MA.A.1 10(b)(3)   CAAHEP I.P (13)

OBJECTIVE: To perform a blood glucose test from skin puncture using a One Touch Ultra device following manufacturer's directions.

STANDARD: This task takes 5 minutes or less.

EQUIPMENT AND SUPPLIES: Automatic lancet; soap; water; cotton balls; sterile 2 × 2 gauze squares; gloves; patient's record; pen; biohazard waste container.

STEPS:

1. Check patient's record for tests ordered. Check for patient allergies.
2. Assemble equipment and supplies (Figure 16-1A).
3. Perform hand hygiene, and don gloves.
4. Identify patient, and explain procedure.

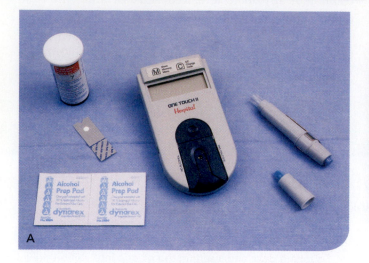

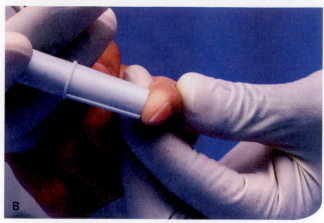

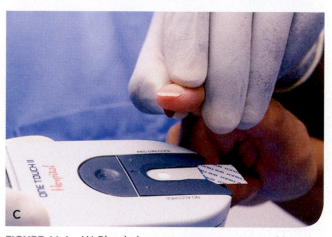

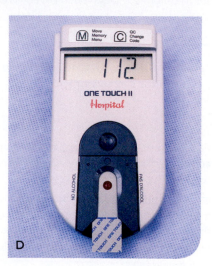

FIGURE 16-1 (A) Blood glucose meter, test strips, and lancet injector; (B) place injector against the site; (C) gently squeeze a large drop of blood onto the reagent strip; (D) the glucose meter will display the glucose reading.

5. Wash area for skin puncture on finger or heel (for infant) with soap and water, then dry. (Alcohol dries skin especially if repeated skin punctures are necessary.)

6. Insert test strip into monitor. Test must be performed within 30 seconds after strip is inserted.

7. Gently massage area to stimulate blood flow.

8. Adjust automatic lancet to depth needed.

9. Place automatic lancet on side of finger, and release so lancet punctures skin immediately (Figure 16-1B).

10. Gently massage finger from base upward to increase blood flow, and wipe off first drop.

11. Place a large drop of blood on test strip (Figure 16-1C).

12. Wait 30 seconds, and read results on device monitor (Figure 16-1D).

13. Wipe site with cotton ball.

14. Discard biohazard waste in proper container.

15. Clean area. Remove and dispose of gloves in biohazard waste container.

16. Perform hand hygiene.

17. Document patient's record with results.

NOTE: Remember to choose alternate finger if repeated testing necessary.

CHARTING EXAMPLE: 11/13/XX 8:00 A.M. FBG done using One Touch Ultra, middle finger (L) hand. FBG = 230 mg/dL.

· J. McWilliams, CMA (AAMA)

PERFORMING QUALITY CONTROL FOR BLOOD GLUCOSE TESTING USING SureStep FLEXX GLUCOSE MONITOR

ABHES VII.MA.A.1 10(b)(3); VII.MA.A.1 10(b)   CAAHEP I.P (11); I.P (13)

OBJECTIVE: To perform quality control for blood glucose using a SureStep Flexx Monitor and following manufacturer's directions.

STANDARD: This test takes 10 minutes or less.

EQUIPMENT AND SUPPLIES: SureStep Flexx blood glucose monitor with test strips, controls, and directions; gloves; biohazard waste container; QC log.

STEPS:

1. Turn on the meter. (Figure 16-2 shows SureStep Flexx blood glucose monitoring equipment.)
2. Perform hand hygiene, and don gloves.
3. Check battery status to ensure adequate power.
4. Press "Continue" button.
5. Select "Quality Control (QC) Test" from main menu by touching correct area on screen.
6. Select Control Test by touching "High" or "Low" area on screen to indicate which control test is to be done.
7. Enter operator ID assigned by specific facility.
8. Select control solution lot number from list displayed, or enter it manually. Verify lot number on control solutions.
9. Select test strip lot number (and code) from list displayed, or enter it manually. Verify lot number (and code) on test strips.
10. Shake control solution vial gently. Check confirmation dot on back of test strip to ensure it is completely blue.
11. Apply 1 drop of control solution to pink test square on test strip.
12. Insert test strip into test holder within 2 minutes of applying control solution. White side of test strip tip should be facing up.
13. Firmly push strip into meter.
14. Check result, which appears in about 30 seconds.
15. Control solution test results should fall within expected ranges printed on test strip bottle. If control solution test results fall outside expected control range, select "Enter Note" and follow recommendations.
16. Remove and dispose of test strip and gloves in biohazard waste container.
17. Perform hand hygiene.
18. Both "High" and "Low" controls must be completed and fall in range printed on test strip bottle before proceeding with patient testing. Log QC as appropriate in facility.

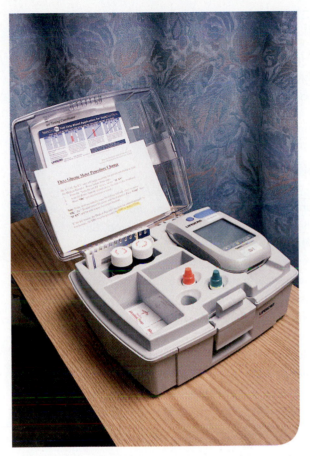

FIGURE 16-2 SureStep Flexx blood glucose monitoring system.

MONITORING BLOOD GLUCOSE WITH
A SureStep FLEXX MONITOR

ABHES VII.MA.A.1 10(b)(3)   CAAHEP I.P (13)

OBJECTIVE: To monitor blood glucose using a SureStep Flexx Monitor and following manufacturer's directions.

STANDARD: This task takes 10 minutes or less.

EQUIPMENT AND SUPPLIES: SureStep Flexx blood glucose monitor with test strips, controls, and directions; blood lancet; 2 × 2 sterile gauze; alcohol pads or other antimicrobial skin preparation pad; gloves; biohazard waste container; sharps container; pen.

STEPS:

1. Complete quality control procedure (Procedure 16-3). If control results are within range, proceed as follows.
2. Check patient's record for tests ordered. Check for patient allergies.
3. Press power button to turn on meter.
4. Check battery status as status screen appears.
5. Assemble equipment and supplies.
6. Perform hand hygiene, and don gloves.
7. Press "Continue."
8. Select "Patient Test" on main menu.
9. Enter operator ID, and press "OK."
10. Check to ensure code number displayed on meter matches code number on test strip bottle.
11. Enter patient's ID (medical record number or SS), and press "OK."
12. Select test strip lot number (and code) from list displayed, or enter it manually. Verify lot number and code displayed on screen.
13. Follow directions for performing skin puncture (Chapter 13).
14. Apply drop of blood to test strip by carefully touching pink test square on test strip. Check confirmation dot on back of test strip to verify that it turned completely blue.
15. Use 2 × 2 gauze pads, and apply direct pressure to puncture site to control bleeding.
16. Insert test strip completely into test strip holder within 2 minutes of applying blood. Strip must be completely inserted to receive accurate results.
17. Check results, which appear in approximately 30 seconds.
18. Evaluate patient results that fall above or below the critical lab values limit.
    - Press "Enter Note," and choose one to three comments, if indicated, that correspond to patient's current situation.
    - Follow appropriate actions as determined by facility policy and procedure.
19. Press "OK," and remove test strip from meter.
20. Remove and dispose of gloves and test strip according to facility policy.
21. Perform hand hygiene.

CHARTING EXAMPLE: 11/14/XX 3:00 P.M. SureStep Flexx B. Gluc. ring finger R hand. B. gluc. = 132 mg/dL · · · · C. Ryan, RMA

PERFORMING A GLYCOSYLATED HEMOGLOBIN TEST
USING A BAYER DCA 2000+ ANALYZER

ABHES VII.MA.A.1 10(b)(3)   CAAHEP I.P (13)

OBJECTIVE: To perform a glycosylated hemoglobin test using a Bayer DCA 2000+ Analyzer with quality control following manufacturer's directions.

STANDARD: This task takes 10 minutes.

EQUIPMENT AND SUPPLIES: DCA 2000+ Analyzer; DCA 2000 Reagent Kit with capillary holder, reagent cartridge, calibration code; DCA 2000 Hemoglobin A1C normal, abnormal control kit with reconstitution fluid; dropper can assemblies and normal; abnormal control card (double sided); optical test cartridge; alcohol pads; 2 × 2 sterile gauze; lint-free tissue; lancet or vacuum tubes (EDTA, heparin, citrate, fluoride/oxalate only) for blood; gloves; pen; patient's record or laboratory requisition; biohazard waste and sharps containers.

NOTE: Blood that has been refrigerated in tubes containing correct anticoagulant may be used within 1 week. Blood vacuum tubes should be brought to room temperature and be well mixed before using.

STEPS:

1. Check patient's record or laboratory requisition for tests ordered. Check for patient allergies.

2. Verify that name on patient's vacuum tube and laboratory requisition match.

3. Assemble equipment (Figure 16-3A) and supplies.

4. Perform hand hygiene, and don gloves.

5. Perform quality control as follows:
   - Perform optics check. Locate barcode on optical test cartridge; with barcode facing right, insert cartridge into barcode track, then quickly and smoothly slide cartridge down past blue dot on instrument. A beep signals a successful scan. (If no beep sounds after repeating scan check, see troubleshooting section of operator's manual.) Open cartridge compartment, hold optical test cartridge so barcode faces right, insert cartridge until a subtle snap is heard or felt, and close door. After 6 minutes of transmittance, standard deviation (SD) and drift are displayed. Remove cartridge, record results on Optical Test form provided, and compare. If results are not within specified range, rerun test or contact company.
   - Calibrate as follows each time a new shipment or a new lot number of reagent cartridges is used or a new operator performs the test: Remove calibration card from reagent box and locate barcode. With barcode facing right, insert calibration card into barcode track. Hold card gently against right side of track, and slide card down past blue dot. A beep indicates a successful scan. (See troubleshooting section of manual if beep does not sound after repeating scan). Document all information on HgA1C cartridge inventory and calibration form. Label reagent box with date of calibration. Proceed to perform quality control.
   - For quality control, run both N and ABN controls each day patient samples are run and with each new lot number of reagent cartridges.
   - Reconstitute controls as follows: Remove controls from refrigerator just before reconstituting. Tap bottom of each bottle. Carefully remove caps from each (N and ABN) bottle. Holding reconstitution dropper bottle vertically, dispense 1 (first) drop into tissue; while still holding vertically, add 6 drops to control bottle. Replace cap, swirl to mix several times, and let stand 15 minutes at room temperature. Repeat with other control bottle. Write expiration date on reconstituted controls. After 15 minutes rotate bottles well, then invert each to ensure controls are well mixed. Discard cap, and replace with eyedropper cap.
   - For control procedure, same procedure is used for N and ABN controls: Remove capillary holder from plastic wrap. Insert tip of eyedropper into control bottle, and aspirate a small amount of solution without bubbles. Hold capillary tube to eyedropper and fill with 1 µL (microliter) of control. (Do not allow control solution to make contact with any part of capillary holder except tip of capillary.) Recap control bottle. With lint-free tissue wipe sides of capillary tube without touching tip. Insert capillary holder into a reagent cartridge until it snaps into place. Hold control card so correct barcode for correct control faces right. (Barcodes are on both sides: one side for N, and one side for ABN.) Insert control card above blue dot into barcode track, and slide it down past blue dot quickly and smoothly. A beep will sound if scanned successfully. Open cartridge compartment door. With barcode facing right, insert cartridge into compartment until a snap is heard or felt. Using a smooth and slow continuous motion, pull flexible pull tab completely out of reagent cartridge, and close door. Record value displayed on control sheet before removing cartridge. Check to make sure result is within acceptable range. If not, press "Escape" and record out-of-range results. Repeat with second control. Log QC as per facility protocol. Patient tests cannot be run if controls do not check out with manufacturer's expected values. (See Box 16-1 for other steps to follow.)

6. If necessary, perform skin puncture per steps previously provided, or use correct whole blood specimen from patient's tube.

7. Touch tip of capillary tube into blood until filled (Figure 16-3B).

8. Wipe sides of capillary tube with tissue.

9. Insert capillary holder into cartridge (flat side toward cartridge) until holder snaps into place.

10. Scan barcode on cartridge through barcode reader on left side of analyzer. (With barcode facing right, insert into barcode track above blue dot and slide it down quickly. A beep and change in display indicate a successful scan.) If unsuccessful, repeat process.

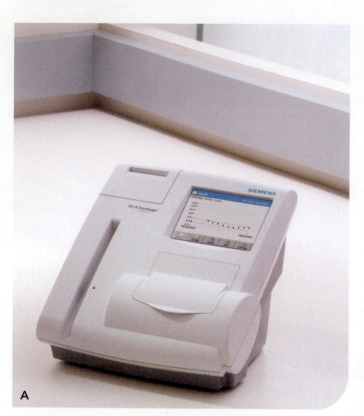

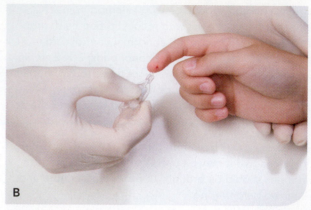

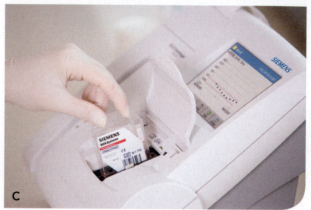

FIGURE 16-3 (A) Bayer DCA 2000+ Analyzer is used to perform HbA1c tests to monitor glucose levels over time; (B) one microliter of whole blood is collected in a capillary holder; (C) the reagent cartridge is inserted into the analyzer, the pull tab is removed, and the instrument door is closed to initiate the analysis.
© 2009 Siemens Healthcare Diagnostics Inc. Photo Courtesy of Siemens Healthcare Diagnostics.

11. Hold cartridge so barcode faces to right and insert it into compartment until a "click" is heard (Figure 16-3C).

12. Slowly and firmly pull plastic tab while holding down cartridge.

13. Close door.

14. Read results from display and record.

15. Remove cartridge by holding down button on right side of compartment with right hand. With left hand gently push plastic tab on cartridge to right to unlock it. Then pull upward.

16. Dispose of all biohazard waste. Clean area. Remove and dispose of gloves properly.

17. Perform hand hygiene.

18. Document results in patient's record or on laboratory requisition.

CHARTING EXAMPLE: 11/14/XX 5:00 P.M. HgbA1c done from EDTA specimen. Pt. results = 8.4%. Physician notified of results. · D. Korski, RMA

Lipid Testing

Lipids or fats, such as cholesterol, are essential to proper functioning of the body. Fats are stored in the body as adipose tissue, which helps insulate and protect organs and provides an alternative source of energy during times of decreased levels of glucose. Cholesterol, one type of lipid, is manufactured in part by the liver and is an important component of cell walls. Cholesterol also is necessary for the production of hormones and bile. It is accepted as fact that cardiovascular disease is linked to elevated lipid levels. The epidemic of obesity and cardiovascular disease in the United States makes it essential to have more frequent lipid screenings. Heart attacks are the number one cause of death in the United States. The American Heart Association and other groups recommend that fats make up no more than 30% of the total daily caloric intake and that total cholesterol levels in blood not exceed 200 mg/dL. A cholesterol of 240 mg/dL or greater is considered high risk for heart disease. Health assessments help to identify those with increased risk of developing cardiac disease. A lipid panel, blood pressure, height, weight, and social habits such as smoking and alcohol consumption provide the information needed to assess a patient's risk of cardiac disease.

CHOLESTEROL

Cholesterol is a saturated fatty acid. (*Saturated* refers to the number of hydrogen ions attached to the molecule. The more saturated a fat, the more solid it is at room temperature.) Saturated fats tend to increase blood cholesterol levels. Thus animal fats and butter are solid, whereas corn, safflower, and olive oils are liquid at room temperature and tend not to affect cholesterol levels.

Cholesterol and triglycerides are two routinely measured plasma lipids. (Triglycerides are any combination of glycerol with 3 to 5 different fatty acids; in the bloodstream, triglycerides combine with proteins to form lipoproteins.) Because they are not soluble in plasma, which is mostly water, they must be attached to proteins to travel through the blood. Lipids are categorized by the way they are transported in the bloodstream as **lipoproteins**. These lipoproteins are broken down as follows:

- **High-density lipoproteins (HDL).** This "good cholesterol" protects against the formation of plaque (abnormal accumulation of lipids and sometimes calcium deposited in blood vessels and leading to blockages). It also takes cholesterol from the blood vessel walls to the liver for excretion.

- **Low-density lipoproteins (LDL).** This "bad cholesterol" forms plaque and causes atherosclerosis. Some individuals have a genetic predisposition to make large amounts of LDL. LDL is also elevated upon consumption of saturated fats and trans fats (unsaturated fatty acids formed by hydrogenation of vegetable oils that have been linked to increase in blood cholesterol).

- **Very low-density lipids (VLDL).** These lipids are linked to triglycerides and to the formation of plaque.

The ratio of total cholesterol (TC) to high-density lipids provides an assessment for patients at risk of atherosclerosis and cardiac risk. Total cholesterol is the sum of HDL and LDL. The ratio of TC/HDL should be under 4.5. Exercise as well as diet modifications to reduce fat intake and refined carbohydrates will raise HDL levels and lower the TC/HDL ratio. Triglycerides become elevated in patients that consume refined carbohydrates (cakes, cookies) and alcohol. Excessive triglycerides in the blood causes lipemic serum (a serum that is milky white in appearance), which interferes with many chemistry tests. Patients should fast at least 12 to 14 hours prior to testing for triglycerides.

CLIA Waived chemistry tests are available for point of care testing, community-based health clinics, and physician's offices. POC units such as the Cholestech LDX (Figure 16-4) and ProAct Cholesterol Device provide quantitative results for cholesterol. The Cholestech is also approved for two liver enzyme tests (alanine aminotransferase [ALT] and aspartate aminotransferase [AST], levels of which may become elevated when patients are taking statin-type drugs to lower cholesterol.)

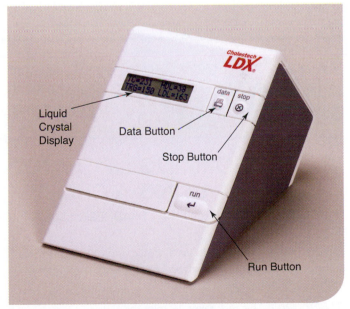

Liquid Crystal Display

Data Button

Stop Button

Run Button

FIGURE 16-4 The Cholestech LDX Analyzer has a 32-character display screen and three buttons that control all the steps needed for operation: RUN, DATA, STOP.
Photo Courtesy of Inverness Medical.

PROCEDURE 16-6

PERFORMING A CHOLESTEROL TEST USING A ProAct TESTING DEVICE

ABHES VII.MA.A.1 10(b)(3)   CAAHEP I.P (13)

OBJECTIVE: To obtain a blood cholesterol level using a ProAct testing device and following manufacturer's directions.

STANDARD: This task takes 15 minutes.

EQUIPMENT AND SUPPLIES: ProAct testing device and supplies; heparinized capillary tubes; lancet; 2 × 2 sterile gauze pads; gloves; biohazard waste container; patient's record; pen.

STEPS:

1. Check patient's record or laboratory requisition for tests ordered. Check for patient allergies.
2. Check expiration date of test kits, supplies, and storage requirements of reagents.
3. Perform hand hygiene, and don gloves.
4. Perform controls as indicated by manufacturer and facility protocol.
5. Assemble equipment and supplies.
6. Identify patient, and explain procedure.
7. Perform skin puncture according to previously described procedure.

8. Fill capillary tube with patient's blood without bubbles. If bubbles are present, fill another tube and discard previous tube.
9. Remove test strip from container, and recap container. Unwrap and remove strip from foil, and place it on paper towel on a clean, dry, hard surface.
10. Without touching strip with capillary tube, place 1 drop of blood in center of application zone.
11. Place strip into port of ProAct Device. Unit will immediately start to count down for 160 seconds.
12. Check strip to ensure no uneven color is present. If uneven color is present, repeat test.
13. Discard test strip and other waste into biohazard waste container.
14. Document patient's record with test results displayed. Report elevated results to physician.

CHARTING EXAMPLE 11/15/XX 9:00 A.M. ProAct cholesterol test done (middle finger R hand). Results 252 mg/dL. Notified physician and provided pamphlets on managing cholesterol per physician's orders. · · · · · · · · · · · · · · I. Rodriguez, CMA (AAMA)

PROCEDURE 16-7

PERFORMING LIPID PROFILE AND GLUCOSE TESTING USING A CHOLESTECH LDX ANALYZER

ABHES VII.MA.A.1 10(b)(3)   CAAHEP I.P (13)

OBJECTIVE: To perform a lipid profile and glucose analysis using a Cholestech LDX Analyzer using quality control and following manufacturer's directions.

STANDARD: This task takes 10 minutes.

EQUIPMENT AND SUPPLIES: Cholestech Analyzer and printer; Level 1, Level 2 controls; optics check container and

cassette; foil-wrapped test cassettes; Cholestech capillary tubes and black plungers; MiniPet Pipette and tips; lancets; 2 × 2 sterile gauze; alcohol pads; gloves; biohazard waste container; patient's record; QC log; pen.

- *Make note of the following:* Only a fresh skin puncture sample or a green top tube with lithium heparin may be used.

- Patients must fast 12 to 14 hours prior to testing and refrain from alcohol for 2 days.
- Optics check must be run daily and recorded. If results are out of range, no patient tests may be run until cause is determined.
- Liquid Cholestech controls must be run monthly, whenever a new set of cassettes is opened.
- It is always prudent to have first-time users run controls to observe their technique.

STEPS:

1. Check patient's record or laboratory requisition for tests ordered. Check for patient allergies.
2. Turn on analyzer to warm up.
3. Check expiration date on test kit and storage requirements.
4. Remove test cassette from refrigerator 10 minutes before using it.
5. Perform optics check by inserting cassette in drawer of analyzer, and log and compare numbers.
6. Assemble other equipment and supplies as needed.
7. Perform hand hygiene, and don gloves.
8. Identify patient, and explain procedure. If venous blood in lithium heparin green top tube is available, compare name on tube with patient's record and confirm a match.
9. If cassettes have been refrigerated, allow them to come to RT before opening. Remove cassette from foil packet without touching black bar or brown magnetic strip.

10. Press "Run," analyzer will perform a self-test, and screen will display "Self-Test OK." Drawer will open, and display will say, "Load Cassette and Press Run." Drawer will remain open 4 minutes. If test is not run in 4 minutes, "System Time out" message will appear. "Press Run to Continue" message will appear. Push "Run" within 15 seconds or screen will go blank and self-test must be run again.
11. Insert black plunger into red end of Cholestech LDX capillary tube.
12. Perform skin puncture observing steps previously described. Collect blood into Cholestech LDX capillary tube with plunger in place. Or use MiniPet pipette provided with analyzer with a disposable tip to collect blood from green top lithium heparin tube.

    Dispense blood or control sample into cassette well within 5 minutes; otherwise, blood may clot (Figure 16-5A).
13. Place filled cassette into drawer of analyzer, keeping it level and with black bar facing analyzer (brown magnetic strip is on right). (See Figure 16-5B.)
14. Press "Run." Drawer will close, and a beep will sound when testing is complete. Printer attached to analyzer will print results on self-adhesive paper, which can then be placed directly in patient's chart. Press "Data" to display calculated result of a panel of tests and questions to be answered to assess cardiac risks.
15. Reference values with Cholestech LDX Analyzer are as follows:
    - TC 200 mg/dL or less
      200–239 mg/dL   Low risk

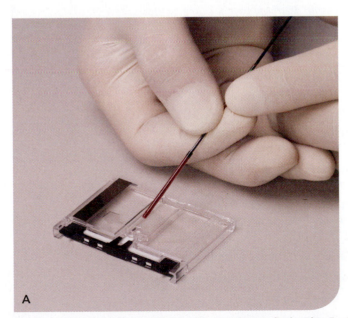

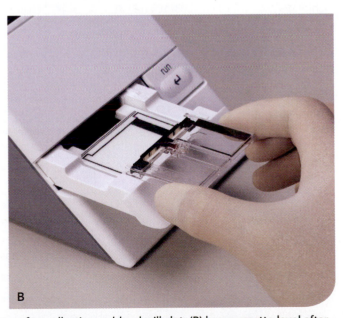

FIGURE 16-5 (A) A fingerstick sample must be applied within 5 minutes after collection or blood will clot; (B) keep cassette level after sample is applied, and immediately place the cassette into the drawer of the analyzer with black bar facing the analyzer and brown strip on the right.
Photo Courtesy of Inverness Medical.

| 240–300 mg/dL | Moderate risk |
| Over 300 mg/dL | High risk |

The following are also desirable results:

- HDL over 40 mg/dL
- LDL under 100 mg/dl if other risk factors present
- Triglycerides under 150 mg/dL
- TC/HDL 4.5 or less

16. Dispose of sharps and biohazard waste in correct containers. Clean area.

17. Remove and dispose of gloves properly. Perform hand hygiene.

18. Document patient's record.

CHARTING EXAMPLE: 11/15/XX 1:00 P.M. Cholestech lipid panel and Gluc performed from NaLi green tube. Results attached. · C. Ames, RMA

Other Chemistry Tests

Many chemistry tests are available through reference and hospital laboratories—in fact, too many to go into detail about each in this text. Because chemistry tests are important in helping to diagnose many diseases, the number of POC tests available is likely to increase. Table 16-3 provides normal values and the clinical significance of abnormal results of some commonly ordered chemistry tests.

TABLE 16-3 Normal Values and Clinical Significance of Out of Range Results

Tests	Normal Values	Clinical Significance
Albumin	3.5–5.5 g/dL	Decreases in kidney disease, severe burns
Bilirubin (total)	0.3–1.4 mg/dL	Increases in liver disease, RBC destruction, obstruction of bile ducts
Calcium (Ca)	4.3–5.3 mEq/L	Increases in hyperparathyroidism Decreases in hypoparathyroidism, malnutrition
Chloride (Cl)	98–108 mEq/L	Decreases in sever diarrhea, severe burns, acidosis
Cholesterol	Under 200 mg/dL	Increases in atherosclerosis
Creatinine	0.6–1.5 mg/dL	Increases in kidney disease
Globulins	2.3–3.5 g/dL	Increases in chronic infection
Carbon dioxide (CO_2)	35–45 mm Hg	Increases in pulmonary disease Decreases in acidosis, kidney disease
pH	7.35–7.45	Increases in hyperventilation, alkalosis Decreases in acidosis, hypoventilation
Phosphorus (P)	1.8–4.1 mEq/L	Increases in kidney disease, hypoparathyroidism Decreases in hyperparathyroidism
Potassium (K)	3.5–5.0 mEq/L	Increases in severe cellular destruction Decreases in diarrhea, kidney disease
Sodium (Na)	136–142 mEq/L	Increases in dehydration Decreases in kidney disease, diarrhea, severe burns
Urea nitrogen (BUN)	8–25 mg/dL	Increases in kidney disease, high-protein diet
Uric acid	3.0–7.0 mg/dL	Increases in kidney disease, gout

17 Diagnostic Imaging

PROCEDURES

Procedure 17-1 Performing a General X-ray Examination

Procedure 17-2 Sequencing Multiple Radiographic/Diagnostic Imaging Examinations

Procedure 17-3 Maintaining and Loaning Radiographic Records

TERMS TO LEARN

fluoroscopy

computed tomography (CT)

magnetic resonance imaging (MRI)

sonography

dosimeter

Radiology uses radiant energy—X-rays—to view body parts and functions. Several modalities are used to visualize the human body through diagnostic imaging. They include radiography, contrast studies, **fluoroscopy**, **computed tomography (CT)**, **magnetic resonance imaging (MRI)**, **sonography**, and nuclear medicine. Although MRIs and sonography do not involve radiation energy, their administration is usually considered part of the radiology department. Specialists in the diagnostic imaging field are known as radiologists.

X-rays are high-energy waves that are invisible to the naked eye and able to penetrate dense material such as the human body. X-ray images or radiographs are produced by projecting X-rays through organs or structures of the body onto photographic film. Radiopaque substances such as bone allow fewer X-rays to pass through, and as a result they appear light on the film. Radiolucent materials such as soft tissue (e.g., lungs) permit greater penetration of X-rays and leave a dark, shadowy image on the film. If X-rays are permitted to penetrate the body for longer periods of time they can change the structure of cells. This property is useful in the treatment of tumors using radiation.

Radiologic procedures are performed in hospital radiology departments or outpatient facilities designated as diagnostic imaging centers. Some offices, ambulatory care clinics, and urgent care centers have basic X-ray machines to take simple X-rays such as flat chest plates. State medical practice acts govern who can perform radiography and limited scope radiography. Health care providers must always function within their own scope of practice and be aware of county and state regulations. In most states in the United States, licensure is required to take X-rays. State licensure often requires completion of a set period of educational classes culminating in an examination. Medical assistants in some states are permitted to take limited scope X-rays. However, medical assistants are more frequently involved in patient education, patient preparation, positioning of the patient, and scheduling diagnostic imaging procedures.

Staff and patients must adhere to radiation safety protocols. A film badge or **dosimeter** must be worn on the outer clothing of all personnel working with or near radiologic equipment. The dosimeter contains a strip of film that reacts to X-ray exposure, and it records the level and intensity of radiation exposure. Radiation exposure is cumulative; therefore, each exposure to radiation is added to the effect of all previous exposures. The dosimeter must be read on a regular basis by the radiation safety supervisor and records maintained as designated by safety guidelines. A lead apron or shield must be worn by all female patients of childbearing age. Female patients of appropriate age should be asked if they are pregnant. Technicians must wear a lead shield or stand behind a lead-lined wall when taking X-rays.

This chapter covers the following procedures:

- Performing a general X-ray examination
- Sequencing multiple radiographic procedures
- Maintaining and loaning radiographic records

Patient Positions

For most radiologic examinations, the patient is asked to disrobe and wear a gown. Many of the diagnostic imaging procedures involve positions and interventions that may be embarrassing to the patient. All articles of clothing or jewelry containing metal must be removed. As in all procedures, assisting the patient and providing for his or her safety and privacy are essential. The elderly, children, and patients who are mentally challenged require special attention. (Table 17-1 lists and describes various radiology positions. Figure 17-1

TABLE 17-1 Radiology Positions

Position	Description
Anteroposterior (AP)	The X-ray beam is directed from front to back. Patient may be standing or supine. The patient's anterior surface (front) faces the X-ray equipment, and the patient's posterior surface (back) faces the film plate.
Posteroanterior (PA)	The X-ray beam is directed from back to front. The patient stands upright with his or her back to the X-ray equipment and his or her front facing the film plate.
Oblique	The patient is angled in relation to the film plate so that the X-ray beam can be directed at the areas that would be hidden on an AP, PA, or lateral X-ray.
Lateral	The X-ray beam is directed toward one side of the body. In right lateral (RL) position, the patient's right side is near the film plate and the left side faces the X-ray equipment.
Axial	The X-ray beam is angled to direct a ray along the axis of the body or body part. Cephalad angulation means the X-ray is beamed at an angle from the feet toward the head. Caudal angulation means the X-ray is beamed from the head toward the feet.

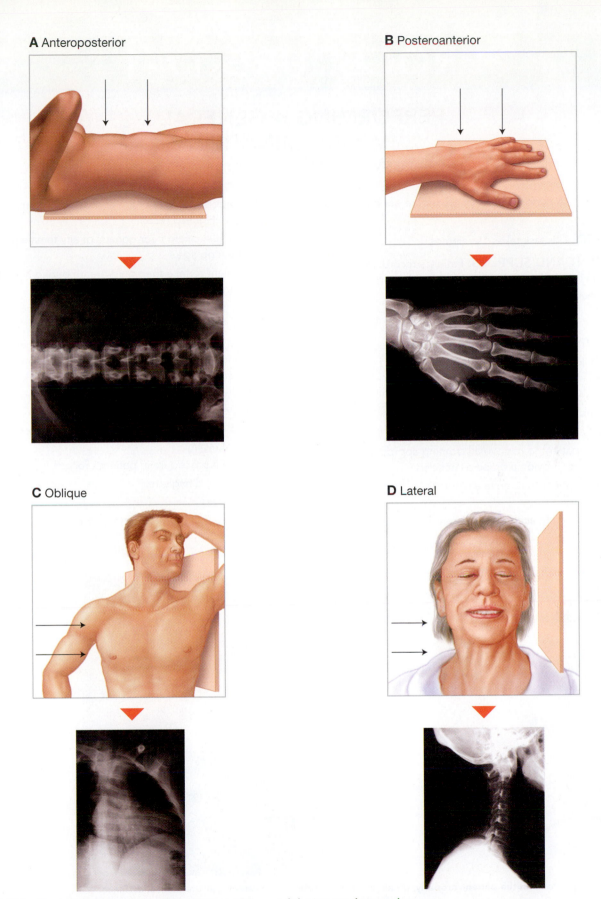

FIGURE 17-1 Examples of the most common X-ray positions and the images they produce.

PROCEDURE 17-1

PERFORMING A GENERAL X-RAY EXAMINATION

ABHES VII.MA.A.1 9(m)   CAAHEP I.P (10)

OBJECTIVE: To perform an X-ray procedure per physician's orders.

STANDARD: This task takes 15 minutes.

EQUIPMENT AND SUPPLIES: Patient's record; dosimeter badge; X-ray machine; X-ray film; X-ray film holder; processing machine; lead aprons; drapes; pen.

STEPS:

1. Perform hand hygiene.
2. Check patient's record for physician's orders. Check for patient allergies.
3. Check X-ray machine.
4. Assemble equipment and supplies.
5. Identify patient, and explain procedure.
6. Instruct patient to remove all clothing appropriate for procedure. Provide a drape as needed.
7. Instruct patient to remove all metallic articles and jewelry for procedure.
8. Position patient according to X-ray view required (Figure 17-2A).

9. Set controls with X-ray tube and cassette at appropriate distance (Figure 17-2B).
10. Place a lead shield over gonads of any female patient of childbearing age.
11. Ask patient to take then hold breath during X-ray (unless X-raying an extremity).
12. Take a position behind a lead wall or shield before taking X-ray.
13. Ask patient to remain in examination room without dressing until films are reviewed by physician or radiologic technician.
14. If films are satisfactory, instruct patient to dress, assisting if necessary.
15. Label X-ray and X-ray sleeve according to procedure and policy of facility.
16. Document procedure in patient's record.
17. Perform hand hygiene.

CHARTING EXAMPLE: 05/05/XX 7:00 A.M. Chest X-ray done. · M. King, CMA (AAMA)

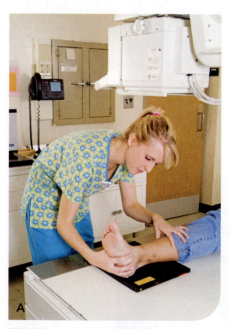
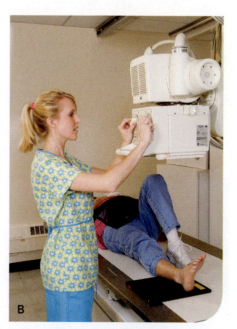

FIGURE 17-2 (A) Position the patient properly; (B) align the X-ray tube to the cassette at the correct distance.

illustrates the X-ray pathways and the images produced when the patient is placed in position for the specific procedure.)

Contrast Studies

Various radiologic procedures involve the use of contrast media. Contrast media is radiopaque. It can be administered by mouth, by enema, by injection through intravenous lines, or by catheter. Contrast media may be a gas, such as oxygen or carbon dioxide; a heavy metal, such as barium sulfate; organic iodine; or either oil based or water soluble. Table 17-2 provides examples of various commonly ordered contrast studies. Most contrast medium studies require specific patient preparation prior to the procedure.

Patient preparation for upper GI series (barium swallow)

Prior to procedure:

- Light evening meal.
  1. NPO 12 hours prior to procedure.
  2. No smoking immediately before procedure.

Postprocedure:

- Drink plenty of liquids to flush out barium.
- Take laxative if prescribed.

Patient preparation for lower GI Series (barium enema)

Prior to procedure:

- Clear liquids only (coffee, tea, broth, carbonated drinks, clear gelatin; no milk products).
- Approximately 4:00 P.M. drink cathartic ordered, such as magnesium citrate or castor oil.

- Early evening enemas if ordered until return is clear. Check facility policy regarding the number of enemas limited to 24-hour period and advise the patient.
- NPO for 12 hours except water.

Postprocedure:

- Increase fluid intake.
- Laxative if needed after 24 hours or as ordered.
- Inform patient stools may be whitish in color for 24 to 48 hours.
- Gas pains may be present for a few hours.

Patient preparation and instructions for intravenous pyelogram (IVP)

Prior to procedure:

- Check on allergy to iodine or shellfish.
- Warn patient of the flushed warm sensation produced by iodine medium.
- Light evening meal.
- Take laxative as prescribed.
- NPO except water for 12 hours prior to procedure.
- Enema in A.M. of procedure if ordered.

Postprocedure:

- Increase fluid intake.

Patient preparation for cholecystogram (gallbladder)

Prior to procedure:

- Check patient for allergy to shellfish or iodine.
- Light, fat-free meals for 24 hours before.
- Take iodine tablets as prescribed with water after evening meal unless iodine is administered by IV.

TABLE 17-2 Common Contrast Studies

Procedure Ordered	Organs Examined	Reasons for Examination
Cholecystogram or gallbladder series	Gallbladder	To diagnose disease or disorders of gallbladder such as tumors, stones, inflammation and obstructions
Intravenous pyelogram (IVP)	Urinary tract, including kidneys, ureters, urinary bladder, and urethra	To diagnose disease or disorders such as strictures, obstructions, tumors, stones; to study the size and shape of the organs involved
Lower GI, air contrast colon study, barium enema	Large intestines	To look for diseases or disorders of the large intestines and conditions such as polyps, diverticula, obstructions, tumors, and lesions
Upper GI, small bowel, barium swallow	Upper GI tract: esophagus, stomach, small intestines	To diagnose ulcers, tumors, hiatal hernia, obstructions, or esophageal varices; to study the size and shape of organs

TABLE 17-3 Flat-Plate Radiographic Procedures

Abdomen	Flat plate survey of abdomen for tumors, obstructions, ascites, hematomas, enlarged organs, abscesses
Bone	X-ray studies to detect abnormal shape, size, structure, fractures, bone growth, osteomyelitis, arthritis
Chest	Routine chest X-ray to detect abnormalities, TB, pneumonia, atelectasis, pneumothorax, tumor, abscess
Kidney, ureters, bladder (KUB)	X-ray to detect normal size, shape, renal calculi, obstructions, tumors, abscesses
Skull	X-ray of sinuses for signs of infection, intracranial pressure, cranial fractures, congenital anomalies, bone defects

- Take laxative if prescribed.
- NPO, except for water, after iodine tablets are taken.
- NPO day of procedure.

Postprocedure:

- Increase fluid intake.

Failure to properly instruct the patient regarding preprocedure preparation or incorrect preparation by the patient will result in the procedure being rescheduled, thus delaying diagnosis and treatment. Instructions should be given to patients verbally and in writing so they may refer to them at home. (Table 17-3 lists the common flat-plate radiographic procedures that do not require contrast medium.)

Sequencing Multiple Radiographic Procedures

Scheduling diagnostic imaging procedures requires contacting the facility, obtaining an appointment, and completing the procedures. Precertification by the patient's insurance company might be required; if so, obtaining the permission is the first step. Each facility should have a policies and procedures manual containing the required patient preparation guidelines for each procedure required by specific diagnostic imaging centers. Once the appointment is scheduled, review with the imaging center the current patient preparation. If a discrepancy between your manual and the imaging center's requirements is identified, obtain a new copy of the required preparation. Next, call the patient and provide information about the date and time of the procedure, the address and telephone number of the imaging center, and verbal information about patient preparation. Send the patient a printed copy of all the information given verbally over the telephone, and document it in the patient's chart.

Special attention must be paid to the type of procedure ordered and what other procedures may be performed on the same day. For example, if contrast medium is required for one procedure, it may interfere with other tests. Moreover, the patient may not be able to tolerate multiple procedures on the same day. In general, procedures not requiring contrast medium are performed before those that do require it. Thus, fiber-optic procedures such as gastroscopy or sigmoidoscopy should be performed before examinations requiring barium; and thyroid assessment tests requiring iodine uptake should be performed after blood work for T3, T4, or nuclear medicine thyroid scans because the iodine remains in the thyroid for several weeks and affects other test results. Another consideration in scheduling examinations is to try to schedule fasting patients in the morning and nonfasting patients in the afternoon.

Maintaining Radiographic Records

X-ray records of radiologic procedures must be kept in special storage containers that protect the film from damage from light. They also should be kept in a cool, dry place. Radiographic images belong to the site where the procedure was performed. Many times the radiographic studies are performed at one location and used as part of a consultation at another site. The original report of the procedure is kept at the facility where the procedure was performed. A copy of the report is sent to the primary and consulting physicians.

X-rays are loaned to consulting physicians, and each facility has its own policies governing the loan procedures. The general procedure includes verbal and written consent of the patient. X-rays are generally loaned for 30 days. X-rays may be copied for another facility, and some facilities charge

SEQUENCING MULTIPLE RADIOGRAPHIC/DIAGNOSTIC IMAGING EXAMINATIONS

ABHES VII.MA.A.1 8(c)   CAAHEP V.P (2)

OBJECTIVE: To schedule multiple procedures taking into consideration the patient preparation guidelines, patient tolerance for procedures, requirements of radiology centers, and physician preferences.

STANDARD: This task takes 15 minutes.

EQUIPMENT AND SUPPLIES: Radiology center guidelines for patient preparation; physician's orders; patient's record; pen; telephone.

STEPS:

1. Check physician's orders for radiographic procedures. Check for patient allergies.

2. Check manual provided by radiology center performing procedure for guidelines on patient preparation and sequencing multiple procedures.

3. Review patient's record to determine how soon physician needs examination performed.

4. Keep in mind physician's preferences for sequencing procedures based on patient's suspected diagnosis and history.

5. Call radiology center to schedule appointments; schedule procedures requiring fasting as early in day as possible.

6. Schedule all procedures that do not require contrast media or iodine uptake first.

WHY? Contrast media and iodine will interfere with other testing protocols.

7. Draw blood for tests for thyroid function before CT procedures or other procedures that require iodine as contrast media.

8. Schedule CT scans of abdomen and pelvis before procedures requiring barium.

9. Schedule procedures of urinary tract, liver, and gallbladder next.

10. Schedule lower and upper GI series next.

NOTE: These are suggested sequences. Each facility may have slightly different requirements.

11. Call patient and review schedule of appointments, making sure that patient or caregiver is writing down information. Provide date and time of procedure, as well as name, location, and telephone number of testing facility. Specify exactly what preparations patient must perform. Also send this information to patient in writing. (On day before procedure, testing facility should call to remind patient about procedure. If not, primary physician's office must do this to increase patient compliance in keeping appointments.)

12. Encourage patient to ask questions.

13. Document patient's record.

CHARTING EXAMPLE: 09/26/XX 11:00 A.M. Scheduled CT of abdomen on 9/30/XX at 9:00 A.M.; lower GI series on 10/2/XX at 10:00 A.M. Pt. given verbal and written preparation information and Memorial Radiology's location, telephone number, directions. · · · · · · · · · · · · · · · · Z. Dina, CMA (AAMA)

for those copies. Generally, the site borrowing the records is responsible for returning them. A log is kept at the lending site, and date, time, and to whom the X-rays were given are recorded.

With advances in teleradiology, many institutions use information systems to archive X-rays. Digital images can then be transmitted to distant locations via intranets, the Internet, CDs, DVDs, and such.

Other Diagnostic Imaging Procedures

As mentioned in the beginning of this chapter, numerous types of examinations can provide physicians with vital diagnostic information. It is beyond the scope of this text to go into details about each one; however, a summary of procedures and brief definition of each follows in Box 17-1.

PROCEDURE 17-3

MAINTAINING AND LOANING RADIOGRAPHIC RECORDS

ABHES VII.MA.A.1 8(b)   CAAHEP V.P (8)

OBJECTIVE: To maintain and loan radiographic records correctly.

STANDARD: This task takes 5 minutes.

EQUIPMENT AND SUPPLIES: Patient consent form; labels; X-ray film; large envelope or film jacket; log; patient's record; pen.

STEPS:

1. Locate the films in questions in on-site filing system.
2. Place the films in a large envelope labeled with patient's name and DOB, date of procedure, and physician's name.
3. Check patient's record for signed consent form needed to release records to another facility.
4. Document in patient's record where films are to be taken, including name of physician, address, and telephone number.
5. Before handing out film, record transfer transaction in a log or file with date, patient's name, destination, and physician receiving films.
6. Tell patients date by which films are to be returned and that receiving physician is responsible for returning them.

CHARTING EXAMPLE: 09/26/XX 2:15 P.M. Upper GI X-rays released to patient after consent form signed. Films are to be reviewed by Dr. Ellis Cook, 890 Main St. Haverhill, CT 06990, 203-483-9929. · V. Learned, RMA

BOX 17-1 Definitions of Diagnostic Imaging Procedures

Procedure	Description
Angiography	An X-ray visualization of the internal anatomy of blood vessels after radiopaque material has been injected into the blood vessels
Arthrography	A diagnostic procedure used to produce an arthrogram or image inside a joint
Cholangiography	An examination of the vessels associated with the gallbladder using a contrast medium such as iodine
Fluoroscopy	Use of a continuous beam of X-rays to observe movement within the body or specific organs
Mammography	An X-ray examination of the breast to screen for cancer
Myelography	An examination of the spinal cord
Nuclear medicine	Injection or placement of radioactive isotopes that concentrate in specific areas of the body for short periods of time to provide for examination or scan of an organ or system
Radiation therapy	High-energy radiation used to destroy cancer cells in an exactly marked area
Retrograde pyelogram	Insertion of a catheter into the urinary tract through the bladder to the ureters to evaluate the function of the ureters
Sonography/ ultrasound	Use of high-frequency sound waves to produce images of internal structures

18 Pharmacology

PROCEDURES

Procedure 18-1 Preparing for Medication Administration

Procedure 18-2 Following Administration of Medication Protocol

Procedure 18-3 Preparing Oral Medications

Procedure 18-4 Preparing a Prescription for the Physician's Signature

Procedure 18-5 Administering Oral Medication to Adults

Procedure 18-6 Administering Oral Medication to a Child

Procedure 18-7 Applying Topical Medication

Procedure 18-8 Applying Transdermal Medication

Procedure 18-9 Administering Rectal Suppositories

Procedure 18-10 Administering a Vaginal Suppository

Procedure 18-11 Reconstituting Powdered Medication

Procedure 18-12 Withdrawing Medication from a Vial

Procedure 18-13 Withdrawing Medication from an Ampule

Procedure 18-14 Preparing for Injection by Combining Medications in One Syringe Using Two Different Vials

Procedure 18-15 Preparing Two Medications in Two Syringes and Combining into One Syringe

Procedure 18-16 Setting Up a Prefilled Disposable Medication Cartridge Syringe

Procedure 18-17 Administering an Intradermal Injection

Procedure 18-18 Administering a Subcutaneous Injection

Procedure 18-19 Administering an Intramuscular Injection

Procedure 18-20 Administering a Z-Track Injection

TERMS TO LEARN

parenteral

nomogram

pharmacodynamics

agonists

antagonists

pharmacokinetics

absorption

distribution

action

metabolism

excretion

contraindicated

adverse reactions

side effects

synergism

antagonism

potentiation

idiosyncratic

teratogenic

Pharmacology is the study of the origins, uses, and actions of drugs and their effects on the body. Drugs are found in nature in plants, animals, and foods and are produced synthetically in pharmaceutical laboratories. Drugs have four names:

- **Chemical name.** That describes the actual chemical molecular formula used to make the drug
- **Official name.** That is listed in official publications
- **Generic or nonproprietary name.** That is the name assigned during development and is given to the manufacturer that discovers the chemical compound of the drug (written in lowercase letters and must be used by any company that produces the drug)
- **Trade or brand name.** That is given to the drug by the manufacturer with the approval of the U.S. Food and Drug Administration (FDA; first letter is capitalized with official trademark symbol (™) of the U.S. Patent Office; remains under patent agreement for 20 years).

Drug Safety

In the United States the Food and Drug Administration (FDA) regulates the manufacture and distribution of drugs and food products to ensure that the products actually include the ingredients listed on the labels. The Controlled Substances Act (1970) was enacted to regulate drugs that may be abused or cause dependency. Any manufacturer of controlled substances must register them with the U.S. attorney general and the Bureau of Narcotics and Dangerous Drugs (BNDD). The Drug Enforcement Agency (DEA), part of the Department of Justice, regulates the drugs listed by the Bureau of Narcotics and Dangerous Drugs (BNDD). All physicians who prescribe, dispense, or administer controlled substances are required to register with the DEA. Physicians are registered for 3 years and are issued DEA numbers that must be listed on each prescription that is written by the physician. The DEA is required to revise the drugs listed on the Controlled Substances Schedule (list) as new drugs emerge.

Drug References

The *U.S. Pharmacopeia–National Formulary* (USP–NF) and the *Physicians' Desk Reference* (PDR) are two widely used drug references. The *USP–NF* is the official list of all accepted therapeutic drugs and their chemical formulas. Revision takes place every 5 years, and supplements are published as needed. The *PDR* is updated annually and is divided into sections to make it easier to look up drugs. The *American*

Hospital Formulary Service (AHFS) is distributed to physicians and provides information on drugs arranged by classification. The *Compendium of Drug Therapy* is published annually and distributed to physicians. It contains drug information, photographs of drugs, and telephone numbers for pharmaceutical companies and poison control centers.

Package inserts prepared by the manufacturer with each prescribed drug follow FDA guidelines and provide complete information about the drug. Patients should be encouraged to keep package inserts, to read the information, and to bring any questions to the attention of their health care provider.

The numerous online references include Medline and WebMD. However, not every Web site can be trusted. Government, university, and professional organization Web sites usually provide up-to-date credible information.

Familiarity with references is vital because it is impossible to remember details about each of the vast number of drugs available today. In any case, the motto when working with drugs should be "When in doubt, look it up." It takes some practice to look up medications quickly and become accustomed to the names, many of which sound alike.

Drug Classifications

Drugs are classified as prescription drugs and over-the-counter drugs (OTC). Drugs are also classified by their addictive ability and according to their effect in the body.

Prescriptions for drugs may be written or ordered verbally by licensed professionals, including physicians, physician's assistants, dentists, and advanced practice nurses. Pharmacists receive prescriptions either verbally or in writing from licensed professionals or their designated agents, and they are charged with filling prescriptions exactly as ordered.

Nonprescription (OTC) drugs are found today on the shelves of a variety of stores. OTC drugs are regulated by the FDA and include medications such as aspirin, antacids, and various cold medications. OTC drugs are dangerous if taken incorrectly and may interact with other OTC drugs and prescription medications. Patients or caregivers should inform physicians about all medications being taken including OTC, prescriptions, vitamins, and herbal substances.

Controlled substances have the potential for addiction or abuse. Controlled substances, also known as schedule drugs, are divided into five categories according to their potentially addictive capabilities. Table 18-1 lists the categories of controlled substances and examples in each category.

Controlled substances must be inventoried daily and verified by a second person. If controlled substances are

TABLE 18-1 Schedule for Controlled Substances

Schedule I substances (C-1) have no accepted medical use in the United States; have high potential for abuse; cannot be prescribed or obtained legally in the United States; and may be used in controlled research experiments:

- Narcotics (e.g., heroin)
- Stimulants such as amphetaminelike drugs (e.g., Ecstasy)
- Hallucinogens (e.g., LSD, mescaline, peyote)
- Cannabis (e.g., marijuana)

Schedule II substances (C-II) have an acceptable medical use; have high potential for addiction and abuse; cannot be refilled without a new prescription written by a physician; and must be stored under lock and key. A 2-year record of dispensing must be kept. Prescriptions must contain the DEA number of the physician:

- Narcotics (e.g., morphine, codeine, cocaine, opium, Oxycodone)
- Amphetamines (e.g., Ritalin, Dexedrine)
- Cocaine
- Barbiturates/depressants (short acting; e.g., Phenobarbital, Seconal, Amobarbital)

Schedule III Substances (C-III) have an acceptable medical use; lower abuse potential; do not require assignment of a DEA number; do require a handwritten order from a physician; and are refillable five times in six months.

- May contain small amounts of narcotics with nonnarcotic compounds (e.g., Tylenol with codeine, anabolic steroids, hydrocodone, butabarbital)

Schedule IV Substances (C-IV) have medically accepted use and less potential for abuse than Schedule III substances; may be refilled five times in 6 months with authorization from physician by telephone and physician's signature:

- Antianxiety drugs (e.g., Xanax, Valium, Librium)
- Sedative hypnotics (e.g., Ambien, Halcion, Dalmane, Versed)

Schedule V Substances (C-V) have a medically accepted use and limited abuse potential; a prescription must be authorized by a physician, and the patient must be over age 18 years and must show ID:

- Cough medicines with codeine
- Antidiarrheal medications (e.g., Lomotil)

stolen or misplaced, the police must be notified immediately. The prescribing, dispensing, administering, and disposing of controlled substances must be documented. The type of paperwork required varies from state to state.

General classifications of drugs are based on their actions in the body. Table 18-2 provides a list of drug classifications and their main functions.

Drug Prescriptions

The physician is responsible for deciding which medication a patient requires. A prescription is a legal document, and it should be written legibly in ink or typed on a prescription pad or hospital form. Prescription pads are usually preprinted forms that include the physician's name, address, telephone number, and DEA number. State medical practice acts govern who can write out a prescription on verbal orders from a physician. In any case, the physician must sign the prescription for any controlled substance in categories II, III, or IV. A prescription authorizes pharmacists to provide the prescribed dose of medication and corresponding instructions

to the patient who will ingest or use the medication. In most states prescriptions are valid for 1 year after they are written and signed by the physician. Controlled drugs are written for one drug per prescription and cannot be refilled. Figure 18-1 is an example of a completed prescription. The following are the parts of a prescription:

- **Physician information.** Name, address, telephone/fax number
- **Patient information.** Patient's name and address
- **Date of prescription**
- **Superscription.** Symbol *Rx*, which means "Take thou"
- **Inscription.** Main part of prescription, including drug name, form, and strength
- **Subscription.** Directions to pharmacist for amount of drug to be dispensed
- **Signature (Sig).** Patient instructions to be placed on the label
- **Refill information.** "Repetatur 0, 1, 2, 3, 4" ("Let it be repeated 0, 1, 2, 3, 4")

TABLE 18-2 Drug Classifications, Examples, and Main Functions

Classes of Drugs	Examples	Main Functions/Effects
Alzheimer's treatment	Aricept, Cognex	Stimulate neurotransmitters to improve behavior and memory
Analgesics (narcotics)	Morphine, Darvon, Demerol	Relieve severe postop pain, pain from trauma, and pain from terminal illness
Analgesics (nonnarcotic)	Aspirin, acetaminophen, ibuprofen	Relieve minor pain
Anesthetics (general)	Thiopental, Versed, Brevital	Produce loss of sensation for surgical and dental procedures
Anesthetics (local)	Lidocaine, procaine (Novocaine)	Produce regional or local loss of sensation
Antianxiety	Valium, Xanax, Ativan	Relieve anxiety, muscle tension, nausea, and vomiting
Antiarrhythmics	Tenormin, propanolol (Inderal), Toprol	Restore normal heartbeat, treat arrhythmias
Antibiotics	Penicillin, cephalosporins (Keflex), aminoglycosides (Garamycin), sulfonamides	Treat bacterial infections
Anticoagulants	Dicumarol, warfarin sodium (Coumadin), heparin sodium	Prevent blood clots, treat thrombosis conditions
Anticonvulsants	Dilantin, Tegretol, phenobarbital	Prevent seizures, halt seizures
Antidepressants: tricyclic antide-pressants (TCAs) and selective serotonin reuptake inhibitors (SSRIs)	Elavil, Pamelor Prozac, Paxil, Zoloft	Treat depression, mood elevators
Antiemetics	Compazine, Phenergan, Tigan	Stop vomiting, relieve nausea
Antifungals	fluconazole (Diflucan), tolnaftate (Tinactin)	Treat yeast, fungal infections
Antihistamines	Diphenhydramine (Benadryl), chlorpheniramine (Chlor-Trimeton), cetirizine (Zyrtec)	Reduce histamine production, treat allergy and hay fever
Antihyperlipidemics	simvastatin (Zocor), atorvastatin (Lipitor)	Reduce and treat elevated lipid levels, high cholesterol
Anti-HIV	zalcitabine, delavirdine	Treat HIV
Anti-hypertensives	Altace, clonidine (Catapres), Adore	Reduce blood pressure
Anti-inflammatory agents	NSAIDs, aspirin, acetaminophen, naproxen sodium (Aleve)	Reduce inflammation of muscles and joints
Antineoplastics	methotrexate (Folex), fluorouracil (5-FU), Cytoxan	Chemotherapy to treat cancer and inhibit growth of neoplasms
Antiparasitics	Vermox, Mintezol, Antiminth	Treat worm infestations
Anti-Parkinson agents	Artane, Sinemet, Cogentin	Increase level of dopamine, reduce tremors
Antipruritics	Calamine lotion, diphenhydramine, corticosteroid ointments	Treat itching
Antipyretics	Acetaminophen, aspirin	Lower elevated body temperature
Antispasmodics	Belladonna, atropine, Bentyl	Reduce motility in the GI tract
Antitussives	Codeine sulfate, dextromethorphan (Robitussin DM), Triaminic	Treat or suppress cough

Anti-ulcer	Biaxin, Amozil	Treat ulcers by eliminating *H. pylori* from stomach
Antivirals	Amantadine (Symmetrel), acyclovir (Zovirax), rimantadine (Flumadine)	Treat viral infections such as respiratory syncytial virus (RSV), cytomegalovirus (CMV), influenza
Asthma prophylactics	cromolyn sodium	Used before exposure to allergen
Bronchodilators	Proventil, Theo-Dur	Relaxes smooth muscle in bronchi to open airways
Cardiac glycosides	digitoxin, digoxin	Slow and strengthen heartbeat, treat congestive heart failure (CHF)
Cathartics (laxatives)	Mineral oil, citrate of magnesia, Dulcolax	Stimulate bowel to evacuate feces
Coagulants	Vitamin K, menadiol sodium	Increase ability to coagulate blood, treat hemorrhage
Contraceptives	Ovral, Triphase	Prevent pregnancy
Decongestants	Afrin, pseudoephedrine	Constricts nasal membrane to open airways
Diuretics	Lasix, Bumex, hydrochlorothiazide	Increase urination, reduce fluid retention, treat CHF and hypertension
Expectorants	Robitussin, Organidin	Increase respiratory secretions, thin secretions
Histaminic II blockers	Tagamet, Zantac, Pepcid	Reduce gastric acid secretions
Hormone replacement therapy	Premarin, Provera, Prempro	Treat menopausal symptoms
Hypoglycemics	Glucophage, Glucotrol	Stimulate production of insulin
Insulin	NPH, Humulin	Replace insulin not produced by pancreas
Thrombolytics	Streptokinase, alteplase	Dissolve blood clots in myocardial infarctions (MIs) and cerebrovascular accidents (CVAs)
Thyroid medications	Synthroid, Levoxyl	Replacement therapy when secretions decreased
Antithyroid	Tapazole	Inhibit production of hormone in cases of overproduction
Proton pump inhibitors (PPIs)	Prilosec, Nexium, AcipHex	Reduce gastric secretions by blocking enzyme that causes secretions
Vasoconstrictors	Norepinephrine, epinephrine (Adrenalin)	Constrict blood vessels to treat shock
Vasodilators	Nitroglycerin (Nitro-stat)	Dilate blood vessels, treat angina

- **Physician's signature**
- **"Dispense as written" or "Substitute generic medication"**
- **DEA number**

Abbreviations are widely used in medicine. Pharmacology abbreviations include those associated with metric, apothecary, and household measurements. Appendix I presents common abbreviations, many of which are associated with prescriptions and administering medications. The Institute for Safe Medication Practices states that many medical errors result from unclear or unapproved abbreviations, illegible writing, misplaced or overlooked decimals, misunderstood verbal orders, or incomplete orders. Medication errors are a growing problem. Some of the most common problems reported are giving the wrong dose of a medication,

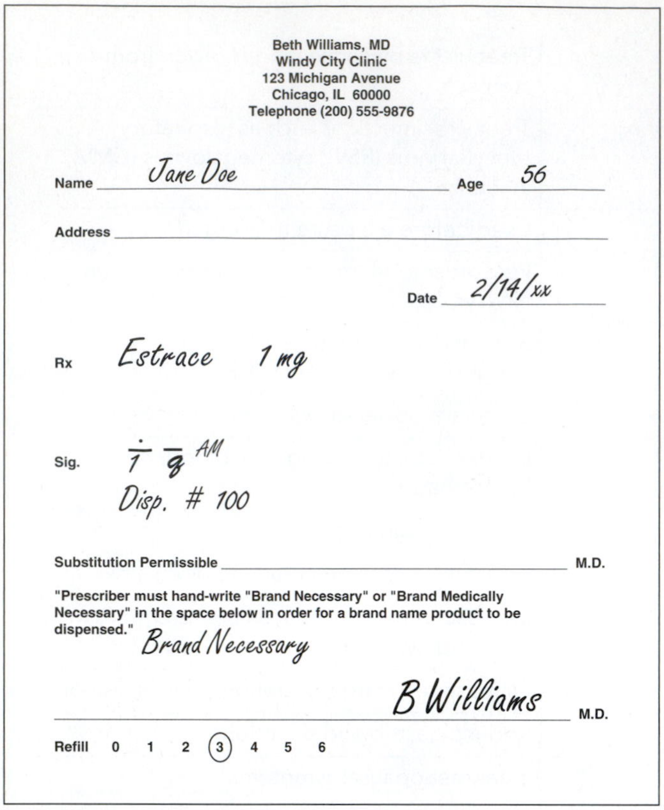

Beth Williams, MD
Windy City Clinic
123 Michigan Avenue
Chicago, IL 60000
Telephone (200) 555-9876

Name *Jane Doe* Age *56*

Address

Date *2/14/xx*

Rx *Estrace 1 mg*

Sig. *ī q̄ AM*
Disp. # 100

Substitution Permissible ______ M.D.

"Prescriber must hand-write "Brand Necessary" or "Brand Medically Necessary" in the space below in order for a brand name product to be dispensed." *Brand Necessary*

B Williams M.D.

Refill 0 1 2 (3) 4 5 6

FIGURE 18-1 An example of a prescription.

dispensing the wrong drug, and specifying the wrong route of administration. Some of these errors result in patient deaths. The Joint Commission issued a "Do Not Use" list of abbreviations in May 2005 for the purpose of reducing the number of medical errors associated with terminology and abbreviations. (See Appendices I and II.) If there is any confusion about the name or dose of a verbally ordered medication, or any other question about it, ask immediately. If a written prescription or order is illegible, ask the physician to review it before proceeding.

Medication Measurement and Conversion

Different measuring systems are used to prepare and administer medications. In the past, both metric and apothecary systems were used. Today the metric system is most widely used for medications, and the apothecary system is seldom used. The terms of measurement in the apothecary system are minim or drop, grain, and dram (a grain is based on the weight of 1 grain of wheat). The metric system uses units of length (meter), volume (liter), and weight (gram). It is important to become familiar with the units and their numerical meanings. The metric system is based on multiples of 10 and uses decimals in place of fractions. In descending order the abbreviations and their numerical equivalents are listed in Box 18-1.

BOX 18-1 Metric Prefixes and Their Numerical equivalents

kilo	1,000	one thousand times
hecto	100	one hundred times
deca	10	ten times
deci	0.10	one-tenth (1/10)
centi	0.010	one-hundredth (1/100)
milli	0.001	one-thousandth (1/1,000)
micro	0.000001	one-millionth (1/1,000,000)
nano	0.000000001	one-billionth (1/1,000,000,000)

Converting from one metric unit to another is easy. It involves moving the decimal to the right or to the left, depending on whether you are converting from a smaller unit to a larger unit or vice versa:

- To go from a larger unit to a smaller unit, move the decimal to the right; in other words, multiply by 1,000.

$$2 \text{ grams} = 2{,}000 \text{ mg}$$

- To go from a smaller unit to a larger unit, move the decimal point to the left; in other words, divide by 1,000.

$$500 \text{ mg} = 0.5 \text{ g}$$

Occasionally, household measurements are used for teaspoon, tablespoon, and ounce. It is difficult to standardize these measurements, and their use should be avoided. When pharmacies do fill a prescription with the instruction for giving "2 tsp," a special measuring device is included to standardize the amount of medication to be taken.

The avoirdupois system is widely used in the United States and is based on the pound. When weighing a patient, the scale provides weight in pounds and ounces and an additional scale for metric weight in grams and kilograms. Recall from Chapter 10 that 1 kg = 2.2 lb. or 1 lb. = 0.45 kg. Conversion among the metric, apothecary, avoirdupois, and household systems is possible. The terms and their equivalents are presented in Table 18-3.

TABLE 18-3 Metric and Apothecary Equivalents

Metric System	Apothecary System
Weight	
30 grams (gm)	1 ounce (oz)
1 gram (gm)	15 grains (gr)
60 milligrams (mg)	1 grain (gr)
30 milligrams (mg)	½ grain (gr)
Volume	
4,000 milliliters (mL)	1 gallon (4 quarts)
1,000 milliliters (mL)	1 quart (2 pints or 32 fl. ounces)
500 milliliters (mL)	1 pint (16 fl. ounces)
250 milliliters (mL)	1 cup (8 fl. ounces)
30 milliliters (mL)	1 fluid ounce (8 fluidrams)
4 milliliters (mL)	1 fluidram (60 minims)
1 milliliter (mL)	15 minims

CALCULATING DOSAGES

At times the order for a drug calls for a dose of drug that is not on hand. For instance, the physician orders 500 mg of a medication, and only 250 mg tablets are on hand. It cannot be stressed too emphatically how important it is to calculate doses correctly. Misplacing a decimal or making a mathematical error may be life threatening. To calculate doses when different systems are involved, it is necessary to refer to conversion tables or to memorize equivalencies (Table 18-3).

1. **Oral Doses**

   If the oral prescription and the medication on hand are in the same units, then the following formula may be used:

   Dosage ordered ÷ Dosage on hand = Dose to be given

   For example:

   500 mg ordered ÷ 250 mg tablets on hand = Dose is 2 tablets of 250 mg each

2. **Liquid Doses**

   Dose desired ÷ Dose on hand × Quantity = Amount to be given

   For example, the physician orders 0.35 g of medication, and on hand is a liquid containing 700 mg/L. The units have to be the same before doses can be figured out. Change 0.35 g to mg by moving the decimal three places to the right or multiply by 1,000 = 350 mg. Then use the formula:

   350 mg ÷ 700 mg × 1 L = Dose is 0.5 mL

3. **Parenteral Doses**

   To calculate **parenteral** (introduced otherwise than by way of the intestines) doses, use the same formula as for liquid doses:

   Dose desired ÷ Dose on hand × Quantity = Amount to be given

   The patient is to be given 40 mg of medication, and medication on hand is a vial containing multiple doses of the medication with the strength 80 mg/2 mL. Using the formula:

   40 mg ÷ 80 mg × 2 mL = Dose is 1 mL

4. **Doses for Children**

   Calculating medication administration for children uses either body surface area (BSA), which can be calculated from a patient's height, weight, and a scale known as a nomogram. A **nomogram** is similar to the charts used to calculate the growth percentile for a child. Once the BSA is found on the nomogram, the following formula is used:

   BSA × Adult dose ÷ 1.7 = Child's dose

   Clark's rule is also used to calculate a child's dose. This formula is as follows:

   Child's weight in pounds ÷ 150 × Average adult dose = Pediatric dose

Medication administration involving pediatric patients is also governed by facility protocols that should be studied prior to the calculation or administration of a drug to a child.

Legal Implications

Administration of medications, as previously stated, is governed by federal laws and state medical practice acts. Licensed medical professionals are allowed to prescribe and administer medications under state law. Unlicensed assistive personnel, such as medical assistants who are trained to administer medications, may be delegated to do so by physicians. In some states, advanced practice nurses and registered nurses may delegate this responsibility. However, in some states it is illegal for medical assistants or other assistive personnel to administer medications. Individuals employed in health care facilities should be familiar with the medical practice acts of the state in which they are employed. No one should perform a task that they do not know how to do or that is legally outside their scope of practice.

Ignorance of the law is not an excuse. If in doubt, ask questions and request further training before complying with the order given.

Monitoring Medications

Controlled substances must be kept in a safe or locked box or cabinet. Access to keys should be limited to individuals directly involved in administering or prescribing these substances. Controlled substances are monitored in the medical facility by rules established by the DEA. Specific inventory forms must be used and may be ordered from pharmaceutical suppliers. Special tamper-resistant forms are available from the federal government for writing prescriptions for controlled substances. Still, every health care facility may be a target for theft of medications and prescription pads by health care professionals and patients who are substance abusers. Prescription forms or pads should not be left where staff or patients have easy access to them; rather, they must be locked up until needed.

A specific in-house inventory sheet must be used to track all incoming substances, and copies must be retained for 2 years. Inventory sheets must document when controlled substances are administered, dispensed, or disposed of as waste. Drug inventories are often checked when shifts change or at the end of a day.

Disposal of outdated medications must follow federal, state, and local regulations. Drugs may be incinerated or shipped to a DEA office for disposal. A special inventory sheet made out in quadruple and signed by the physician is required. It is illegal for any health care professional to use or divert controlled substances. Legally, these incidents must be reported. Any suspicions should be documented and evidence gathered before contacting authorities. Local police are usually the first to be contacted, and if a physician is involved the DEA and American Medical Association (AMA) are notified as well. If the suspected individual is not a physician, the supervisor or the physician in charge in the facility must be notified of the suspicions.

Facility protocols should be established and telephone calls carefully documented and monitored when requests for any type of prescriptions are made. Patients who resort to "doctor shopping" to obtain additional prescriptions for controlled substances may be identified through these records.

Pharmacodynamics

Pharmacodynamics is the study of the actions of a drug on the cells and tissues of the body. Every drug causes either temporary or permanent physiologic changes. Drugs that are **agonists** cause change in the cell's behavior. **Antagonists** affect cells by blocking a cellular change from happening. Other drugs change the behavior of enzymes, and still others alter biochemical actions in the cell or change the ability of the cell walls to let ions in or out. (Table 18-2 lists drug classes and their effects on the body.)

Pharmacokinetics is the study of the five processes involved in the action of medications: **absorption**, **distribution**, **action**, **metabolism**, and **excretion**.

- *Absorption* is the process of getting the drug into the bloodstream and ultimately into the cells where it produces its action. The route of administration (oral, IV, etc.) affects absorption.
- *Distribution* refers to the movement of the drug through the body to the bloodstream and finally into the cells. Distribution can be impeded by conditions such as cardiovascular disease.
- *Action* refers to the pharmacodynamic processes of absorption and distribution.
- *Metabolism* is the physical and chemical breakdown of the drug by the body. The first-pass effect through the liver is important, particularly in the metabolism of oral drugs. Much of this process takes place in the liver; thus, if liver function is impaired so will be the metabolism of the drug.
- *Excretion* refers to the elimination of the by-products of the drug by the kidneys, skin, lungs, and intestinal tract. Impairment in any of these systems impacts the body's ability to excrete the drug. Accumulation of a drug can be toxic.

Routes of Administration of Drugs

Drugs act either locally or systemically. For example, calamine lotion applied to poison ivy on the hand exhibits a local effect. Drugs that have a systemic effect enter the body and go into the bloodstream to be transported throughout the body. Penicillin given by injection to combat ear infection is an example of a systemic medication. The systemic effect of medications can be obtained by administering drugs through the following routes:

- Oral
- Sublingual
- Buccal
- Vaginal

TABLE 18-4 Factors Affecting Drug Actions

Factors	Effects on Drug Action
Age	Children react more quickly to drugs and must be monitored closely. The elderly have slower metabolisms, and drugs may take longer to clear from their system.
Weight	The larger the patient, the larger the dose of medication needed to cause a therapeutic effect. Children's doses must be carefully calculated according to their height and weight.
Gender	Women may react differently than men to medications due to hormonal and ratio-of-fat-to-muscle differences.
Pathological state	The presence of other disease conditions affecting the liver and kidneys will affect the action of medication. Absorption, distribution, metabolism, and excretion may be compromised.
Time of day	Oral medications are absorbed more quickly on an empty stomach. Other drugs cause gastric irritation and must be given with food.
Tolerance	Repeated treatment with certain drugs can cause the body to become resistant to their effects. Larger doses may be required to obtain the desired result.

- Rectal
- Transdermal
- Inhalation
- Parenteral (by injection)
  - Intradermal
  - Subcutaneous
  - Intramuscular
  - Intravenous

In addition to considering the effects of drugs and their route of administration, other factors influence the behavior of drugs in the patient. Table 18-4 lists some of the factors and their influence on the action of drugs. Sensitivity to a drug may cause an allergic reaction or failure of the drug to act in the expected manner in the patient. Certain drugs are **contraindicated** (not recommended for use) due to certain preexisting medical conditions or allergies. These drugs should be documented in the patient's record.

Adverse Reactions to Drugs

Adverse reactions are unintended, undesirable effects produced by a drug. These secondary effects can occur along with the desired therapeutic effect. **Side effects** are adverse reactions that cause harmless reactions to a drug and are tolerated to obtain the therapeutic effect. For example, dry mouth and drowsiness from antihistamines may be tolerated to relieve symptoms of severe hay fever. When drugs are used simultaneously, interactions may produce undesirable or harmful effects or greater effects than either drug alone. Drugs interactions fall into three categories: **synergism** (two drugs working together), **antagonism** (one drug working against another causing a decreased effect), and **potentiation** (multiplying or prolonging the effect of one drug by another drug). An example of a positive effect of potentiation is the use of muscle relaxants and pain medication to reduce discomfort from muscle trauma. Some drug interactions have negative effects, such as taking antacids with certain antibiotics, such as tetracycline. Several foods taken with certain drugs may decrease or increase a drug's effect. Examples of interaction among foods and drugs are Lipitor and grapefruit; Coumadin and green leafy vegetables; and MAO inhibitors and alcohol. Careful reading of labels and a thorough patient history are important to reduce the chances of negative drug interactions. Unpredictable or **idiosyncratic** reactions occasionally occur. This type of reaction is not considered an allergy but an abnormal, unexpected reaction to a medication, as some individuals have to specific types of anesthesia. Some medications are considered **teratogenic**, which means the risk level for fetal or maternal health problems is high. An aging population brings with it greater challenges to families and health care providers. Older patients tend to take more medications and often are not supervised carefully when living alone. Box 18-2 provides information that must be considered when working with the elderly.

Routes of administration are discussed in more detail later in this chapter. Prior to administering any medication by any method, specific safety precautions must be taken.

BOX 18-2 Life Span Considerations

Many elderly Americans live alone, and many of these individuals take at least one medication that could be harmful if taken incorrectly. Over-the-counter medications taken with other drugs also may cause side effects. The following factors must be taken into consideration to protect this vulnerable population:

- **Multiple medications.** Taking many drugs increases the risk of drug interactions and adverse reactions.
- **Medication errors.** Multiple prescriptions increase the risk of taking the wrong drug at the wrong time or in the wrong dose.
- **Noncompliance.** Not taking the drug or not taking it at the right time can be problematic.

- **Drug cost.** Without prescription insurance, many cannot afford to fill the prescriptions given by physicians and may be a compliance issue.
- **Inadequate monitoring.** Many elderly live alone and far away from loved ones, and thus drug problems are not identified.
- **Drug toxicity.** This can be due to reduced metabolism and excretion or to increased sensitivity to central nervous system (CNS) medications that regulate brain function.

Administering Medications Safely

Each time a drug is to be administered, safety rules known as the "Six Rights" must be carried out. Other important "Rights" have been added here to help prevent medication errors. The following are the "Ten Rights":

1. **Right Medication.** Compare—three times—the drug container label to the order on the medication administration record (MAR) used in hospitals. Note the expiration date, and know all pertinent information about the medication: action, dosage, route, side effects, patient allergies. If in doubt, check a drug reference book. Only administer medication you have prepared yourself. Check the label when removing a drug from a shelf, before taking it from a container, and before shelving the container.

2. **Right Patient.** Use two methods of identification other than room or bed number, such as the patient's name, date of birth, identification number, or identification band.

3. **Right Dose.** Confirm if an adult or child dose is prescribed. Calculate the dosage, and have calculations verified by another clinical staff person who is permitted to administer drugs. Be familiar with the usual dose, and be prepared to question any unusual dose.

4. **Right Time.** Check the order. Plus or minus 30 minutes is acceptable unless facility protocol states otherwise.

5. **Right Route.** Check the order. For injections, use the correct site.

6. **Right Documentation.** Document the date, drug name, dose, route (site if by injection), time, patient's response, and your signature. If a drug is not administered, document that information and the reason, and report it to the physician.

7. **Right Patient Education.** Be certain the patient understands what and he or she is taking, what precautions are needed, and what to expect.

8. **Right to Refuse.** Any competent adult has the right to refuse medication. The patient must be fully informed, and the refusal must be documented.

9. **Right Assessment.** Certain medications require specific assessment (e.g., pulse, respiratory rate, test results) prior to being administered. Some orders specify that evaluations be performed prior to administration of medications.

10. **Right Evaluation.** Follow up after administering medication to monitor side effects or reactions.

Medication administration in a hospital involves protocols established by the facility. In addition, most facilities use a medication administration record (MAR; Figure 18-2) and carts for transporting medications from room to room. Pharmacy staff restock the carts, and automated dispensing systems may require different procedural steps. The procedures that follow apply to smaller facilities, not hospitals: mainly ambulatory care centers and physician's offices. Only licensed personnel may administer narcotics; thus, all protocols for controlled substance

MEDICATION ADMINISTRATION RECORD

PRN#:

MRN#: AGE:

ADM: 08-04-09 SEX:

DOB: HT:

DR. HT:

VERIFIED BY: _____ DATE: _____

DIAGNOSIS: ALOC
PNEUMONIA

ALLERGIES: NO KNOWN DRUG ALLERGIES

GENERATED: 08-07-09 07:32
FOR PERIOD: 08-07-09 08:00
THROUGH: 08-08-09 07:59

START	STOP	MEDICATION/I.V./IVPB/IRRIGATION		0800-1559	1600-2359	0000-0759
08-06	09-05	FERROUS SULFATE 300MG=5ML TWICE A DAY PO (FESO4)	(973539)	09	17	
08-06	09-05	DOCUSATE SODIUM 100MG=1UDCUP TWICE A DAY PO (COLACE) 100MG/30ML UD HOLD FOR LOOSE STOOL	(973532)	09	17	
08-05	09-04	ASCORBIC ACID 500MG=1TAB TWICE A DAY PO (VITAMIN C) 500MG TAB	(972096)	09	17	
08-05	09-04	LEVOTHYROXINE 0.05MG=1TAB DAILY PO (SYNTHROID) 0.05MG TAB	(972095)	09		
08-05	09-04	ASPIRIN 325MG=1 TAB DAILY PO (ASPIRIN) 325MG TAB *W/FOOD TO AVOID GI UPSET	(972094)	09		
08-04	08-14	CEFUROXIME ADDV. 1.500GM=1VIAL EVERY 8 HOURS IV (KEFUROX) 1.5GM ADDV *ATTACH TO D5W 50ML ADDV BAG *ACTIVATE BEFORE INFUSION* * INFUSE OVER 30 MINS*	(971776)	14	22	06
		——— **PRN ORDERS** ———				
08-04	09-03	ACETAMINOPHEN 650MG=1SUPP EVERY 4 HOURS AS NEEDED PR (TYLENOL) 650MG SUPP	(971779)			

INITIALS	SIGNATURE	SHIFT	INITIALS	SIGNATURE	SHIFT	INITIALS	SIGNATURE	SHIFT

SITE CODES:

A. Right Upper Outer Quadrant Gluteus
B. Left Upper Outer Quadrant Gluteus
C. Right Outer Aspect Arm
D. Left Outer Aspect Arm
E. Right Ventrogluteal
F. Left Ventrogluteal
G. Abdomen
H. Right Thigh
I. Left Thigh

FIGURE 18-2 Sample medication administration record.

administration in a facility must be adhered to completely. All narcotics or controlled substances must be documented on appropriate inventory sheets, and cabinets must be kept locked.

In some facilities, medications are administered using barcode scanners. The person administering the medication scans his or her barcode or ID, the patient's wrist band, and the prepackaged medication to be given.

PROCEDURE 18-1

PREPARING FOR MEDICATION ADMINISTRATION
ABHES VII.MA.A.1 (6)(a); VII.MA.A.1 (6)(b); VII.MA.A.1 9(j)   CAAHEP II.P (1); II.A (1)

OBJECTIVE: To prepare to administer medication(s) as ordered by physician.

STANDARD: Time is dependent on type and number of medications ordered.

EQUIPMENT AND SUPPLIES: Patient's record; physician's order if not written in record; drug reference resource; calculator if needed; pen.

STEPS:

1. Check physician's order for medication to be administered to patient (drug, dose, route, time). Check for patient allergies.
2. Research any medication that is unfamiliar to you. (Discover generic name, trade name, classification, major uses, pharmacologic actions, safe dosage, route and time, side effects, adverse reactions).
3. Check patient's record for allergies, contraindications to drug ordered, and other relevant factors such as weight, age, and so on.
4. Check for any "discontinue" order that contradicts order on hand.
5. Obtain medication from storage, checking name three times: when taken from shelf, when preparing dosage, and when returning to shelf. Check expiration date.
6. Check label to ensure that drug is indicated for route ordered.
7. Calculate dosage. Have another clinical staff member permitted to administer medication check calculations if necessary.
8. Prepare medication(s) for administration. Check drug label before and after preparation. Check one more time before administration.
9. Perform hand hygiene. Don gloves if required.

PROCEDURE 18-2

FOLLOWING ADMINISTRATION OF MEDICATION PROTOCOL
ABHES VII.MA.A.1 9(j)   CAAHEP II.P (1); II.A (1)

OBJECTIVE: To follow exactly the administration of medication protocol established by facility.

STANDARD: This task takes 5 minutes.

EQUIPMENT AND SUPPLIES: Gloves if indicated; prepared medication; patient information or patient's record; pen; sharps container; biohazard waste container.

STEPS:

1. Check patient's name, age, and DOB against order.
2. Check for patient allergies.
3. Identify patient using two identifiers other than room or bed number. For example, ask patient to state name and date of birth.
4. Explain procedure and purpose of medication to patient.
5. Provide privacy as needed. Assist patient into proper position for administering medication.
6. If indicated, measure vital signs before administering medication.
7. Perform hand hygiene, and don gloves if needed.
8. Administer medications by correct route and following "Ten Rights" of administration of medications.
9. Dispose of equipment appropriately. Remove and dispose of gloves properly.
10. Perform hand hygiene.
11. Observe patient, and check vital signs if required.
12. Document administered medication in patient's record, including time, drug, dose, route (including site of injection), and patient's reaction.

CHARTING EXAMPLE: 11/25/XX 2:10 P.M. 2 tab Tylenol 3 given for pain in R ankle per Dr. Lee. ·········· R. Stein, RMA

ORAL MEDICATIONS

Oral medications (pill, tablet, capsule, or liquid) are the easiest to administer and are preferred by patients. Oral medication is slowly absorbed into the body because it goes through the digestive tract before being absorbed into the bloodstream.

Oral medication cannot be given to an unconscious patient, one with nausea and vomiting, or one who is NPO. Some oral medications are produced in unit doses (prewrapped single dose) and are easy to administer. Sample unit doses may be given by the physician to the patient to begin home treatment.

PROCEDURE 18-3

PREPARING ORAL MEDICATIONS

ABHES VII.MA.A.1 9(j)   CAAHEP II.P (1)

OBJECTIVE: To correctly prepare ordered oral medication from medications on hand.

STANDARD: This task takes 5 minutes.

EQUIPMENT AND SUPPLIES: Oral medication in tablet, capsule, or liquid form; patient's record or physician's order; pen; beverage or substance to assist swallowing based on patient's preference; pill cutter; mortar and pestle; measuring device needed (spoon, medicine cup, calibrated dropper syringe); straw; waste container.

STEPS:

Liquid medication:

1. Follow Procedure 18-1 to prepare for medication administration and Procedure 18-2 for medication administration protocol.
2. Perform hand hygiene.
3. Remove lid from bottle and place top with inside of cap facing up to avoid contamination. Check label.
4. Hold bottle with label facing up to avoid dripping.
5. Place medication cup on flat firm surface (Figure 18-3).

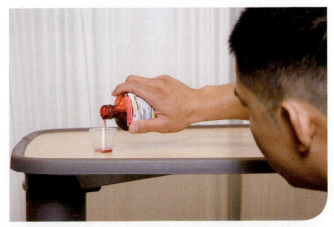

FIGURE 18-3 Pouring a liquid medication from a bottle at eye level.

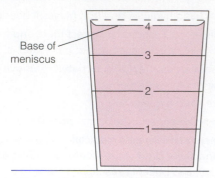

FIGURE 18-4 Place medication on a flat surface at eye level, fill to the desired level, and read, using the bottom of the meniscus aligned with the markings on the container.

6. Pour liquid medication and read at eye level at the lowest point of meniscus (Figure 18-4). Check label.

7. Wipe bottle lip before recapping. Check medication label again.

Crushing or altering medications:

NOTE: Enteric-coated, extended-release, or sustained-release pills cannot be cut or crushed.

1. Follow steps for medication administration (Procedure 18-2).

2. Perform hand hygiene.

3. Prepare medication as follows:

Pill

- Leave pill in packaging if a unit dose is on hand to limit losing any of dose.
- Pound pill with pestle or other tool to crush it, or place pill between two medication cups, one inside the other, to avoid losing any during crushing.
- Mix crushed medication in a small amount of soft food (jelly, applesauce, pudding) to make swallowing easier.

Tablet

- Check orders for partial dosage needed. Place tablet in pill cutter, or break tablet if scored.

Capsule

- If capsule is on hand, open capsule and sprinkle medication in small amount of soft food. Remind patient not to chew "beads," if present, because they contain timed-released dose.
- Make sure that all medication was consumed.
- Offer water or other liquid as appropriate.
- If multiple doses of tablet, capsule, or pill are needed, uncap bottle and shake number of tablets, capsule, or pills needed for dosage ordered into cap. Then transfer to a medicine cup for administration to patient.

PROCEDURE 18-4

PREPARING A PRESCRIPTION FOR THE PHYSICIAN'S SIGNATURE

ABHES VII.MA.A.1 (6)(c); VII.MA.A.1 (6)(d)   CAAHEP IX.P (2)

OBJECTIVE: To prepare a prescription ordered by the physician for his or her signature.

STANDARD: This task takes 10 minutes

EQUIPMENT AND SUPPLIES: Order for medication; pen; blank prescription; drug reference; patient's record.

STEPS:

1. Assemble equipment and supplies.

2. Check patient's record for physician's order for medication.

3. Check for patient allergies.

4. If unfamiliar with medication, look it up in drug reference.

5. If unable to read physician's writing or unsure of any portion of prescription, ask physician.

6. On blank prescription, include the following information in appropriate areas:
   - Patient's name, address, age
   - Date

- Name of medication correctly spelled. If generic, use lowercase letters; if trade name, capitalize first letter.
- Dosage. Use a zero before decimal and no trailing zero for fractional doses (e.g., 0.6 mg).
- Quantity to be dispensed. Should be numerical and written (e.g., #20; twenty). Number of pills should equal length of treatment.
- Clearly written directions for taking medication. Follow facility policy for using abbreviations or writing it out fully (e.g., Sig: take 2 tab 3 times a day for 7 days.). Use only approved abbreviations.
- Refills. Write number clearly. Write "0" if no refills ordered. Never leave this section blank. Some prescription pads have preprinted numbers and "NR" to indicate "No Refills."
- Check the "Dispense as Written" category if substitution with generic form is not ordered.
- Check DEA number, which is usually printed on prescription form. Make sure it is clearly visible.

- Group practices. Circle prescribing physician's name in case signature is difficult to read.
7. Give prescription to physician to review and sign.
8. Document prescription order in patient's record. Make a copy for office files if required by office policy.
9. Give prescription to patient, and explain how medication is to be taken.
10. Answer any question patient may have about medication. Refer questions to physician if necessary.

CHARTING EXAMPLE: 11/25/XX 3:00 P.M. Prescription given to patient per physician's orders for Ambien 10 mg #30. Pt. to take 1 Tab. PO ½ hour before bed PRN. No refills. Pt. instructed to watch for side effects. · C. Walsh, CMA (AAMA)

PROCEDURE 18-5

ADMINISTERING ORAL MEDICATION TO ADULTS

ABHES VII.MA.A.1 9(j)   CAAHEP I.P (8); II.A (1)

OBJECTIVE: To administer oral medication to an adult patient per physician's orders.

STANDARD: This task takes 5–10 minutes.

EQUIPMENT AND SUPPLIES: Oral medication; liquid to assist swallowing; measuring devices; pill cutter or mortar and pestle; patient's record; pen.

STEPS:

1. Follow Procedure 18-1 to prepare for medication administration and Procedure 18-2 for medication administration protocol.
2. Prepare oral medications following procedural steps in Procedure 18-3.
3. Identify patient by checking patient's name and birth date.
4. Explain procedure and type of medicine and purpose.
5. Help patient assume a sitting position.
6. Measure vital signs if indicated.
7. Hand medication cup to patient, and offer water to aid swallowing.
8. Make sure patient swallows medication.
9. Discard medication cup.
10. Document patient's record with medication given.
11. Observe patient for possible side effects or adverse reactions.

CHARTING EXAMPLE: 11/25/XX 1:00 P.M. Pt. given 2 tab. 250 mg/tab acetaminophen per physician's orders for headache. · S. Ramirez, RMA

Never give oral medication to an unconscious patient.

Split or cut tablets, unless:

- They are extended release.
- They crumble when cut.

Chewable medications may be crushed.

Liquid capsules can be opened by making a needle hole and squeezing out the contents.

Remember the following:

- Do not crush gel or enteric-coated tablets.
- Do not try to open sealed capsules.
- Do not crush capsules.
- Do not give oral medicines sublingually.

(See Box 18-3 for guidelines for administering oral medications.)

OTHER ROUTES OF ADMINISTRATION

Sublingual medications are placed under the patient's tongue, not swallowed (Figure 18-5). The medication dissolves and is absorbed through the oral mucosa. For example, nitroglycerin tablets are given sublingually to relieve angina pain and dilate blood vessels. Medications are fairly rapidly absorbed by this route. Instruct the patient not to eat or drink until the medication is completely dissolved.

For buccal administration of medication, the dose is placed between the cheek and gum and slowly dissolves (Figure 18-6). It is then absorbed through the oral mucosa. Sometimes medications are given by the buccal route for

PROCEDURE 18-6

ADMINISTERING ORAL MEDICATION TO A CHILD

ABHES VII.MA.A.1 9(j)   CAAHEP I.P (8); II.A (1)

OBJECTIVE: To administer oral medication to a child per physician's orders.

STANDARD: This task takes 5–10 minutes.

EQUIPMENT AND SUPPLIES: Oral medication; liquid to assist swallowing; measuring devices; pill cutter or mortar and pestle; patient's record; pen.

STEPS:

1. Follow Procedure 18-1 to prepare for medication administration and Procedure 18-2 for medication administration protocol.
2. Prepare oral medications following procedural steps in Procedure 18-3.
3. Identify patient by asking patient's name and birth date, checking identification band, or checking with parent or caregiver who is present.
4. Speak to child in age-appropriate manner. Explain that it is time to take her medicine. Explain purpose of medication to family present.
5. Assess vital signs if indicated.

6. Administer Medication as follows:

   Pill:

   - Ask family if child can swallow medicine or would prefer it in soft food.
   - Administer medication in age-appropriate manner.
   - Follow with liquids of child's choice to assist swallowing.
   - Make sure that patient swallowed all medication.
   - Praise child in age-appropriate manner for taking medication.

   Liquid medication:

   - Aspirate prescribed dose into dropper or syringe and place it in buccal area of mouth aiming at cheek.
   - Allow child to suck medication or squeeze it slowly into mouth. If an infant allow her to suck medication from a nipple.

7. Document medication given in patient's record.

CHARTING EXAMPLE: 11/25/XX 9:00 A.M. 1 mL ampicillin 250 mg/mL given by mouth per physician's orders. Pt. swallowed full dose of medication ordered. · · · · · · · · · · · · D. Lacy, RMA

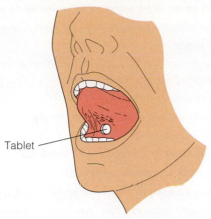

FIGURE 18-5 Sublingual administration of a tablet.

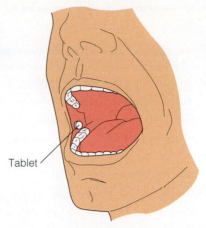

FIGURE 18-6 Buccal administration of a tablet.

topical relief, as with throat lozenges, thus providing a local rather than systemic effect.

Instillation of medications refers to administering drops or ointments or sprays to eyes, ear, and nose. These were discussed in Chapter 5. To review these procedures see the following:

- Procedure 5-26 (Instilling Eye Medication)
- Procedure 5-30 (Instilling Ear Medication)
- Procedure 5-31 (Instilling Nasal Medication)

Inhalation refers to medications that are inhaled as sprays, gases, or vapors. To review these procedures see the following:

- Procedure 21-6 (Instructing a Patient to Use a Metered-Dose Inhaler)
- Procedure 21-7 (Administering a Nebulized Breathing Treatment)
- Procedure 21-8 (Administering Oxygen by Nasal Cannula or Face Mask)

TOPICAL MEDICATIONS

Topical medications include creams, lotions, sprays, ointments, and liniments. These medications are applied to skin, to a wound, or to both. Antibiotics, moisturizers, sunscreen, and medications to relieve itching are typical topical medications.

Transdermal medications are administered in the form of a patch applied to the skin. The location of the patch depends on the manufacturer's directions and the patient's conditions. A transdermal patch releases medication onto the skin. The medication is then absorbed through the skin and eventually into the bloodstream for slow, steady release of medication. A transdermal patch should never be cut because the entire dose of medication is released immediately. Accidental overdose or death may result. Patches can remain in place for varying periods, depending on the medication. Some are left on for several hours, days or weeks. This route of administration eliminates the need for the patient to remember to take frequent oral doses and assists with noncompliance problems. Medications prescribed in this form include pain medication, hormone replacement therapy, angina medication, and birth control. The procedures for applying topical and transdermal medications follow.

SUPPOSITORIES

Suppositories are capsule-shaped medications covered with a substance such as cocoa butter that melts at body temperature.

PROCEDURE 18-7

APPLYING TOPICAL MEDICATION

ABHES VII.MA.A.1 9(m)   CAAHEP II.P (1); II.A (1)

OBJECTIVE: To correctly apply topical medication ordered by physician.

STANDARD: This task takes 5–10 minutes.

EQUIPMENT AND SUPPLIES: Medication (tube, jar, bottle); soap and water; gloves; gauze or dressing as ordered; tape; pen; biohazard waste container; patient's record.

STEPS:

1. Follow Procedure 18-1 to prepare for medication administration and Procedure 18-2 for medication administration protocol.
2. Assemble other equipment and supplies.
3. Identify patient, and explain procedure.
4. Provide privacy as needed, and explain purpose of medication.
5. Perform hand hygiene.
6. Don gloves.
7. Cleanse skin in area with soap and water. Dry thoroughly.
8. Squeeze medication from tube, or apply medication to tongue blade.
9. Using a gloved hand, apply medication smoothly over area.
10. Apply dressing if ordered.
11. Remove and dispose of gloves properly.
12. Perform hand hygiene.
13. Return medication to proper storage area.
14. Document procedure in patient's record.

CHARTING EXAMPLE: 11/27/07 10:20 A.M. Bacitracin oint. Applied to wound area on L forearm. WD area was dry with no disc. · S. Campo, RMA

PROCEDURE 18-8

APPLYING TRANSDERMAL MEDICATION

ABHES VII.MA.A.1 9(m)   CAAHEP II.P (1); II.A (1)

OBJECTIVE: To correctly apply transdermal medication following manufacturer's directions.

STANDARD: This task takes 10 minutes.

EQUIPMENT AND SUPPLIES: Medication patch or tube; gloves; soap and water; premeasured medication administration paper; pen; plastic wrap (optional); pen; patient's record; biohazard waste container.

STEPS:

1. Follow Procedure 18-1 to prepare for medication administration and Procedure 18-2 for following medication administration protocol.
2. Obtain transdermal patch or premeasured paper provided with medication. Read manufacturer's directions thoroughly.
3. Assemble other equipment and supplies.
4. Identify the patient, and explain procedure.

Safety Alert! Remind patient not to place heating pad over patch area. Heat may increase absorption of medication.

5. Provide privacy as needed, and explain purpose of medication.
6. Perform hand hygiene, and don gloves.
7. Administer medication as follows:

   Patch:
   - Remove previous patch, and discard in biohazard waste container. Rotate application areas to prevent skin irritation.
   - Cleanse area before applying new patch.
   - Remove protective cover from patch (Figure18-7A), and apply to clean, dry, hairless area. Press firmly for 30 seconds to ensure good adhesion (Figure 18-7B).

   Premeasured paper:
   - Squeeze required dose on paper. Apply paper to skin and spread medication using paper over two inch area.
   - Cover paper with plastic wrap or tape. Label with date time and initials.

8. Remove and dispose of gloves in biohazard waste container. Perform hand hygiene.
9. Document administration of medication in patient's record.

CHARTING EXAMPLE: 11/27/XX 10:00 A.M. 2% nitroglycerin ointment applied in transdermal patch to L. thorax. · O. Campo, CMA (AAMA)

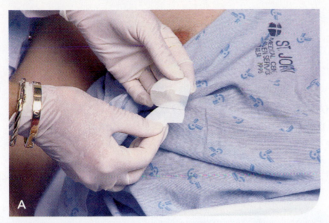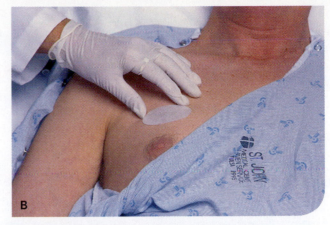

FIGURE 18-7 (A) Remove the protective coating from the patch; (B) apply patch immediately to clean, dry, hairless skin and label with date, time, and initials.

These medications are usually stored in a cool place or in the refrigerator until needed. Suppositories are inserted into the rectum or vagina. Patients may administer them at home for constipation, vaginal yeast infection, and to reduce fever in adult patients and smaller children who are unable to swallow tablets or are suffering from nausea and vomiting. Procedures for administering rectal and vaginal suppositories follow.

PROCEDURE 18-9

ADMINISTERING RECTAL SUPPOSITORIES

ABHES VII.MA.A.1 9(m)   CAAHEP I.P (10)

OBJECTIVE: To correctly insert rectal suppository per physician's orders.

STANDARD: This task takes 5 minutes.

EQUIPMENT AND SUPPLIES: Suppository as ordered; gloves; tissues; paper towel; pen; patient's record; biohazard waste container; lubricant.

STEPS:

1. Check medication order. Check expiration date of order. Check for patient allergies. Follow Procedure 18-1 to prepare for medication administration and Procedure 18-2 for medication administration protocol.
2. Perform hand hygiene.
3. Assemble equipment and supplies.
4. Remove prescribed dose of suppository from refrigerator if necessary.
5. Identify patient, and explain procedure and purpose of medication.
6. Provide privacy, and assist patient into Sims' position.
7. Squeeze lubricant onto paper towel.
8. Remove foil wrapper from suppository.
9. Moisten suppository tip with lubricant or warm water to ease insertion.
10. Don gloves, inspect anal area for hemorrhoids, and expose anal area with care.
11. Ask patient to bear down to help open anus. Insert suppository about 1½ inches (for adult, less for child) into rectal canal (Figure 18-8).
12. Ask patient to lie still for 15 minutes to allow coating of suppository to begin to melt. Medication begins to work in about 1 hour.
13. Dispose of gloves in biohazard waste container, and perform hand hygiene.

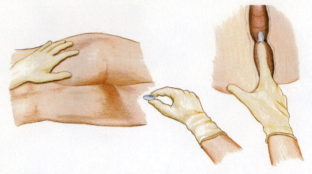

FIGURE 18-8   Inserting a rectal suppository.

14. After 15 minutes has elapsed, assist patient into comfortable position. Explain what effect medication should have and what patient should expect.

15. Document administration of medication in patient's record.

CHARTING EXAMPLE: 11/27/XX 11:00 A.M. glycerin rectal supp. administered for constipation. Pt. reported BM after 1 hour. · M. Dennehey, CMA (AAMA)

PROCEDURE 18-10

ADMINISTERING A VAGINAL SUPPOSITORY

ABHES VII.MA.A.1 9(m)   CAAHEP I.P (10)

OBJECTIVE: To correctly insert a vaginal suppository per physician's order.

STANDARD: This task takes 10 minutes.

EQUIPMENT AND SUPPLIES: Vaginal suppository ordered; suppository applicator; gloves; patient's record; pen; biohazard waste container.

STEPS:

1. Check patient's record for order. Check for patient allergies. Follow Procedure 18-1 to prepare for medication administration and Procedure 18-2 for medication administration protocol.

2. Check expiration date of suppository.

3. Perform hand hygiene.

4. Assemble equipment and supplies.

5. Identify patient, and explain procedure and purpose of medication.

6. Provide privacy.

7. Don gloves, and assist patient into Sims' or dorsal recumbent position.

8. Remove wrapper from suppository and insert into applicator.

9. Insert applicator with suppository into vaginal canal about 2 inches.

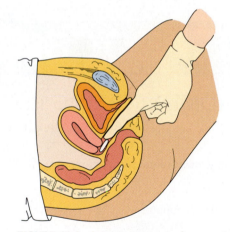

FIGURE 18-9   Inserting a vaginal suppository.

10. Ask patient to lie still for about 15 minutes until absorption of suppository takes place.

11. Discard equipment. Remove and dispose of gloves in biohazard waste container.

12. Perform hand hygiene.

13. Document administration of vaginal suppository in patient's record.

CHARTING EXAMPLE: 11/27/XX 11:45 A.M. Vag. suppository (Monistat) given. No discharge or odor noted. · G. Calitas, RMA

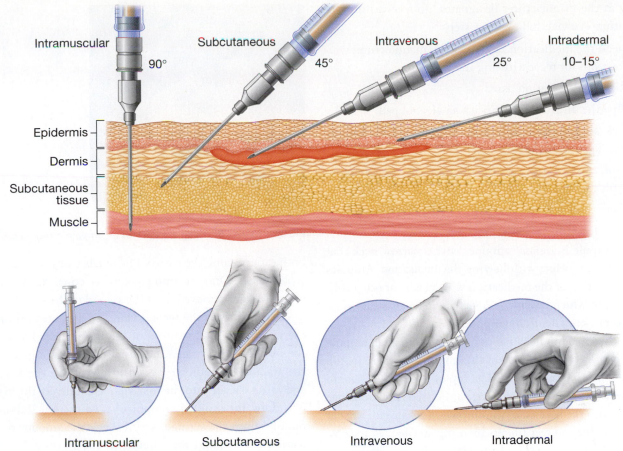

FIGURE 18-10 Angle of needle insertion for four types of injections.

PARENTERAL MEDICATIONS

Parenteral medications are administered through injection. The routes include intradermal, subcutaneous, intramuscular, and intravenous. (Figure 18-10 illustrates the angle of insertion for the four types of injections.) Generally, medications administered by injection reach the bloodstream more quickly than those administered by other routes. Some parenteral medications may be targeted to a particular area, such as a local anesthetic prior to excision of a cyst.

Injections are named for the tissue into which they are administered. Individuals performing injections must have training and be approved for these procedures under current federal and state medical practice acts.

Parenteral Medication Equipment

Several types of syringes are available in a variety of sizes. The size of the syringe and the gauge and length of the needle depend on the type of medication to be given. (Figure 18-11 shows a syringe with all its parts labeled.) Federal legislation requires health care facilities to provide equipment to protect against accidental needlesticks.

Injectable medications are supplied in a variety of containers. They may be supplied in vials, ampules, prefilled cartridges, and powders that need to be reconstituted. Vials are glass or plastic containers sealed by a stopper. Once the plastic or metal cap is removed, the stopper must be cleaned with 70% alcohol before using the medication. To aspirate medication from the vial, an equal amount of air must be injected into the container. To withdraw medication, the vial is turned upside down and the needle inserted with the syringe held at eye level so the barrel can be read accurately.

Vials may contain a single dose or multiple doses. Once a multiple dose vial is opened, the date and time of opening must be noted on the container. It is strongly recommended that a filtered needle or filter straw be used for medications supplied in vials or ampules. This prevents particles of glass or rubber being withdrawn from the these containers.

Medications in vials in powder form must be reconstituted with a specific sterile diluent (sterile water or saline)

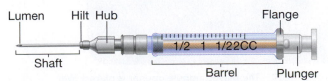

FIGURE 18-11 A hypodermic needle, with parts labeled.

exactly as the manufacturer designates. To reconstitute dry medication in a vial, follow these steps:

- Check the medication label and the manufacturer's directions for reconstituting instructions.
- Check the expiration date.
- Wipe the diluent vial top with an alcohol pad.
- Insert sterile syringe, and withdraw designated amount.
- Wipe the top of the powdered medication vial with alcohol, and insert the needle; dispense the exact amount of diluent into the powder.
- To mix, roll vial between palms to dissolve. Avoid shaking vial and causing bubbles.

An ampule is a glass container with a narrow neck that must be broken before withdrawing the medication. Ampules prevent reaction of the medication with plastic or other substances from which other containers are made. Care must be taken to prevent cuts from ampules.

To open an ampule, a safety device known as an ampule opener is placed over the top of the ampule and then the top is broken off (Figure 18-12). The top of the ampule should be tapped before opening to release fluid from the top above the neck into the bottom of the ampule. If an ampule opener is not available, protect fingers by using sterile 2 × 2 gauze to cover the top and neck of the ampule before breaking it (Figure 18-13).

A filtered needle is used to withdraw medication from the ampule to prevent small particles of glass from entering the syringe. The needle should be discarded and replaced with a sterile needle before injecting. The ampule may be inverted to withdraw medication without causing it to spill.

If ordered by the physician, medications may be combined in one syringe using two vials. The medications are removed from the vials in a specific order, and contamination of either medication must be avoided. Determine the total medication volume to be injected. After removing

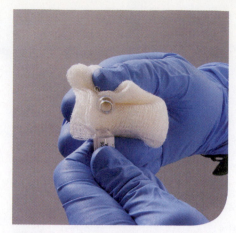

FIGURE 18-13 Breaking the neck of an ampule using gauze.

both caps, cleanse the tops of both vials using separate antiseptic wipes. Draw air into the syringe equal to the amount of liquid to be removed from the second of the two vials, and inject the air into the second vial. (This creates pressure in the vial that allows removal of the liquid later.) Withdraw the needle and syringe, draw air into the syringe equal to the amount of liquid to be withdrawn from the first vial, and inject the air into the first vial. Then invert the vial and withdraw the ordered amount of medication. Remove all bubbles from the syringe, and recheck the amount of medication ordered and the amount in the syringe. Insert the needle into the second vial, and withdraw the prescribed amount of medication, removing bubbles and rechecking as before. (Some facilities require the use of a filter needle to draw up medication, then needles are changed prior to administration.) Proceed to administer medications as ordered. If in doubt about whether two medications may safely be combined, check with the pharmacist on call.

Medications may be drawn up in two separate syringes from two different vials and then combined into the first syringe. After medications are drawn into two separate syringes, the needle is removed from the first syringe and the plunger is pulled back far enough to accommodate all the medication from the second syringe. The needle from the second syringe is then inserted into the hub of the first, and medication is slowly injected from the second syringe into the first. A new sterile needle is then attached to the first syringe to administer the medications ordered.

Medications may be available in prefilled cartridge syringes. The following procedures are presented here: reconstituting powered medication; withdrawing medication from a vial; withdrawing medication from an ampule; preparing for injection by combining medications in one syringe using two different vials; preparing medications in two syringes and combining medications into one syringe; and setting up a prefilled medication cartridge syringe.

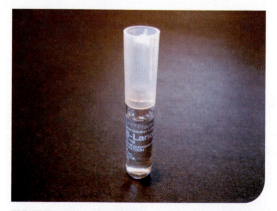

FIGURE 18-12 The plastic ampule opener is placed over the top of the ampule.

PROCEDURE 18-11

RECONSTITUTING POWDERED MEDICATION

ABHES VII.MA.A.1 9(j)   CAAHEP II.P (1); II.A (1)

OBJECTIVE: To correctly reconstitute powdered medication prior to parenteral administration following manufacturer's directions.

STANDARD: This task takes 5 minutes.

EQUIPMENT AND SUPPLIES: Physician's orders; medication; two sterile syringes; reconstituting diluent; sharps container; marker.

STEPS:

1. Check physician's orders, and check for patient allergies.
2. Perform hand hygiene.
3. Assemble equipment and supplies.
4. Obtain medication, and recheck physician's orders to confirm medication matches order.
5. Check expiration date of medication.
6. Check manufacturer's directions for amount and type of diluent to use.
7. Remove caps from both diluent and medication, and cleanse tops of vials with antiseptic.
8. Insert needle of first sterile syringe into diluent, and inject amount of air equal to amount of diluent needed.
9. Withdraw required amount of diluent, and inject diluent into powdered medication vial.
10. Roll vial between palms to enhance mixing. Avoid shaking vial and causing bubbles.
11. Wait required time for medication to completely dissolve.
12. Label vial with date and time of reconstitution.
13. Discard first syringe in sharps container. Use a second sterile syringe to administer medication as ordered by physician.

PROCEDURE 18-12

WITHDRAWING MEDICATION FROM A VIAL

ABHES VII.MA.A.1 9(j)   CAAHEP II.P (1); II.A (1)

OBJECTIVE: To correctly withdraw medication from a vial prior to parenteral administration.

STANDARD: The time this task takes is less than 5 minutes.

EQUIPMENT AND SUPPLIES: Antiseptic wipes; vial of medication; physician's orders; marking pen; sharps container; appropriate-size syringes and needles.

STEPS:

1. Check physician's order for medication. Check for patient allergies.
2. Perform hand hygiene.
3. Assemble equipment and supplies.
4. Obtain medication, and recheck physician's orders to confirm medication matches order.
5. Check expiration date of medication.
6. Remove cap from vial if necessary, and wipe top of vial with antiseptic wipe.
7. Select syringe and needle appropriate to route and type of medication to be given.
8. Pull plunger back equal to amount of medication to be withdrawn from vial.
9. Insert needle into upright vial, and inject air while keeping needle above surface of medication (Figure 18-14).
10. With syringe at eye level, invert vial and pull plunger to exact amount of medication to be given, keeping needle bevel in liquid (Figure 18-15).
11. Leave needle in place in inverted vial, and expel air bubbles by tapping side of syringe with finger below air bubble. Recheck amount of medication in syringe.

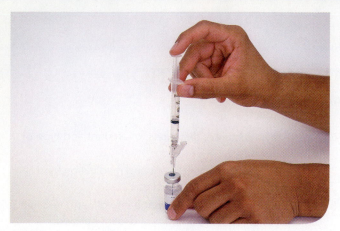

FIGURE 18-14   Injecting air into a vial.

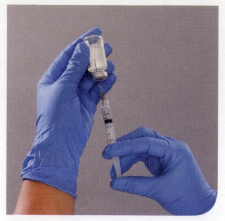

FIGURE 18-15   Withdrawing a medication from an inverted vial.

12. Turn vial upright, and remove needle.

13. Replace needle guard to prevent accidental sticks, or follow facility policy regarding changing needles.

14. Recheck medication and amount against order.

15. Place multiple-dose vials in correct storage area. Mark vial with date, time opened. Medication is ready to be administered to patient.

PROCEDURE 18-13

WITHDRAWING MEDICATION FROM AN AMPULE

ABHES VII.MA.A.1 9(j)   CAAHEP II.P (1); II.A (1)

OBJECTIVE: To correctly open and withdraw medication from an ampule prior to parenteral administration.

STANDARD: This task takes less than 5 minutes.

EQUIPMENT AND SUPPLIES: Physician's orders; ampule of medication; 2 × 2 gauze squares; antiseptic wipe; biohazard waste container; syringes and needles.

STEPS:

1. Check physician's orders, and check for patient allergies.

2. Perform hand hygiene.

3. Assemble equipment and supplies.

4. Obtain medication, and recheck physician's orders to confirm medication matches order.

5. Check expiration date of medication.

6. Tap neck of ampule to move any medication down into body of container.

7. Use ampule opener, or score neck with a file if it is not already marked. Use a gauze pad to grasp neck of ampule between thumb and forefinger of one hand. Hold body of ampule with other hand. Break stem away from body to prevent injury.

8. Set ampule upright on firm surface.

9. Insert filtered needle into ampule, and if needle is long enough withdraw medication. (Figure 18-16A illustrates withdrawing medication from an ampule on a flat surface, and Figure 18-16B illustrates withdrawing medication from an inverted ampule.) If shorter needle is used, invert ampule and withdraw exact amount of medication.

10. Place ampule upright, and withdraw needle.

11. Tap syringe to remove bubbles. Expel air with syringe in upright position. Recheck amount of medication.

12. Cover needle with guard to prevent stick, or follow facility policy regarding changing needles.

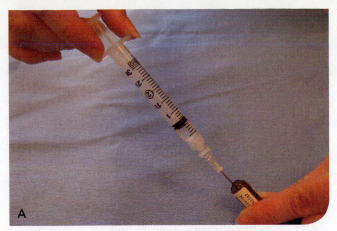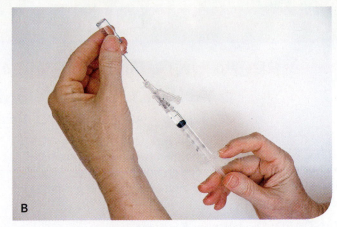

FIGURE 18-16 (A) Withdrawing a medication from an ampule on a flat surface; (B) withdrawing medication from an inverted ampule.

PROCEDURE 18-14

PREPARING FOR INJECTION BY COMBINING MEDICATIONS IN ONE SYRINGE USING TWO DIFFERENT VIALS

ABHES VII.MA.A.1 9(j)   CAAHEP II.P (1); II.A (1)

OBJECTIVE: To correctly combine two medications from two different vials in the same syringe for parenteral administration.

STANDARD: This task takes 5 minutes.

EQUIPMENT AND SUPPLIES: Physician's orders; two medication vials; appropriate-size needles and syringes; marker; sharps container; antiseptic wipes.

STEPS:

1. Check physician's orders, and check for patient allergies.
2. Perform hand hygiene.
3. Assemble equipment and supplies.
4. Obtain medication, and recheck physician's orders to confirm medication matches order.
5. Check expiration date of medication.
6. Remove cap from vials if necessary. Wipe tops of vials with separate antiseptic wipes. If multiple-dose vials are used, mark with date and time of opening.
7. Select syringe and needle appropriate to route and type of medication to be given. Use filtered needles or filter straw whenever possible.
8. Pull plunger back equal to amount of medication to be withdrawn from second vial.
9. Insert needle into second upright vial and inject air, keeping needle above surface of medication. Withdraw needle but not medication at this time.
10. Draw air into syringe equal to amount of medication to be obtained from first vial, and inject it into first vial in same manner as above.
11. Without removing needle, invert first vial and withdraw prescribed amount of medication. Expel all air bubbles.
12. Recheck amount of medication, and remove syringe.
13. Insert needle into second vial, invert vial, and carefully withdraw exact amount of medication ordered.
14. Cover needle with guard to protect against sticks, or follow facility policy regarding changing needles. Avoid contamination until ready to administer to patient.

PROCEDURE 18-15

PREPARING TWO MEDICATIONS IN TWO SYRINGES AND COMBINING INTO ONE SYRINGE

ABHES VII.MA.A.1 9(j)   CAAHEP II.P (1); II.A (1)

OBJECTIVE: To correctly prepare two medications in two syringes to combined into one syringe prior to injecting patient. (This is an alternative method to the one presented in Procedure 18-14.)

STANDARD: This task takes 5 minutes.

EQUIPMENT AND SUPPLIES: Two medication vials; two syringes of appropriate size with correct-size needles; antiseptic wipes; sharps container; marker; gloves.

STEPS:

1. Check physician's orders, and check for patient allergies.
2. Perform hand hygiene.
3. Assemble equipment and supplies.
4. Obtain medication, and recheck physician's orders to confirm medication matches order.
5. Check expiration date of medications.
6. Remove cap from vials if necessary. Wipe tops of vials with separate antiseptic wipes. If multiple-dose vials are used, mark with date and time of opening.
7. Select syringe and needle appropriate to type of medication to be given.
8. First syringe must be large enough to contain entire volume of medication ordered.
9. Prepare each syringe by drawing up dose ordered from each vial or ampule, as indicated in previous procedures.
10. After preparing syringes, remove needle from first syringe.
11. Pull back plunger on first syringe enough to allow second medication to be added to first syringe.
12. Insert needle of second syringe into hub of first syringe, and slowly inject medication from second syringe into first syringe. Recheck total amount.
13. Attach a new needle of appropriate gauge and length to first syringe. Cover needle with guard to protect against contamination and needlestick until time of administration.

PROCEDURE 18-16

SETTING UP A PREFILLED DISPOSABLE MEDICATION CARTRIDGE SYRINGE

ABHES VII.MA.A.1 9(j)   CAAHEP II.P (1); II.A (1)

OBJECTIVE: To set up a prefilled disposable medication syringe in a reusable cartridge holder for parenteral administration of medication.

STANDARD: This task takes 5 minutes.

EQUIPMENT AND SUPPLIES: Physician's orders; prefilled medication cartridge; cartridge holder syringe; biohazard waste container; sharps container.

STEPS:

1. Check physician's orders, and check for patient allergies.
2. Perform hand hygiene.
3. Assemble equipment and supplies.
4. Obtain medication and recheck physician's orders to confirm medication matches order.
5. Check expiration date of medications.

6. Hold reusable cartridge syringe (e.g., tube) in one hand, and pull plunger back with other hand.

7. Insert prefilled medication cartridge needle first into cartridge holder.

8. Twist flange of reusable cartridge syringe clockwise until it is secure.

9. Screw plunger rod onto screw at bottom of medication cartridge until in place in rubber stopper.

10. Remove needle guard, and expel any bubbles.

11. Recheck amount of medication in syringe and amount ordered. If amount in syringe is greater than needed, expel excess medication while taking care not to contaminate needle.

NOTE: If the needle becomes contaminated, the cartridge must be discarded.

12. After injecting patient, remove entire cartridge from holder and discard in sharps container. Holder may be reused after cleaning with alcohol or according to facility protocol.

Administering Parenteral Medication

The term *parenteral* means "not through the gastrointestinal tract." The common parenteral injection routes are intradermal, subcutaneous, intramuscular, and intravenous. Previous sections of this chapter presented the types of syringes, needles, and how to draw up medications into a syringe from various types of medication containers. In addition, identification of the patient and safety precautions are covered. The remainder of this chapter is devoted to how, why, where, and what to give when administering intradermal, subcutaneous, and intramuscular injections. Intravenous methods and techniques are covered in Chapter 19.

The maximum amount of medication that can safely be administered in each of the following routes is as follows:

- Intradermal: 0.01 to 0.1 mL
- Subcutaneous: 0.5 to 1.0 mL
- Intramuscular: 1 to 2 mL in an adult (except into the deltoid, which is a smaller muscle: 0.5 to 1.0 mL)

Legal Alert! Many states view the skill of medication administration as nondelegable to assistive personnel in acute care settings. Every professional caregiver must be aware of the federal, state, and local ordinances governing administration of medications and the ability to delegate that task.

ADMINISTERING INTRADERMAL INJECTIONS

Intradermal injections are administered just below the surface of the skin. This route allows for slower absorption of medication because the intradermal area is less enriched with blood vessels than deeper tissues. A typical intradermal medication is the Purified Protein Derivative Antigen (PPD) for tuberculin (TB) testing. Allergy testing, mentioned in Chapter 5, also involves intradermal injections. Small amounts of medication are injected (0.01–0.10 mL) by this route. The most common sites for intradermal injections are the forearm and the upper back. Any site used for injection should be free of irritation, lesions, and excess hair (Figure 18-17). A small syringe with a ¼- to ½-inch fine gauge needle (26–27) is generally used. The needle is inserted into the skin at angles of 10° to 15° with the bevel up. The steps for performing an intradermal injection are given in Procedure 18-17.

ADMINISTERING SUBCUTANEOUS INJECTIONS

The subcutaneous route is used when medication must be absorbed more slowly than if given intramuscularly. (Muscle tissue has a richer blood supply and thus allows for more rapid distribution of medication than does the fatty subcutaneous tissue.) The subcutaneous route is used for insulin, heparin, tetanus toxoid, allergy medications, epinephrine, and vaccines such as measles, mumps, and rubella (MMR). Small doses of nonirritating, water-soluble, nonviscous medication are given by this route. If large amounts of irritating substances are administered, a sterile abscess could form and cause a painful, hard lump. Irritating substances are administered intramuscularly because they will be absorbed more quickly.

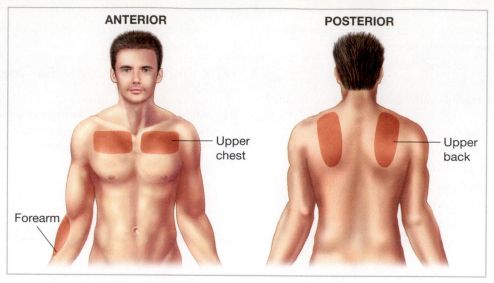

FIGURE 18-17 Body sites commonly used for intradermal injections.

PROCEDURE 18-17

ADMINISTERING AN INTRADERMAL INJECTION

ABHES VII.MA.A.1 9(j)   CAAHEP II.P (9); II.A (1)

OBJECTIVE: To correctly administer an intradermal injection and document procedure properly.

STANDARD: This procedure takes 5 minutes.

EQUIPMENT AND SUPPLIES: Physician's orders; medication; tuberculin syringe with small needle; antiseptic wipes; gauze pads; gloves; pen; patient's record; sharps container; biohazard waste container.

STEPS:

1. Follow steps for preparing for medication administration (Procedure 18-1), following administration of medication protocol (Procedure 18-2), and preparing injections from a vial or ampule (Procedure 18-12 or 18-13).
2. Identify patient, and explain procedure.
3. Select a site free of lesions and excess hair for injection.
4. Perform hand hygiene, and don gloves if required.
5. Cleanse area with antiseptic wipe, and allow to dry.
6. Remove needle cover.
7. Pull skin taut in selected area.
8. Holding syringe almost parallel to skin, insert needle at a 10° to 15° angle with bevel up. Bevel should be visible through skin (Figure 18-18A).
9. Do not aspirate.
10. Slowly inject medication to produce a wheal under skin (Figure 18-18B). If no wheal develops, medication was injected into deeper tissue.
11. Withdraw needle at same angle it was inserted. Do not rub or massage area.
12. Use needle safety device. Dispose of needle and syringe in sharps container.
13. Mark area for easy identification during future evaluation.
14. Assess patient and make him or her comfortable.
15. Dispose of gloves, and perform hand hygiene.
16. Document patient's record with date, time, route, site, and type and amount of medication given.
17. Observe patient for 15 minutes in case of allergic testing. For PPD testing, instruct patient to return in 48 to 72 hours for test reading.

CHARTING EXAMPLE: 01/08/XX 8:15 A.M. PPD test given (L) forearm 0.10 mL/D. Pt. instructed to return in 48 hours for recheck. · N. Dow, RMA

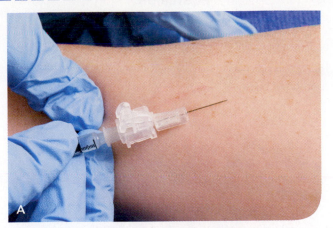
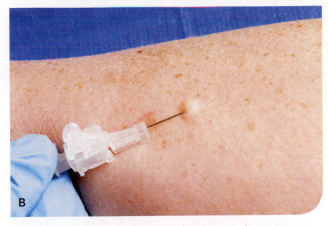

FIGURE 18-18 (A) For a subcutaneous injection, insert the needle bevel up at an angle of less than 15°; (B) when a subcutaneous injection is properly administered, the medication forms a bleb or wheal under the epidermis.

The most common sites used for subcutaneous injections are the outer portion for the upper arm, the abdomen away from the umbilicus, the anterior part of the thigh, and the back below the scapular area (Figure 18-19). Rotation of injection sites is necessary to avoid injury to the tissue. A patient may be required to administer medications by injection at home to regulate glucose levels, in which case patients should be taught to keep a chart of sites used for daily injections.

Generally a 1, 2, or 3 mL syringe with a ⅜- to ⅝-inch-long 25 to 27 gauge needle is used for subcutaneous injections. Insulin syringes are marked in units and are available in sizes of 30, 50, and 100 units. The syringe is held like a dart, and the needle is inserted at a 45° to 90° angle. A 90° angle is used with short needles; however, the angle depends on the amount of subcutaneous tissue at the site used. The skin at the site should be grasped so about 1 inch of tissue is "pinched." Once the needle is inserted, depending on the medication and the recommendations of the pharmacy, the plunger should be pulled back to aspirate and make sure that the needle is in a blood vessel. If blood is returned, the needle should be withdrawn and discarded, and a new injection should be prepared. Injecting medication into a blood vessel may be dangerous because it is absorbed more quickly than is safe. Aspiration is not recommended with certain medications.

Tissue at a subcutaneous injection sites may be "spread" with fingers if there is considerable fatty tissue. The CDC has no regulations about wearing gloves during injections. If the danger of blood contact is great, then gloves should be worn. The facility protocol should dictate the gloving policy.

ADMINISTERING INTRAMUSCULAR INJECTIONS

Intramuscular (IM) injections are used when more rapid absorption of medication is desired. This is the route used for injecting hormones, pain medications, and some vaccines.

BOX 18-4 TB Tests

There are two types of tests for tuberculosis in use: the tine test and the Mantoux test. To administer the tine test, the forearm is cleansed and the an applicator consisting of four prongs or tines containing purified protein derivative (PPD) is pressed firmly on the clean area. The Mantoux test, considered more accurate by the CDC, consists of injecting PPD by intradermal injection. In either case, the patient must return for evaluation 48 to 72 hours later. A hard raised area at the site larger than 10 mm is considered a positive reaction. The patient who tests positive will need follow-up testing and a complete history and physical.

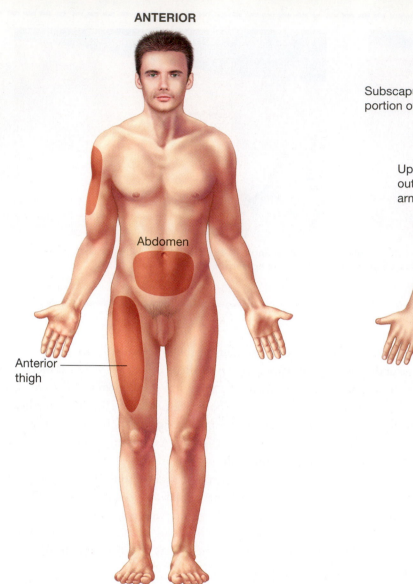

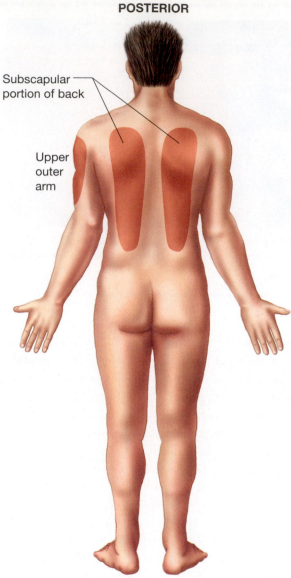

ANTERIOR

POSTERIOR

Subscapular portion of back

Upper outer arm

Abdomen

Anterior thigh

FIGURE 18-19 Body sites commonly used for subcutaneous injections.

PROCEDURE 18-18

ADMINISTERING A SUBCUTANEOUS INJECTION

ABHES VII.MA.A.1 9(j)   CAAHEP II.P (9); II.A (1)

OBJECTIVE: To correctly administer a subcutaneous injection and document procedure properly.

STANDARD: This task takes 5–10 minutes.

EQUIPMENT AND SUPPLIES: Physician's orders; medication; tuberculin syringe with small needle; antiseptic wipes; gauze pads; gloves; pen; patient's record; sharps container; biohazard waste container; patient's record.

STEPS:

1. Follow steps for preparing for medication administration (Procedure 18-1), administration of medication protocol (Procedure 18-2), and preparing injections from a vial or ampule (Procedure 18-12 or 18-13).

2. Identify patient, and explain procedure.

3. Select a site that is free of irritation, infection, edema, or bruises. Avoid those that have been recently used for injection. Select a needle that is one-half the length of skinfold when grasped.

4. Assist patient into comfortable position.

5. Perform hand hygiene, and don gloves if required.

6. Cleanse area with antiseptic wipe, and allow to air-dry. Hold antiseptic wipe between fingers of nondominant hand.

7. Remove needle guard and "pinch an inch" of skin between forefinger and thumb of nondominant hand (Figure 18-20).

8. Holding syringe like a dart, insert needle at a 45° to 90° angle. If indicated, aspirate by pulling back plunger with thumb of dominant hand.

9. If no blood appears, inject medication slowly; wait a few seconds, then remove needle at same angle of insertion.

10. Use needle safety device to protect against needlesticks.

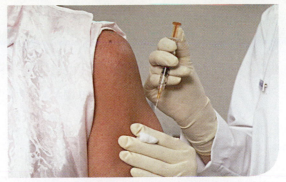

FIGURE 18-20 Administering subcutaneous injection into pinched tissue.

11. Massage injection site to promote absorption of medication, unless contraindicated by pharmacy directions.

12. Assist patient into a comfortable position. Discard syringe and needle in sharps container.

13. Remove and dispose of gloves in biohazard waste container. Perform hand hygiene.

14. Document patient's record with date, time, route, site, and amount and type of medication.

CHARTING EXAMPLE: 01/09/XX 9:00 A.M. Insulin 20 U given subcutaneously into anterior (L) thigh. · · · · · · · · · · · · · ·
· I. Haverstad, CMA (AAMA)

Syringes up to 5 mL with needles varying in length, depending on the age and condition of the patient, are used for IM injections. Generally needles are 1 to 2 inches long with gauges between 19 and 23. The selection of a site also depends on the age and weight of the patient, the viscosity of the medication, and patient preference whenever possible. The following are the commonly used sites:

- **Deltoid muscle.** Only a small amount of medication may be injected into this triangular muscle in the upper arm. Locate the site by placing your hand on the patient's shoulder, palpating the acromion process, and coming down 2 to 3 inches. This muscle is not well developed in children.

- **Vastus lateralis muscle.** This muscle is located in the anterior, lateral part of the thigh. It is the preferred site for injecting infants and children intramuscularly and is used for all ages because it is away from major blood vessels and nerves.

- **Ventrogluteal muscle.** To locate this part of the gluteus medius muscle, place the palm on the greater trochanter of the femur with the index finger on the anterior portion of the superior iliac spine and the middle finger spread out posteriorly as far as possible. The injection site is the middle of this triangular area.

- **Dorsogluteal muscle.** This injection site is in the upper outer quadrant of the buttocks. To inject here, place your hand on the iliac crest, locate the superior iliac spine, and place a mark. Then locate the greater trochanter of the femur, place a mark, and draw an imaginary line between the two marks you have made.

When administering large amounts of medication at one time it is better to split the doses and inject into two different sites.

ADMINISTERING Z-TRACK INJECTIONS

Administering medications using the Z-track method prevents the medication from leaking out through the needle "track" just created. Some medications are irritating or cause staining in the surrounding tissue, thus the Z-track method should be used. If in doubt, consult a drug reference

PROCEDURE 18-19

ADMINISTERING AN INTRAMUSCULAR INJECTION

ABHES VII.MA.A.1 9(j)   CAAHEP II.P (9); II.A (1)

OBJECTIVE: To correctly administer an intramuscular injection and document the procedure properly.

STANDARD: This task takes 5–10 minutes.

EQUIPMENT AND SUPPLIES: Physician's orders; medication; syringe and needle appropriate for patient and medication; antiseptic wipes; gauze pads; gloves; pen; patient's record; sharps container; biohazard waste container.

STEPS:

1. Follow steps for preparing for medication administration (Procedure 18-1), administration of medication protocol (Procedure 18-2), and preparing injections from a vial or ampule (Procedure 18-12 or 18-13).

2. Identify patient, and explain procedure.

3. Select a site that is free of irritation, infection, edema, or bruises. Use identifying landmarks to locate correct site. Avoid sites that have been used recently for injection. When selecting a site, consider the patient's age and size. When choosing a needle and syringe, consider the amount and viscosity of medication and the injection site.

4. Assist patient into comfortable position. Positions that may be used, depending on the route of administration, are deltoid (standing, sitting, or supine with arm relaxed; Figure 18-21); vastus lateralis (infant, supine; Figure 18-22); ventrogluteal (lying on side or back with knee and hip slightly flexed; Figure 18-23); and dorsogluteal (prone with feet turned inward, or on side with upper knee and hip flexed and in front of lower leg).

5. Perform hand hygiene, and don gloves if required.

6. Cleanse area with antiseptic wipe, and allow to air-dry. Hold antiseptic wipe between fingers of nondominant hand.

7. Remove needle guard. Spread skin taut between thumb and forefinger. In children and some geriatric patients with less fatty tissue, grasping of muscle is permitted.

8. Holding syringe like a dart, insert needle at a 90° angle. Aspirate by pulling back plunger with thumb of dominant hand.

9. If no blood appears, inject medication slowly. Wait a few seconds, then remove needle at same angle of insertion.

10. Use needle safety device to protect against needlesticks.

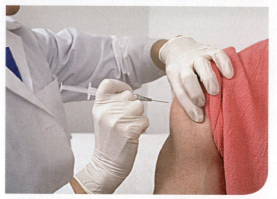
FIGURE 18-21 Administering an intramuscular injection into the deltoid site.

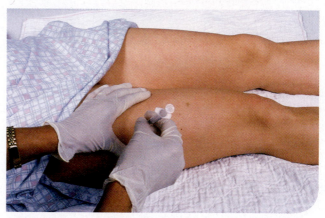
FIGURE 18-22 Administering an intramuscular injection into the vastus lateralis site of an adult.

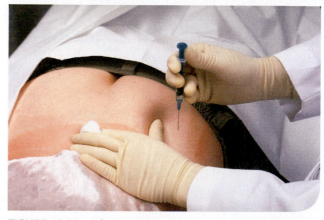
FIGURE 18-23 Administering an intramuscular injection into the ventrogluteal site.

11. Massage injection site to promote absorption of medication unless contraindicated by pharmacy directions.

12. Assist patient into a comfortable position. Discard syringe and needle in sharps container.

13. Remove and dispose of gloves in biohazard waste container. Perform hand hygiene.

14. Document patient's record with date, time, route, site, and amount and type of medication.

CHARTING EXAMPLE: 01/09/XX 10:00 A.M. Demerol 75 mg given in (L) deltoid per physician's orders. Pt. indicated relief of pain in 35 minutes. · · · · · · · · · · · · · · · C. Corso, CMA (AAMA)

book such as the PDR or ask the pharmacist on duty. This method is similar to an intramuscular method, except that the skin is pulled to one side before injecting and then released to effectively seal off the "track" made by the needle. When injecting irritating medications, change the needle after drawing up the medications to prevent tissue discomfort.

An air lock injected after the medication has been administered helps to seal off the area and prevent medication leakage. To create an air lock after the medication is drawn up, aspirate 0.2 mL of air. The air will rise above the medication during injection, enter the tissue last, and seal off the injection track.

PROCEDURE 18-20

ADMINISTERING A Z-TRACK INJECTION
ABHES VII.MA.A.1 9(j)   CAAHEP II.P (9); II.A (1)

OBJECTIVE: To administer a Z-track injection and document properly.

STANDARD: This task takes 5–10 minutes.

EQUIPMENT AND SUPPLIES: Physician's orders; medication; syringe and needle appropriate for patient and medication; antiseptic wipes; gauze pads; gloves; pen; patient's record; sharps container; biohazard waste container.

STEPS:

1. Follow steps for preparing for medication administration (Procedure 18-1), administration of medication protocol (Procedure 18-2), and preparing injections from a vial or ampule (Procedure 18-12 or 18-13).

2. Identify patient, and explain procedure.

3. Select a site that is free of irritation, infection, edema, or bruises. Use identifying landmarks to locate correct site. Avoid those that have been recently used for injection. When selecting a site, consider the patient's age and size. When choosing a needle and syringe, consider the amount and viscosity of medication and the injection site.

4. Assist patient into comfortable position. (Prone position makes it easier to identify landmark for dorsogluteal injection.)

5. Perform hand hygiene, and don gloves.

6. Cleanse area with antiseptic wipe, and allow to air-dry. Hold antiseptic wipe between fingers of nondominant hand.

7. Remove needle guard, and pull skin 1 to 1½ inches to side away from site (Figure 18-24).

8. Holding syringe like a dart, insert needle at a 90° angle. If indicated, aspirate by pulling back plunger with thumb of dominant hand.

9. If no blood appears, inject medication and air bubble slowly; wait 10 seconds, then remove needle and release tissue (Figures 18-25A and 18-25B).

10. Use needle safety device to protect against needlesticks.

11. Apply light pressure with wipe; do not massage injection site. (Massaging area may cause irritating medication to enter subcutaneous tissue and cause tissue irritation.)

12. Assist patient into comfortable position. Discard syringe and needle in sharps container.

13. Remove and dispose of gloves in biohazard waste container. Perform hand hygiene.

14. Document patient's record with date, time, route, site, and amount and type of medication.

CHARTING EXAMPLE: 01/10/XX 11:00 A.M. 30 mcg Interferon given IM (L dorsogluteal muscle) using Z-track. Pt. tolerated inj. well. · · · · · · · · · · · · · · L. Monahan, CMA (AAMA)

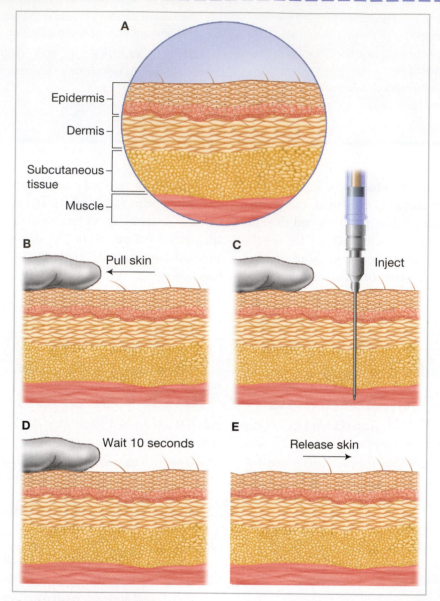

FIGURE 18-24 An example of the Z-track method of injection.

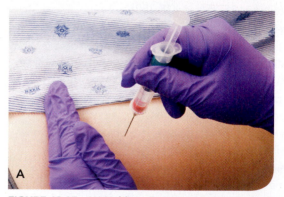

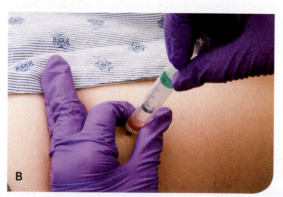

FIGURE 18-25 (A) Holding the syringe between the thumb and forefinger. Note the other hand is using the Z-track technique; (B) in addition to pulling the skin to the side, the nondominant hand is holding the barrel of the syringe to avoid moving it while the dominant hand aspirates by pulling back on the plunger.

19 Intravenous Therapy

PROCEDURES

Advanced Procedure 19-1 Preparing an IV Infusion

Advanced Procedure 19-2 Preparing the Venipuncture Site for IV

Advanced Procedure 19-3 Starting an IV with a Winged Needle

Advanced Procedure 19-4 Inserting an Over-the-Needle Catheter

Advanced Procedure 19-5 Adding Extension Tubing to an IV Set

Advanced Procedure 19-6 Monitoring an Intravenous Infusion

Advanced Procedure 19-7 Changing the IV Solution

Advanced Procedure 19-8 Converting an IV to an Intermittent Infusion Lock

Advanced Procedure 19-9 Administering Medication to an IV Line by Injection "Push"

Advanced Procedure 19-10 Administering Medication Using a Secondary ("Piggyback") Bag

Advanced Procedure 19-11 Administering Medication Using a Peripheral Saline Lock

Advanced Procedure 19-12 Discontinuing an IV

TERMS TO LEARN

infiltration

solvent

solutes

intravascular fluid

osmolarity

total parenteral nutrition (TPN)

peripheral parenteral nutrition (PPN)

bolus

peripheral catheters

central vascular devices (CVADs)

peripheral insertion of central catheter (PICC)

vesicants

IV administration set

electronic infusion devices (EIDs)

iontophoresis

patient-controlled analgesia (PCA)

epidurals

patency

cannula

Note: This chapter covers advanced intravenous therapy procedures. No ABHES or CAAHEP medical assisting standards or guidelines exist for these procedures.

The intravenous (IV) route of administering medications is used when a drug is too irritating to the tissues, a patient is unable to take substances orally, or when immediate action of a drug is desired. Introducing a sterile solution of a drug directly into the bloodstream is a fast and accurate means of administering medication. IV therapy helps to accomplish the following:

- Maintain proper balance of fluids and electrolytes in the body

- Provide nutrition to patients who are unable to eat

- Transfuse blood and blood products to those who have lost blood through accident or illness or lack specific blood products, such as platelets and serum albumin

- Deliver medications

IV therapy is not without risks, like any invasive procedure. Risks include infection, phlebitis, **infiltration** (fluid enters the tissue instead of the bloodstream), overdose, adverse reactions from mixing incompatible drugs, and blood vessel and nerve damage. Aids to daily living are more difficult to use for patients with an IV. IV therapy is more costly than other methods of administering medications.

Legal Regulations

IV treatments are ordered by licensed professionals, such as physicians (MDs), physician's assistants (PAs), doctors of osteopathy (DOs), and advanced practice nurses (APNs). The administration of the IV to the patient is usually performed by a nurse (RN), although some states also permit a licensed practical nurse (LPN) or licensed vocational nurse (LVN) to administer it. Medical and nurse practice acts in each state define the scope of practice for nurses and other professionals in that particular state. Some states permit medical assistants to set up, administer, and regulate IV treatment under the direct order of a physician. Countless facilities require medical assistants to be able to set up an IV tray, to monitor the IV site for signs of infection and infiltration, and to remove an IV when the order to discontinue is given. This chapter covers those facets of IV treatment, as well as setting up and administering an IV and administering medication through an IV. Although the nurse may start the infusion, the medical assistant is an important member of the IV team.

Although medical assistants are not licensed, they do sit for national examinations, RMA and CMA (AAMA), and are registered with their organizations as holding current certification. AAMA-certified medical assistants must earn 60 continuing education units in a 5-year period to maintain their active status. All health care providers should be conversant with the state medical practice acts affecting their particular occupation and should never perform any function outside their particular scope of practice. Ignorance of the law is never an excuse.

Federal and hospital guidelines must be followed closely. Guidelines cover the use of IV equipment, selection of a site, use of the correct-size equipment, proper monitoring of the IV, and knowledge of side effects and complications. Guidelines are established by the CDC, the Joint Commission, and the Infusion Nurses Society (INS) with regard to maintaining IV sites, catheter placement, and applying a dressing to an IV site. Every facility should have IV therapy protocols in place, and employees must be kept up to date with changes to guidelines issued by federal and state agencies.

Intravenous Therapy for Fluid and Electrolyte Balance

The goal of this text is to provide clinical competencies and not to cover the physiology of fluid and electrolyte balance; however, a brief discussion of fluid balances is warranted. The body is composed mainly of fluid. The fluids in the body are composed of water (**solvent**) and dissolved substances (**solutes**). The solutes are electrolytes such as sodium and potassium and nonelectrolytes such as proteins. For a person to be healthy, balance or internal equilibrium (homeostasis) must be maintained in the body. Body fluids help regulate body temperature, transport nutrients and gases, and remove cellular waste products. The fluid in the body is either extracellular (outside the cell) or intracellular (inside the cell). Extracellular fluid (ECF) is found in two forms: interstitial fluid (within tissues) and **intravascular fluid** (blood plasma). Each day fluids are gained and lost in several different ways. The average daily intake of fluid through food and drink is about 2,500 mL, and the daily output through urine, respiratory gases, perspiration, and feces is about the same. Fluid amounts are regulated by hormones, including antidiuretic hormone (ADH) and aldosterone.

Six major electrolytes are found in body fluids: sodium (Na), potassium (K), calcium (Ca), chloride, (Cl), phosphorus (P), and magnesium (Mg). Electrolytes in water come apart to form ions, which are electrically charged particles that conduct current. This electrical current is essential for normal cell function and thus normal body functions. Some electrolytes are found mainly inside the cell (intracellular [ICF] K and P). Sodium (Na) and chloride (Cl) are found mainly outside the cell (extracellular [ECF]). The cell membranes that separate ICF and ECF are semipermeable, meaning that only certain components move freely back and forth. Large molecule substances such as proteins cannot pass easily through the walls, but electrolytes may pass back and forth freely. Body fluids are in constant motion, moving back and forth between fluid areas.

IV infusions are given to correct fluid imbalances. The three types of IV fluids are isotonic, hypotonic, and hypertonic solutions. An isotonic solution has the same **osmolarity** as blood and body fluids, thus it stays where it is infused in the bloodstream. Hypotonic solutions have a lower osmolarity than blood, and fluid will move out of the bloodstream into the cells and interstitial spaces. Thus, a hypotonic solution brings fluid to the cells while decreasing the amount of fluid in the circulatory system. A hypertonic solution has higher osmolarity than blood, thus fluid moves from the cells and interstitial spaces to the bloodstream to reduce edema and stabilize blood pressure.

The following are examples of the three types of IV solutions:

Hypotonic solutions

0.33% sodium chloride

2.5% dextrose in water

half normal saline

Hypertonic solutions

5% dextrose in half normal saline

5% dextrose in normal saline

3% albumin

Isotonic solutions

Ringer's solution

Lactated Ringer's solution

Normal saline

5% dextrose in water

Patients should be assessed for signs of fluid imbalance. A decrease in body fluids is evidenced by decreased weight, decreased blood pressure, dry mouth, cracked lips, decreased urine output, increased thirst, increased electrolyte levels, and decreased tearing. Signs of excess fluid are weight gain, edema (either generalized or in the feet and ankles and fingers), difficulty breathing, elevated blood pressure, distention of the jugular vein, puffy eyelids, and decreased serum electrolytes.

Other Uses of Intravenous Therapy

IV administration of drugs is an effective means of providing rapid treatment. Drugs such as antibiotics, cardiovascular drugs, anticonvulsants, antineoplastics, and thrombolytics are given by this route. The drugs may be given in a continuous infusion over a short time or in one single dose.

Blood and blood products are given by IV to maintain homeostasis, to prevent shock from blood loss, and to maintain adequate blood volume. Whole blood is composed of three formed elements (WBCs, RBCs, platelets) and plasma. Blood may be administered as whole blood or as packed red blood cells (some plasma removed), as an infusion of WBCs, or as platelets. Plasma or albumin may also be administered by IV.

Essential nutrients may be given by the IV route if the patient is unable to absorb nutrients in the normal manner. **Total parenteral nutrition (TPN)** is designed for each patient individually to meet their own requirements and contains proteins, carbohydrates, lipids, electrolytes, vitamins, minerals, and water. Long-term use of TPN can cause liver damage. It is administered by a central line. **Peripheral parenteral nutrition (PPN)** is administered through an IV when limited nutritional therapy is required. The mixture contains fewer nonprotein calories and less amino acid concentration than TPN. PPN may contain lipid emulsions and can be given for about 3 weeks. PPN can cause vein damage and infiltration. Any patient receiving IV nutritional supplements must be monitored closely for intake, output, and electrolyte balance.

Intravenous Delivery Methods

IV solutions may be delivered either by the peripheral route or by the central vein route. Concentrated solutions are given through a central vein, such as concentrated parenteral nutrition with high levels of proteins and dextrose, solutions with pH of less than 5 or more than 9, or chemotherapy that would be irritating to the peripheral tissues. The following are the three basic means for delivering IV therapy:

- Continuous infusion—solutions given over a long period
- Intermittent infusion—solutions given over short periods or at set intervals
- Direct injection (also called IV push or **bolus**)—single dose

The method and site of delivery used for IV therapy depend on the patient's age and condition and the purpose of the therapy. The decision is made by the ordering physician.

CENTRAL VASCULAR ACCESS DEVICES

IV therapy is administered through a variety of catheters and devices. **Peripheral catheters** are the most common type. They are inserted into the veins of the hands, arms, and antecubital area. These are short catheters used for short-term treatments, usually no longer than 5 days. They need to be changed frequently (every 48 to 72 hours), according to the policy of the facility. Peripheral catheters are discussed more fully later in this chapter.

Midline catheters are longer than peripheral catheters and are normally inserted an inch or so above or below the antecubital fossa and into one of the proximal veins of the arm. They are shorter than peripheral insertion of central catheter (PICC) lines (see below) in that they are used for long-term treatments but are shorter in length. Midline catheters are used for administration of nonirritating solutions or medications. Problems of phlebitis, clotting, and thrombosis that occur with a midline catheter are more difficult to access than problems that occur with a shorter peripheral catheter.

Long-term IV therapy generally requires **central vascular devices (CVADs)** that must be medically positioned. These include subcutaneous ports, catheters, and central vascular catheters. CVADs allow repeated access to the patient's vascular system without venipuncture. Patients can to be active while protecting their veins from sclerosis and infection.

Central venous catheters fall into three categories: central catheters, peripheral insertion of central catheter lines, and subcutaneously implanted vascular access ports. Central venous catheters are medically inserted through the chest wall into the jugular or subclavian vein. They are used for administering fluids or blood, obtaining blood specimens, and administration of medications. Catheters can be tunneled and nontunneled. A tunneled catheter is designed for long-term use, is radiopaque, and is most likely made of silicon because silicon is less likely to cause thrombosis than polyurethane. Being radiopaque allows the catheter's placement to be checked by X-ray. A tunneled catheter has a cuff that encourages tissue growth within the tunnel to help stabilize the catheter and keep organisms out of the circulatory system. A nontunneled catheter is designed for short-term use, is also radiopaque, and must be changed according to facility policy.

A **peripheral insertion of central catheter (PICC)** line is inserted in the basilic vein, and the tip rests in the lower one-third of the superior vena cava. This type of central catheter is used to administer **vesicants** (drugs that cause blistering), other irritating medications, blood products, and TPN. Fewer complications occur with a PICC line than with a central venous catheter; however, the PICC's small diameter can occlude frequently. A PICC line does require a peripheral vein large enough to accept the larger bore needle used to introduce the catheter.

The third type of central catheter is the subcutaneously implanted vascular access port (VAP). This type of central access is used when the patient needs long-term IV therapy. It is similar to other central venous catheters except that it has no external parts. Access is gained by inserting a special needle through the skin. This type of venous catheter lessens the chance of infection, is less noticeable, and is less restrictive for the patient.

Peripheral Vascular Access Devices

Note: The following presentation provides advanced information about central venous therapy so the reader will have some familiarity with the terms and definitions related to this important type of IV treatment.

Once the physician's order is written for IV treatment, the selection of a suitable site is made before bringing any equipment to the patient. The procedure and the purpose of treatment are explained to the patient. At this time, a preliminary inspection of the patient's veins and possible site assessment is done. The sites generally used for peripheral IV therapy are the metacarpal, cephalic, and basilic veins and their branches. The more distal veins are preferred over the proximal veins. If the distal vein is damaged, then the more proximal one can be used. The superficial veins on the back of the hand and forearm are good choices. The back of the hand has small superficial veins that are easily dilated. The dorsum (upper surface) of the forearm has long straight veins with larger diameters. The veins of the foot and leg are used as a last resort. Placing IVs on the affected side in mastectomy patients should be avoided. Areas with edema, infection or scarring, cellulitis, a shunt or fistula, or sclerotic veins should be avoided. Scalp veins are suitable for infants because the veins are easily visible. (See Table 19-1 for a list of the peripheral sites and their advantages and disadvantages.)

Intravenous Containers and Administration Sets

Plastic infusion containers are generally used for IV administration. They are soft, flexible bags or semirigid containers that are easy to store, transport, and discard. However, glass

TABLE 19-1 Peripheral Sites for Intravenous Therapy

Site	Location	Advantage	Disadvantage
Digital veins	Lateral and dorsal portions of fingers	Used as last resort for short-term therapy	Requires splinting of fingers; cannot accommodate large volumes
Metacarpal veins	Dorsum of hand	Easily accessible bones of hand	Painful insertion due to nerve endings in hand; wrist movement limited with longer catheter
Accessory cephalic vein	Continuation of metacarpal veins of thumb along radial bone	Large vein, good for venipuncture	May be difficult to position catheter even with skin
Cephalic vein	Radial side of forearm and upper arm	Large vein, good for large-gauge needle	May decrease joint movement due to proximity of device to elbow
Median ante-brachial vein	Emerging from palm on ulnar side of forearm	Satisfactory for winged needles; last resort if nothing else available	Painful insertion; high risk of infiltration
Basilic vein	On ulnar side of forearm and upper arm	Accepts large-bore needles; straight vein good for venipuncture	Inconvenient position for patient during insertion; painful; difficult to stabilize vein
Antecubital veins	In antecubital fossa	Large veins, good for VP, easily visible	May be difficult to stabilize; infiltration risk from fragile veins
Dorsal venous veins	On dorsal portion of foot	Acceptable for infants and toddlers	Increased risk for deep vein thrombosis (DVT); difficult to stabilize and walk
Scalp veins	Bilateral superficial temporal veins (above the ear); metopic vein (mid forehead)	Acceptable for infants, easily visible, may be used as last resort	Difficult to stabilize, increased risk of infiltration from vein fragility

containers are used to deliver medications that are absorbed by plastic, such as nitroglycerin. Glass bottles require venting to allow air in to permit the fluid to flow out. Plastic containers collapse as fluid flows out and do not require venting.

An **IV administration set** includes the tubing that carries the fluid from the container to the patient. Every administration set also has a spike insert that fits into the opening on the infusion container. All types also have drip chambers (vented or nonvented) through which the fluid flows before entering the tubing. All sets have some form of clamp (screw, roller, slide) that provides a means of regulating the flow of the infusion. In addition, all sets end with some form of sterile-capped adapter to which a catheter or other peripheral access device is attached.

Drip chambers are either macrodrip or microdrip systems. Macrodrip systems deliver the infusion in large volumes at a rapid rate, whereas microdrip systems deliver smaller volumes of infusion at a slower rate. The microdrip system is used for pediatric patients and adults requiring small amounts of IV solutions. The drop factor is the number of drops required to deliver 1 mL of medication. Macrodrip systems deliver 10 to 20 drops/mL, and microdrip

systems deliver 60 drops/mL. The rate of drip is determined by the physician and regulated by the appropriate caregiver. Each administration set has the drop factor stated on the set. Some infusion administration sets are used only with **electronic infusion devices (EIDs)**.

The following are the three major types of IV administration sets:

- Basic or primary sets (Figure 19-1A)
- Secondary line or add-a-line sets (Figures 19-1B and 19-1C)
- Volume control sets (Figure 19-1D)

Primary administration sets connect a single container to carry fluid directly to the patient. At the distal end, the set is connected to the catheter with an adapter. A primary administration set may have injection ports through which secondary sets of tubing are added. The Y-type of primary infusion sets are not vented and have two tubes of equal length, each with its own clamp and possibly its own drip chamber. One drip chamber may be placed higher than the other; thus, two infusions can be given at the same time or individually by clamping off one. Check valves or one-way valves are found in many primary sets and are used when

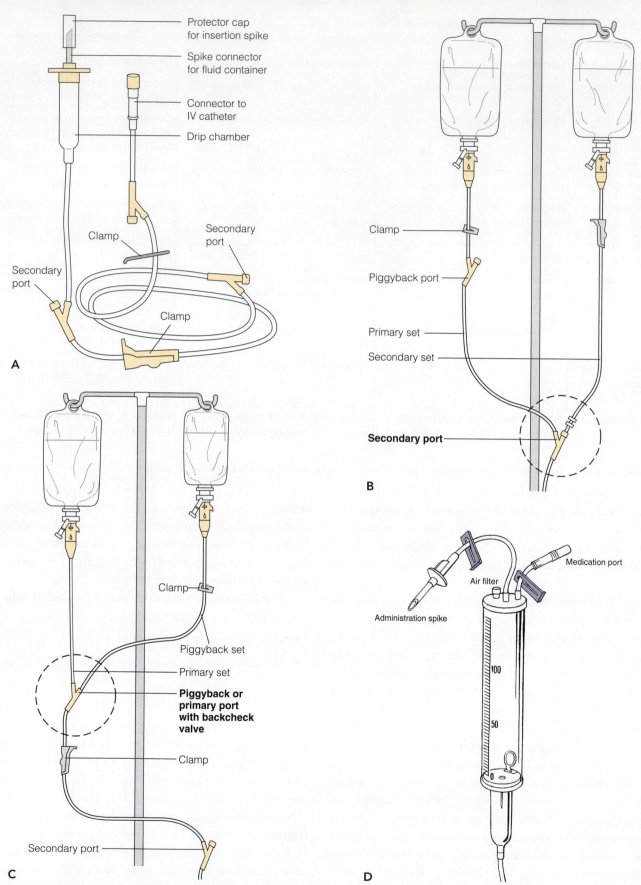

FIGURE 19-1 (A) Standard IV administration set; (B) secondary intravenous lines, a tandem alignment; (C) secondary intravenous lines: "piggyback" set; (D) a volume-control infusion set.

secondary lines are attached to prevent the second infusion from flowing into the primary one. Blood administration sets are Y-type sets. Y-type administration sets can only be used with collapsible containers.

Secondary administration sets, or piggyback sets, are used when either continuous or intermittent flow is required. These sets eliminate the need for a separate venipuncture, and thus the primary infusion does not have to be interrupted.

Volume-control sets deliver exact volumes of infusion and medication and are calibrated in milliliters. The volume control set is used for pediatric patients and others who cannot tolerate large volumes of fluid. Volume-control sets are attached at the top of the administration set above the drip chamber. They may be attached to a Y-site and are available in macro or micro drip systems. Whatever type of administration set is used, a venous access device (catheter or needle) is required to enter the vein.

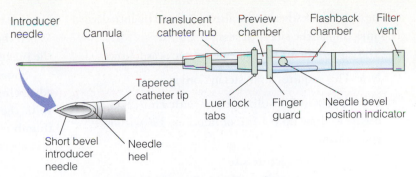

FIGURE 19-2 Schematic of an over-the-needle catheter.

VENOUS ACCESS DEVICES

The most commonly used peripheral venous access devices are catheter sets and winged infusion or butterfly sets. These devices are available in varying lengths and gauges and may be made of a variety of materials (e.g., silicone, polyurethane, Teflon, polyethylene). Plastic catheters are less prone to infiltration than sets with steel needles. Straight steel needles are rarely used to today, except for direct administration of medication to the IV because they tend to dislodge and infiltrate easily.

Winged infusion sets have butterflylike wings attached to the needle on one end and tubing on the other that terminates in a capped hub. The wings make it easier to grip the needle when inserting it. After the insertion the wings are flattened and taped down to secure the device. Before the winged infusion set is inserted, it should be primed with sterile normal saline to remove air and prevent air from entering the vascular system. Winged infusion sets are available in varying gauges and lengths and are used on pediatric patients or for short-term infusions.

The over-the-needle catheter is widely used for venous access. (See Figure 19-2.) It is a flexible catheter and a rigid needle or stylet that is slightly longer than the catheter and that punctures the vein. Generally over-the-needle devices are available in 1- to 1¼-inch lengths and gauges of 14 to 26. These devices are left in place for 2 to 3 days, depending on the facility policy. Once the needle enters the vein, the catheter is threaded into the vein carefully and the needle or stylet is withdrawn. Entrance to the vein can be confirmed by the flow of blood into the chamber just behind the hub. Winged

infusions are also available in over-the-needle sets. The hub is replaced by flexible wings for easier insertion and taping.

Any venous access device that has a catheter can be changed into an intermittent type of administration set by placing a sterile access cap (lock) over the adapter end of the catheter. The lock must be flushed with normal saline to ensure it remains open.

Puncturing the Vein

Chapter 13 described finding the vein, applying the tourniquet, cleansing the area, and entering the vein and should be reviewed at this time. The steps for completing the venipuncture, attaching the IV infusion, and securing the site with a dressing are covered in the following sections. Preparation to set up and attach an IV differs in a few ways from the preparation for a normal venipuncture. Specifically, the tourniquet should be placed 5 to 6 inches above the venipuncture site. Arterial flow should still be present when the tourniquet is in place. The area should be cleaned with 2% chlorhexidine, 10% povidone-iodine solution, or 70% alcohol according to CDC recommendations. The site is cleansed with a swab starting in the center and moving outward without going over areas already cleaned.

All antiseptics must be allowed to air-dry before proceeding with the venipuncture. Local anesthetics are sometimes ordered to reduce pain during a venipuncture. Analgesic cream (e.g., EMLA) is applied at least 30 minutes before the procedure is to be done and lasts about 60 minutes. This form of local anesthesia is good when dealing with children. EMLA is a 5% emulsion preparation of 2.5% lidocaine and 2.5% prilocaine that it is applied to unbroken skin under a patch-type dressing. It must be applied at least 30 minutes to 1 hour prior to performing the venous access.

Another technique, **iontophoresis**, delivers local analgesia to the skin at the site. A small device with two electrodes uses a mild electric current to deliver ions of 2% lidocaine and epinephrine 1:100,000 solution into the skin. This numbs the area and should be administered 10 to 20 minutes ahead of time. A local anesthetic may also be ordered by intradermal (ID) injection at the site of access.

The procedure for ID local anesthetic is as follows:

Note: This requires a physician's order.

- Use a U-100 mL insulin syringe with a fine 27G needle to draw up 0.1 mL of lidocaine 1% without epinephrine.
- Clean the venipuncture site.
- Insert the needle (30° angle) into the skin next to the vein. If vein is deep, inject on top of vein.
- Inject lidocaine without aspirating until a wheal appears. The entire amount may not be required to form a wheal.
- Withdraw the syringe, and massage the wheal to distribute the medication. The area should remain numb for about 30 minutes.

Normal saline produces the same type of anesthetic effect as lidocaine, but it does not sting like lidocaine. Normal saline is injected over and on either side of the vein with a fine needle inserted with the bevel down.

With the infusion and administration set readied (this is covered in detail later in Procedure 19-1), all equipment and supplies at the patient's bedside, and the patient in a comfortable position, the insertion and advancement of the venous access device may begin. After applying the tourniquet and cleansing the site, the device is inserted bevel up at a 5° to 15° angle (deeper veins require larger angle). Once the vein is accessed, blood is visible in the "flashback" chamber. The device should be almost parallel with the skin. To advance the catheter into the vein, begin by releasing the tourniquet. Next stabilize the vein with one hand and with the other hand advance the catheter up to the hub. Do not advance the needle (the vein could be punctured). Next remove the inner needle. Apply pressure with a finger to the catheter (helps prevent blood leakage while removing the needle and advancing the catheter), and attach the primed IV administration set tubing. Alternatively, advance the catheter while the IV is running. To do this, begin by releasing the tourniquet and then remove the needle. Next, using aseptic technique, attach the IV tubing and begin the infusion. As the vein is stabilized with one hand, thread the catheter into the vein with the other. This method reduces the risk of puncturing the vein wall because the needle is removed before the catheter is advanced.

Using a steel needle winged set, insert the needle fully while holding the wings. While holding it in place, release the tourniquet, open the administration set clamp slightly, and check for free flow or infiltration. Tape the infusion set in place using the wings as an anchor to prevent movement. When the infusion set is an over-the-needle set, use either of the previously mentioned catheter advancement techniques.

Some IV therapists prefer the one-handed method of advancing the catheter. In this case, one hand anchors the vein, the skin is punctured, and with the index finger or thumb of that hand the catheter is advanced off the needle into the vein and the needle is withdrawn.

Securing the Venous Access Device

The CDC recommends that the dressing used to cover the skin around the venous access device be either sterile gauze or sterile transparent semipermeable dressing. Transparent dressings of this type also permit air flow, deter bacteria, and allow visual evaluation of the site. Transparent membrane dressings (TMDs) are available in various sizes and thicknesses. Some are one piece with dressing and tape in one unit. Whatever type of dressing is used, the most important factor is that the site can be evaluated often. In addition, any type of dressing should cover only the IV site, not the hub or connections of the administration set tubing. The patient may shower with the sterile transparent semipermeable dressing. If blood is oozing from the site, a sterile gauze dressing may be preferable.

When securing the IV site, tape should never encircle the extremity. Impairment of circulation may result. In a pediatric or disoriented patient of any age, self-adhering wrap is often used to secure and protect the site without restricting blood flow. Check the protocol for IV therapy in the facility for use of arm boards; generally, they are used only if absolutely necessary.

Tape is used to secure the IV device. The hub and IV device can be kept from moving by using several different taping techniques (chevron, U, or H methods). Whatever the method, as little tape as possible is used. Sterile tape is preferred since it is placed in close proximity to the IV site. (Figures 19-3A and 19-3B illustrate the three types of taping methods.)

To use the chevron method, a long strip of ½-inch tape is cut and placed sticky side up under the hub. The ends are then crossed over the hub and fastened to the patient's arm. A piece of 1-inch tape is placed across each of the end of the chevron, and the tubing is looped and secured with another piece of the 1-inch tape.

The U method is similar in that the tape is placed sticky side up under the hub, then each piece of the tape is folded over the wings of the butterfly catheter parallel to the hub. Then the catheter is stabilized and dressing secured.

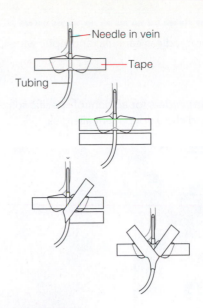

Needle in vein
Tape
Tubing

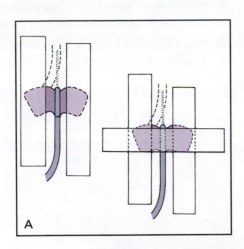

A

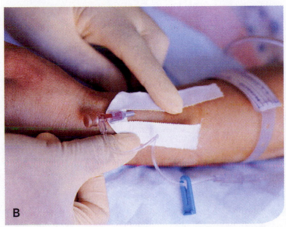

B

FIGURE 19-3 (A) Taping the butterfly needle with the H and chevron methods; (B) U method of securing a venous access device.

The H method involves three strips of ½-inch tape. One strip is placed over each wing of the butterfly parallel to the catheter, and the third is placed across the first two to make an H. The dressing is then applied.

Once the site is secured and the dressing is in place, a label is applied showing the date, time of insertion, type and gauge of needle, and your initials.

Preparing the IV Infusion

Before the actual IV is brought to the patient, the infusion system must be set up according to the physician's orders. The following procedure demonstrates the steps required to prepare an IV infusion system.

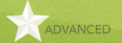 ADVANCED

PROCEDURE 19-1

PREPARING AN IV INFUSION

OBJECTIVE: To prepare an IV infusion correctly following physician's orders.

STANDARD: This task takes 10 minutes or less.

EQUIPMENT AND SUPPLIES: Physician's order; patient's record; administration tubing set compatible with orders; label; pen; correct IV solution; IV pole or electronic pump device; adapters or needless cannula; antiseptic wipes; pen.

STEPS:

1. Verify physician's orders for amount of specific solution to be given, and check for patient allergies.

2. Perform hand hygiene.
3. Assemble equipment and supplies necessary.
4. Compare IV solution label with physician's orders.
5. Check expiration date on IV solution, and inspect bag for leaks by pressing gently on bag (Figure 19-4A).

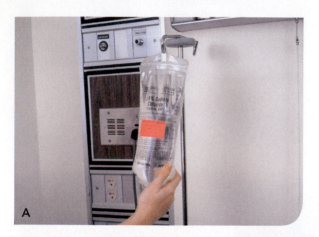

A

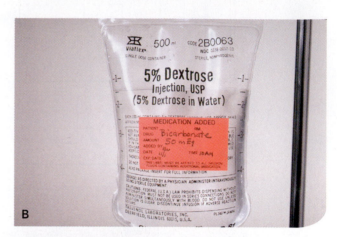

B

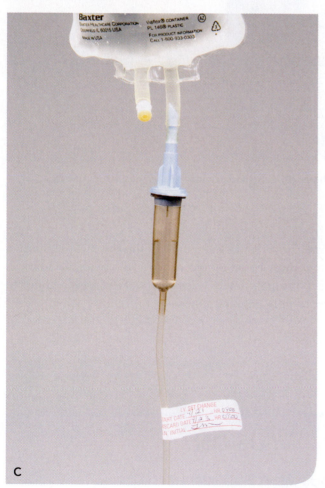

C

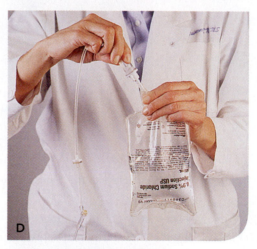

D

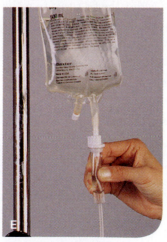

E

FIGURE 19-4 (A) Examine intravenous fluid container before setup; (B) label medication added to IV infusion; (C) attach label to tubing with date, time, and initials; (D) insert the spike into the IV bag. Photographer: Elena Dorfman; (E) squeeze the drip chamber. Photographer: Elena Dorfman.

6. Allow IV bag to come to room temperature if stored in refrigerator.

7. Look at bag carefully against a light and dark background for cloudiness, color change, or particles. If anything is abnormal, bag should be discarded and a new one obtained.

8. Hang IV container on IV pole.

9. Remove administration set from package, and close clamp.

10. Attach time label to bag (Figures 19-4B and 19-4C) and a label containing patient's name, room number, identification number, in addition to date and time IV hung, amount of any additives, drip rate, expiration date, time of infusion, and your name. Place information label on bag away from bag label with name of solution.

11. Remove covering from tubing spike (end closest to drip chamber).

12. Remove cover from port on end of bag, and avoid contaminating spike and port.

13. Insert spike into insertion site (Figure 19-4D).

14. Release pressure on drip chamber until it is half full (Figure 19-4E).

15. Attach filter if indicated. (Filters are used when giving lipids, blood, TPN, **patient-controlled analgesia (PCA)**, or **epidurals**.)

16. Prime tubing by opening clamp and allowing fluid to flow through tubing to displace air.

17. Close tubing clamp after priming.

18. Drape filled tubing over IV pole until ready to perform venipuncture. If electronic infusion device is used, make sure to check manufacturer's requirements for type of tubing needed and how to load tubing into pump.

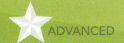
ADVANCED

PROCEDURE 19-2

PREPARING THE VENIPUNCTURE SITE FOR IV

OBJECTIVE: To prepare the venipuncture site prior to starting an IV.

STANDARD: This task takes 5–7 minutes.

EQUIPMENT AND SUPPLIES: Prepared infusion system with administration tubing; IV administration setup; antiseptic; swabs (2% chlorhexidine); gloves, sterile or clean depending on facility policy; sterile tape; IV pole or electronic infusion pump; patient's record; pen; disposable tourniquet (latex free); sterile venous access device of appropriate size; gauge for the patient; transparent semipermeable dressing.

STEPS:

1. Check physician's order, and check for patient's allergies.

2. Identify patient using two methods of identification.

3. Assemble equipment and supplies. Prepare infusion per steps in Procedure 19-1.

4. Greet patient, and explain procedure and purpose of IV.

5. Position patient, and provide privacy.

6. Allay patient's fears as much as possible.

7. Inspect patient, and determine best site for IV. Choose a site on patient's nondominant side if possible. Also consider patient's activity level. Inspect both arms and hands, and palpate veins. Choose an area free of infection, scarring, and away from joints (antecubital fossa is used as last resort). Do not use a vein below an infiltration or phlebitis area. To preserve more proximal sites for later infusions, use most distal end possible of a vein. Avoid arm on side of mastectomy. Use vein of lower extremity as last resort and with permission of physician.

8. Perform hand hygiene, and don gloves.

9. Place tourniquet 4 to 6 inches above site selected.

10. Tap vein to increase blood flow. Ask patient to open and close fist a few times. If vein still difficult to palpate, apply warm compress for a few minutes after releasing tourniquet. Then replace tourniquet, and check vein again.

11. Swab site vigorously with 2% chlorhexidine over a 2- to 4-inch area.

12. Let prep solution air-dry before continuing. Do not touch site again before venipuncture.

13. Continue as appropriate with type of venous access device used (butterfly, steel needle, over-the-needle catheter).

BOX 19-1 IV Reminders

- Do not shave IV sites. Shaving can facilitate infection through minor cuts in skin.
- Use scissors to clip hairy areas prior to IV infusion.
- Use latex-free tourniquets, and discard after use.
- Follow facility policy for number of times to try to insert IV (usually 2).

- IVs started outside hospital in an emergency should be restarted in hospital as soon as possible to ensure proper asepsis.
- Be familiar with the scope of practice as it applies to unlicensed personnel performing IV therapy.

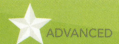ADVANCED

PROCEDURE 19-3

STARTING AN IV WITH A WINGED NEEDLE

OBJECTIVE: To successfully start an IV using a winged (butterfly type) needle.

STANDARD: This task takes 5–10 minutes.

EQUIPMENT AND SUPPLIES: Prepared infusion system; IV administration setup; antiseptic; swabs (2% chlorhexidine); gloves, sterile or clean depending on facility policy; tape; IV pole or electronic infusion pump; patient's record; pen; disposable tourniquet (latex free); sterile winged needle of appropriate size and gauge for the patient; tubing or short tubing to attach an administration tubing set; transparent semipermeable dressing; sterile tape; biohazard waste container.

STEPS:

1. Follow steps in previous procedure for preparing venipuncture site (Procedure 19-2).

2. Choose appropriate-size winged needle for patient (infant, child, adult with fragile veins).

3. Attach end of winged-needle tubing to end of IV administration tubing set.

4. Carefully remove cover from needle, and prime tubing by letting fluid from IV infusion run through it. Replace needle cover to preserve sterility.

5. Apply tourniquet, and select appropriate vein.

6. Cleanse site, and allow to air-dry.

7. Remove needle cover again, and hold needle by its wings. Anchor vein, and pull skin taut with thumb of nondominant hand below vein (Figure 19-5).

8. With bevel up at about 30° angle, insert needle into skin either next to or alongside vein, then enter vein from side; or insert needle through skin below vein site, then enter vein. (Either method protects fragile veins from hematoma more than if needle enters directly through skin into vein.)

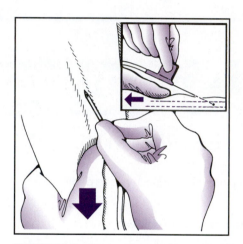

FIGURE 19-5 Grasp wings and insert needle at 30° angle.

9. After vein is entered, observe for "flashback" of blood in tubing.

10. Carefully advance needle until it reaches hub. Release tourniquet.

11. Attach IV tubing, open clamp, and observe drip chamber. Flow should enter easily with no sign of infiltration at site; if not, inject normal saline for a saline lock to keep tubing open.

12. Slow drip rate while securing needle in place.

13. To secure needle, place ½-inch-wide sterile tape, sticky side up, under needle and crossed over to form chevron wings. Do not place tape directly on insertion site.

14. Make a short loop with IV tubing to prevent it from being pulled out, and tape IV tubing a short way from needle site. (See Figure 19-6A.)

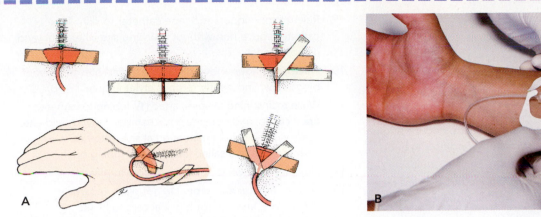

FIGURE 19-6 (A) Use the chevron method to secure winged needle. Then apply transparent dressing over the infusion site; (B) apply transparent dressing over infusion site.

15. Apply transparent dressing over infusion site (Figure 19-6B).
16. Remove and dispose of gloves in biohazard waste container.
17. Label dressing with date, time, your initials, and size of catheter.
18. Adjust drip rate to rate prescribed by physician.

NOTE: Dressing should be changed every 48 to 72 hours or according to facility policy.

19. Document procedure in patient's record.

BOX 19-2 Times Changes for Various Types of Tubing

Always check facility policy regarding tube changes.

- TPN and lipids every 24 hours
- Blood and blood products every 4 hours after 2 units of blood

- Primary and secondary tubing every 96 hours
- Primary intermittent tubing every 24 hours
- Extension tubing whenever the venous access device is replaced

---

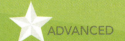ADVANCED # PROCEDURE 19-4

INSERTING AN OVER-THE-NEEDLE CATHETER

OBJECTIVE: To successfully insert an over-the-needle catheter for infusion therapy.

STANDARD: This task takes 5–10 minutes.

EQUIPMENT AND SUPPLIES: Prepared infusion container; IV administration setup; antiseptic; swabs (2% chlorhexidine); gloves; sterile or clean, depending on facility policy; sterile tape; IV pole or electronic infusion pump; patient's record; pen;

disposable tourniquet (latex free); over-the-needle (OTN) catheter set of appropriate size and gauge for the patient; transparent semipermeable dressing; biohazard waste container.

STEPS:

1. Prepare IV system as in Procedure 19-1, and follow steps in Procedure 19-2.
2. Select appropriate size over-the-needle catheter.

3. Perform hand hygiene, and don gloves.

4. Position arm for venipuncture.

5. If vein is not distended, ask patient to hang arm over side of bed to increase dilation of vein.

6. Hold catheter with bevel up, and stabilize vein.

7. Insert needle/catheter at a 45° angle into patient's skin either next to vein or a bit below vein site. Reduce angle to 30°, and enter vein observing for blood flow in hub (Figure 19-7A).

8. While holding needle and using one- or two-handed technique, advance catheter unit until hub touches skin.

9. Release tourniquet, and tape catheter to skin. Tape catheter above hub without touching site where hub and catheter meet.

10. Place one finger above distal end of catheter to prevent blood flow, and gently remove stylet (Figure 19-7B).

11. While maintaining asepsis, attach IV tubing to catheter, open clamp, and observe drip chamber. Flow should enter easily with no sign of infiltration at site. Alternatively, inject normal saline or a saline lock to keep tubing open.

12. Slow drip rate while securing needle in place.

13. Secure catheter and tape. Do not place tape over connectors, and do not block access to IV site.

14. Cover site with sterile transparent dressing. Loop tubing once, and tape tubing to patient's arm.

15. Remove and dispose of gloves in biohazard waste container.

16. Label dressing with date, time, your initials, and size of catheter (Figure 19-8).

17. Adjust drip to rate prescribed by physician.

NOTE: Dressing should be changed every 96 hours or according to facility policy.

18. Document procedure in patient's record.

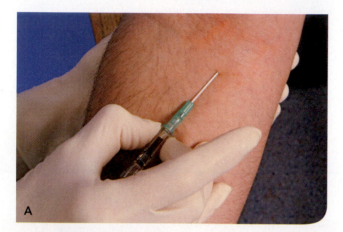

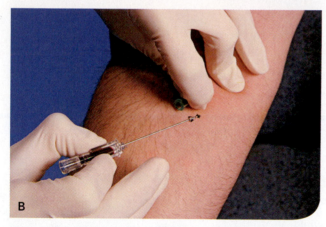

FIGURE 19-7 (A) Blood is noted in the flashback chamber once the stylet has entered the vein; (B) occlude the vein with one finger while removing the stylet.

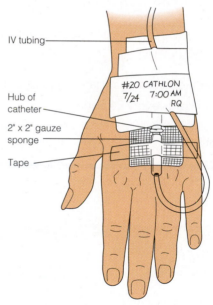

IV tubing

Hub of catheter

2" x 2" gauze sponge

Tape

#20 CATHLON
7/24   7:00 AM
       RQ

FIGURE 19-8 Labeled tape for IV dressing.

Adjusting the Flow Rate of an Infusion

Usually the individual who initiates the infusion adjusts the flow rate based on the rate prescribed by the physi- cian. The IV then must be monitored and regulated, and the patient's responses must be monitored as well. The drop factor is indicated on the label of the infusion set. To calculate the flow rates, the amount of fluid to be given and the length of time for the infusion must be known. Flow rates are designated by the number of milliliters to be given in an hour and by the number of drops per milliliter. The formula for determining these flow rates is as follows:

- **Hourly Rates.** Divide the total volume of the IV by the total time of the IV

For example:

$$\frac{3000 \text{ mL (total infusion)}}{24 \text{ hours (total IV time)}} = 125 \text{ mL/hour}$$

- **Drops per Minute.** Multiply the total amount of IV by the drop factor divided by the total time of IV in minutes

$$\frac{\text{mL per hour} \times \text{drop factor}}{60 \text{ minutes}} = \text{drops per minute}$$

For example, if 1000 mL is to be given over 8 hours and the drip factor is 20 drops/mL:

$$\text{Drops per minute} = \frac{1000 \text{ mL}}{8 \text{ hrs (480 min)}} \times \frac{20 \text{ gtt}}{\text{min}}$$
$$= 41 \text{ gtt/min}$$

The rate in the preceding example is rounded off to 40 drops per minute. The IV therapist then adjusts the rate and counts the drops for 1 minute. The infusion rate is checked at least every hour to maintain the correct flow and to evaluate for infiltration. The flow rate is influenced by the height of the IV bag above the patient's arm. The bag should be about 36 inches (91 cm) above the IV site. The higher the bag is raised, the greater the pressure and the faster the rate. The position of the patient's arm or change in position may decrease or increase the flow. Tubing position and **patency** (openness) may affect the rate. For example, the flow would decrease if the patient leans on the tubing.

Electronic infusion devices (EIDs) regulate the infusion according to preset controls. An alarm may be triggered when the IV solution is low or when the tubing is too low. Figure 19-9 is an example of an EID. Always follow the manufacturer's directions when using an EID. Many require that specific administration sets be used with their instruments. Some infusion sets have one or more ports to attach second infusion sets or administer injections. Needleless systems consist of a blunt **cannula** (tube with a channel or lumen) that is inserted into a special injection port or adapter (Figure 19-10A) on IV tubing to administer injections or secondary infusions sets (Figure 19-10B).

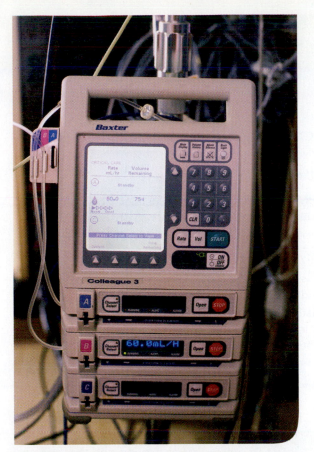

FIGURE 19-9 An intravenous infusion pump.

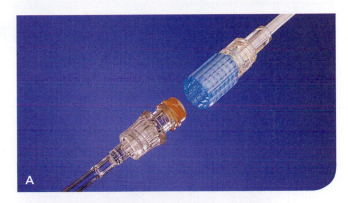

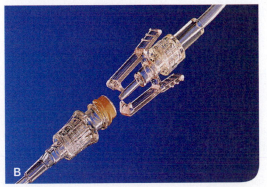

FIGURE 19-10 (A) Threaded-lock cannula used to connect tubing of added set to primary infusion; (B) lever-lock cannula used to connect tubing of added set to primary infusion.

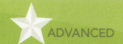
PROCEDURE 19-5

ADDING EXTENSION TUBING TO AN IV SET

OBJECTIVE: To add extension tubing to an existing IV correctly.

STANDARD: This task takes 5 minutes.

EQUIPMENT AND SUPPLIES: Extension tubing; antimicrobial swab; needless cannula; adapter with cap; syringe cannula; 2 syringes with 1 mL normal saline; gloves; patient's record; pen.

STEPS:

1. Check patient's record for orders for additional infusion and for allergies.
2. Gather equipment and supplies appropriate for type of IV in use. Attach extension tubing directly to IV catheter. Check type of cap.

3. Swab tubing's injection cap and insert syringe cannula.
4. At other end of extension tubing, remove protector and prime with 1 mL normal saline.
5. Add needless cannula to tubing if attaching to capped catheter.
6. Swab cannula of patient's IV, and connect extension tubing.
7. Add primed tubing directly to IV catheter.
8. Flush with 1 mL normal saline per facility policies. (Some policies require 2 mL or more to flush.)

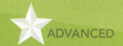
PROCEDURE 19-6

MONITORING AN INTRAVENOUS INFUSION

OBJECTIVE: To maintain the correct infusion drop rate and monitor for signs of complications associated with IV therapy.

STANDARD: This task takes 10 minutes or less.

EQUIPMENT AND SUPPLIES: Patient's record; patient with IV running; gloves; gauze; transparent dressing; sterile tape; tubing appropriate for IV device; pen; biohazard waste container.

STEPS:

1. Check orders for IV therapy. Check for patient allergies.
2. Perform hand hygiene.
3. Identify patient, and explain procedure.
4. Check that correct IV solution is being given. Check flow rate, volume given, and any additives (Figure 19-11).
5. Check tubing for kinks and tightness of connections.
6. Every 8 hours, or according to facility policy, inspect site for signs for edema, infiltration, and phlebitis (redness along vein, warmth, pain).

7. Check dressing for leakage and bleeding.
8. Reposition needle if IV is not flowing.

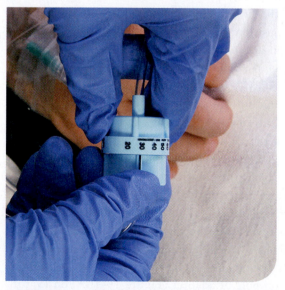

FIGURE 19-11 Dial-A-Flo in line IV rate control device.

9. Instruct patient on ways to maintain IV so it is running smoothly:
   - Avoid putting tension on tubing.
   - Avoid sudden twisting and yanking on tubing.
   - Notify caregiver if rate changes, blood is seen in IV tubing, or pain or swelling occurs at site.

10. Remove and dispose of gloves properly, and perform hand hygiene.

11. Document information in patient's record and bedside information sheet if necessary.

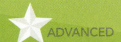

PROCEDURE 19-7

CHANGING THE IV SOLUTION

OBJECTIVE: To hang a new IV infusion bag 1 hour before previous bag is finished and maintain flow of prescribed fluids.

STANDARD: This task takes 5–10 minutes.

EQUIPMENT AND SUPPLIES: Patient's record; IV solution ordered; IV administration set and tubing; timing label; gauze squares; antiseptic swab; gloves; pen.

STEPS:

1. Check physician's orders for name, concentration, volume, and drip rate of infusion.

2. Check for patient allergies.

3. Read label of new container, and verify that it matches orders.

4. Perform hand hygiene.

5. Prepare new container with timing label and additives ordered. Prime tubing. Make sure drip chamber is half full.

6. Identify patient, and explain procedure.

7. With drip chamber half full, hang new bag an hour before previous bag is finished.

8. Stop flow of fluid, remove old bag, and hang new one.

9. Spike new bag, and set prescribed flow rate. Inspect tubing for signs of bubbles. Flick tubing to dislodge bubbles. Dispose of old bag, after draining old fluid if necessary.

10. Remove gloves. Perform hand hygiene.

11. Attach label with all pertinent information (date, time, type of solution).

12. Instruct patient how to help maintain IV so it is running smoothly.
    a. Avoid putting tension on tubing.
    b. Avoid sudden twisting and yanking on tubing.
    c. Notify nurse if rate changes, blood is seen in IV tubing, or pain or swelling occurs at site.

13. Document patient's record.

Converting IV to Saline Lock

A saline lock or heparin lock is a small device with a self-sealing rubber stopper that is screwed onto the hub of the IV catheter or butterfly needle already in place. It is a "cap" for an IV when the IV must remain open without infusing fluids into the patient. Historically heparin was used to keep these "locks" patent, or open. Saline is used often now instead of heparin. The facility protocol dictates which to use. These saline locks are used when intermittent administration of fluids is necessary or to maintain access to a vein for medication administration when large volumes of IV fluid are not needed. In either case the "lock" preserves the vein and avoids another venipuncture. (Procedure 19-8 lists the steps to follow to convert an IV to intermittent infusion or saline lock.)

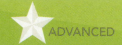
PROCEDURE 19-8

CONVERTING AN IV TO AN INTERMITTENT INFUSION LOCK

OBJECTIVE: To change an IV to an intermittent infusion lock to permit IV administration of medications or fluids when needed.

STANDARD: This task takes 5 minutes.

EQUIPMENT AND SUPPLIES: Gloves; 3 to 5 mL syringe; sterile 25 G needles; antiseptic swab; sterile 2 × 2 gauze; sterile saline (without preservative) or heparin flush solution (10 units/mL or 100 units/mL) in a prefilled syringe; a 3 mL syringe with needleless infusion device; intermittent infusion cap or lock; patient's record; pen.

STEPS:

1. Check patient's record for physician's orders and allergies.
2. Identify patient, and explain procedure.
3. Assemble equipment and supplies.
4. Perform hand hygiene.
5. Examine IV site. If any signs of infiltration or inflammation appear, discontinue IV and find another site.
6. Evaluate whether infusion is running properly.
7. Expose IV catheter hub.
8. Prime extension tubing with saline.
9. Clamp IV tubing to stop IV.
10. Place piece of sterile piece gauze under connection.
11. Don gloves. While stabilizing catheter, twist IV tubing adapter to loosen and remove from IV catheter. Insert

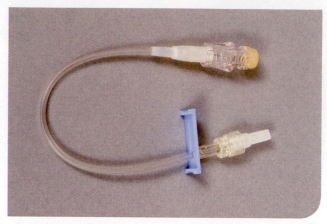

FIGURE 19-12 Intermittent infusion device with injection port.

new infusion plug into IV catheter or engage Luer lock. (See Figure 19-12 for an example of an intermittent infusion device with an injection port.)

12. Flush with saline or heparin per facility policy. Some policies require 2 mL or more.
13. Tape infusion plug in place using chevron or H taping method.
14. Instruct patient about protecting and maintaining IV lock.
15. Document patient's record.

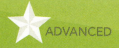
PROCEDURE 19-9

ADMINISTERING MEDICATION TO AN IV LINE BY INJECTION "PUSH"

OBJECTIVE: To administer medication directly to the patient through an existing IV line by injecting medication by direct push.

STANDARD: This task takes 5–10 minutes.

NOTE: Patient should be monitored for adverse reactions.

EQUIPMENT AND SUPPLIES: Medication prepared in syringe with needleless cannula; antimicrobial swab; blood pressure equipment; gloves; syringe with heparin or saline for flushing; watch; patient's record; pen.

STEPS:

1. Check patient's record for physician's order and patient's allergies.
2. Assemble equipment and supplies.

3. Perform hand hygiene.

4. Prepare medication according to pharmacy recommendations, or check package insert or PDR for instructions. If instructions require, flush line before and after medication is administered.

5. Check medication using "Ten Rights."

6. Identify patient, and explain procedure and its purpose.

7. Check IV site for signs of redness, infiltration, edema, or leakage.

8. Don gloves.

9. Clean IV port closest to IV site with antiseptic wipe.

10. Insert cannula of medication syringe into port (Figure 19-13A).

11. Pinch main tubing between port and infusion bag while injecting medication slowly at timed 20-second intervals (Figure 19-13B).

12. Observe patient closely during administration of medication for adverse reactions.

13. Administer and time remaining amount of medication according to instructions.

14. When administration is complete, withdraw cannula.

15. Discard equipment.

16. Remove and dispose of gloves properly. Perform hand hygiene.

17. Measure patient's vital signs if required.

18. Document patient's record completely. Include name and amount of medication administered, date and time administered, flush if performed, type of flushing solution, appearance of IV site, patient's reaction, and your name.

Legal Alert! Adding medication directly to the IV solution container is usually done by the pharmacist according to regulations established by the American Society of Health Systems Pharmacists (ASHP) and the Occupational Safety and Health Administration (OSHA). Check policy and procedure manuals governing this procedure.

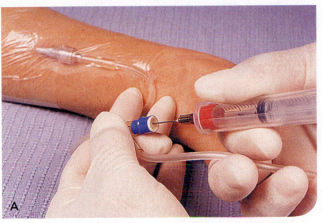
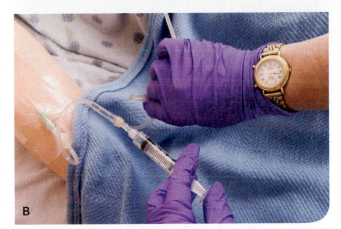

FIGURE 19-13 (A) Inserting a needle through the injection port of an IV lock; (B) using a watch to time the rate of medication injection.

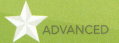 ADVANCED

PROCEDURE 19-10

ADMINISTERING MEDICATION USING A SECONDARY ("PIGGYBACK") BAG

OBJECTIVE: To administer intermittent medication by infusion using a secondary container placed at a higher level than the primary infusion container.

STANDARD: This task takes 5–10 minutes.

EQUIPMENT AND SUPPLIES: Prepared medication/infusion bag with label; secondary administration set;

IV pole extension hook; antimicrobial swab; patient's record; pen.

STEPS:

1. Check patient's record for physician's orders and patient's allergies.
2. Assemble equipment and supplies.
3. Perform hand hygiene.
4. Check medication using "Ten Rights." Check that medication is compatible with existing IV solution.
5. Identify patient, and explain procedure and its purpose.
6. Check IV site for signs of redness, infiltration, edema, or leakage.
7. Spike medication bag with secondary set. Attach needleless cannula to end of it.
8. Clean injection port of primary infusion set with antimicrobial swab.
9. Insert needleless cannula of "piggyback" tubing into primary tubing port.
10. Hang second IV bag on IV pole. Attach extension hook to primary bag and hang it lower than secondary bag (Figure 19-14A).
11. To back prime, hold secondary bag below primary bag and open clamp on secondary bag to clear tubing (Figure 19-14B). This allows primary solution to flow into line into secondary bag (back priming). Continue until chamber of secondary bag is half full.
12. Reclamp secondary bag. Rehang bag.
13. Open secondary bag clamp, and allow infusion to flow at correct drip rate.
14. When "piggyback" bag is empty, reset rate of primary infusion to correct drip rate, then close clamp on secondary bag. Remove bag.
15. To administer a new secondary bag, check to see that it contains same medication, then spike new bag and proceed as above.
16. Document procedure in patient's record.

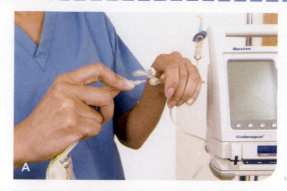

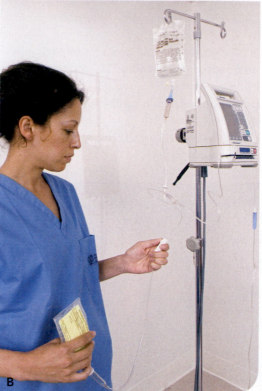

FIGURE 19-14 (A) Insert the needleless cannula of the secondary line into the primary tubing port; (B) lower the medication bag to back prime the secondary.

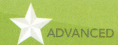ADVANCED

PROCEDURE 19-11

ADMINISTERING MEDICATION USING A PERIPHERAL SALINE LOCK

OBJECTIVE: To successfully administer prescribed medication using a peripheral saline lock.

STANDARD: This task takes 10 minutes.

EQUIPMENT AND SUPPLIES: Gloves; drug solution in its container; administration set; needleless device or 22G 1-inch needle; antiseptic swab; 2 prefilled normal saline syringes (1 mL) each; blood pressure equipment if required; patient's record; pen; biohazard waste container.

STEPS:

1. Check patient's record for physician's order and patient's allergies.
2. Assemble equipment and supplies.
3. Perform hand hygiene.
4. Check medication using "Ten Rights." Check that medication is compatible with existing IV solution.
5. Prepare medication according to manufacturer's directions, and draw up ordered amount into a syringe.

NOTE: Joint Commission guidelines require all syringes with medication be labeled with patient's name, drug, and time of preparation.

6. Fill each of 2 syringes with 1 mL normal saline.
7. Identify patient, and explain procedure and its purpose.
8. Check IV site for signs of redness, infiltration, edema, or leakage.
9. Measure patient's blood pressure as required when giving certain types of medication.
10. Cleanse injection port with antimicrobial swab.
11. Insert first saline syringe into port, and aspirate slightly to check for patency, then flush with saline. Watch surrounding tissue for signs of swelling. If blood was aspirated and no swelling occurs after saline flush, needle is in vein.
12. Insert medication syringe into port and time administration of drug according to manufacturer's directions.
13. Observe patient during administration for signs of adverse reactions.
14. When administration is finished, remove syringe and flush with other saline syringe to maintain patency.
15. Flush line.
16. Dispose of equipment and gloves in appropriate biohazard waste container.
17. Perform hand hygiene.
18. Check patient's blood pressure if indicated.
19. Document patient's record.

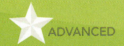

ADVANCED

PROCEDURE 19-12

DISCONTINUING AN IV

OBJECTIVE: To successfully discontinue patient's IV per physician's order and apply sterile dressing to site.

STANDARD: This task takes about 5 minutes.

EQUIPMENT AND SUPPLIES: Sterile 2 × 2 gauze pads; sterile tape; gloves; patient's record; pen; biohazard waste container.

STEPS:

1. Check patient's record for a "Discontinue IV" order.
2. Assemble equipment and supplies.
3. Perform hand hygiene. Don gloves.
4. Identify patient, and explain procedure.
5. Turn off IV.
6. Loosen transparent dressing by loosening edges and pulling toward middle of site on each side and then lifting off.
7. Hold needle/catheter steady while removing dressing. Hold sterile gauze over site as needle is removed. Pull out needle/catheter along line of vein.
8. Immediately apply pressure, and hold firmly for 2 to 3 minutes until bleeding stops. Do not ask patient to bend arm to hold gauze in place. (Bleeding may still occur in this position. Elevation of arm may help stem flow and hasten clotting at site.)
9. Apply sterile pad and tape in place.

10. Observe area for signs of redness, swelling, and hematoma.

11. Dispose of equipment in biohazard waste container. Remove and dispose of gloves in similar manner. Perform hand hygiene.

12. Recheck site in about 15 minutes.

13. Document procedure, including volume infused and date, time, condition of site, patient's reaction to procedure, and if catheter was intact.

Safety Alert! Be sure to determine if patient has received anticoagulant therapy. If he or she has been on this type of medicine, be sure to apply extra pressure to the site after the catheter is removed.

20 Nutrition and Patient Education

PROCEDURES

Procedure 20-1 Teaching a Patient to Read a Food Label

Procedure 20-2 Developing a Teaching Plan to Encourage an Increase in Daily Fiber

Procedure 20-3 Teaching Wellness and Disease Prevention to a Patient

TERMS TO LEARN

scurvy

rickets

Recommended Dietary Allowance (RDA)

glycemic index

hyperinsulinemia

enzymes

saturated fats

unsaturated fats

trans fat

catalysts

compliance

noncompliance

vegan

Nutrition is the study of the intake and processing of food and the utilization of the component food substances for growth, repair, and maintenance of the body. Lack of proper nutrition can lead to many illnesses and disorders. For example, **scurvy** is the result of a lack of vitamin C, and **rickets** is the result of a lack of vitamin D.

Food is psychologically important in people's lives, as evidenced by the many social events centering on food. Different cultures eat a diverse range of foods and may refrain from eating some foods altogether. Thus, health care providers must be mindful of cultural factors when instructing patients to make dietary changes recommended by the physician.

Teaching patients to make life changes to improve their health and reduce the consequences of disease are important competencies. In health care settings patient education and health promotion facts often are effective when presented to the patient in a teaching session. Whenever a patient education session is provided for a patient, it must be documented in the patient's record.

Essential Nutrients for Health

The body requires six classes of nutrients to maintain health: carbohydrates, fats, proteins, vitamins, minerals, and fiber. Water is essential for homeostasis, but strictly speaking it is not a nutrient. The body can make many but not all of the nutrients. Therefore, a balanced diet is important to maintain health and promote repair to body tissues.

Standards are established that suggest the daily requirements of each nutrient to promote a healthy lifestyle. These are called Dietary Reference Intakes (DRIs). The DRI guidelines specify the **Recommended Dietary Allowance (RDA)** (the goal individuals should strive for to meet nutritional requirements). These guidelines are based on what the average healthy person of a specific age, height, and weight and activity level would require. The following paragraphs explain each class of nutrient and the importance of an adequate daily intake of water. Figure 20-1 presents the classes of nutrients, with examples of foods in each class, the function of each nutrient in the body, and examples of sources of the nutrient.

NUTRIENT CLASS	BODILY FUNCTIONS	FOOD SOURCES
CARBOHYDRATES 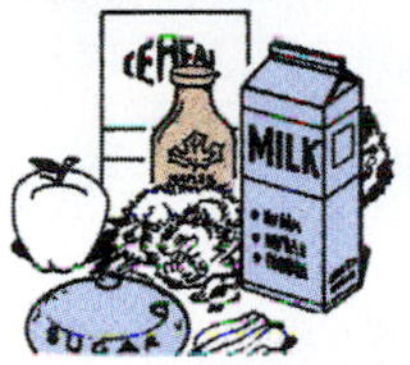	Provides work energy for body activities, and heat energy for maintenance of body temperature.	Cereal grains and their products (bread, breakfast cereals, macaroni products), potatoes, sugar, syrups, fruits, milk, vegetables, nuts.
PROTEINS 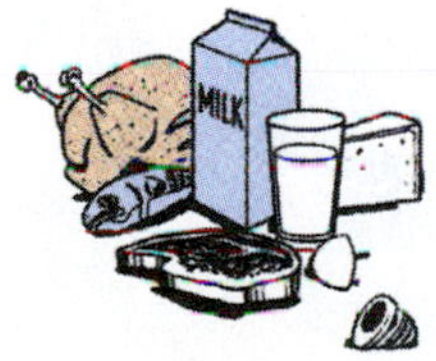	Build and renew body tissues; regulate body functions and supply energy. Complete proteins; maintain life and provide growth. Incomplete proteins; maintain life but do not provide for growth.	Complete proteins: Derived from animal foods—meat, milk, eggs, fish, cheese, poultry. Incomplete proteins: Derived from vegetable foods—soybeans, dry beans, peas, some nuts and whole grain products.
FATS 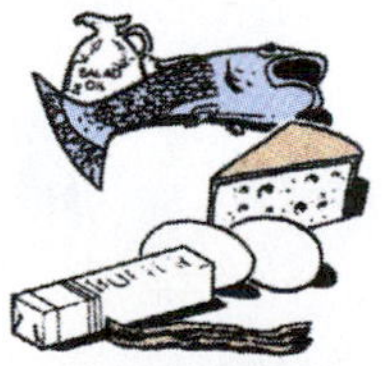	Give work energy for body activities and heat energy for maintenance of body temperature. Carrier of vitamins A and D, provide fatty acids necessary for growth and maintenance of body tissues.	Some foods are chiefly fat, such as lard, vegetable fats and oils, and butter. Many other foods contain smaller proportions of fats—nuts, meats, fish, poultry, cream, whole milk.
MINERALS Calcium 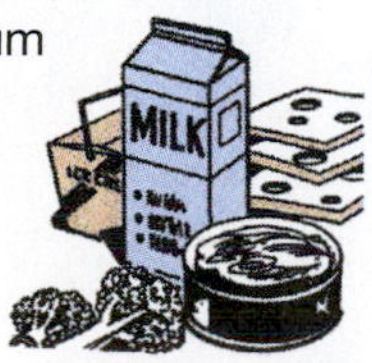	Builds and renews bones, teeth, and other tissues; regulates the activity of the muscles, heart, nerves; and controls the clotting of blood.	Milk and milk products except butter; most dark green vegetables; canned salmon.

FIGURE 20-1   A balanced diet begins with eating foods from the basic food groups.

NUTRIENT CLASS	BODILY FUNCTIONS	FOOD SOURCES
Phosphorus 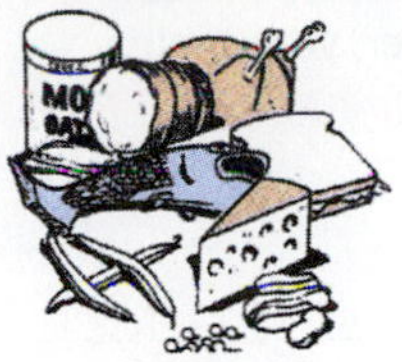	Associated with calcium in some functions needed to build and renew bones and teeth. Influences the oxidation of foods in the body cells; important in nerve tissue.	Widely distributed in foods; especially cheese, oat cereals, whole wheat products, dry beans and peas, meat, fish, poultry, nuts.
Iron 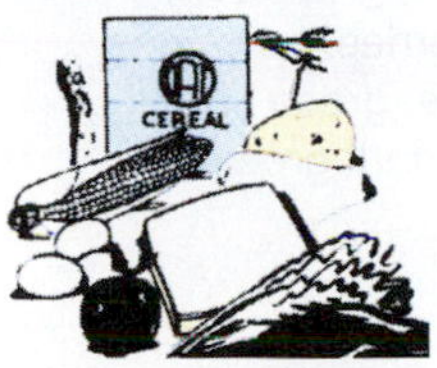	Builds and renews hemoglobin, the red pigment in blood which carries oxygen from the lungs to the cells.	Eggs, meat, especially liver and kidney; deep-yellow and dark green vegetables; potatoes, dried fruits, whole-grain products; enriched flour, bread, breakfast cereals.
Iodine 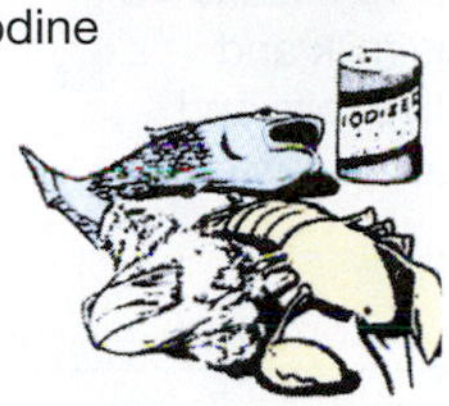	Enables the thyroid gland to perform its function of controlling the rate at which foods are oxidized in the cells.	Fish (obtained from the sea), some plant-foods grown in soils containing iodine; table salt fortified with iodine (iodized).
VITAMINS A 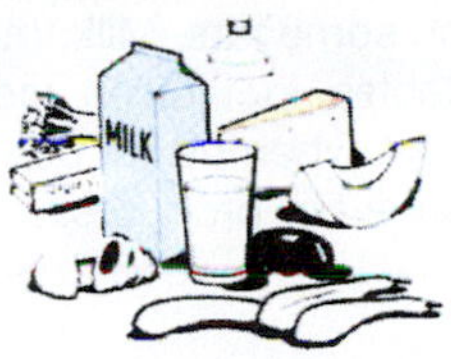	Necessary for normal functioning of the eyes, prevents night blindness. Ensures a healthy condition of the skin, hair, and mucous membranes. Maintains a state of resistance to infections of the eyes, mouth, and respiratory tract.	One form of vitamin A is yellow and one form is colorless. Apricots, cantaloupe, milk, cheese, eggs, meat organs, (especially liver and kidney), fortified margarine, butter, fish-liver oils, dark green and deep yellow vegetables.
B Complex B_1 (Thiamine) 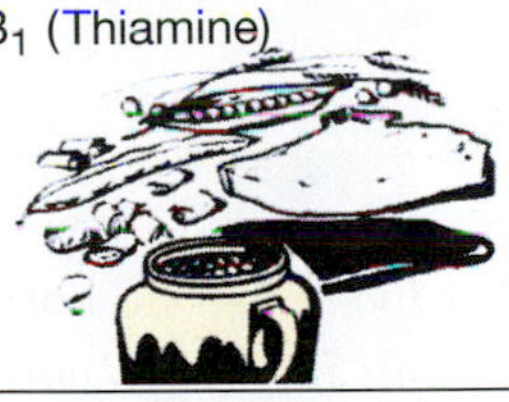	Maintains a healthy condition of the nerves. Fosters a good appetite. Helps the body cells use carbohydrates.	Whole grain and enriched grain products; meats (especially pork, liver and kidney). Dry beans and peas.
B_2 (Riboflavin) 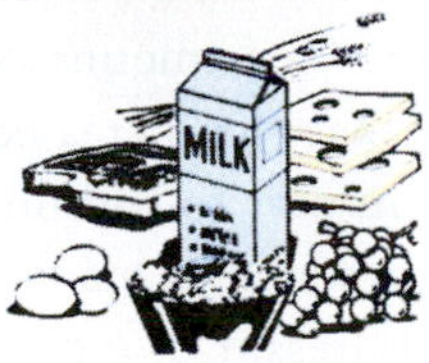	Keeps the skin, mouth, and eyes in a healthy condition. Acts with other nutrients to form enzymes and control oxidation in cells.	Milk, cheese, eggs, meat (especially liver and kidney), whole grain and enriched grain products, dark green vegetables.
Niacin 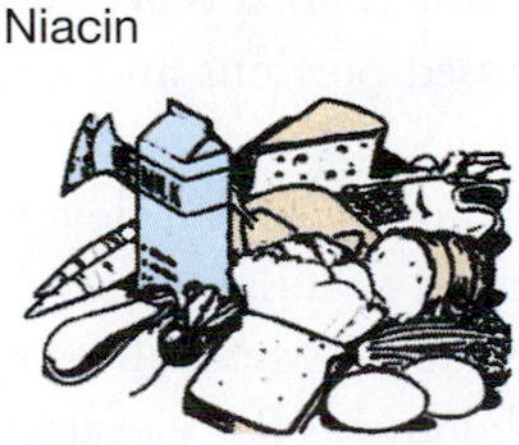	Influences the oxidation of carbohydrates and proteins in the body cells.	Liver, meat, fish, poultry, eggs, peanuts; dark green vegetables, whole grain and enriched cereal products.

FIGURE 20-1 (Continued)

NUTRIENT CLASS	BODILY FUNCTIONS	FOOD SOURCES
VITAMINS (continued) B₁₂ 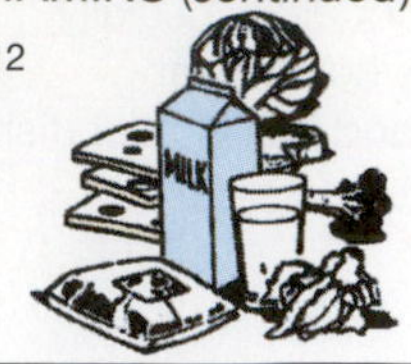	Regulates specific processes in digestion. Helps maintain normal functions of muscles, nerves, heart, blood—general body metabolism.	Liver, other organ meats, cheese, eggs, milk, leafy green vegetables.
C (Ascorbic Acid) 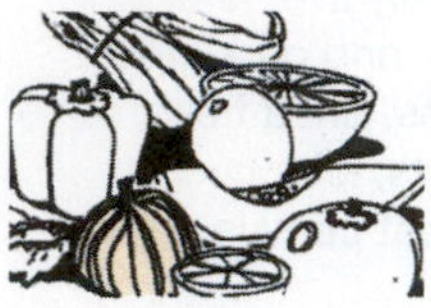	Acts as a cement between body cells, and helps them work together to carry out their special functions. Maintains a sound condition of bones, teeth, and gums. Not stored in the body.	Fresh, raw citrus fruits and vegetables—oranges, grapefruit, cantaloupe, strawberries, tomatoes, raw onions, cabbage, green and sweet red peppers, dark green vegetables.
D 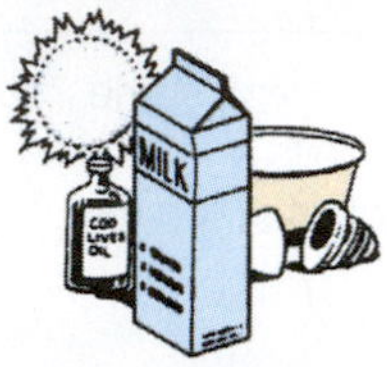	Enables the growing body to use calcium and phosphorus in a normal way to build bones and teeth.	Provided by vitamin D fortification of certain foods, such as milk and margarine. Also fish-liver oils and eggs. Sunshine is also a source of vitamin D.
WATER 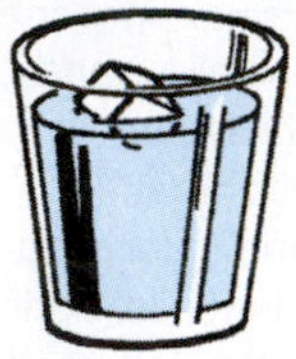	Regulates body processes. Aids in regulating body temperature. Carries nutrients to body cells and carries waste products away from them. Helps to lubricate joints. Water has no food value, although most water contains mineral elements. More immediately necessary to life than food—second only to oxygen.	Drinking water, and other beverages; all foods except those made up of a single nutrient, as sugar and some fats. Milk, milk drinks, soups, vegetables, fruit juices. Ice cream, watermelon, strawberries, lettuce, tomatoes, cereals, other dry products.

FIGURE 20-1   (Continued)

CARBOHYDRATES

Carbohydrates are a main source of energy for the body. They include simple sugars (white sugar, white four, white rice), starches (whole grains, some fruits and legumes), and cellulose (fiber-rich fruits and vegetables). Simple sugars raise the blood glucose level quickly and cause a rapid rise in insulin. Excess glucose is stored in the body as glycogen until needed for energy.

Experts recommend that no more than 10% of the daily intake of calories be in the form of simple or refined carbohydrates. It is suggested that 45% to 60% of the daily caloric intake be in the form of complex carbohydrates, which take longer to break down and do not raise blood glucose levels as quickly. Most white foods, including rice, pasta, flour, and sugar, have a high **glycemic index** (a numerical index given to a carbohydrate-rich food that is based on the average increase in blood glucose levels occurring after the food is eaten). Refined carbohydrates include such items as

cookies, cake, donuts, and other foods that do not contain whole grains and have high glycemic indices. Whole grains, fiber-rich vegetables, and fruits have lower glycemic indices and are recommended, as is limiting amounts of white foods. Some researchers suggest that the increased obesity rate in the United States is due in part to consumption of high fructose corn syrup, which is added to many commercially prepared foods (e.g., salad dressings, many types of crackers and cereals, and even some canned vegetables), and large quantities of pasta. Increased portions and sedentary lifestyles are also factors.

Hyperinsulinemia (high blood insulin levels) and reduced insulin function are linked to inflammatory disease (heart disease) and metabolic syndrome. Metabolic syndrome is characterized by increased abdominal fat, elevated blood glucose levels, elevated blood pressure, elevated triglycerides, and reduced levels of HDL (good cholesterol). Obesity is also linked to insulin resistance and type 2 diabetes.

PROTEINS

Proteins are composed of amino acids, which are the building blocks of the body. The body requires amino acids to produce new proteins, repair body tissues, and produce hormones and **enzymes** (proteins that speed up the rate of biochemical reactions). When proteins are digested, they are broken down into 20 amino acids, all but 9 of which are produced by the body. These 9 must be ingested in the diet.

Dietary sources of protein are meats, eggs, cheese, milk, grains, and legumes. A protein deficiency interferes with many body processes, can cause decreased mental capacity, and affects the entire body.

FATS

Fats or lipids are substances composed of fatty acids. They are either saturated or unsaturated and are not water soluble. When broken down, they produce large amounts of energy. They also are carriers for vitamins A, D, E, and K. Excessive amounts of fat in the diet lead to obesity, atherosclerosis, high blood pressure, and heart disease.

Saturated fats in the human diet come mainly from animals, eggs, and coconut and palm oils. They are solid at room temperature. Experts recommend that saturated fat intake should not be more than 10% of daily calories. **Unsaturated fats** come from nuts, seeds, and vegetables. They are generally liquid at room temperature. When hydrogen is added to unsaturated fat, it forms **trans fat**, which prolongs shelf life and stability. Trans fat is found in shortening, margarine and many snack foods. Trans fats and saturated fats raise the levels of LDL (bad) cholesterol.

VITAMINS

Vitamins are organic food substances essential for growth and numerous body functions. Most vitamins are not made in the body and thus must be obtained from the diet. The following vitamins can be produced in the body: vitamin A (made from carotene), vitamin D (from sunlight), and vitamin K (produced by bacteria in the large intestines). Vitamins have no caloric value but are necessary to maintain homeostasis. The fat-soluble vitamins A and E can be toxic if ingested in large amounts. The water-soluble vitamins (the B-complex vitamins, vitamin C, and bioflavonoids) are measured in milligrams and are more easily excreted from the body.

MINERALS

Minerals are inorganic elements that are prevalent in nature and form about 75% of the inorganic material found in the body. They are found, for example, in bones, teeth, and blood (iron). They are classified into macrominerals and microminerals. The macrominerals are calcium, magnesium, phosphorous, sodium, potassium, chlorine, and sulfur. These minerals are required in larger amounts than the trace minerals iron, zinc, copper, manganese, molybdenum, cobalt, fluorine, selenium, chromium, nickel, tin, and vanadium. None of the minerals have caloric value.

Minerals work as **catalysts** (substances like enzymes that speed up the metabolic processes) in metabolic processes; therefore, a deficiency in one type of mineral affects the actions of others. A mineral deficiency can cause serious health conditions. When foods are refined, many of the vitamins and minerals are lost in the processing. Today many processed foods are "enriched" with minerals such as iron, thiamin, riboflavin, niacin, and folate. A balanced diet that includes a wide variety of foods can provide most of the vitamins and minerals required by the body.

FIBER

Dietary fiber is found in fruits and vegetables that are rich in cellulose. Fiber is classified as water soluble or non–water soluble. The main function of fiber in the diet is to provide bulk to feces and promote elimination. For example, the skins of many fruits, such as plums and apples, are a source of insoluble fiber, and the pulp of the fruit is soluble fiber. The insoluble fiber attracts water, bulks up stool, and aids in elimination. Some other sources of insoluble fiber are whole wheat, celery, potato skins, and wheat and corn bran.

The average American consumes less than half the amount of dietary fiber required for good health. The prevalence of fast foods rich in fats and carbohydrates and low in fiber are considered factors contributing to obesity by many experts. The American Dietetic Association (ADA) recommends consumption of at least 25 to 30 grams of fiber a day for a healthy adult.

WATER

Water is critical to health. Individuals may survive long periods without food but only several days without water. Water makes up about 70% of the human body and is the major solvent in which biochemical reactions occur. Every cell in the body requires water to perform its functions adequately. Many experts recommend that the intake of water should be between 2 to 3 liters per day, or more, depending on the individual's size and amount of physical exertion, the temperature of the environment, and other factors. Roughly 20% to 25% of daily water intake comes from food, and the remainder comes from drinking a variety of beverages including water.

Calories

Carbohydrates, fats, and proteins are energy-producing nutrients. Energy released during metabolism is measured in kilocalories with 1 kilocalorie (kcal) equaling 1,000 calories in food intake. The term *kilocalorie* is used interchangeably with the term *calorie*. A kilocalorie is a measure of the amount of heat required to raise the temperature of 1 kilogram of water 1° Celsius.

When proteins and carbohydrates are broken down in the body, they release 4 kcal per gram consumed, whereas fats release 9 kcal per gram eaten. When excess calories are consumed, they are stored as fat. Thus there must be a balance between the number of calories taken in daily and the amount of calories burned in order to maintain body weight. To lose weight, more calories/energy must be burned than taken in as food. For weight loss, physicians generally recommend that a person consume 500 calories less each day than needed to maintain their weight.

Daily caloric requirements for an individual depend on the sex, age, activity level, and size of the person. A pregnant woman or nursing mother needs more calories per day than they would normally consume. Nutrition experts in general recommend the following ranges to provide adequate energy and nutrients:

- 50–60% of calories from carbohydrates
- 20–30% of calories from fats
- 10–20% of calories from protein

Food Pyramid Guidelines

The U.S. Department of Agriculture (USDA) published a revised Food Pyramid in 2005. Instead of making specific recommendations about the amounts of each of the food groups that are to be consumed each day, the Food Pyramid recommends a personalized approach to food intake and exercise. Figure 20-2 illustrates the Food Pyramid with six

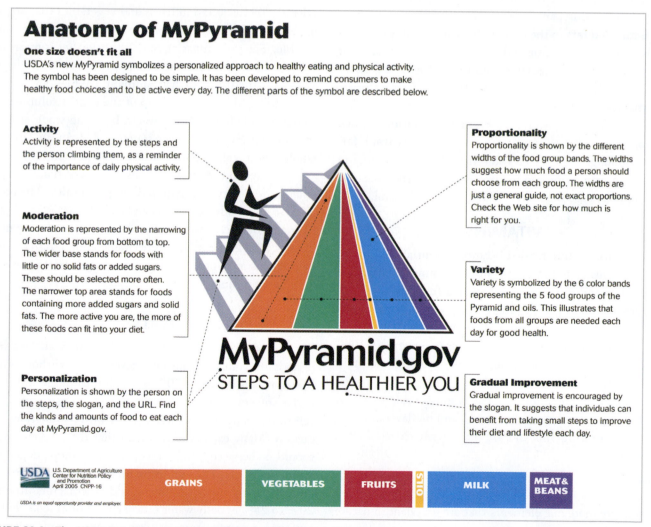

FIGURE 20-2 The USDA Food Pyramid: a personalized approach to healthy eating.
Source: www.MyPyramid.gov.

different color bands that are wide at the bottom representing foods with little or no solid fats or added sugars. The foods represented by the narrow bands of color contain more solid fats and added sugar and should be selected less frequently; it is advised that these foods comprise a larger percentage of the daily diet. The color bands represent grains (orange), vegetables (green), fruits (red), oils (yellow), milk (blue), and meat and beans (purple). On the left side of the pyramid is a figure walking up stairs, which represents the need for daily exercise.

The USDA has developed a Web site, www.MyPyramid .gov, that provides personalized recommendations for food choices and physical activity for a healthy balanced diet. The recommendations take into consideration age, size, and activity level. Interactive activities and printed materials are available at the Web site. In addition, you will find a tracking sheet for daily journaling of food intake, as well as an interactive food group game for children.

Reading a Food Label

Before a patient can begin to make dietary changes, he or she must be able to read and understand a food label. The ability to read a food label correctly is an important tool to help maintain a healthy lifestyle. Figure 20-3 is an example of a food label listing nutritional value:

- **Serving size *and* servings per container.** A food label lists the serving size. The number of servings in this example is 10 per container.

- **Amount per serving.** This heading applies to the rest of the information on the label, except the ingredients.

- **Calories.** The label lists the calories per serving. This label denotes 130 calories per serving. The serving size is 6 crackers, and if the person consumes 12 crackers that doubles the amount of calories eaten. Next the label lists the number of calories from fat. In this example, 40 calories of the total 130 calories per serving are from fat.

- **% Daily value.** The next category of information quantifies the nutrients obtained from eating one serving (6 crackers). The percentages given are based on a diet of 2,000 calories a day.

- **Total fat.** Listed next is the total fat as mentioned and the percentage of the daily value. Thus, this product contains a total of 5 grams of fat per serving, and that is 7% of the daily value of fat that should be consumed that day. The total fat is further divided into saturated fat, trans fat, polyunsaturated fat, and

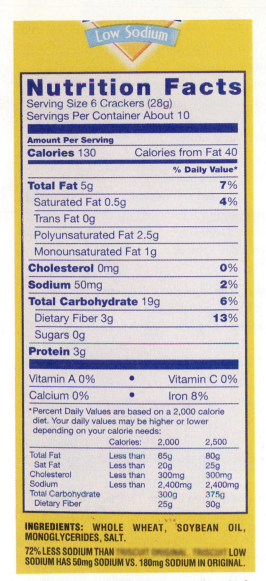

FIGURE 20-3 Food label listing nutritional information.

monounsaturated fat. In our example, the saturated fat amount is .05 g and 4% of the daily value. (Saturated fat comes from animal sources and contains more cholesterol than unsaturated fat.)

- **Cholesterol.** The amount of cholesterol in one serving is presented in milligrams and as a percentage. In this case both amounts are 0.

- **Sodium.** In this example, the amount of sodium is 50 mg, which is 2% of the daily value that should be eaten. (Patients on low-sodium diets must pay close attention to this listing.)

- **Total carbohydrates.** The label lists the total amount of carbohydrates in a serving and the amounts from dietary fiber and simple sugar. On this label, those values are 19 g total carbohydrate (6%), 3 g fiber (13%), and 0 g sugar.

- **Protein.** Protein is the amount of protein per serving, in this case 3 g.

- **Vitamins and minerals.** This is a listing of the amount of vitamins and minerals per serving. This label lists Vitamin A, Vitamin C, Calcium, and Iron. The product in the example contains only 8% of the Percent Daily Value of iron.

- **Other information.** Below the vitamin/minerals listing is an explanation of the Percent Daily Value. It provides the suggested amounts of total fat, saturated fat, cholesterol, sodium, total carbohydrates, and calcium based on a 2,000 and a 2,500 calories per day plan. An individual's daily values may be higher or lower than these, based on their total caloric requirement.

- **Ingredients.** The ingredients are listed with the ingredient in the largest amount present in the food listed first, followed by other items in descending order. Preservatives, artificial coloring agents, and flavors are also listed. This part of the label is essential to patients who have life-threatening allergies to such ingredients as food dyes, nuts, and specific chemicals.

The 1994 Nutrition Labeling and Education Act requires that any specific claims made on the label must conform to USDA guidelines and definitions, such as the following:

- **Reduced or low fat** must have 25% less fat per serving than the regular food product.

- **Low fat** means that the product may have no more than 3 grams of fat per serving.

- **Fat free** means that the product may have no more than 0.5 gram of fat per serving.

- **Light/Lite** means that the product must have at least ⅓ fewer calories per serving than the regular product.

Terms such as *natural, best choice,* or *right* are not covered by these guidelines.

Dietary Guidelines

In the United States nutritional standards and recommendations are controlled by the USDA. The field of dietetics also is regulated, and dieticians are registered with the national Commission for Dietetic Registration and the American Dietetic Association. Registered dietitians (RDs) hold advanced college degrees and have extensive training in a variety of health care settings. The term *nutritionist* can be used by anyone and is mainly unregulated.

Once a patient has seen the physician and a thorough physical examination has been completed, the patient may be advised to make changes in his or her eating habits. A recommendation to see an RD may also be made. In some facilities medical assistants and other health care providers may be asked to give basic information to the patient and reinforce the physician's dietary recommendations. Many food plan modifications can be made to treat a variety of health problems. These are considered in this chapter after a brief presentation of the suggested food guidelines the average individual should be following.

The USDA and the Department of Health and Human Services (HHS) have released guidelines for Americans for a healthy way of life. These guidelines may be found on the Web site http://www.health.gov/dietaryguidelines. These guidelines are based on the Food Pyramid and are adjusted specifically to the patient's size, age, and activity level. In

---

BOX 20-1 Food Group Substitutions and Equivalent Servings

- **Grains.** 1 serving equals ½ cup cooked rice, pasta, or cooked cereal; 1 ounce dry pasta or rice; 1 slice bread; 1 small muffin; 1 cup ready-to-eat cereal. Half of all grains each day should be whole grains.

- **Fruits and Vegetables.** 2 servings = 1 cup; 1 cup cut-up raw or cooked fruit or vegetables; 1 cup fruit or vegetable juice; 2 cups leafy salad greens. Choose canned fruits packed in water. Less than half of fruit eaten daily should be in juice form. Select vegetables of a variety of colors.

- **Meats and Beans.** 1 ounce = 1 serving of lean meat, poultry, or fish; 1 egg; ¼ cup cooked dry beans or tofu; 1 tablespoon (tbsp) peanut butter; ½ ounce (oz) nuts or seeds. Avoid beef with high fat or excess marbling.

- **Milk.** 1 serving = 1 cup of milk or yogurt; 1½ ounces (oz) natural cheese or 2 ounces (oz) processed cheese. Use reduced-fat or low-fat milk and dairy products. Avoid margarines and cream.

- **Oils.** 1 serving = 1 tablespoon (tbsp) regular salad dressing; 1 tablespoon (tbsp) mayonnaise. ½ serving = 1 teaspoon (tsp) vegetable oil; 1 teaspoon (tsp) margarine; 1 tablespoon (tbsp) low-fat dressing. 0 serving = 1 tablespoon (tbsp) fat-free dressing.

BOX 20-2 Sizes of Portions

Simple rules to size up portions:

- 1 cup of salad greens = about the size of a fist
- 1 ounce of cheese = about the size of both thumbs
- 1 portion meat = the size of a fist or deck of cards

---

general terms, the following dietary guidelines should be followed for a healthy lifestyle:

- Make good choices from every food group on the Food Pyramid.
- Achieve a balance between your food intake and activity level.
- Select foods that are low in fat, saturated fat, and cholesterol.
- Limit the amount of salt.
- Use moderation in the amount of refined sugar.
- Use alcohol in moderation.
- Read food labels.
- Use realistic portion control.

Each group on the Food Pyramid allows substitutions for items recommended and for an equivalent amount of a different item substituted from the same food group. For example, a patient may choose 1 slice of bread or ¾ cup of cereal. (Refer to Box 20-1 for Food Group Substitutions and Equivalent Servings.)

Many people have difficulty with portion control when trying to adopt a healthier life style. See Box 20-2 for some suggestions for sizing up portions without measuring. The USDA Food Guide for a 2,000 calories/day healthy eating program is illustrated in Table 20-1. A similar table is available from the USDA for eating plans that require fewer or greater numbers of calories per day. In addition, the DASH food plan to stop hypertension for varying calorie requirements is also available on the USDA Web site.

Dietary Modifications

A diet that is modified for health reasons is known as a therapeutic diet. An eating program can be modified in a number of ways for a variety of reasons. Examples of therapeutic diets are available from a variety of sources. Registered dietitians may be asked to meet with patients to modify their eating plan for therapeutic reasons. It is important to be familiar with the different types of therapeutic diets and the reasons they are used. (Table 20-2 lists the reasons a diet change is necessary and briefly describes each type of diet.)

To assist patients with food plan modifications, health care providers may find an important tool is to write down their own food intake for several days and then to evaluate where they stand nutritionally. Individuals who use a food journal daily are often more successful in making life changes than those who do not write down their intake

TABLE 20-1 2,000 Calorie/Day Food Guide

Food Groups	Servings
Fruits	2 cups
Vegetables	2.5 cups
Grains	6 ounces
Meats and Beans	5.5 ounces
Milk	3 cups
Oils	6 teaspoons
Discretionary Calorie Allowance* (the remaining amount of calories in a food intake pattern after accounting for calories needed for all food groups and using forms of foods that are fat free or low fat with no added sugar)	267 calories

TABLE 20-2 Therapeutic Diets

Type of Diet	Foods Eliminated	Modifications	Disease/Disorder
Clear liquid diet	No solid food or milk products	Clear soup, broth, plain tea, coffee, carbonated beverages	Prior to surgery, certain diagnostic or blood tests or examinations, postsurgery
Full liquid diet	No solids	Clear diet plus fruit and vegetable juices, strained soup, milk or milk shakes, ice cream (melted)	Patients unable to chew or digest solids due to GI problems, infections, oral surgery
Soft diet	No hard-to-chew or hard-to-swallow foods	All soups and liquids, cooked or canned fruits and vegetables, ground meat, soft fish, poultry	Patients with dental problems or difficulty swallowing, postsurgery
Bland diet	No seasonings, irritating fibers	Low fiber, mild foods, milk products, cooked fruits, noncitrus juices	GI problems, allergies
BRAT diet	No foods except those listed	Bananas, rice, applesauce, toast	Vomiting, diarrhea in small children
Elimination diet	No foods specifically named by physician	For example, nuts, dairy products	Severe allergies
Low sodium diet	Reduce sodium intake < 2,000 mg/day or 1 tsp table salt	Increase intake of fresh vegetables and fruits; reduce intake of processed foods and snacks	Hypertension, kidney disease
High-fiber diet	Eat less dairy, animal products	Increase fresh vegetables, fruits, high-fiber cereals, whole wheat breads, legumes	Constipation, diverticular disease
Diabetic diet	Reduce amount of refined sugars, carbohydrates, baked goods, candy, etc.	Balanced diet from Food Pyramid groups with specific exchanges to keep glucose levels in control	Diabetes mellitus types 1 and 2
Low-residue diet	No fried foods, no raw fruit except bananas, no high-fiber foods, no dairy products	Cooked vegetables, fruits, eggs, cooked cereal, lean meats, poultry	Diarrhea, colitis, colostomy
Weight-reduction diet	Reduce amount of refined sugars, carbohydrates, baked goods, candy, etc.; reduce fat intake	Exercise, balanced food plan from food groups with a calorie limit established by size, age, activity level	Obesity, diabetes, heart disease
Pregnancy, lactation	Avoidance of junk food with "empty calories," minimized sodium intake, avoidance of processed foods and certain fish	Balanced food plan from food groups with increased protein and caloric values, per physician; folate-rich foods; vitamin supplements	Pregnancy, nursing

daily. In addition, keeping track of water intake and daily exercise is beneficial when trying to make changes.

Patient Education

Patient education is an important element in a health care plan. Most individuals comply with treatment plans more if they understand their illness and how the plan will help them achieve their health goals. Treatment plans for children are usually taught to them by the parent; however, adults may require educational sessions and activities to learn a skill. Adult patients' learning abilities are affected by factors such as their illness, years of education, reading and vocabulary levels, time constraints, and family situations. Learning styles among people differ. Some learn better by listening, some by visual cues, and others by hands-on activities. Many of us learn through a combination of all the pathways. To be effective, a learning process has to consider all the factors influencing a patient's learning ability as well as the way they learn most easily. Good communication skills on the part of the health care provider are important, as is an understanding of human behavior.

EFFECTIVE TEACHING PLANS

Developing a teaching plan involves six steps:

Assess the patient. The first step is to determine the patient's ability to learn, willingness to change, prior understanding, and any other factors that could interfere with the learning process.

Set the goal. Determine what the patient should learn from the teaching session. What information will be covered in the teaching session?

Define the learning objectives. What steps or procedures must a patient understand and demonstrate in the teaching session?

Gather tools and materials. What tools, equipment, written materials, audiovisual aides, diagrams, and models are needed to achieve the objectives?

Implement the plan. Teach the patient using the previously taken steps. Be clear, demonstrate, and ask the patient to demonstrate a skill or verbalize in return. Use other materials as needed.

Evaluate the goal. Ask the patient to verbalize or demonstrate the goal set. Ask open-ended questions and get feedback. Document the teaching session, including comments about any circumstances that may have interfered or prevented the patient from achieving the goal.

Compliance is a term used to describe a patient's adherence to the health plan the physician has recommended. Whether the health plan refers to taking daily medication, following a food plan, or going to physical therapy, **noncompliance** can be a problem. Failure to follow the recommended health guidelines should be documented in a patient's record.

Health care providers must consider cultural customs in every phase of patient relations. When assisting with food recommendations based on the physician's orders, ethnic and dietary habits must be understood. The www .mypyramid.gov Web site has suggestions for dietary plans suitable for many ethnic groups, including Native Americans, Hispanics, and African Americans. A basic familiarity with some examples of various ethnic food choices is helpful when developing a nutritional teaching plan. Vegetarian food regimes are fairly common today, and a basic familiarity with the food choices also can be developed at the mypyramid .gov Web site. Some vegetarians eat fish or eggs, and others eat only fruits and nuts. A **vegan** does not eat any product associated with animals, including eggs and dairy products. (Procedure 20-1 outline steps for teaching a patient to read a food label. Procedures 20-2 and 20-3 explain how to develop teaching plans focused on nutrition and patient behavior.)

PROCEDURE 20-1

TEACHING A PATIENT TO READ A FOOD LABEL

ABHES VII.MA.A.1 2(a); VII.MA.A.1 9(r)   CAAHEP IV.P (5); IV.P (9)

OBJECTIVE: To teach a patient to read a food label and use nutritional information to make better food selections for a healthier lifestyle.

STANDARD: The time this task takes is 20 minutes or longer, depending on patient's ability and previous knowledge.

EQUIPMENT AND SUPPLIES: Variety of food products; diagram of food label; pencil or pen; paper; Food Pyramid chart; appropriate brochures; audiovisual aids; handouts; patient's record.

STEPS:

1. Check patient's record for physician's orders, and check for allergies.

2. Review patient history to gather overall idea of patient's background, lifestyle, cultural origins, and physical problems.

3. Assemble equipment and supplies.

4. Identify and greet patient. Explain procedure and purpose.

5. Display foods and other materials. Give paper and pencil to patient or caregiver if patient needs assistance.

6. Ask patient about use of food labels to date. Assess whether or not patient has used labels before. If they are unfamiliar with labels, use a diagram to illustrate information listed.

7. Ask patient to explain their idea of size of a serving of ice cream or meat or potato chips. Then show patient what

½ cup ice cream, 3 ounces meat, or 1 serving of chips looks like. (Use whatever food example is pertinent to patient's cultural background.)

8. Ask patient to select one food product you have exhibited, and ask patient to explain what each label listing means. Encourage patient with positive statements, such as "That's right." Provide positive feedback.

9. Select another food product with a healthier list of ingredients than item the patient selected. Ask patient to compare the two items and to write down or verbalize nutritional facts listed in each category. Ask patient to identify which is healthier food.

10. To evaluate patient's understanding, ask how food label would help in shopping or preparing foods. Provide positive feedback. Give patient printed information to take home as a reference. Remind patient to call with questions.

11. Document patient's record.

CHARTING EXAMPLE: 02/06/XX 11:00 A.M. After discussing food label and nutritional information on food labels, Pt. was able to demonstrate understanding by verbalizing nutritional facts on label. Pt. given printed label material, copy of low-carbohydrate, low-fat diet that Dr. Lowe discussed with him. Pt. to call with questions if needed. · · · · · · · · · S. Mendoza, RMA

PROCEDURE 20-2

DEVELOPING A TEACHING PLAN TO ENCOURAGE AN INCREASE IN DAILY FIBER

ABHES VII.MA.A.1 2(a); VII.MA.A.1 9(r)   CAAHEP IV.P (5); IV.P (9)

OBJECTIVE: To develop a teaching plan to encourage a patient to increase daily fiber intake.

STANDARD: The time this task takes is 15–20 minutes, depending on the learning ability and condition of patient.

EQUIPMENT AND SUPPLIES: Patient's record; physician's orders; high-fiber foods or photos of them; diagram of colon; Food Pyramid; printed list of high-fiber foods; daily journal; pen.

STEPS:

1. Check patient's record for physician's orders, and check for allergies.

2. Review patient history to gather overall idea of patient's background, lifestyle, cultural origins, and physical problems.

3. Assemble equipment and supplies.

4. Greet patient, and explain goal (to increase amount of fiber in patient's daily diet to relieve constipation) of teaching session.

5. Ask patient to describe an average daily dietary plan and amount of water intake. Smile, be encouraging. Ask about bowel habits and frequency.

6. Show patient USDA Food Pyramid with food groups. Ask patient to name one or two types of food that would be found in each food group. Provide positive reinforcement.

7. Ask patient to explain what types of foods he or she believes are high in fiber.

8. Display high-fiber food or photos of foods. Give paper and pencil to patient (or to caregiver if patient needs assistance). Ask patient to make a list of all high-fiber foods shown and any others that come to mind.

9. Speak in terms appropriate to patient's level of understanding. Be positive and supportive.

10. Keeping in mind patient's cultural preferences and other factors, ask patient to make another list of preferred foods from high-fiber lists provided by you and written by patient.

11. Show food label, and evaluate patient's comprehension of label's nutritional information. Pay attention to fiber content of label. See if patient can name several other food products that would have more fiber. Provide positive feedback.

12. Explain need for adequate daily amounts of water and exercise within scope of patient's individual abilities.

13. Encourage patient to make a daily food plan, including water intake.

14. Give patient daily food plan sheets, and explain how to record what patient eats and drinks.

15. To evaluate understanding, ask patient to plan next day's meals with you. Modify plan with patient as needed.

16. Provide patient with printed material. Suggest Web sites and other information appropriate for patient's abilities that can be accessed at home.

17. Encourage patient to call with questions after implementing program changes for a few days.

18. At conclusion of session, summarize goals, learning objectives, and session content.

19. Document patient's record with copies of educational materials provided and evaluation of session.

CHARTING EXAMPLE: 02/06/XX 1:00 P.M. Met with Pt. for education session to encourage increase in amount of high-fiber foods, water to relieve constipation. Pt. identified high-fiber foods from Food Pyramid groups. Pt. able to describe present daily food plan. Agreed with need to alleviate constipation and seemed positive about trying to increase daily fiber intake. Pt. verbalized correct foods to add over the next week, amount of water to drink. Pt. given printed materials about high fiber and daily journal pages for week. Pt. to call with any questions. Pt. appeared positive toward making changes. · · · · · · · · · · M. Morris, CMA (AAMA)

Wellness and Prevention

With a greater push toward preventive medicine and making life changes to promote wellness, teaching strategies are increasingly important. Community programs provide many services related to disease prevention and health promotion free of charge. Hospitals clinics and public health offices offer services as well.

A list of preventive screenings and health services should be available in each facility. Free public health brochures are available from many government agencies and are great resources for patient education. Box 20-3 is a list of Internet resources to help reinforce patient education. (Procedure 20-3 lists the steps to develop a plan to teach wellness and disease prevention to a patient.)

PROCEDURE 20-3

TEACHING WELLNESS AND DISEASE PREVENTION TO A PATIENT

ABHES VII.MA.A.1 2(a); VII.MA.A.1 9(r)   CAAHEP IV.P (5); IV.P (9)

OBJECTIVE: To teach wellness care and disease prevention to a patient with elevated cholesterol and LDL levels as ordered by physician.

STANDARD: The time this task takes depends on the development of the plan and the ability of the patient to comprehend the information.

EQUIPMENT AND SUPPLIES: Patient's medical record; physician's orders; examples of low-fat foods; diagrams of atherosclerotic arteries; normal lipid levels versus patient's levels; relevant handouts and brochures, if available.

STEPS:

1. Check patient's record for physician's orders and allergies.

2. Review patient history to gather overall idea of patient's background, lifestyle, cultural origins, and physical problems. Determine what factors may interfere with patient's learning.

3. Collect material and supplies geared to lowering fat intake. Keep in mind patient's lifestyle and health problems.

4. List goals and learning objectives to be covered with patient. The following are points to be included in reducing dietary fats:
   - Read food labels. Select food with less than 3 grams of fat per serving.
   - Grill, broil, and bake foods instead of frying.
   - Limit high-calorie/high-fat foods, such as candy and ice cream.
   - Use skim milk or 1% milk.

- Use less butter and margarine.
- Remove fat from meat and skin from poultry before cooking.
- Use low-fat dressings on salads.
- Eat less red meat and more fish.
- Eat beans as a source of protein.

5. Greet patient, and explain goal of teaching session and purpose.

6. Ask patient to describe his or her daily dietary plan and water intake. Smile. Be encouraging.

7. Determine that patient understands different types of fats (saturated fat, unsaturated fat, trans fat) and a few foods in which each is found.

8. Speak in terms appropriate to patient's level of understanding. Be positive and supportive.

9. Keep patient's cultural preferences in mind. Ask patient to list food choices he or she would be willing to make based on your list of suggestions.

10. Encourage patient to make a food plan each night for the next day.

11. Give patient daily food plan forms, and explain procedure to write down what patient eats and drinks.

12. Provide patient with appropriate printed material. If appropriate for patient's abilities, suggest Web sites and other information that can be accessed at home or at the library.

13. Encourage patient to call with questions after implementing program changes for a few days.

14. At conclusion of session, summarize goals, learning objectives, and session content.

15. Document patient's record with copies of educational materials provided and evaluation of session.

CHARTING EXAMPLE: 02//15/XX 5:00 P.M. Instructed Pt. on low-fat food program; covered dangers of elevated cholesterol and explained HDL/LDL. Pt. able to verbalize information. Gave weekly food journal sheets and reading info from AHA. Web site info demonstrated. Pt. able to demonstrate in return. · L. Lopez, RMA

BOX 20-3 Health Resources for Reinforcing Patient Education

National Institute of Arthritis and Musculoskeletal and Skin Diseases (NIAMS)	www.niams.nih.gov	National Center for Complementary and Alternative Medicine	www.nccam.nih.gov
National Library of Medicine	www.nlm.nih.gov	American Academy of Pediatrics	www.aap.org
National Institute of Drug Abuse	www.nida.nih.gov		
		American Cancer Society	www.cancer.org
Food and Nutrition Information	www.usda.gov	American Heart Association	www.americanheart.org
Alcoholics Anonymous	www.aa.org	Food Pyramid	www.MyPyramid.gov

21 Cardiology and Pulmonology

PROCEDURES

Procedure 21-1 Performing a 12-Lead Single-Channel or Multichannel Electrocardiogram

Procedure 21-2 Applying a Holter Monitor

Procedure 21-3 Assisting with Treadmill Stress Testing

Procedure 21-4 Performing Spirometry Testing

Procedure 21-5 Teaching Peak Flow Measurement

Procedure 21-6 Instructing a Patient to Use a Metered-Dose Inhaler (MDI)

Procedure 21-7 Administering a Nebulized Breathing Treatment

Procedure 21-8 Administering Oxygen by Nasal Cannula or Face Mask

Procedure 21-9 Collecting a Sputum Specimen

TERMS TO LEARN

artifacts

electrodes

leads

syncope

forced vital capacity (FVC)

chronic obstructive pulmonary disease (COPD)

metered-dose inhalers

nebulizers

nares

expectorate

Cardiology

The circulatory system consists of the heart, blood vessels, and blood. Disorders of the cardiovascular system are the number one cause of death in the United States. Lifestyle factors such as lack of exercise, stress, obesity, and genetics all play a part in cardiovascular disease. The symptoms of cardiovascular disease and disorders are varied due to the wide range of precipitating causes, such as poor circulation, defective heart valves, and blood clots. Blood tests and other diagnostic procedures are among the most common tests health care workers perform. Procedures for performing 12-lead and 3-lead electrocardiograms, applying a Holter monitor, and assisting with treadmill testing follow.

PERFORMING A 12-LEAD ELECTROCARDIOGRAM

Electrical charges created by the cardiac conduction system can be sensed throughout the body. Electrodes placed in specific areas can detect those charges and transmit them to an electrocardiogram (ECG or EKG) machine for amplification and recording on paper. The ECG is one of the most valuable diagnostic tools for evaluating the electrical system of the heart. It can relate changes that have taken place in the heart, although it cannot predict what will happen in the future. The physician can assess the ECG recording for cardiac problems. Interpretation of ECG recording is the duty only of the physician or other licensed personnel. However, effective interpretation depends on the quality of the recording provided by the individual performing the ECG.

If no energy is sensed by the ECG machine, a flat line will be recorded. Deflections from the baseline follow a fundamental rule in electrocardiography: current flowing toward a positive electrode creates an upright deflection, while current flowing toward a negative electrode creates a downward deflection.

Each cardiac cycle (the mechanical events that occur to pump blood) is represented on an ECG by wave patterns called P, QRS, and T. Figure 21-1 illustrates each part of one normal cardiac cycle and the corresponding area of the heart that triggers the complex. Figure 21-2 shows how time is represented by each small block on ECG paper.

Patient preparation for an ECG is fairly simple and noninvasive. It is most important that the patient be comfortable and calm to obtain an artifact-free result. **Artifacts** are abnormal signals that do not reflect the electrical activity of the heart. They may be caused by

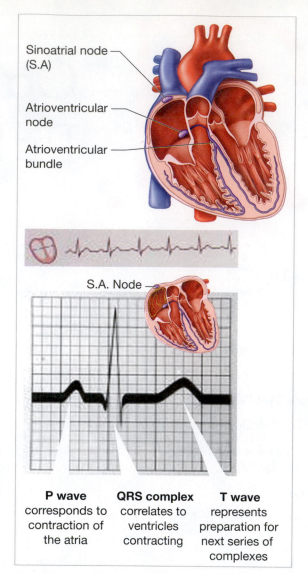

P wave	QRS complex	T wave
corresponds to contraction of the atria	correlates to ventricles contracting	represents preparation for next series of complexes

FIGURE 21-1 The heart and an electrocardiogram tracing.

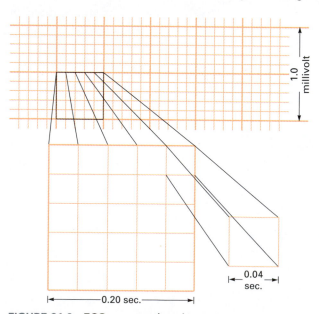

FIGURE 21-2 ECG paper and markings.

patient movement (Figure 21-3A), electrical interference (Figure 21-3B), or improperly attached electrodes (Figure 21-3C).

Many types of ECG machines are in use. A conventional 12-lead single-channel electrocardiograph may be operated either manually or in automatic mode. In a single-channel machine, each lead is recorded separately, one after the other. These recordings must be cut and mounted onto special mounting paper, then placed in the patient's chart.

A multichannel ECG machine records several different leads simultaneously. The 3-channel ECG machine is widely used and records Leads I, II, III; next aVR, aVL, and aVF; then V1, V2, V3; and last V4, V5, and V6. Multichannel machines provide results more quickly and do not require cutting strips to mount them. Interpretive software is built in on some ECG machines, as are telephone or fax transmission capabilities.

Electrodes, or sensors, may be made of metal or other types of conductive material. They pick up the electrical

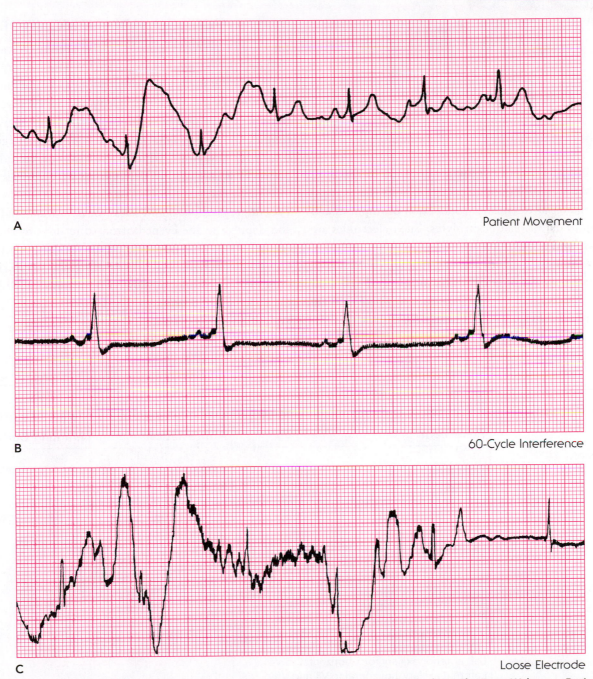

A   Patient Movement

B   60-Cycle Interference

C   Loose Electrode

FIGURE 21-3   Types of interface: (A) patient movement; (B) 60 cycle interference; (C) loose electrode. From Walraven, *Basic Arrhythmias, 6e.*

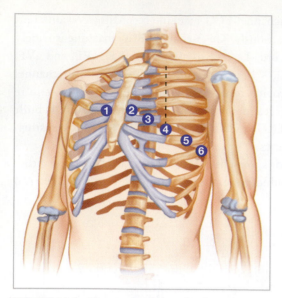

FIGURE 21-4 Placement of chest leads.

right leg (RL), and left leg (LL). The chest leads, or precordial leads, are abbreviated with V and numbered V1, V2, V3, V4, V5, and V6. Figure 21-4 illustrates the placement of the precordial leads. Each lead is coded on the recording automatically using a series of dots and dashes. Table 21-1 gives the location of each sensor and matching marking code.

The physician may request a rhythm strip (lead II is run for 20 seconds) to help diagnose the patient's problem. This is handed to the physician to review before proceeding with the rest of the ECG.

APPLYING A HOLTER MONITOR

The Holter monitor records cardiac activity for at least a 24-hour period while the patient is ambulatory. Holter monitoring is performed when the ECG is not conclusive, fatigue is a factor, or an irregularity was not captured on the tracing. It is helpful to try to coordinate symptoms such as fatigue, chest pain, **syncope** (faintness), and vertigo (dizziness) with cardiac arrhythmias. A small tape recorder and a patient diary are used to detect heart irregularities that are infrequent and not detected on the standard 12-lead ECG. Patient preparation should stress the importance of the diary and depressing the event button to record any distress or "event" when any symptoms occur. Patients should maintain normal activity level, but during the test period they must exclude bathing or showering, swimming, sleeping on the abdomen, and using electric blankets. They also should avoid high-voltage areas.

impulses and relay them over wires or **leads** to the ECG machine. Many facilities use disposable sensors that contain electrolyte material to enhance conduction of impulses and do not require additional electrolytes. Such electrodes are self-adhesive and disposable.

Lead wires coming from the machine are connected to the sensors by means of small alligator clips. These lead wires are color coded or labeled according to where they are to be attached—for example, left arm (LA), right arm (RA),

TABLE 21-1 Sensor/Lead Placement and Marking Codes

Lead	Placement	Abbreviation	Marking Code
Limb Leads:			
Lead I	Right arm to left arm	RA–LA	.
Lead II	Right arm to left leg	RA–LL	..
Lead III	Left arm to left leg	LA–LL	...
Augmented Leads:			
aVR	RA–midpoint LA–LL	(LA–LL) RA	-
aVL	LA–midpoint (RA–LL)	(RA–LL) LA	--
aVF	LL–midpoint (RA–LA)	(RA–LA) LL	---
Chest Leads			
V1	4th intercostal space, right sternal border		_ .
V2	4th intercostal space, left sternal border		_ ..
V3	Midway between V2 and V4		_ ...
V4	5th intercostal space, midclavicular left		_ ....
V5	Left anterior axillary fold, horizontal to V4		_ .....
V6	Left mid axillary, horizontal to V4 and V5		_ ......

PROCEDURE 21-1

PERFORMING A 12-LEAD SINGLE-CHANNEL OR MULTICHANNEL ELECTROCARDIOGRAM

ABHES VII.MA.A.1 9(o)(l)   CAAHEP I.P (5)

OBJECTIVE: STANDARD: This task takes 10 minutes.

EQUIPMENT AND SUPPLIES: Quiet room; ECG machine with cable and lead wires; alligator clips; ECG paper; disposable electrodes; electrolyte if needed; alcohol; patient gown; patient's record; pen; mounting form.

STEPS:

1. Review physician's orders.
2. Perform hand hygiene.
3. Assemble equipment.
4. Attach and plug in power cord.

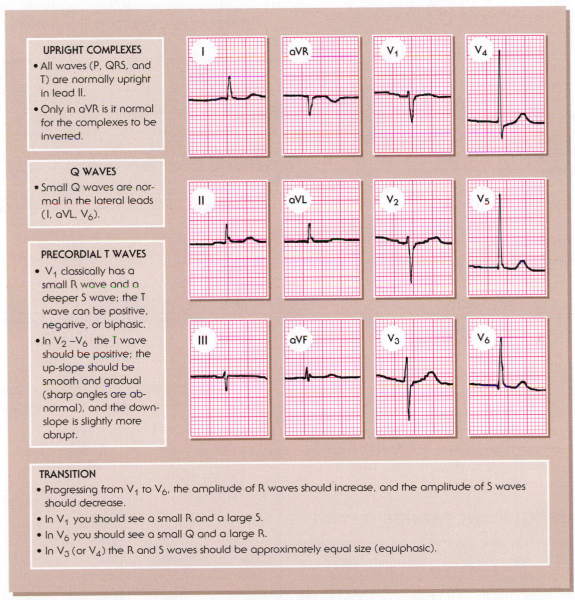

UPRIGHT COMPLEXES
- All waves (P, QRS, and T) are normally upright in lead II.
- Only in aVR is it normal for the complexes to be inverted.

Q WAVES
- Small Q waves are normal in the lateral leads (I, aVL, V₆).

PRECORDIAL T WAVES
- V₁ classically has a small R wave and a deeper S wave; the T wave can be positive, negative, or biphasic.
- In V₂–V₆ the T wave should be positive; the up-slope should be smooth and gradual (sharp angles are abnormal), and the downslope is slightly more abrupt.

TRANSITION
- Progressing from V₁ to V₆, the amplitude of R waves should increase, and the amplitude of S waves should decrease.
- In V₁ you should see a small R and a large S.
- In V₆ you should see a small Q and a large R.
- In V₃ (or V₄) the R and S waves should be approximately equal size (equiphasic).

FIGURE 21-5   Features of a normal 12-lead ECG. From Walraven, *Basic Arrhythmias*, 6e.

5. Verify that machine is operational and positioned properly.

6. Identify and greet patient, and explain procedure.

7. Provide a gown for privacy. Instruct patient to disrobe above waist. Offer assistance as needed. Explain that gown opening must be in front. Female patients should be told to remove their stockings/panty hose.

8. Position patient in supine position, and provide pillows and draping for comfort and privacy as needed.

9. Enter patient data: name, sex, date, identification number, height, weight, cardiac medications, and other identifying data as needed.

10. Prepare skin at electrode sites by wiping away skin oils with alcohol pads. Shave or clip extra hair to provide good contact.

11. Apply electrodes on fleshy portions of upper arms and lower legs. Arm sensors should have tabs pointing down, and leg sensors should have tabs pointing up. Apply chest electrodes V1 through V6 as shown in Figure 21-4, with tabs pointing down.

12. Connect lead wires at all sites. Recheck each to ensure that they are firmly and correctly attached. (Leads are color coded as follows: RA = white; LA = black; RL = green; LL = red. Chest electrodes are brown or multicolored, depending on machine.)

13. Remind patient not to talk or move while ECG is being performed.

14. Set sensitivity at 1 and paper speed at 25 mm per second.

15. Depress Auto Run button, and record 12-lead ECG. If artifacts are present, use problem-solving skills to correct problems.

16. When ECG is completed, check for artifacts and standardization mark. (With standardization set on 1, normal standardization mark should be 10 mm high and 2 small squares wide; set on ½, standardization mark should be 5 mm high; and set on 2, standardization mark should be 20 mm high.)

17. If single-lead ECG machine used, carefully roll up entire strip appropriately labeled with patient information, and secure without paper clips for later mounting.

18. Disconnect lead wires, and remove sensors. Wipe off electrolyte, if used, from patient's skin.

19. Politely dismiss patient, assisting patient in stepping down from examination table and dressing if necessary.

20. Mount information if necessary, and record data in patient's record. (Figure 21-5 is an example of a normal 12-lead electrocardiogram.)

21. Clean examination room.

22. Perform hand hygiene.

CHARTING EXAMPLE: 3/9/XX 2:35 P.M. 12-lead ECG obtained and given to Dr. Lopez for evaluation. · M. Negri, CMA (AAMA)

The leads for a Holter monitor are placed in different locations than for a resting ECG (see Table 21-2). Disposable electrodes, special adhesive, and electrolyte gel are used. The Holter monitor remains in place for at least 24 hours, and the patient should return to the office to have it disconnected and removed.

EXERCISE TOLERANCE STRESS TESTING

At times patients will have symptoms that are not obvious on a resting ECG. A stress test is an evaluation of the heart's response to exercise while a 12-lead ECG is being performed. Faster heart rates make it easier to detect decreased blood flow. Stress testing is helpful to detect early cardiac

TABLE 21-2 Placement of Holter Monitor Electrodes

Electrode	Lead	Location
A (yellow)	mV1	4th intercostal space at right sternal border
B (white)	mV5	Right clavicle just lateral to sternum
C (blue)	mV1	Left clavicle just lateral to sternum
D (red)	mV5	5th intercostal space left of axillary line
E (green)	Ground	Lower right chest wall

PROCEDURE 21-2

APPLYING A HOLTER MONITOR

ABHES VII.MA.A.1 9(m)   CAAHEP I.P (5); IV.P (5)

OBJECTIVE: To apply a Holter monitor and provide patient instruction on wearing the monitor for 24 hours and recording information and symptoms in the diary.

STANDARD: This task takes 15 minutes.

EQUIPMENT AND SUPPLIES: Holter monitor with sensors; patient cable; patient activity diary; fresh batteries; blank recording tape; adhesive tape; razor; alcohol.

STEPS:

1. Review physician's orders.
2. Perform hand hygiene.
3. Assemble equipment. Install new batteries and a blank tape. Verify machine is operational.
4. Greet and identify patient, and explain procedure.
5. Provide gown (with opening in front for female patients). Ask patient to disrobe from waist up and then sit on examination table. Provide assistance as needed.
6. Prepare electrode sites and attach electrodes. Attach sensors in these locations: (A) 4th intercostal at right sternal edge; (B) right clavicle just lateral to sternum; (C) left clavicle just lateral to sternum; (D) 5th intercostal space left of axillary line; (E) lower right chest wall.
7. Attach wires to electrodes, and connect to patient cable. Perform a baseline recording.
8. Show patient Event, Clear, and Low Battery buttons (Figure 21-6).
9. Place recorder in carrying case, and attach to patient's belt or to shoulder strap. Check for excessive tension on wires. Record starting time in diary.

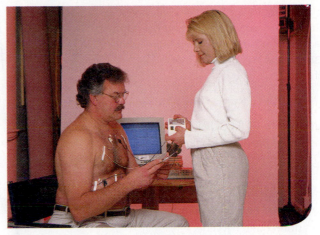

FIGURE 21-6 **Explain to the patient the Event button and how the monitor works.**

10. Confirm that patient understands all instructions.
11. Inform patient of time and date to return to have monitor removed.
12. Record information in patient's record.
13. Clean examination room.
14. Perform hand hygiene.

CHARTING EXAMPLE: 03/20/XX Holter monitor set up and started at 4:05 P.M. Patient given written and verbal instructions on diary, Event button, and activities of daily living. Pt. to return at 3:45 on 03/21/XX for removal of monitor. · D. Martinez, CMA (AAMA)

disease, evaluate results of cardiac rehabilitation, and assess those at high risk for developing heart disease. The treadmill test is a noninvasive ECG recording performed while the patient is closely monitored.

Frequent blood pressure readings are taken while the patient exercises on a treadmill at prescribed rates of speed and increased inclination. The test continues until the heart rate hits a predetermined level or the patient experiences fatigue or chest pain. Electrodes are applied to the chest only. Male patients with hairy chests should be shaved to promote adherence of the electrode.

After the exercise portion of the test is concluded the patient will rest while monitoring blood pressure and heart rate continue until both return to normal. Complications may occur and emergency carts appropriately stocked should be on hand.

Nuclear stress testing is helpful to determine which parts of the heart muscle have decreased blood flow. Although similar to treadmill testing, the patient is given an injection of a radioactive substance such as thallium and then exercises while BP and ECG monitoring take place.

PROCEDURE 21-3

ASSISTING WITH TREADMILL STRESS TESTING

ABHES VII.MA.A.1 9(m)   CAAHEP I.P (10)

OBJECTIVE: To apply patient electrodes to monitor and record ECG, BP, and heart rate while patient is exercising on treadmill with adjustments to treadmill as ordered by physician.

STANDARD: This task takes 30 minutes.

EQUIPMENT AND SUPPLIES: Treadmill; electrodes; blood pressure; monitor; emergency cart.

STEPS:

1. Review physician's orders.
2. Assemble necessary supplies.
3. Perform hand hygiene.
4. Identify, interview, and instruct patient.
5. Offer female patients a gown with opening in front. Shave male patients' chests as needed to allow for better adhesion of sensors.
6. Plug in power cord, and turn on machine.
7. Perform a baseline ECG (see Procedure 21-1).
8. Disconnect patient cable from ECG machine.
9. Attach sphygmomanometer to patient's arm.
10. Permit patient to walk on slow-moving treadmill to get feel of it.
11. Connect patient to all recording devices.
12. Check with physician to determine pace and incline of treadmill.
13. Record BP, ECG, and pulse (P), and respiration (R) periodically while observing patient for difficulty breathing, chest pain, redness, and signs of distress (Figure 21-7).

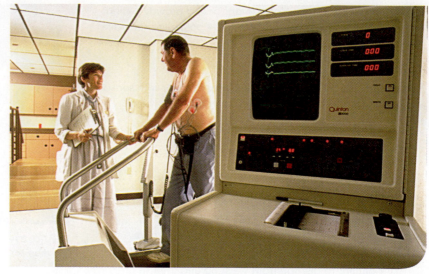

FIGURE 21-7   The patient must be observed very closely during a stress test.

14. When test is complete, clean patient's skin and assist as needed.
15. Document information in patient's record.
16. Clean area.
17. Perform hand hygiene.

CHARTING EXAMPLE: 3/20/XX 3:10 P.M. Treadmill stress test performed. Patient observed for 15 minutes after testing. Pt. says "I feel fine." Pt. tolerated procedure well. · M. Shapiro, RMA

Pulmonology

Pulmonology is the study and treatment of diseases of the respiratory system. The respiratory system includes the trachea, bronchial tubes, lungs, and alveoli. The primary function of the respiratory system is to conduct oxygen to the lungs for transportation via the bloodstream to all the cells in the body and to carry waste products, namely carbon dioxide and water, to the outside of the body for elimination. Pulmonary function tests are performed to evaluate lung volume and capacity, to assist in the differential diagnosis of patients with suspected obstructive or restrictive pulmonary disease processes, and to assess the effectiveness of drug therapies.

SPIROMETRY TESTING

One pulmonary function test frequently performed in medical offices is spirometry. A spirometer measures the amount of air that normally moves in and out of lungs and how

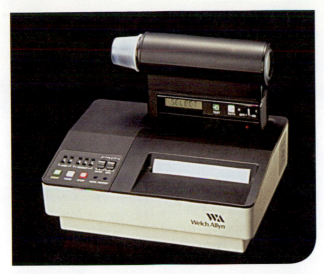

FIGURE 21-8 One type of spirometer.

much lung space is available after the patient normally inhales and exhales.

A diagnostic spirometer is employed to evaluate the patient's ability to ventilate during a maximum forced exhale. (See Figure 21-8 for an example of one type of spirometer.) This device measures and records the volume exhaled within a specific length of time (1 second, 3 seconds, etc.). The air movement is recorded on special paper with a vertical mark for each second and a horizontal mark for each liter of oxygen. **Forced vital capacity (FVC)** is the maximum volume of air expelled when the patient exhales as forcibly and quickly as possible. The patient must exhale as much air as possible and continue to exhale it for 6 seconds to be considered a satisfactory test. At least three efforts at exhaling must be demonstrated. Forced expiratory volume after 1 second (FEV^1) is the volume of air in liters that is forcefully exhaled in the first second of exhalation. In patients with healthy lungs, about 70% to 75% of air is exhaled in the first second. These values are often reported as a ratio—FEV^1/FVC;

patients with normal lungs often have a ratio close to 90%, whereas patients with **chronic obstructive pulmonary disease (COPD)** may have a ratio that falls below 70%.

Proper patient preparation for a spirometry procedure is essential. Patients should be told the following:

- To refrain from eating a heavy meal for 8 hours before testing to prevent a full stomach from interfering with diaphragm muscles.
- To refrain from using a bronchodilator for 4 hours before testing.
- To refrain from smoking for 8 hours before testing.
- To refrain from strenuous activity for 4 hours before testing.
- To wear loose-fitting clothing to permit easier breathing during testing.

Spirometers must be calibrated every day to ensure accurate test results. Each manufacturer provides directions for calibration; however, calibration essentially involves injecting a specified amount of air (usually 3 liters) into the machine. The output results should equal the amount injected within manufacturers' limits. The output results should be documented each day.

Performing Spirometry Testing

When the patient arrives, the procedure should be explained and demonstrated in detail, and the patient should be allowed time to repeat the demonstration. The test should be performed three times, with the two best results used to calculate pulmonary function. Results are considered normal if the patient's best result is 80% of pretest calculated values based on patient demographic information. The patient's best effort requires coaching and encouragement by the tester. The effectiveness of bronchodilator medication may be tested 10 to 15 minutes after administration of the ordered dose by repeating the spirometry test. (Procedure 21-4 lists the steps for performing a spirometry test.)

PROCEDURE 21-4

PERFORMING SPIROMETRY TESTING

ABHES VII.MA.A.1 9(m)   CAAHEP I.P (10)

OBJECTIVE: To perform pulmonary function test to measure lung volume and capacity.

STANDARD: This task takes 15–30 minutes.

EQUIPMENT AND SUPPLIES: Spirometry machine; nose clip; patient mouthpiece; disinfectant; biohazard waste container; paper; pen; patient's record; scale for height and weight; vital sign equipment.

STEPS:

1. Review physician's orders.
2. Perform hand hygiene.
3. Assemble all equipment.
4. Calibrate spirometer as necessary according to manufacturer's directions.
5. Identify patient.
6. Confirm proper patient preparation (see list above). Have patient loosen or remove any tight clothing, such as girdles, bras, and belts that could impede test. If patient has ill-fitting dentures, ask that they be removed to permit a tight seal around mouthpiece.
7. Ask about present general health, and document.
8. Explain and demonstrate procedure. Ask patient to demonstrate in return to confirm understanding.
9. Weigh and measure patient, and record results.
10. Measure patient's vital signs, and record results.
11. Start machine, and enter needed patient information.
12. Seat patient near machine with feet flat on floor, legs uncrossed, head and chin slightly elevated.
13. Review procedure again.
14. Apply nose clip.
15. Have patient inhale forcibly.
16. Place mouthpiece in patient's mouth and have patient seal lips around mouthpiece.

NOTE: New mouthpiece and tubing should be used for each patient.

17. Push Start button, and encourage patient to exhale as forcibly as possible for as long as possible. Coach by saying "Keep blowing . . . more, more . . . that's good" or something similar.
18. Make recommendations to improve outcomes, and repeat procedure until three acceptable efforts are obtained. Computerized machines will select best three efforts and print results. As many as eight attempts may be needed to obtain satisfactory results.
19. Remove nose clip, and ask patient to remain until physician reviews results and speaks to patient. Patient may feel lightheaded and slightly dizzy and should remain seated for a while.
20. Record test result in patient's chart.
21. Clean spirometer according to manufacturer's directions. Clean nose clip.
22. Clean exam room and perform hand hygiene.

CHARTING EXAMPLE: 05/16/XX 10:00 A.M. Spirometry test performed with 3 acceptable results obtained. Pt. felt "slightly dizzy" after testing · · · · · · · · · · · A. J. Campo, CMA (AAMA)

PEAK FLOW MEASUREMENT

Peak flow meters measure the patient's ability to move air into and out of the lungs. Peak flow meters measure the fastest rate at which the patient exhales (PEFR: Peak expiratory flow rate) after taking a maximum inhalation.

Keeping a record of peak flow either daily or when asthma attacks occur helps the physician develop a treatment plan. Patients, family members, or both need instruction on the proper use of a peak flow meter and how to maintain a diary or chart of results. Instructional steps for teaching the use of peak flow meter follow.

PROCEDURE 21-5

TEACHING PEAK FLOW MEASUREMENT

ABHES VII.MA.A.1 9(r); VII.MA.A.1 8(cc)   CAAHEP IV.P (5); I.A (2)

OBJECTIVE: To instruct patient to correctly monitor peak flow and record results.

STANDARD: This task takes 5 minutes.

EQUIPMENT AND SUPPLIES: Peak flow meter; documentation diary/chart; diagram of lungs and breathing processes; pen; patient's record.

STEPS:

1. Review physician's orders.

2. Perform hand hygiene.

3. Assemble peak flow meter with disposable mouthpiece or individual peak flow meter for patient use at home. (In Figure 21-9, a medical assistant is fitting a mouthpiece into a peak flow meter.)

4. Identify patient, and explain procedure. Include an explanation of breathing processes and importance to overall health.

5. Demonstrate how mouthpiece fits, and explain what numbers on side mean. Peak flow meter should always be set on zero to start.

6. Have patient place mouthpiece in mouth and form a tight seal. Explain that better results may be obtained if patient stands for test.

7. Instruct patient to stand, take as deep a breath as possible, place mouthpiece in mouth without biting down on

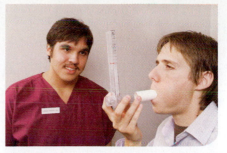

FIGURE 21-10 Ask the patient to exhale as hard and as fast as possible.

it, and exhale as completely and forcibly as possible (Figure 21-10).

8. Instruct patient to note number on machine where sliding gauge stopped and to record it. Reset to zero. Repeat three times.

9. Patient should follow physician's orders for number of times a day and time of day to perform this procedure. "Best" result should be documented on chart or in diary.

10. Demonstrate how to wash mouthpiece with soap and water without submerging peak flow meter.

11. Document instruction.

12. Perform hand hygiene.

CHARTING EXAMPLE: 05/16/XX 9:30 A.M. Pt. instructed on use of peak flow meter and recording of results. Returned demonstration easily, verbally confirmed understanding. Peak flow charting form given. Pt. to perform peak flow measured 3× twice/day in A.M. and P.M. Results today: 380 LPM. · R. Negri, CMA (AAMA)

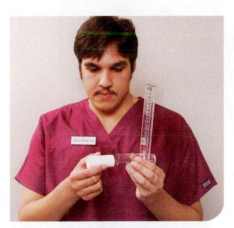

FIGURE 21-9 Peak flow meter.

PULMONARY INHALATION TREATMENTS

Inhalation treatments are used to introduce moisture and medication to the lungs. Nebulizer treatments and **metered-dose inhalers** (MDI) are used to treat asthma and other respiratory conditions. The patient breathes in a fine mist containing fine droplets of medication. **Nebulizers** deliver medications to deeper areas of the lungs. The steps to teach a patient how to use a metered-

dose inhaler and to administer nebulizer treatments follow.

Metered-Dose Inhalers

A metered-dose inhaler holds about 200 doses of medication in a pressurized container with an attached mouthpiece. If MDIs are misused, inadequate treatments result, therefore proper instruction is important. Use of an MDI with a spacer or plastic chamber is believed to improve the amount of medication reaching the small airways.

INSTRUCTING A PATIENT TO USE A METERED-DOSE INHALER (MDI)

ABHES VII.MA.A.1 9(r); VII.MA.A.1 8(cc)   CAAHEP IV.P (5); I.A (2)

OBJECTIVE: To instruct a patient to correctly use a metered-dose inhaler (MDI).

STANDARD: This task takes 5–10 minutes.

EQUIPMENT AND SUPPLIES: Prescribed medication canister; metered-dose inhaler (MDI) dispenser; spacer if ordered; pen; patient's record.

STEPS:

1. Perform hand hygiene.
2. Verify physician's order, and assemble equipment.
3. Check of name of medication, dose, expiration date, and patient's name three times.
4. Explain and demonstrate procedure.
5. Instruct patient to insert correct medication container into mouthpiece. If spacer is ordered, fit it onto plastic holder, remove cap from MDI, and shake gently. (See Figure 21-11 for examples of a metered-dose inhaler and one with an extender spacer.)
6. Instruct patient to inhale deeply and exhale as much as possible in preparation for medication.
7. Instruct patient to hold inhaler upright, place mouthpiece in mouth, and close lips around mouthpiece without biting down on it (Figure 21-12). (Figure 21-13 shows a patient using a metered-dose inhaler with an extender spacer.)

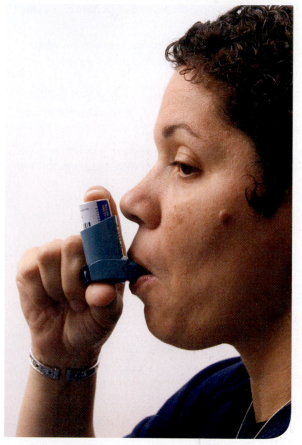

FIGURE 21-12 Placing MDI in mouth with lips sealed around mouthpiece.

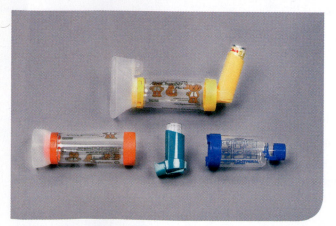

FIGURE 21-11 Metered-dose inhaler and metered-dose inhaler with and without spacer.

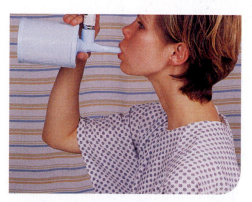

FIGURE 21-13 An extender spacer attached to a mouthpiece placed in mouth.

8. Instruct patient to depress inhaler and slowly and deeply inhale through mouth (3–5 seconds) and hold breath for 10 seconds. Exhale slowly. If repeat dose ordered, patient should be told to wait 1 minute.

9. Patient should be instructed to wash mouthpiece after use and dry thoroughly.

10. Emphasize overuse of MDI could have potentially serious side effects.

11. If steroid medication administered, patient should rinse mouth without swallowing after dose.

12. Instruct patient to wash and dry hands after dose is complete.

13. Instruct patient to assess breathing and reaction to medication after dose. Make patient is aware that certain drugs may increase heart rate, palpitations, tremors, and nervousness.

14. Document procedure.

15. Perform hand hygiene.

CHARTING EXAMPLE: 05/16/XX 2:00 P.M. Pt. instructed in use of MDI. Able to demonstrate accurately and verbalized understanding. 2 puffs Albuterol given as directed. No Pt. reaction noted. · · · · · · · · · · · · · · · E. Lendhart, CMA (AAMA)

PROCEDURE 21-7

ADMINISTERING A NEBULIZED BREATHING TREATMENT

ABHES VII.MA.A.1 9(m)   CAAHEP I.P (10); II.A (1)

OBJECTIVE: To set up and administer a nebulized breathing treatment.

STANDARD: This task takes 15 minutes.

EQUIPMENT AND SUPPLIES: Nebulizer; nebulizer disposable setup; physician's order; inhalation medication; normal saline; pen; patient's record; biohazard waste container.

STEPS:

1. Perform hand hygiene.

2. Verify orders and check medication label three times for dose, medication name, and expiration date. Check that medication and dosage match physician's order in patient's chart.

3. Assemble equipment.

4. Identify patient, and explain procedure.

5. Remove nebulizer treatment cup. Dilute medication as ordered with saline, and place exact amount in nebulizer chamber.

6. Keep cup vertical, and connect top of chamber to mask or T-piece sidearm. Attach mouthpiece to one end of T-piece.

7. Attach one end of corrugated tubing to other end of T-piece and other end to connector on nebulizer machine.

8. Instruct patient to place mouthpiece in mouth and to seal around it with lips without biting. Ask patient to breathe normally during the treatment occasionally taking a deep breath.

9. Turn on machine. Monitor patient's pulse before, during, and after treatment.

10. When medication cup is empty, turn off machine and ask patient to remove mouthpiece.

11. Disconnect all disposable parts, and discard in biohazard waste container. Store machine.

12. Perform hand hygiene.

13. Document procedure, including pulse values.

CHARTING EXAMPLE: 05/16/XX 1:00 P.M. Pt. given 2 mg Albuterol with 3 mL of NS by nebulizer. Tolerated procedure well. Pt. states "breathing easier." Pre Rx P 70, P 88 during, post Rx P 100. Notified Dr. Fox. · · · · · · C. Negri, CMA (AAMA)

Safety Alert! Be sure patients understand the difference between the effects of a bronchodilator (opens airways) and other respiratory medication, such as steroids (reduce inflammation in airways)

ADMINISTERING OXYGEN BY NASAL CANNULA

Oxygen levels may be decreased in patients with certain respiratory conditions. The procedure for correctly administering oxygen based on physician's orders follows.

PROCEDURE 21-8

ADMINISTERING OXYGEN BY NASAL CANNULA OR FACE MASK

ABHES VII.MA.A.1 9(m) CAAHEP I.P (10); II.A (1)

OBJECTIVE: To administer oxygen by cannula or face mask as ordered by physician.

STANDARD: This task takes 5 minutes.

EQUIPMENT AND SUPPLIES: Oxygen in portable tank or wall unit; oxygen mask with strap or nasal cannula with strap; flow meter; humidifier if ordered; pen; patient's record.

STEPS:

1. Verify physician orders.
2. Identify patient, and explain procedure.
3. Assemble equipment.
4. Insert oxygen flow meter into wall outlet, and connect cannula tubing to flow meter.
5. Place disposable humidifier unit between flow meter and cannula if ordered.
6. Perform hand hygiene.
7. Perform vital signs. Perform pulse oximetry if ordered. Record all results.
8. Place prongs of cannula into **nares**, loop tubing behind ears, and adjust to hold securely (see Figure 21-14); or place mask comfortably on patient's face covering nose and mouth.
9. Adjust flow rate as specified in order. (Flow rate should be less than 6 L/min for cannula and at least 6 L/min for mask.)
10. Check patient after 5 minutes. Monitor pressure around ears, and pad tubing as needed.
11. Document procedure.
12. Perform hand hygiene.

CHARTING EXAMPLE: 05/16/XX 5:00 P.M. Oxygen administered by nasal cannula at 3 L/min per order Dr. Liu. Pt. says "breathing easier." P 82, R 22, BP 142/88, T 99°F. .... M. Mendoza, RMA

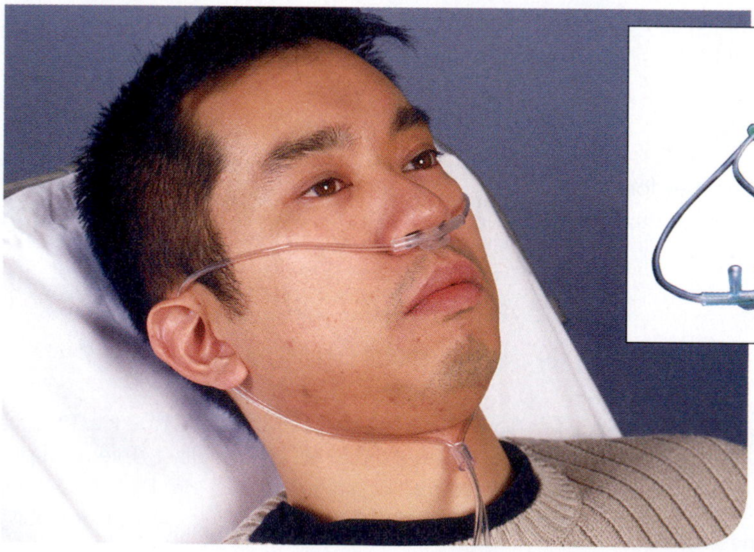

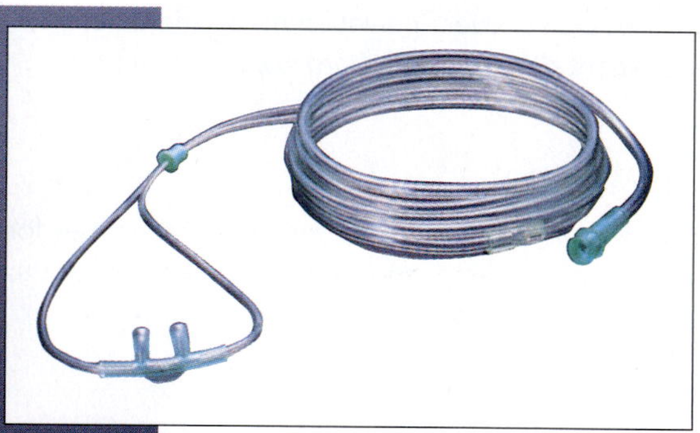

FIGURE 21-14 Nasal cannula.

COLLECTING A SPUTUM SPECIMEN

Microorganisms can cause a variety of respiratory conditions. Physicians may order a sputum collection for culture and sensitivity. Often it is repeated several times at specified times of the day or night. Sputum results from a "productive" cough and should not be a saliva specimen. The procedure for collecting a sputum specimen follows.

COLLECTING A SPUTUM SPECIMEN
ABHES VII.MA.A.1 10(d)   CAAHEP I.P (7)

OBJECTIVE: To collect and process a sputum specimen without contamination.

STANDARD: This task takes 5 minutes.

EQUIPMENT AND SUPPLIES: Sterile labeled sputum specimen container; gloves; mask; lab requisition form; biohazard waste container; tissue; pen; patient's record.

STEPS:

1. Review physician's orders.
2. Perform hand hygiene.
3. Identify patient, and explain procedure. Give written instruction to patient if other specimens are to be collected at home.
4. Assemble equipment.
5. Don gloves and mask and other PPE as required.
6. Ask patient to cough and **expectorate** directly into specimen container without contaminating top or sides. First morning specimen is best if possible. Avoid having saliva or nasal secretions in specimen.
7. Secure lid tightly, and place container in specimen bag.
8. Complete lab request, and attach.
9. Clean area, and dispose of gloves and mask in biohazard waste container.
10. Perform hand hygiene.
11. Document procedure.

CHARTING EXAMPLE: 05/16/XX 7:00 A.M. sputum for C&S obtained and sent to Abbey Lab. · · · · · · · · R. Mendoza, RMA

Appendix A

COMMON MEDICAL ABBREVIATIONS

AAO	alert, awake, and oriented		DOA	dead on arrival
A&O	alert and oriented		DTR	deep tendon reflexes
ABD	abdomen		DVT	deep venous thrombosis
ABG	arterial blood gas		DX	diagnosis
abs	absent		ECG	electrocardiogram
AC	before eating		EMG	electromyogram
ACLS	advanced cardiac life support		ENT	ears, nose, and throat
ADH	anti-diuretic hormone		FBS	fasting blood sugar
adm	admission		FTT	failure to thrive
ADR	adverse drug reaction		FU	followup
ad lib	as much as needed		Fx	fracture
AFP	alpha-fetoprotein		GI	gastrointestinal
amb	ambulatory		GSW	gunshot wound
amt	amount		GTT	glucose tolerance test
ant	anterior		HA	Headache
ante	before		HBP	high blood pressure
AOB	alcohol on breath		HCG	human chorionic gonadotropin
AP	anteroposterior		HCT	hematocrit
ASAP	as soon as possible		HDL	high density lipoprotein
BCP	birth control pills		HEENT	head, eyes, ears, nose, throat
BE	barium enema		Hgb	hemoglobin
bid	twice a day		HIV	human immunodeficiency virus
BM	bowel movement		HO	history of
BMR	basal metabolic rate		H&P	history and physical examination
BP	blood pressure		HR	heart rate
BPH	benign prostatic hypertrophy		HS	at bedtime
BPM	beats per minute		HSV	herpes simplex virus
BS	bowel or breath sounds		HTN	hypertension
BX	biopsy		Hx	history
c̄	with		I&D	incision and drainage
CA	cancer		ICU	intensive care unit
Ca	calcium		ID	infectious disease
CAD	coronary artery disease		IG	immunoglobulin
CAT	computerized axial tomography		IM	intramuscular
CBC	complete blood count		INF	intravenous nutritional fluid
CC	chief complaint		IV	intravenous
CHF	congestive heart failure		L	left
CNS	central nervous system		LLL	left lower lobe
C/O	complaining of		LMP	last menstrual period
COPD	chronic obstructive pulmonary disease		LOC	loss of consciousness or level of consciousness
CP	cerebral palsy		LPN	licensed practical nurse
CPAP	continuous positive airway pressure		MAO	monoamine oxidase
CPR	cardiopulmonary resuscitation		MBT	maternal blood type
CT	computerized tomography		MI	myocardial infarction or mitral insufficiency
CVA	cerebrovascular accident		mL	milliliter
CXR	chest X-ray		MMR	measles, mumps, rubella
DC	discontinue or discharge		MRI	magnetic resonance imaging
DNR	do not resuscitate		MRSA	methicillin resistant staph aureus

MS	multiple sclerosis	RTC	return to clinic
MVA	motor vehicle accident	s̄	without
NG	nasogastric	SOAP	subjective, objective, assessment, plan
NKA	no known allergies	SOB	shortness of breath
NKDA	no known drug allergies	SQ	subcutaneous
NMR	nuclear magnetic resonance	STAT	immediately
NPO	nothing by mouth	Sx	symptoms
NSAID	nonsteroidal anti-inflammatory drugs	T&C	type and cross
NSR	normal sinus rhythm	TB	tuberculosis
OB	obstetrics	tid	three times a day
OPV	oral polio vaccine	TIG	tetanus immune globulin
OR	operating room	TMJ	temporo mandibular joint
PA	posteroanterior	TNTC	too numerous to count
PC	after eating	TO	telephone order
PDR	*Physician's Desk Reference*	TPN	total parenteral nutrition
PE	physical exam	TSH	thyroid stimulating hormone
PKU	phenylketonuria	TT	thrombin time
PMH	previous medical history	Tx	treatment
PO	by mouth	UA	urinalysis
PR	by rectum	UAO	upper airway obstruction
PRN	as needed	UBD	universal blood donor
PT	prothrombin time, or physical therapy	URI	upper respiratory infection
Pt	patient	US	ultrasound
PTT	partial thromboplastin time	UTI	urinary tract infection
PUD	peptic ulcer disease	VO	verbal order
q	every (e.g., q6h = every 6 hours)	WBC	white blood cell
qd	every day	WD	well developed
qh	every hour	WF	white female
qid	four times a day	WM	white male
qod	every other day	WNL	within normal limits
R	right	WO	written order
RA	rheumatoid arthritis	yo	years old
RBC	red blood cell	YOB	year of birth
R/O	rule out	yr	year
ROM	range of motion	ytd	year to date
ROS	review of systems		

Appendix B

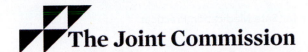

Official "Do Not Use" List[1]

Do Not Use	Potential Problem	Use Instead
U (unit)	Mistaken for "0" (zero), the number "4" (four) or "cc"	Write "unit"
IU (International Unit)	Mistaken for IV (intravenous) or the number 10 (ten)	Write "International Unit"
Q.D., QD, q.d., qd (daily)	Mistaken for each other	Write "daily"
Q.O.D., QOD, q.o.d, qod (every other day)	Period after the Q mistaken for "I" and the "O" mistaken for "I"	Write "every other day"
Trailing zero (X.0 mg)* Lack of leading zero (.X mg)	Decimal point is missed	Write X mg Write 0.X mg
MS	Can mean morphine sulfate or magnesium sulfate	Write "morphine sulfate" Write "magnesium sulfate"
MSO_4 and $MgSO_4$	Confused for one another	

[1] Applies to all orders and all medication-related documentation that is handwritten (including free-text computer entry) or on pre-printed forms.

*Exception: A "trailing zero" may be used only where required to demonstrate the level of precision of the value being reported, such as for laboratory results, imaging studies that report size of lesions, or catheter/tube sizes. It may not be used in medication orders or other medication-related documentation.

Additional Abbreviations, Acronyms and Symbols
(For possible future inclusion in the Official "Do Not Use" List)

Do Not Use	Potential Problem	Use Instead
> (greater than) < (less than)	Misinterpreted as the number "7" (seven) or the letter "L" Confused for one another	Write "greater than" Write "less than"
Abbreviations for drug names	Misinterpreted due to similar abbreviations for multiple drugs	Write drug names in full
Apothecary units	Unfamiliar to many practitioners Confused with metric units	Use metric units
@	Mistaken for the number "2" (two)	Write "at"
cc	Mistaken for U (units) when poorly written	Write "mL" or "ml" or "milliliters" ("mL" is preferred)
µg	Mistaken for mg (milligrams) resulting in one thousand-fold overdose	Write "mcg" or "micrograms"

Updated 3/5/09

Appendix C

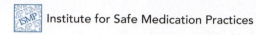

Institute for Safe Medication Practices

ISMP'S LIST OF *ERROR-PRONE ABBREVIATIONS, SYMBOLS, AND DOSE DESIGNATIONS*

The abbreviations, symbols, and dose designations found in this table have been reported to ISMP through the USP-ISMP Medication Error Reporting Program as being frequently misinterpreted and involved in harmful medication errors. They should NEVER be used when communicating medical information. This includes internal communications, telephone/verbal prescriptions, computer-generated labels, labels for drug storage bins, medication administration records, as well as pharmacy and prescriber computer order entry screens.

The Joint Commission (TJC) has established a National Patient Safety Goal that specifies that certain abbreviations must appear on an accredited organization's do-not-use list; we have highlighted these items with a double asterisk (**). However, we hope that you will consider others beyond the minimum TJC requirements. By using and promoting safe practices and by educating one another about hazards, we can better protect our patients.

Abbreviations	Intended Meaning	Misinterpretation	Correction
µQ	Microgram	Mistaken as "mg"	Use "mcg"
AD, AS, AU	Right ear, left ear, each ear	Mistaken as OD, OS, OU (right eye, left eye, each eye)	Use "right ear," "left ear," or "each ear"
OD, OS, OU	Right eye, left eye, each eye	Mistaken as AD, AS, AU (right ear, left ear, each ear)	Use "right eye," "left eye," or "each eye"
BT	Bedtime	Mistaken as "BID" (twice daily)	Use "bedtime"
cc	Cubic centimeters	Mistaken as "u" (units)	Use "mL"
D/C	Discharge or discontinue	Premature discontinuation of medications if D/C (intended to mean "discharge") has been misinterpreted as "discontinued" when followed by a list of discharge medications	Use "discharge" and "discontinue"
IJ	Injection	Mistaken as "IV" or "intrajugular"	Use "injection"
IN	Intranasal	Mistaken as "IM" or "IV"	Use "intranasal" or "NAS"
HS hs	Half-strength At bedtime, hours of sleep	Mistaken as bedtime Mistaken as half-strength	Use "half-strength" or "bedtime"
IU**	International unit	Mistaken as IV (intravenous) or 10 (ten)	Use "units"
o.d. or OD	Once daily	Mistaken as "right eye" (OD-oculus dexter), leading to oral liquid medications administered in the eye	Use "daily"
OJ	Orange juice	Mistaken as OD or OS (right or left eye); drugs meant to be diluted in orange juice may be given in the eye	Use "orange juice"

Per os	By mouth, orally	The "os" can be mistaken as "left eye" (OS-oculus sinister)	Use "PO," "by mouth," or "orally"
q.d. or QD**	Every day	Mistaken as q.i.d., especially if the period after the "q" or the tail of the "q" is misunderstood as an "i"	Use "daily"
qhs	Nightly at bedtime	Mistaken as "qhr" or every hour	Use "nightly"
qn	Nightly or at bedtime	Mistaken as "qh" (every hour)	Use "nightly" or "at bedtime"
q.o.d. or QOD**	Every other day	Mistaken as "q.d." (daily) or "q.i.d. (four times daily) if the "o" is poorly written	Use "every other day"
q1d	Daily	Mistaken as q.i.d. (four times daily)	Use "daily"
q6PM, etc.	Every evening at 6 PM	Mistaken as every 6 hours	Use "6 PM nightly" or "6 PM daily"
SC, SQ, sub q	Subcutaneous	SC mistaken as SL (sublingual); SQ mistaken as "5 every"; the "q" in "sub q" has been mistaken as "every" (e.g., a heparin dose ordered "sub q 2 hours before surgery" misunderstood as every 2 hours before surgery)	Use "subcut" or "subcutaneously"
ss	Sliding scale (insulin) or ½ (apothecary)	Mistaken as "55"	Spell out "sliding scale;" use "one-half" or "½"
SSRI	Sliding scale regular insulin	Mistaken as selective-serotonin reuptake inhibitor	Spell out "sliding scale (insulin)"
SSI	Sliding scale insulin	Mistaken as Strong Solution of Iodine (Lugol's)	
i/d	One daily	Mistaken as "tid"	Use "1 daily"
TIW or tiw	3 times a week	Mistaken as "3 times a day" or "twice in a week"	Use "3 times weekly"
U or u**	Unit	Mistaken as the number 0 or 4, causing a 10-fold overdose or greater (e.g., 4U seen as "40" or 4u seen as "44"); mistaken as "cc" so dose given in volume instead of units (e.g., 4u seen as 4cc)	Use "unit"

Dose Designations and Other Information	Intended Meaning	Misinterpretation	Correction
Trailing zero after decimal point (e.g., 1. 0 mg)**	1 mg	Mistaken as 10 mg if the decimal point is not seen	Do not use trailing zeros for doses expressed in whole numbers
"Naked" decimal point (e.g., .5 mg)**	0.5 mg	Mistaken as 5 mg if the decimal point is not seen	Use zero before a decimal point when the dose is less than a whole unit
Drug name and dose run together (especially problematic for drug names that end in "l" such as Inderal40 mg; Tegretol300 mg)	Inderal 40 mg Tegretol 300 mg	Mistaken as Inderal 140 mg Mistaken as Tegretol 1300 mg	Place adequate space between the drug name, dose, and unit of measure

Dose Designations and Other Information	Intended Meaning	Misinterpretation	Correction
Numerical dose and unit of measure run together (e.g., 10mg, 100mL)	10 mg 100 mL	The "m" is sometimes mistaken as a zero or two zeros, risking a 10- to 100-fold overdose	Place adequate space between the dose and unit of measure
Abbreviations such as mg. or mL. with a period following the abbreviation	mg mL	The period is unnecessary and could be mistaken as the number 1 if written poorly	Use mg, mL, etc. without a terminal period
Large doses without properly placed commas (e.g., 100000 units; 1000000 units)	100,000 units 1,000,000 units	100000 has been mistaken as 10,000 or 1,000,000; 1000000 has been mistaken as 100,000	Use commas for dosing units at or above 1,000, or use words such as 100 "thousand" or 1 "million" to improve readability

Drug Name Abbreviations	Intended Meaning	Misinterpretation	Correction
ARA A	vidarabine	Mistaken as cytarabine (ARA C)	Use complete drug name
AZT	zidovudine (Retrovir)	Mistaken as azathioprine or aztreonam	Use complete drug name
CPZ	Compazine (prochlorperazine)	Mistaken as chlorpromazine	Use complete drug name
DPT	Demerol-Phenergan-Thorazine	Mistaken as diphtheria-pertussis-tetanus (vaccine)	Use complete drug name
DTO	Diluted tincture of opium, or deodorized tincture of opium (Paregoric)	Mistaken as tincture of opium	Use complete drug name
HCl	hydrochloric acid or hydrochloride	Mistaken as potassium chloride (The "H" is misinterpreted as "K")	Use complete drug name unless expressed as a salt of a drug
HCT	hydrocortisone	Mistaken as hydrochlorothiazide	Use complete drug name
HCTZ	hydrochlorothiazide	Mistaken as hydrocortisone (seen as HCT250 mg)	Use complete drug name
MgSO$_4$**	magnesium sulfate	Mistaken as morphine sulfate	Use complete drug name
MS, MSO$_4$**	morphine sulfate	Mistaken as magnesium sulfate	Use complete drug name
MTX	methotrexate	Mistaken as mitoxantrone	Use complete drug name
PCA	procainamide	Mistaken as patient controlled analgesia	Use complete drug name
PTU	propylthiouracil	Mistaken as mercaptopurine	Use complete drug name
T3	Tylenol with codeine No. 3	Mistaken as liothyronine	Use complete drug name
TAC	triamcinolone	Mistaken as tetracaine, Adrenalin, cocaine	Use complete drug name
TNK	TNKase	Mistaken as "TPA"	Use complete drug name
ZnSO$_4$	zinc sulfate	Mistaken as morphine sulfate	Use complete drug name

Stemmed Drug Names	Intended Meaning	Misinterpretation	Correction
"Nitro" drip	nitroglycerin infusion	Mistaken as sodium nitroprusside infusion	Use complete drug name
"Norflox"	norfloxacin	Mistaken as Norflex	Use complete drug name
"IV Vanc"	intravenous vancomycin	Mistaken as Invanz	Use complete drug name

Symbols	Intended Meaning	Misinterpretation	Correction
℥	Dram	Symbol for dram mistaken as "3"	Use the metric system
ℳ	Minim	Symbol for minim mistaken as "mL"	Use the metric system
×3d	For three days	Mistaken as "3 doses"	Use "for three days"
> and <	Greater than and less than	Mistaken as opposite of intended; mistakenly use incorrect symbol; "< 10" mistaken as "40"	Use "greater than" or "less than"
/ (slash mark)	Separates two doses or indicates "per"	Mistaken as the number 1 (e.g.,"25 units/ 10 units" misread as "25 units and 110" units)	Use "per" rather than a slash mark to separate doses
@	At	Mistaken as "2"	Use "at"
&	And	Mistaken as "2"	Use "and"
+	Plus or and	Mistaken as "4"	Use "and"
°	Hour	Mistaken as a zero (e.g., q2° seen as q 20)	Use "hr," "h," or "hour"

ISMP 2007

**These abbreviations are included on TJC's "minimum list" of dangerous abbreviations, acronyms and symbols that must be included on an organization's "Do Not Use" list, effective January 1, 2004. Visit www.jointcommission.org for more information about this TJC requirement.

Institute for Safe
Medication Practices
www.ismp.org

Appendix D

NORMAL BLOOD VALUES/DISEASE CONDITIONS EVALUATED FOR ABNORMAL VALUES

Test	Normal Value Range	Normal Value Range (SI)	Possible Indications
Ammonia (NH_3)–diffusion	20–120 mcg/dl	12–70 mcmol/L	Abnormal levels of ammonia in the body are used to investigate severe changes in mood and consciousness and to help diagnose the cause of a coma of unknown origin.
Ammonia nitrogen	15–45 µg/dl	11–32 µmol/L	The test for ammonia nitrogen is non-specific and does not indicate a cause. Higher-than-normal levels simply indicate the body is not effectively metabolizing and eliminating ammonia.
Amylase	35–118 IU/L	0.58–1.97 mckat/L	The normal level of amylase will depend on the method used to collect the data. An increased level may indicate several disorders of the digestive and reproductive systems or cancer of the pancreas. Tubal pregnancies will also cause a rise in the amylase levels. Decreased amylase levels may indicate damage to the pancreas and kidneys.
Anion gap (Na^+—[Cl^- + HCO_3^-]) (P)	7–16 mEq/L	7–16 mmol/L	A determination of electrolytes in the blood fluid. Abnormal readings indicate a variety of factors. The test is nonspecific and only tells the physician that there is cause for additional testing. Some factors that cause an abnormal anion gap reading are uncontrolled diabetes, starvation, kidney damage, and ingestion of potentially toxic substances such as antifreeze, excessive amounts of aspirin, or methanol.
Bicarbonate Arterial Venous	 21–28 mEq/L 22–29 mEq/L	 21–28 mmol/L 22–29 mmol/L	See *Carbon dioxide content*
Bilirubin Conjugated (direct) Total	 0.2 mg/dl 0.1–1 mg/dl	 4 mcmol/L 2–18 mcmol/L	Increased levels of bilirubin may be an indication of some kind of blockage of the liver or bile duct, hepatitis, trauma to the liver, a drug reaction, or long-term alcohol abuse or some inherited disorders such as Gilbert's, Rotor's, Dubin-Johnson, Crigler-Najjar which will cause an increase in levels. Increased levels of bilirubin in newborns is a critical situation as excessive levels kill developing brain cells and may lead to mental retardation.

Calcitonin	< 100 pg/ml	< 100 ng/L	Increased levels of calcitonin in combination with a thyroid biopsy may be an indication of C-cell hyperplasia.
Calcium, Total Calcium, Ionized	8.6–10.3 mg/dl 4.4–5.1 mg/dl	2.2–2.74 mmol/L 1–1.3 mmol/L	Increased levels of calcium in the body indicate an inability to metabolize the intake. This can be due to several factors: hyperthyroidism, sarcoidosis, tuberculosis, excess vitamin D intake, kidney transplant, and high protein levels (e.g., if a tourniquet is used for too long while blood is collected). In this case, free or ionized calcium remains normal.
Carbon dioxide content (plasma)	21–32 mmol/L	21–32 mmol/L	Higher or lower-than normal CO_2 levels indicate a problem losing or retaining fluid—disrupting the acid-base balance, which can be an indication of several disorders.
Carcinoembryonic antigen	< 3 ng/ml	< 3 mcg/L	CEA is a protein that is found in embryonic tissues. Increased CEA levels can indicate some non-cancer-related conditions of inflammation of internal organs. Pregnant women who smoke tend to have embryos that have increased levels of CEA. In a normally healthy infant all detectable levels of CEA are gone by birth.
Chloride	95–110 mEq/L	95–110 mmol/L	Increased levels of chloride may indicate dehydration or increased blood sodium. Decreased levels of chloride occur with prolonged vomiting, chronic diarrhea, emphysema, or other chronic lung disease, and with loss of acid from the body.

Coagulation screen
  Bleeding time
  Prothrombin time
  Partial thrombo-
    plastin time
    (activated)
  Protein C
  Protein S
	
	3–9.5 min
	10–13 sec
	22–37 sec
	
	0.7–1.4 µ/ml
	0.7–1.4 µ/ml
		
		180–570 sec
		10–13 sec
		22–37 sec
		
		700–1400 U/ml
		700–1400 U/ml
			Indicates an inability of the body to develop adequate clotting factors or the inability to produce the correct amount of clotting factors.

Copper, total	70–160 mcg/dl	11–25 mcmol/L	Indication of liver disease.
Corticotropin (ACTH adreno-corticotropic hormone)—0800 hr	< 60 pg/ml	< 13.2 pmol/L	This test is used in conjunction with cortisol to determine if a patient has Cushing's syndrome or Addison's disease.

Coritsol 0800 hr
    1800 hr
    2000 hr
	5–30 mcg/dl
	2–15 mcg/dl
	50% of 0800 hr
		138–810 nmol/L
		50–410 nmol/L
		50% of 0800 hr
			Abnormal levels in coritsol may indicate Cushing's syndrome or Addison's disease.

Creatine kinase
  Female
  Male
	
	20–170 IU/L
	30–220 IU/L
		
		0.33–2.83 mckat/L
		0.5–3.67 mckat/L
			Creatine kinase is an enzyme found in the heart, brain, skeletal muscle, and other tissues. The body has specific types of CK to indicate which muscles are affected.

Creatinine kinase isoenzymes, MB fraction	0–12 IU/L	0–0.2 mckat/L	Depending on the ratio, the CK-MB fraction will indicate some form of muscle damage. The specific ratio can indicate if the muscle damage is cardiac or skeletal.
Creatinine	0.5–1.7 mg/dl	44–150 mcmol/L	Increased creatinine levels indicate a disorder with kidney function. Creatinine can also increase temporarily as a result of muscle injury.

(continued)

Test	Normal Value Range	Normal Value Range (SI)	Possible Indications
			Low levels of creatinine are not common. They may be seen in persons with decreased muscle mass, such as comatose patients. Normal pregnancy will cause the creatinine levels to drop and are not a cause for concern.

Follicle-stimulating hormone (FSH)
  Female
  Midcycle
  Men
	2–13 mlU/ml
	5–22 mlU/ml
	1–8 mlU/ml
		2–13 IU/L
		5–22 IU/L
		1–8 IU/L
			Increased levels of FSH and LH (luteinizing hormone) are consistent with primary ovarian failure, which is when ovaries themselves fail. In men this may be an indication of testicular developmental defects or injury.
			
			Decreased levels of FSH and LH are an indication of secondary ovarian failure, which results in problems with the pituitary or hypothalamic gland. In men this may be an indication of hypothalamic disorders.

Glucose, fasting	65–115 mg/dl	3.6–6.3 mmol/L	Indicates diabetes or pre-diabetes.
Glucose Tolerance Test (Oral), 2 hour	(mg/dl) Normal fasting		Indicates diabetes or pre-diabetes.
Post-drink: Impaired tolerance Indicates diabetes	65–99 < 140 mg/dl 140–199 mg/dl > 200 mg/dl		
Haptoglobin	44–303 mg/dl	0.44–3.03 g/L	If the haptoglobin levels are decreased in combination with several other tests, it may be an indication of hemolytic anemia. Haptoglobin will be elevated in many inflammatory diseases, such as ulcerative colitis, acute rheumatic disease, heart attack, and severe infection.
Fibrinogen	200–400 mg/dl	2–4 g/L	Lower-than normal fibrinogen levels indicate that the person may not be able to form a stable blood clot after injury. Chronically low levels may indicate an inherited condition such as afibrinogenemia, or to an acquired condition such as liver disease, malnutrition, or some types of cancer. Higher-than normal levels of fibrinogen may indicate: acute infections, breast, kidney, or stomach cancer, chronic DIC, inflammatory disorders, myocardial infarction, stroke, or trauma. Fibrinogen concentrations may rise sharply in any condition that causes inflammation or tissue damage.

Hematocrit (Hct)
  Female
  Male
Hemoglobin A$_{1C}$
	35%–46%
	40.0%–50.0%
	40.0%–50.0% of total
		0.36–0.446
		fraction of 1
		0.4–0.503
		fraction of 1
		0.053–0.075
			Decreased hematocrit level indicates anemia, such as iron deficiency, but may have other causes such as vitamin or mineral deficiencies, recent bleeding, liver cirrhosis, and malignancies.
			
			Abnormally high levels of hematocrit may be an indication of dehydration and can be easily cured by increased fluid intake.
			
			Polycythemia vera—greater-than normal number of red blood cells in a person can also cause a prolonged increase in hematocrit levels. Higher-than normal hematocrit levels are also seen in persons with chronic pulmonary conditions or lung damage. The person's bone marrow will increase production of red blood cells to supply the body with oxygen in response to a lacking pulmonary system.

Hemoglobin (Hb) 　Female 　Male	11.6–15.5 g/dl 13.7–16.7 g/dl	121–153 g/L 138–175 g/L	Low levels of Hb are an indication of anemia. Some types of anemia are treated with iron, folic acid, or vitamin B_{12} or B_6 supplements. It is normal for women of childbearing age to have temporary decreases during menstrual periods and pregnancy.
Leukocyte count (WBC)	3800–9800/mcl	3.8–9.8 ¥ 10^9/L	Infections usually cause increased WBC counts and may be treated with antibiotics. Leukemias (blood cancer) require chemotherapy and other treatments.
Erythrocyte count (RBC) 　Female 　Male	3.8–5.2 ¥ 10^6/mcl 4.3–5.7 ¥ 10^6/mcl	3.8–5.2 ¥ 10^{12}/L 4.3–5.7 ¥ 10^{12}/L	A low ESR can indicate polycythemia, extreme leukocytosis, and some protein abnormalities.
Erythrocyte sedimentation rate (sedrate, ESR) 　Female 　Male	30 mm/hr 20 mm/hr	30 mm/hr 20 mm/hr	Elevated ESR level is an indication of inflammation, anemia, infection, pregnancy, and advanced age.
Leukocytes (WBC)	K/uL		Raised levels may indicate infections, inflammation, or cancer. Decreased levels may indicate autoimmune conditions, some severe infections, bone marrow failure, and congenital marrow aplasia. Decreased levels may also occur with certain medications such as methotrexate.
Lymphocytes of WBC			Chronic high levels may indicate lymphocytic leukemia.
Lipase	7–60 units/L @ 37 C	7–60 units/L @ 37 C	High lipase levels, with abdominal pain, may indicate acute pancreatitis lightly raised levels can indicate kidney disease, salivary gland inflammation, or peptic ulcer disease.
Lipids 　Total Cholesterol 　　Borderline high 　　High 　HDL 　　High 　LDL 　　High	< 200 mg/dl 200–239 mg/dl 240–above > 60 mg/dl < 40 mg/dl (men) < 50 mg/dl (women) < 100 mg/dl > 130 mg/dl		A person with high cholesterol has more than twice the risk of coronary heart disease as someone whose cholesterol is below 200 mg/dL. Low HDL is considered a major risk factor for heart disease. If you don't have coronary heart disease or diabetes and have one or no risk factors, your LDL goal is less than 160 mg/dL. If you don't have coronary heart disease or diabetes and have two or more risk factors, your LDL goal is less than 130 mg/dL. If you do have coronary heart disease or diabetes, your LDL goal is less than 100 mg/dL.
Triglycerides 　High	> 150 mg/dl > 200 mg/dl and above		Normal triglyceride levels vary by age and sex. A high triglyceride level combined with low HDL cholesterol or high LDL cholesterol seems to speed up atherosclerosis (the buildup of fatty deposits in artery walls). Atherosclerosis increases the risk for heart attack and stroke. Info on lipids from the American Heart Association.

(continued)

Test	Normal Value Range	Normal Value Range (SI)	Possible Indications

PSA
  0–54 yrs
  55–59 yrs
  60–64 yrs
  65–69 yrs
  70 plus yrs
	0.00–2.50 ng/ml
	0.00–3.40 ng/ml
	0.00–4.10 ng/ml
	0.00–5.10 ng/ml
	0.00–5.60 ng/ml
			PSA is a test indicating the level of protein cells the prostate is producing. The higher the PSA number, the more likely prostate cancer is present. Age, hormonal factors, and medications can alter the test results so a high PSA alone is not a cancer indicator.

TSH	0.40–5.00 IU/ml		A high TSH result is often due to some type of acute or chronic thyroid dysfunction that causes the thyroid to be underactive. Although rare, a high TSH can be an indication of secondary hyperthyroidism, which is a problem with the pituitary gland. A low TSH result can indicate an overactive thyroid gland.
Urea, plasma (BUN)	8.5–25 mg/dl	2.9–8.9 mmol/liter	Increased BUN levels may be due to acute or chronic kidney disease, damage, or failure. Conditions that result in reduced blood flow to the kidneys, such as a recent heart attack, will also result in an increased BUN. Low BUN levels are rarely detected because they result from diseases or symptoms, such as dehydration or starvation, that do not warrant a BUN test.
Urinalysis pH Specific Gravity	5.0–7.5 1.001–1.030	5.0–7.5 1.001–1.030	Specific gravity is an indication of how well the kidneys are filtering waste products. Reduced specific gravity can indicate diabetes insipidus, certain renal diseases, excess fluid intake, or diabetes mellitus. Raised specific gravity can indicate dehydration, adrenal insufficiency, nephrosis, congestive cardiac failure, or liver disease.

CELSIUS/FAHRENHEIT TEMPERATURE CONVERSIONS

Celsius	Fahrenheit	Celsius	Fahrenheit
34.0	93.2	38.6	101.4
34.2	93.6	38.8	101.8
34.4	93.9	39.0	102.2
34.6	94.3	39.2	102.5
34.8	94.6	39.4	102.9
35.0	95.0	39.6	103.2
35.2	95.4	39.8	103.6
35.4	95.7	40.0	104.0
35.6	96.1	40.2	104.3
35.8	96.4	40.4	104.7
36.0	96.8	40.6	105.1
36.2	97.1	40.8	105.4
36.4	97.5	41.0	105.8
36.6	97.8	41.2	106.1
36.8	98.2	41.4	106.5
37.0	**98.6**	41.6	106.8
37.2	98.9	41.8	107.2
37.4	99.3	42.0	107.6
37.6	99.6	42.2	108.0
37.8	100.0	42.4	108.3
38.0	100.4	42.6	108.7
38.2	100.7	42.8	109.0
38.4	101.1		

To convert Fahrenheit to Celsius: $(F - 32) \times (5/9) = C$
To convert Celsius to Fahrenheit: $C \times (9/5) + 32 = F$

Note: Values in bold indicate normal body temperatures.

Appendix F

MEDICAL TERMINOLOGY WORD PARTS

Medical terms are like individual jigsaw puzzles. Once you divide the terms into their component parts and learn the meaning of the individual parts, you can use that knowledge to understand many other new terms. Four basic component parts are used to create medical terms:

Root — The basic, or core, part that makes up the essential meaning of the term. The root usually, but not always, denotes a body part. Root words usually come from the Greek or Latin languages. For example, *bronch* is a root that means "the air passages in the lungs" or "bronchial tubes." *Cephal* means "head."

Prefix — One or more letters placed before the root to change its meaning. Prefixes usually, but not always, indicate location, time, number, or status. For example, the prefix *bi-* means "two" or "twice." When *bi* is placed before the root *lateral* ("side") to form *bilateral,* the meaning is "having two sides."

Suffix — One or more letters placed after the root to change its meaning. Suffixes usually, but not always, indicate the procedure, condition, disorder, or disease. For example, the suffix *-itis* means "inflammation," that is, damaged tissue that is red and painful. The medical term *bronchitis* means "inflammation of the bronchial tubes." Another example is the suffix *-ectomy,* which means "removal." Hence, *appendectomy* means "removal of the appendix."

Combining vowel — A letter used to combine roots with other word parts. The vowel is usually an *o,* but sometimes it is an *a* or *i.* When a combining vowel is added to a root, the result is called a combining form. For example, in the word *encephalogram,* the root is *cephal* ("head"), the prefix is *en-* ("inside"), and the suffix is *-gram* ("something recorded"). These word parts are joined by the combining vowel *o* to make a word easier to pronounce. *Cephal/o* is the combining form. An *encephalogram* is an X-ray of the inside of the head.

Analyzing a Medical Term

You can often decipher the meaning of a medical term by breaking it down into its separate parts. Consider the following examples:

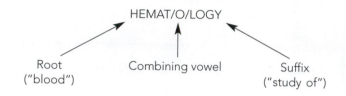

The term *hematology* is divided into three parts. When you analyze a medical term, begin at the end of the word. The ending is called the suffix. Almost all medical terms contain suffixes. The suffix in *hematology* is *-logy,* which means "study of." Now look at the beginning of the word. *Hemat* is the root word, which means "blood." The root word gives the essential meaning of the term.

The third part of this term, which is the letter *o,* has no meaning of its own, but is an important connector between the root (*hemat*) and the suffix (*logy*). It is the combining vowel. The letter *o* is the combining vowel usually found in medical terms.

Putting together the meanings of the suffix and the root, the term *hematology* means "the study of blood."

The combining vowel plus the root is called the combining form. A medical term can have more than one root word; therefore, there can be two combining forms. For example:

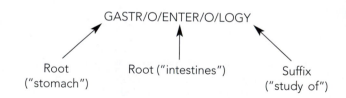

The two combining forms are *gastr/o* and *enter/o.* The entire term (reading from the suffix, back to the beginning of the term, and across) means "the study of the stomach and the intestines."

Rules for Using Combining Vowels

1. A combining vowel is not used when the suffix begins with a vowel (a-e-i-o-u). For example, when *neur/o* (nerve) is joined with the suffix *-itis* (inflammation), the combining vowel is not used because *-itis* begins with a vowel. *Neuritis* (new-RYE-tis) is an inflammation of a nerve or nerves.

2. A combining vowel is used when the suffix begins with a consonant. For example, when *neur/o* (nerve) is joined with the suffix *-plasty* (surgical repair), the combining vowel *o* is used because *-plasty* begins with a consonant. *Neuroplasty* (NEW-roh-plas-tee) is the surgical repair of a nerve.

3. A combining vowel is always used when two or more root words are joined. As an example, when *gastr/o* (stomach) is joined with *enter/o* (small intestine), the combining vowel is used with *gastr/o*. *Gastroenteritis* (gas-troh-en-ter-EYE-tis) is an inflammation of the stomach and small intestine.

Suffixes and Medical Terms Related to Pathology

Pathology is the study of disease, and the following suffixes describe specific disease conditions.

Suffix	Meaning
-algia	pain and suffering
-dynia	pain
-ectomy	surgical removal
-graphy	process of recording a picture or record
-gram	record or picture
-necr/osis	death (tissue death)
-scler/osis	abnormal hardening
-sten/osis	abnormal narrowing
-centesis	surgical puncture to remove fluid for diagnostic purposes or to remove excess fluid
-plasty	surgical repair
-scopy	visual examination with an instrument

The Double RRs Suffixes

The following suffixes are often referred to as the "double RRs"

* -rrhage and –rrhagia	Bursting form; an abnormal excessive discharge or bleeding. *Note: -rrhage* and *-rhagia* refer to the flow of blood.
* -rrhaphy	To suture or stitch.
* -rrhea	Abnormal flow or discharge; refers to the abnormal flow of most bodily fluids. *Note:* Although -rrhea and -rrhage both refer to abnormal flow, they are not used interchangeably.
* -rrhexis	Rupture.

Contrasting and Confusing Prefixes

The following contrasting prefixes can be confusing. Study this list to make sure you know the differences between the contrasting terms.

Ab- means "away from." *Abnormal* means not normal or away from normal.

Ad- means "toward" or "in the direction." *Addiction* means drawn toward or a strong dependence on a drug or substance.

Dys- means "bad," "difficult," "painful." *Dysfunctional* means an organ or body that is not working properly.

Eu- Means "good," normal, well, or easy. Euthyroid (you-THIGH-roid) means a normally functioning thyroid gland.

Hyper- means "excessive" or "increased." *Hypertension* (high-per-TEN-shun) is higher-than-normal blood pressure.

Hypo- means "deficient" or "decreased." *Hypotension* (high-poh-TEN-shun) is lower-than-normal blood pressure.

Inter- means "between" or "among." *Interstitial* (in-ter-STISH-al) means between, but not within, the parts of a tissue.

Intra- means "within" or "into." *Intramuscular* (in-trah-MUS-kyou-lar) means within the muscle.

Sub- means "under," "less," or "below." *Subcostal* (sub-KOS-tal) means below a rib or ribs.

Supra- means "above." *Supracostal* (sue-prah-KOS-tal) means above or outside the ribs.

Singular and Plural Endings

Many medical terms have Greek or Latin origins. As a result of these different origins, the rules for changing a singular word into a plural form are unusual. In addition, English endings have been adopted for some commonly used terms.

GUIDELINES TO UNUSUAL PLURAL FORMS

Guideline	Singular	Plural
1. If the term ends in an *a*, the plural is usually formed by adding an *e*	bursa vertebra	bursae vertebrae
2. If the term ends in *ex* or *ix*, the plural is usually formed by changing the *ex* or *ix* to *ices*	appendix index	appendices indices
3. If the term ends in *is*, the plural is usually formed by changing the *is* to *es*.	diagnosis metastasis	diagnoses metastases
4. If the term ends in *itis*, the plural is usually formed by changing the *is* to *ides*.	arthritis meningitis	arthritides meningitides
5. If the term ends in *nx*, the plural is usually formed by changing the *x* to *ges*.	phalanx meninx	phalanges meninges
6. If the term ends in *on*, the plural is usually formed by changing the *on* to *a*.	criterion ganglion	criteria ganglia

7. If the term ends in *um*, the plural is usually formed by changing the *um* to *a*.

| diverticulum | diverticula |
| ovum | ova |

8. If the term ends in *us*, the plural is usually formed by changing the *us* to *i*.

| alveolus | alveoli |
| malleolus | malleoli |

Basic Medical Terms

The following subsections discuss basic medical terms that are used to describe diseases and disease conditions, major body systems, and body direction.

TERMS USED TO DESCRIBE DISEASES AND DISEASE CONDITIONS

The basic medical terms used to describe diseases and disease conditions are listed here.

- A *sign* is evidence of disease, such as fever, that can be observed by the patient and others. A sign is objective because it can be evaluated or measured by others.

- A *symptom,* such as pain or a headache, can only be experienced or defined by the patient. A symptom is subjective because it can be evaluated or measured only by the patient.

- A *syndrome* is a set of signs and symptoms that occur together as part of a specific disease process.

- *Diagnosis* is the identification of disease. To diagnose is the process of reaching a diagnosis.

- A *differential diagnosis* attempts to determine which of several diseases may be producing the symptoms.

- A *prognosis* is a forecast or prediction of the probable course and outcome of a disorder.

- An *acute* disease or symptom has a rapid onset, a severe course, and relatively short duration.

- A *chronic* symptom or disease has a long duration. Although chronic symptoms or diseases may be controlled, they are rarely cured.

- A *remission* is the partial or complete disappearance of the symptoms of a disease without having achieved a cure. A remission is usually temporary.

- Some diseases are named for the condition described. For example, *chronic fatigue syndrome* (CFS) is a persistent overwhelming fatigue that does not resolve with bed rest.

- An *eponym* is a disease, structure, operation, or procedure that is named for the person who discovered or described it first. For example, Alzheimer's disease is named for Alois Alzheimer, a German neurologist who lived from 1864 to 1915.

- An *acronym* is a word formed from the initial letter or letters of the major parts of a compound term. For example, the acronym AMA stands for American Medical Association.

TERMS USED TO DESCRIBE MAJOR BODY SYSTEMS

The following is a list of the major body systems and some common related combining forms used with each.

Major Structures and Body System	Related Roots with Combining Forms
Skeletal system	bones (oste/o); joints (arthr/o) cartilage; (chondr/o)
Muscular system	muscles(my/o); ligaments (syndesm/o) tendons (ten/o, tend/o; tendin/o)
Cardiovascular system	heart (card/o, cardi/o); arteries (arteri/o); veins (phleb/o, ven/o) blood (hem/o, hemat/o)
Lymphatic and immune systems	lymph, lymph vessels, and lymph nodes (lymph/o); (lymphangi/o); tonsils (tonsill/o); spleen (splen/o) thymus (thym/o)
Respiratory system	nose (nas/o, rhin/o); pharynx (pharyng/o); trachea (trache/o) larynx (laryng/o); lungs (pneum/o, pneumon/o)
Digestive system	mouth (or/o); esophagus (esophag/o); stomach (gastr/o) small intestines (enter/o); large intestines (col/o); liver (hepat/o) pancreas (pancreat/o)
Urinary system	kidneys (nephr/o, ren/o); ureters (ureter/o); urinary bladder; (cyst/o, visic/o); urethra (urethr/o)
Integumentary system	glands (aden/o); skin (cutane/o, dermat/o, derm/o); sebaceous glands (seb/o); sweat glands (hidraden/o)
Nervous system	nerves (neur/o); brain (encephal/o) spinal cord (myel/o) eyes (ocul/o, ophthalm/o) ears (acoust/o, ot/o)
Endocrine system	adrenals (adren/o); pancreas (pancreat/o); pituitary (pituit/o) thyroid (thyr/o, thyroid/o) parathyroids; (parathyroid/o) thymus (thym/o)
Reproductive system	*Male:* testicles (orch/o, orchid/o) *Female:* ovaries (oophor/o, ovari/o) uterus (hyster/o, metr/o, metri/o, uter/o)

TERMS USED TO DESCRIBE BODY DIRECTION

Certain terms are used to describe the location of body parts relative to the trunk or other parts of the anatomy. See Figure F-1.

Ventral (VEN-tral) refers to the front or belly side of the body or organ (*ventr* means "belly side" of the body and *al* means "pertaining to").

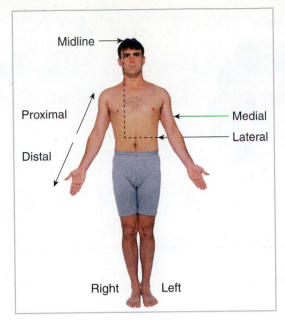
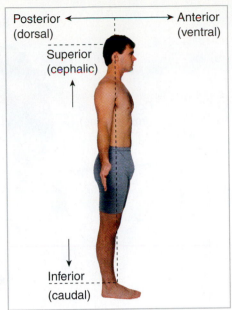

FIGURE F-1 **Directional anatomical terms.**

Dorsal (DOR-sal) refers to the back of the body or organ (*dors* means "back side of the body and *al* means "pertaining to").

Anterior (an-TEER-ee-or) means situated in the front. It also means on the forward part of an organ (*anter* means "front" or "before" and *ior* means "pertaining to"). For example, the stomach is located anterior to (in front of) the pancreas. *Anterior* is also used in reference to the ventral surface of the body.

Posterior (pos-TEER-ee-or) means situated in the back. It also means on the back portion of an organ (*poster* means "back" or "after" and *ior* means "pertaining to"). For example, the pancreas is located posterior to (behind) the stomach. Posterior is also used in reference to the dorsal surface of the body.

Superior means uppermost, above, or toward the head. For example, the lungs are superior to (above) the diaphragm.

Inferior means lowermost, below, or toward the feet. For example, the stomach is located inferior to (below) the diaphragm.

Cephalic (seh-FAL-ick) means toward the head (*cephal* means "head" and *ic* means "pertaining to").

Caudal (KAW-dal) means toward the lower part of the body (*caud* means "tail" or "lower part" of the body and *al* means "pertaining to").

Proximal (PROCK-sih-mal) means situated nearest the midline or beginning of a body structure. For example, the proximal end of the humerus (the bone of the upper arm) forms part of the shoulder. Or, it may be easier for you to think of it as "closer to the origin of the body part or the point of attachment of a limb to the body trunk."

Distal (DIS-tal) means situated farthest from the midline or beginning of a body structure. For example, the distal end of the humerus forms part of the elbow.

Medial means the direction toward or nearer the midline. For example, the medial ligament of the knee is near the inner surface of the leg.

Lateral means the direction toward or nearer the side and away from the midline. For example, the lateral ligament of the knee is near the side of the leg.

Bilateral means relating to, or having, two sides.

PLANES OF THE BODY

Medical professionals often refer to sections of the body in terms of anatomical planes (flat surfaces). These planes are imaginary lines—vertical or horizontal—drawn through an upright body. The following terms are used to describe a specific body part (see Figure F-2):

- Coronal plane (frontal plane): A vertical plane running from side to side; divides the body or any of its parts into anterior and posterior portions.

- Sagittal plane (median plane): A vertical plane running from front to back; divides the body or any of its parts into right and left sides.

- Axial plane (transverse plane): A horizontal plane; divides the body or any of its parts into upper and lower parts.

Prefixes, Root Words, and Suffixes

The most common medical prefixes, root words, and suffixes are listed here. Knowing these common prefixes, roots, and suffixes will help you decipher medical terms.

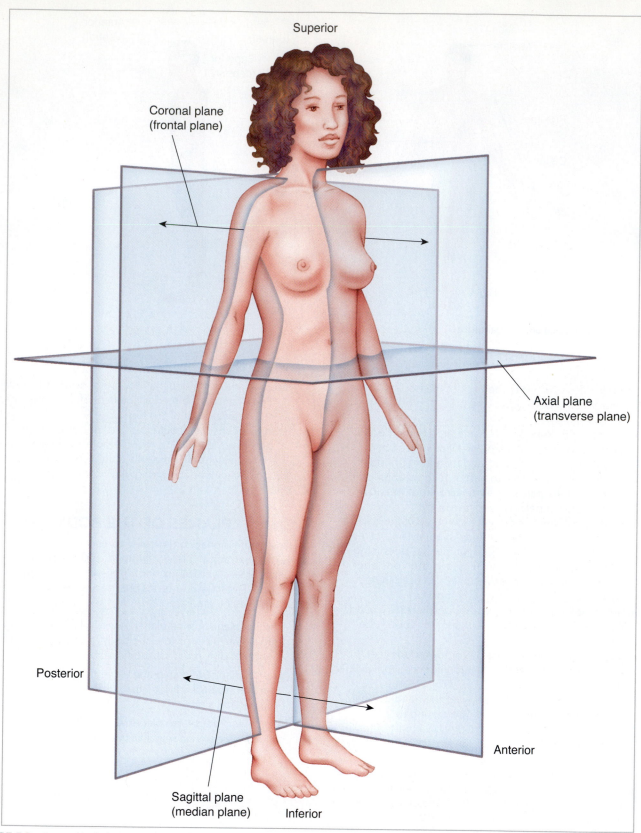

Superior

Coronal plane
(frontal plane)

Axial plane
(transverse plane)

Posterior

Anterior

Sagittal plane
(median plane)

Inferior

FIGURE F-2 **Anatomical planes.**

PREFIXES

a	without or absence of
ab	from; away from
ad	to; toward
an	without or absence of
ante	before
anti	against
bi	two
bin	two
brady	slow
con	together
contra	against
de	from; down from; lack of
dia	through; complete; between; apart
dis	to undo; free from
dys	difficult; labored; painful; abnormal
ec	out
ecto	outside
endo	within
epi	on; upon; over
eso	inward
eu	normal; good
ex	outside; outward
exo	outside; outward
extra	outside of; beyond
hemi	half
hyper	above; excessive
hypo	below; incomplete; deficient
in	in; into; not
infra	under; below
inter	between
intra	within
mal	bad
meso	middle
meta	after; beyond; change
micro	small
multi	many
neo	new
nulli	none
pan	all; total
para	outside; beyond; around
per	through
peri	surrounding (outer)
poly	many; much
post	after
pre	before; in front of
pro	before
quadri	four
re	back
retro	back; behind
semi	half
sub	under; below
super	over; above
supra	above; beyond; on top
sym	together; joined
syn	together; joined
tachy	fast; rapid
tetra	four
trans	through; across; beyond
tri	three
ultra	beyond; excess
uni	one

ROOT WORDS

abdomin	abdomen
aden	gland
adren	adrenal gland
adrenal	adrenal gland
aer	air; oxygen; gas
alveol	alveolus
angi	(blood) vessel; (lymph) vessel
ankyl	crooked; stiff; bent
appendic	appendix
arteri, arter	artery
arteriol	arteriole (small artery)
arthr	joint
ather	yellowish; fatty plaque
aur	ear
aut	self
bil	bile
bio	life
blephar	eyelid
bronch	airway; bronchus
bronchiol	bronchiole
burs	bursa
carcin	cancer
cardi	heart
caud	tail; toward lower part of the body
cephal	head
cerebell	cerebellum
cerebr	cerebrum; brain
cervic	neck; cervix
cheil	lip
chiro	hand
cholangi	bile duct
chole	gall; bile
chondr	cartilage
coccyg	coccyx; tailbone
col	colon; large intestine
conjunctiv	conjunctiva
corne	cornea
coron	heart; crown of the head
cost	rib
crani	cranium; skull
cutane	skin
cyan	blue
cyst	bladder; sac
cyt, cyte	cell
dacry	tears; tear duct
dactyl	fingers or toes
dent	tooth
derm	skin
dermat	skin
dipl	two; double
diverticul	diverticulum
dors	back (of the body)

duoden	duodenum	macr	abnormal largeness
ectop	located away from usual place	mamm	breast
edema	swelling	mast	breast
electr	electricity; electrical activity	meat	opening or passageway
encephal	brain	melan	black
endocrin	endocrine	men	menstruation
enter	intestines (usually small intestine)	mening	meninges
epiglott	epiglottis	ment	mind
epitheli	epithelium	mes, meso	middle
erythr	red	metr	uterus
esophag	esophagus	mon	one
esthesi	sensation; feeling; sensitivity	morbid	disease; sickness
eti	cause (of disease)	muc	mucus
exocrin	secrete out of	my, myos	muscle
faci	face	myc	fungus
fasci	fascia; fibrous band	myel	bone marrow; spinal cord
fract	break; broken	myelon	bone marrow
galact	milk	myring	eardrum
gastr	stomach	narc	stupor; numbness
ger	old age; aged	nas	nose
geront	old age; aged	nat	birth
gingiv	gums	necr	death (cells; body)
glauc	gray	nephr	kidney
gloss	tongue	neur	nerve
gluc	sweetness; sugar	noct	night
glyc	sugar; glucose	nyct	night
glycos	sugar; glucose	nyctal	night
gnos	knowledge; a knowing	ocul	eye
gonad	gonad; sex glands	onc	tumor
gyn	woman	onych	nail
gynec	woman	oophor	ovary
gyr	turning; folding	ophthalm	eye
hem	blood	or	mouth
hemat	blood	orth	straight
hepat	liver	oste	bone
hidr	sweat	ot	ear
hist	tissue	ox	oxygen
hom	same	palpat	touch; feel; stroke
home	sameness; unchanging	pancreat	pancreas
hydr	water	par, part	bear; give birth to; labor
hyster	uterus	parathyroid	parathyroid
ile	ileum	path	disease; suffering
ili	ilium	pector	chest; muscle
immun	immune	ped	child; foot
irid	iris	pelv	pelvis; pelvic bone
kerat	horny tissue; hard	pen	penis
kin	movement	perine	perineum
kinesi	movement; motion	peritone	peritoneum
labi	lips	petr	stone; portion of temporal bone
lacrim	tear duct; tear	phac, phak	lens of the eye
lact	milk	phag	eat; swallow
lapar	abdomen	phalang	finger or toe bone
laryng	larynx	pharyng	pharynx, throat
later	side	phas	speech
lei	smooth	phleb	vein
leuk	white	phot	light
lingu	tongue	phren	mind
lip	fat	physi	nature
lith	stone; calculus	pleur	pleura
lob	lobe	pneum	lung; air
lymph	lymph	pneumat	lung; air

pneumon	lung; air	thorac	thorax; chest
pod	foot	thromb	clot
poli	gray matter	thym	thymus gland
polyp	polyp; small growth	thyr	thyroid gland
poster	back (of body)	thyroid	thyroid gland
prim	first	tom	cut; section
proct	rectum	ton	tension; pressure
pseud	fake; false	tone	to stretch
psych	mind	tonsill	tonsils
pulmon	lung	top	place; position; location
py	pus	tox, toxic	poison; poisonous
pyel	renal pelvis	trach, trache	trachea; windpipe
pylor	pylorus	trachel	neck; necklike
pyr	fever; heat	trich	hair
quadr	four	tubercul	little knot; swelling
rect	rectum	tympan	eardrum; middle ear
ren	kidney	ulcer	sore; ulcer
retin	retina	ungu	nail
rhin	nose	ur	urine; urinary tract
sacr	sacrum fallopian (uterine)	ureter	ureter
salping	tube	urethr	urethra
sanit	soundness; health	uria	urination; urine
sarc	flesh; connective tissue	urin	urine or urinary organs
scler	sclera; white of eye; hard	uter	uterus
scoli	crooked; curved	uvul	uvula; little grape
seb	sebum; oil	vagin	vagina
seps	infection	valv	valve
sept	infection; partition; septum	valvul	valve
sial	saliva	vas	vessel; duct
sinus	inus	vascul	blood vessel; little vessel
somat	body	ven	vein
somn	sleep	versicul	seminal vesicles; blister
son	sound	vertebr	vertebra; backbone
sopor	sleep	vesic	urinary bladder
sperm	sperm, spermatazoa; seed	vir	poison; virus
spermat	sperm, spermatazoa; seed	viril	masculine; manly
spher	round; sphere; ball	vis	seeing; sight
sphygm	pulse	visc	sticky
spin	spine; backbone to	viscer	viscera; internal organs; sternum
spir	breathe	viscos	sticky
splen	spleen	vit	life
spondyl	vertebra; spinal or vertebral column	xanth	yellow
staphyl	grapelike clusters	xen	strange; foreign
stern	breastbone	xer	dry
steth	chest (muscles)	zygot	joined together
stoma	mouth; opening		
stomat	mouth; opening		
strab	squint; squint-eyed		
synovi	synovia; synovial membrane		
system	system		
ten, tend	tendon		
tendin	tendon		
test	testis; testicle		
therm	heat		

Additional Root Words

caus	burning sensation; capable of burning
cusp	point; cusp
flexion	bending
genital	pertaining to birth
lumb	lumbar; loin region
mediastin	mediastinum
tens, tensi	pressure, force, stretching

SUFFIXES

Suffixes Meaning "Pertaining to"

ac

al, ine

ar, ior

ary, ory

eal, ous

ial
ic
ical, tic

Suffixes Meaning "Abnormal Conditions"

ago	abnormal condition, disease
esis	abnormal condition, disease
ia	abnormal condition, disease
iasis	abnormal condition, disease
ion	condition
ism	condition, state of abnormal condition
osis	disease

Common Suffixes Used in Medical Terminology

algia	pain, suffering
asthenia	weakness
cele	hernia, protrusion
centesis	surgical puncture to remove fluid
cidal	killing
clasia	break
clasis	break
clast	break
clysis	irrigating; washing
coccus	berry shaped (a form of bacterium)
crine	separate; secrete
crit	to separate
cyte	cell
desis	fusion; to bind; tie together
drome	run; running
ductor	to lead or pull
dynia	pain
ectasis	stretching out; dilation; expansion
ectomy	excision or surgical removal
ectopia	displacement
emesis	vomiting
emia	blood; blood condition
gen	producing, forming
genesis	producing; forming
genic	producing, forming
gnosis	a knowing
gram	record; X-ray
graph	instrument used to record
graphy	process of recording; X-ray filming
ictal	seizure; attack
ism	state of
itis	inflammation
lepsy	seizure
logist	specialist
logy	study of
lysis	destruction; reduce; separation
malacia	softening
mania	madness; insane desire
megaly	enlargement
meter	instrument used to measure
metry	measurement
morph	form; shape
oid, ode	resembling

oma	tumor; mass
opia	vision (condition)
opsy	to view
oxia	oxygen
paresis	slight paralysis
pathy	disease
penia	abnormal reduction in number; lack of
peps, pepsia	digestion
pexy	surgical fixation; suspension
phagia	eating; swallowing
philia	love
phily	love
phobia	abnormal fear of or adversion to specific objects or things
phonia	sound or voice
phoria	feeling
physis	growth
plasia	formation; development; a growth
plasm	growth; formation; substance
plasty	plastic or surgical repair
plegia	paralysis; stroke
pnea	breathing
porosis	lessening in density; porous condition
praxia	in front of; before
ptosis	drooping; sagging; prolapse
ptysis	spitting
rrhage	bursting forth, an abnormal excessive discharge or bleeding
rrhagia	bursting forth, an abnormal excessive discharge or bleeding
rrhaphy	to suture or stitch
rrhea	abnormal flow or discharge
rrhexis	rupture
schisis	split; fissure
sclerosis	hardening
scope	instrument used for visual exam
scopic	visual exam
scopy	visual exam with an instrument
sepsis	infection
sis	state of
spasm	sudden involuntary muscle contraction
stalsis	contraction; constriction
stasis	control; stop; standing still
stat	to stop
stenosis	narrowing; constriction
stomy	new artificial opening
therapy	treatment
tome	instrument used to cut
tomy	cutting into; surgical incision
tripsy	crushing
trophy	nourishment
ule	little
uria	urine; urination

Source: Adapted from Vines, Deborah, Braceland, Ann, Rollins, Elizabeth, and Miller, Susan. *Comprehensive Health Insurance: Billing, Coding, and Reimbursement.* © 2008. Pearson Education. Upper Saddle River, NJ.

Glossary

abdominal paracentesis: procedure to remove fluid from the abdominal cavity

abdominal ultrasound: high-frequency sound waves used to create outline of organs in the abdomen

abortion: termination of pregnancy before the fetus reaches age of viability (ability to live on own, which is about 28 weeks of gestation or end of second trimester)

absorption: the process of getting a drug into the bloodstream and ultimately into the cells where it produces its action

accuracy: correctness

action: the pharmacodynamic processes of absorption and distribution

adverse reactions: unintended, undesirable effects produced by a drug

aerobes: organisms that require oxygen

agonists: drugs that cause change in the cell's behavior

AIDS: acquired immunodeficiency syndrome

aliquot: a small sample representative of the entire specimen

allergens: substances such as pollen, insect bites, mold, or dust mites that are capable of inducing the productions of antibodies, thus causing an allergic reaction

alpha-fetoprotein (AFP): a fetal blood protein found in amniotic fluid of pregnant women with very low levels associated with Down syndrome in fetus and high levels with neural tube defects (spina bifida) in fetus

amniocentesis: puncturing of the amniotic sac to withdraw amniotic fluid for genetic testing and assessment of fetal development

anaerobes: organisms that grow best in the absence of oxygen

analyte: substances for which the test is being performed, such as glucose or sodium

anaphylactic shock: life-threatening reaction, including respiratory distress, tachycardia, convulsions, and death

anemia: a decrease in the number of red blood cells or amount of hemoglobin in the red blood cells; indicated in a decreased hematocrit and hemoglobin

anoscope: instrument used to examine anal area

antagonism: one drug working against another and causing a decreased effect

antagonists: drugs that affect cells by preventing a cellular change

anthropometry: the science of size, proportion, weight, and height

antibody: protein usually found in serum after the blood has coagulated and fibrinogen has been removed

antigen: a substance that appears foreign to the body and causes production of a specific antibody

antisera: sera that contains antibodies for a specific antigen

anuria: absence of urine

approximated: edges of wound brought together

aquathermic pad: a form of heat therapy in which a pad is applied to a body part and connected by hoses to a pump that causes water to circulate through the pad to provide heat

artifact: abnormal signals on an ECG that do not reflect the electrical activity of the heart

ascites: excess fluid buildup in the abdominal cavity

atherosclerosis: a common form of arteriosclerosis (hardening of arteries) caused by plaque deposits

auscultation: listening to sounds within the body

autolytic: self-dissolution or self-digestion of tissue

bacteremia: bacteria in the blood

biopsy: a diagnostic examination of tissue removed from a growth or organ

bolus: a mass or rounded lump, such as a large pill, wad of chewed food, or large dose of drug introduced intravenously

calibrate: the process of setting an instrument to respond accurately to test a reagent or device

cannula: tube with a channel or lumen

carcinoma in situ: a tumor that has not invaded surrounding tissues

casts: protein structures formed in kidney tubules

catalysts: substance that speeds up a chemical reaction without being permanently altered

catheterization: the process of introducing a sterile tube into the urinary bladder to obtain urine

central vascular devices (CVADs): subcutaneous ports, catheters, and central vascular catheters that allow repeated access to the patient's vascular system without venipuncture

cerumen: foreign material in the ear canal

chorionic villi sampling (CVS): a procedure for obtaining at 8 to 12 weeks of gestation a sample chorionic villi (later part of placenta) through the abdominal wall or through the cervix for chromosomal, DNA, and enzymatic analysis in women who are at high risk for fetal abnormalities

chronic obstructive pulmonary disease (COPD): lung disease in which the airways become narrowed, limiting the flow of air to and from the lungs; chronic bronchitis or emphysema

colony: a macroscopic growth of a microorganism on a culture plate composed of one type of microbe

compliance: term used to describe a patient's adherence to the health plan the physician has recommended

compound microscope: a microscope with two sets of lenses, oculars, and objectives

computed tomography (CT): imaging technique that produces cross-sectional views of the body; X-rays taken at multiple angles and then computerized to produce a cross-section

contact precautions: precautions used when infections are difficult to treat and microorganism transmission among patients and health care providers would be easy; patients isolated, caregivers wear gowns and gloves

contraindicate: to make (a treatment or procedure) inadvisable

control sample: samples that are similar to the testing specimen required, have been previously tested, and have a known value

corpuscle: small rounded body frequently used to describe cells; white or red blood cells

cryotherapy: the practice of using cold for therapeutic purposes

debridement: a method of removing affected wound tissue

desensitization injections: administration of minute amounts of the allergen into the patient's system over an extended period of time to build up a tolerance for the allergen

discretion: the use of tactful communication with patients and coworkers

distribution: movement of the drug through the body to the bloodstream and finally into the cells

dosimeter: device that must be worn by personnel working in radiology; contains a strip of film that reacts to X-ray exposure and records the level and intensity of radiation exposure

droplet precautions: precautions used around patients suspected of being infected with organisms spread by droplets during sneezing, coughing, and talking; mask is worn if the caregiver is within 3 feet of the patient; gown and gloves are worn when contact is possible with the blood or body fluids of suspected patents

dysplasia: signs of infection or cancerous (tumor) cells

dyspnea: difficult or labored breathing

electrocardiogram (ECG): activity of the heart captured by skin electrodes and recorded on an electrocardiographic device

electrocautery: cauterization by electric current

electrodes: sensors used to pick up electrical impulses of the heart and relay them over wires or to the ECG machine

electronic infusion devices (EIDs): devices that regulate the infusion according to pre-set controls; an alarm may be triggered when the IV solution is low or when the tubing is too low

ELISA: a rapid enzyme immunochemical testing method for determining the presence of an antigen or antibody in the blood, during which an antigen or antibody is bound to an enzyme and that molecule can bind specific immunological targets in body fluid samples and highlight their presence enzymatically with color change

empathy: sensitivity to another's feelings and ability to imagine oneself in another's place

enzymes: proteins that speed up the rate of biochemical reactions

epididymis: a soft tubular cord behind the testis that stores and carries sperm

epidural: a form of anesthesia produced by injection of a local anesthetic into the peridural space of the spinal cord

epilepsy: a chronic condition characterized by frequent seizures

epistaxis: nosebleed

erythrocytes: red blood cells

excision: removal of a lesion, such as a mole, wart, or tumor

excretion: elimination of drug by-products by the kidneys, skin, lungs, and intestinal tract

expectorant: an agent that promotes the discharge or expulsion of mucus from the respiratory tract

external controls: liquid positive and negative substances tested before the patient sample to check the reliability of the instrument and testing technique

exudate: discharge

facultative anaerobes: organisms that require a reduced amount of oxygen

fetal heart rate: the heart rate of the fetus, which is different from the heart rate of the mother

fetid: foul smelling

first responders: emergency medical services (EMS) workers who are trained to recognize medical conditions, initiate basic life support, and access other parts of the emergency medical system

fluoroscopy: diagnostic imaging procedure that uses a continuous beam of X-rays to observe movement within the body or specific organs

fontanels: soft spot on a baby's head

forced vital capacity (FVC): the maximum volume of air expelled when the patient exhales as forcibly and quickly as possible

frenulum linguae: fold of tissue beneath the tongue that anchors the tongue to the bottom of the mouth

fundal height: measurement from the top of the uterus to the top of the pubic bone

gait belt: a safety device placed around the patient's waist and held by the caregiver to provide stability

genitalia: external genital organs

gerontology: the study of the aging process and its effects on people

glycemic index: a numerical index given to a carbohydrate-rich food that is based on the average increase in blood glucose levels occurring after the food is eaten

goniometer: a special type of protractor that measures range of motion

gravida: a pregnant woman; also, the number of pregnancies (e.g., gravida 4)

hematoma: mass of clotted blood

hematopoiesis: the formation of blood

hematuria: the presence of red blood cells in urine

hepatitis B: a sometimes fatal form of hepatitis caused by the hepatitis B virus (HBV) and spread by contact with infected blood, needles, or other infected bodily fluids

homeostasis: a balanced state

human immunodeficiency virus (HIV): a retrovirus that causes AIDS

hyperglycemia: elevated blood glucose

hyperinsulinemia: high blood insulin levels

hypersensitivity: exaggerated reactions to allergens

hyperthermia: elevated body temperature due to failed thermoregulation

hypoglycemia: decreased level of blood glucose

hypothermia: body temperature that drops below what is required for normal metabolism

hypothyroidism: decrease in amount of thyroid hormone

hypovolemic shock: state of profound depression of vital body function caused by decrease in the amount of circulating blood

idiopathic: of unknown cause

idiosyncratic: unpredictable reaction to a drug that occurs occasionally

impaired glucose tolerance (IGT): condition in which beta cells in the pancreas become sluggish; decreases insulin production and leads to periods of high and low blood sugar

in utero: in the uterus

in vitro: outside the body

in vivo: in the living body

indices: hematology screening tests that are calculated from hematocrit, hemoglobin, and red blood cell count values

infiltration: fluid enters the tissue instead of the bloodstream

inspection: visual examination

insufflator: a device to blow air, powder, or gas into a body cavity

integrity: connotes that the caregiver is dependable, honest, dedicated to high principles, thorough, and punctual

internal controls: built-in positive control used in qualitative tests to prove the device or test kit is working properly

interstitial fluid (ISF): tissue fluid or fluid among cells of body

intravascular fluid: blood plasma

intubate: introduction of a tube into a hollow organ to open or keep open, as in the trachea or intestine

iontophoresis: delivery of local analgesia to the skin at the site

IV administration set: includes a venous access device, container of solution, and necessary tubing and filters

kyphosis: abnormal increase in the outward curvature of the thoracic spine; also known as hunchback or humpback

lavage: irrigation of the eye

leads: wires used to relay electrical impulses to the ECG machine

leukocytes: white blood cells

leukocytosis: indicates an increase in the number of white blood cells

leukopenia: a decrease in the number of white blood cells

lipemic: high fat content

lipidemia: excess of lipids in the blood

lipoproteins: any of a large class of proteins composed of complex proteins and lipids (fats); high-density lipoprotein (HDL) and low-density lipoprotein (LDL)

lochia: the vaginal discharge consisting of blood, mucus, and white blood cells that occurs during the approximately 3-week-long period after giving birth

logrolling: moving the patient as a single unit to prevent spinal injury

lordosis: abnormal increase in the forward curvature of the spine; also known as swayback

lumen: the cavity or channel within a tubular structure

magnetic resonance imaging (MRI): medical imaging that uses radio-frequency radiation and does not require contrast medium or exposure to ionizing radiation; MRI is useful for visualizing soft tissues

manipulation: passive assessment of the range of motion of a joint

menarche: first menstruation

menses: menstrual flow

mensuration: the use of special tools to measure the body or specific body parts

metabolic syndrome: a syndrome marked by three or more of the following factors—abdominal obesity, elevated triglycerides, low HDL levels, elevated fasting blood glucose

metabolism: the physical and chemical breakdown of the drug by the body

metered-dose inhaler: holds about 200 doses of medication in a pressurized container with an attached mouthpiece; used to treat asthma and other respiratory conditions

mons pubis: fleshy prominence over symphysis pubis

morphology: form and structure

nares: the pair of openings of the nose; the nasal cavity

nebulizer: a machine used to treat asthma and other respiratory conditions; delivers medications to deeper areas of the lungs

nomogram: similar to the charts used to calculate the growth percentile for a child

noncompliance: Failure to follow recommended health guidelines

normal flora: microorganisms that are normally present in or on the body and are usually nonpathogenic

nosocomial infection: an infection acquired in a medical setting

NPO: nothing by mouth (*nils per os*)

obturator: device used to close the end of an instrument to allow easier penetration

oliguria: decreased amounts of urine production

orifices: openings

orthostatic hypotension: drop in blood pressure with change of position from supine to sitting or standing

osmolarity: the concentration of osmotically active particles in a solution

outside laboratory: a hospital-based or independent laboratory capable of handling a large number of specimens and performing tests ranging from simple to complex

palpation: use of the hands to feel the skin and accessible underlying organs

papules: small, solid, round, raised spot on skin

para: number of births after 20 weeks of gestation

paramedics: EMS workers who are licensed to provide more advanced emergency care

parasite: an organism that lives in, with, or on another organism

parenteral: introduced otherwise than by way of the intestines

patency: state of being freely open

patient-controlled analgesia (PCA): anesthesia administered by IV in controlled doses that is administered by the patient as needed to maintain therapeutic serum levels

percussion: use of the fingertips to tap the body lightly but sharply to gain information about the positions and sizes of underlying body parts

periosteum: connective tissue that covers all bones except the articular surfaces

peripheral catheters: most common type of catheter; inserted into the veins of the hands, arms, and antecubital area

peripheral insertion of central catheter (PICC): a catheter inserted into a peripheral vein with tip ending in superior or inferior vena cava and left in place to provide easy access to a vein

peripheral parenteral nutrition (PPN): nutrition administered into a peripheral vein, usually with less caloric content than total parenteral nutrition (TPN)

Petri dish: a glass or plastic dish with a loose cover that is used in culturing bacteria

pharmacodynamics: the study of the actions of a drug on the cells and tissues of the body

pharmacokinetics: the study of the five processes involved in the action of medications

phenylketonuria: genetic disease marked by an inability to metabolize phenylalanine (a type of amino acid); may cause severe mental retardation

pinna: projecting portion of the external ear

plaque: deposits of cholesterol on inner walls of arteries

polycythemia: an overproduction of blood cells as indicated by an elevated hematocrit level

polyuria: excessive amount of urine

potentiation: multiplying or prolonging the effect of one drug by another drug

precision: refers to the reproducibility of laboratory results each time the test is performed

problem-oriented medical record (POMR): type of medical record that is based on identifying patient problems and charting by problems

puerperium: a period of 4 to 6 weeks after childbirth

pulse deficit: the difference between the apical pulse and the radial pulse

pulse pressure: the difference between the systolic and diastolic blood pressure readings

punch biopsy: removal of a small section from a specific location in a lesion

purosanguineous: an exudate containing blood and pus

purulent: a thickish exudate composed of pus; may be greenish yellow, depending on causative agent

pyuria: the presence of white blood cells in urine

qualitative test: test that analyzes specimens for the presence or absence of a substance

quantitative test: test that analyzes for the presence and amount of the analyte and reports results in numerical values or units

quantity not sufficient (QNS): when the specimen obtained from the patient is insufficient for performing the test

Queckenstedt test: a test to evaluate intracranial pressure that involves having the assistant press on the patient's jugular vein (right, left, or both, in the neck) while the physician monitors the cerebrospinal fluid (CSF) pressure

reagents: substances required for a chemical reaction or used to detect the presence of another substance

Recommended Dietary Allowance (RDA): guidelines that are based on what the average healthy person of a specific age, height, weight, and activity level would require

reference laboratory: a laboratory that performs large numbers of complex tests that other laboratories only occasionally perform

rehabilitation: the process of returning a patient as close as possible to the person's normal physical condition after injury or disease

restoration: to bring back to the former state

rhinorrhea: runny nose

rickets: illness that is the result of a lack of vitamin D

Ringer's solution: an aqueous solution of the chlorides of sodium, potassium, and calcium

Romberg test: a test during which patient closes eyes and stands with feet together while attempting to stand without swaying

rule of nines: a simple mathematical calculation used for estimating the amount of body surface affected by burns

sanguineous: a bright to dark red exudate that contains blood

saturated fats: fats that are solid at room temperature; mainly found in the human diet in animal products, eggs, and coconut and palm oils

scapula: shoulder blade

scoliosis: an abnormal lateral curvature of the spine

scurvy: illness that is the result of a lack of vitamin C

sediment: solid material remaining at the bottom of the test tube after centrifugation

seizure: convulsion caused by disorganized electrical activity in the brain

sensitivity: a microbiology term describing the lack of growth of an organism in response to a specific antibiotic

septicemia: pathogenic organisms in the bloodstream

serous: a clear, watery exudate composed mainly of serum

serosanguineous: a clear blood-tinged exudate that contains both blood and serum

serum: liquid portion of blood

side effects: adverse reactions that cause harmless reactions to a drug and are tolerated to obtain the therapeutic effect

Sitz bath: bath taken in a sitting position

SOAP: a charting method comprising *s*ubjective and *o*bjective information, *a*ssessment, and *p*lan of care

solutes: electrolytes such as sodium and potassium and nonelectrolytes such as proteins found in fluids in the body

sonography: diagnostic imaging procedure that uses high-frequency sound waves to produce images of internal structures

specificity: ability of a particular antibody to react with only one antigen

speculum: probing and dilating instrument used to spread apart a body cavity for ease of visualization

squamous cell carcinoma: a type of skin cancer affecting the middle layer of the skin

standard deviation: a statistical term describing the amount of variation from the mean in a set of data

Standard Precautions: new guidelines developed by the Centers for Disease Control and Prevention (CDC) for isolation precautions in hospitals; combine major features of Universal Precautions and body substance isolation precautions into one set of recommendations

stat: without delay

strabismus: lazy eye

supernatant: clear fluid above sediment or precipitate

syncope: fainting

synergism: the increased effect of drugs working together

teratogenic: a medication with a high risk level for fetal or maternal health problems

thrombectomy: removal of a blood clot or thrombus

thrombocytes: platelets

thoracentesis: procedure performed to remove air or fluid from the pleural cavity to improve breathing

total parenteral nutrition (TPN): nutrition provided only through parenteral (outside the intestines) route

trans fat: unsaturated fats to which hydrogen has been added; found in shortening, margarine, and many snack foods

transmission-based precautions: precautions that fall into three categories—airborne, droplet, and contact; followed to reduce the risk of transmitting diseases such as tuberculosis and chicken pox

transudates: substances that pass through membranes

trocar: probing and dilating instrument used to withdraw fluids from cavities

turbid: cloudy or opaque

turnaround time: the time it takes to produce results

ubiquitous: widespread

umbilicus: belly button

Universal Precautions: routine infection control precautions developed in 1985 to prevent the transmission of hepatitis B virus, human immunodeficiency virus (HIV), and other bloodborne pathogens

unsaturated fats: fats that come from nuts, seeds, and vegetables and are generally liquid at room temperature

urinary meatus: where urine is discharged

vegan: a person who does not eat any product associated with animals, including eggs and dairy products

vertex: top, highest point of the head

vertigo: dizziness

vesicants: drugs that cause blistering

vesicle: small fluid-filled, raised, blisterlike spot on skin

vomitus: material ejected from stomach through mouth

xiphoid process: tip of the sternum

Index

A

A antigen, 282
Abbreviations
    common medical, A-1–A-2
    ISMP's list of error-prone, A-4–A-7
    pharmacology, 313, 314
Abdominal paracentesis, 168
Abdominal thrusts
    for choking adults, 175, 178–179
    for choking children, 175, 178–179
    for choking infants, 176–177
Abdominal ultrasound, 80
ABO blood groups
    explanation of, 282, 283
    tests for, 284–285
Abortion, 76
Absorption, drug, 316
Accuracy, of clinical tests, 200
Acetest tablets, 222
Acquired immune deficiency syndrome
        (AIDS), 78. See also HIV/AIDS
Action, drug, 316
Active assist range of motion
        (AAROM), 116
Active range of motion (AROM), 116
Adhesive skin closures, 162
Adoptive equipment/devices
    canes, 127, 128
    crutches, 128–130
    explanation of, 127
    use of, 132–133
Adults
    abdominal thrusts for, 175, 177–179
    administering oral medications to,
        323–324
    airways in, 172
    CPR for, 182–183
    height measurement for, 21, 39
    rescue breathing for, 180
    skin puncture for, 239–240
AED. See Automatic external
        defibrillator (AED)
Aerobes, 230
Agar, 230
Agglutination
    explanation of, 276, 277
    of red blood cells, 282
Agglutination tests
    for ABO blood grouping, 284–285
    guidelines for, 278
    inhibition, 224

Agonists, 316
Airborne precautions, 11
Airway
    blocked, 174 (See also Choking)
    primary assessment of, 171–172
Aldosterone, 344
Allergens, 61
Allergic rhinitis, 62
Allergies
    common types of, 62
    desensitization injections for, 64
    explanation of, 61
Allergy tests
    assisting with, 61
    intradermal, 64, 335
    patch, 63, 64
    radioallergosorbent, 64
    safety guidelines for, 63
    scratch, 62–64
Alpha-fetoprotein (AFP), 80
Ambulatory care centers, 146
American Dietetic Association (ADA), 369
American Hospital Association, Patient's Bill
        of Rights, 3
American Hospital Formulary Service
        (AHFS), 310
American Medical Association (AMA), 316
Amniocentesis, 80
Amplified DNA probe test
    explanation of, 77–78
    obtaining material for, 79–80
Ampules
    explanation of, 330
    withdrawing medication from,
        332–333
Anaerobes, 230
Analgesic cream, 349
Analyte, 198, 300
Anaphylactic emergencies
    assisting patients during, 188–189
    explanation of, 61
    symptoms of, 188
Anaphylactic shock kits, 61
Anaphylaxis, 188
Anemia, 257–258
Aneroid sphygmomanometers, 34, 35
Anesthetics, 147
Angiography, 308
Anoscope, 68
Antagonism, 317
Antagonists, 316
Anteroposterior (AP) position, 302, 303

Anthropometry, 39–40
Antibodies, 276
Anticoagulant therapy, 364
Antidiuretic hormone (ADH), 344
Antigens, 276
Antisera, 283
Antistreptolysin O Test (ASO), 282
Anuria, 216
Apgar scoring, 100
Apical heart rate, 29
Apical pulse (AP)
    explanation of, 29
    measurement of, 31–32, 104
Apical–radial pulse, 29, 32
Appearance, 173
Approximated wound, 160
Aquathermic pads, 120, 121, 123
Arm slings, 141–142
Arm splints, 194
Arterial blood gases (ABG), 253
Arthrography, 308
Artifacts, 380–381
Ascites, 168
Ascorbic acid, 368
Aseptic hand washing, 12–13
Aspiration, of joint fluid, 165–166
Assessment
    primary, 171–172
    secondary, 172–173
Assistive devices
    explanation of, 127
    home safety suggestions for patients
        using, 130
    types of, 127–130
Asthma, 62
Asthma attack, 188
Atherosclerosis, 290
Audiometry, 93, 94
Aural temperature, 26–27
Auscultation, 43
Autoclave
    sterilizing instruments in, 16–17
    wrapping instruments for, 15–16
Autolytic method, 163
Automated cell counter, 208
Automatic external defibrillator (AED)
    method to use, 185–186
    training for use of, 170, 172
Axial position, 302
Axillary crutches, 128, 131
Axillary temperature, 28, 103
Axillary thermometers, 22

B

Back blows
  for conscious infants, 176–177
  for unconscious infants, 177–178
Bacteremia, 253
Bacteria
  explanation of, 231
  shapes of, 230
  urinary tract infections from, 221
Bandages
  explanation of, 147
  figure-eight, 143
  spiral, 142–143
  tubular gauze, 194
B antigen, 282
Barcode scanners, 320
Bayer DCA 2000+ Analyzer, 294–296
Beans, 372
Bed, transferring patient to wheelchair from,
  136–137
Bilirubin, in urine, 223–224
Bioflavonoids, 369
Biopsy
  bone marrow, 164
  cervical, 81–83
  explanation of, 164
BioStar Acceava Mono II test, 278–279
BioStar Acceava Strep A test, 280–281
Bleeding. See Severe bleeding
Bleeding time test, 254–255
Blood. See also Hematology
  coagulation studies of, 273, 274
  components of, 257
Blood agar plate, 232
Blood antigens, 282–283
Blood cells. See Red blood cells (RBCs);
    White blood cells (WBCs)
Blood chemistry tests
  blood glucose, 288–289
  explanation of, 288
  lipid, 296–300
  list of commonly ordered, 300
Blood cultures, 253–254
Blood glucose, 288–289
Blood glucose meter, 291
Blood glucose tests
  CLIA waived, 290–294
  explanation of, 289
  glucose tolerance, 289
  glycosylated hemoglobin, 290, 294–296
  One Touch Ultra device for, 291–292
  postprandial, 289
  SureStep Flexx Monitor for, 294
Blood groups
  agglutination slide testing to determine,
    283–285
  explanation of, 282, 283
Blood pressure
  average normal, 35
  equipment to measure, 34

  explanation of, 34–35
  in infants and children, 104
Blood smears
  differential, 269–271
  peripheral, 267–268, 271
Blood specimens. See Phlebotomy; Skin puncture
Blood values
  normal, A-8–A-12
Body fat, 41
Body fluids, 9, 11
Body mass index (BMI), 21, 39, 40
Body mechanics, 134, 139
Body surface area (BSA), 315
Bolus, 345
Bone marrow biopsy, 164
Brand name, of drugs, 310
Breast cancer, 75
Breast examinations, 75–76
Breathing assessment, 171–172
Buccal medications, 324–325
Bureau of Narcotics and Dangerous Drugs
    (BNDD), 310
Burns
  caring for, 192
  classification of, 189, 191
  rule of nines for, 189, 190
Butterfly infusion sets, 246, 251–252

C

Calcium, 344, 366
Calories
  daily guidelines for, 373
  explanation of, 370
  on food labels, 371
Cancer
  breast, 75
  skin, 65
  testicular, 84
Candidiasis, 78, 221
Canes, 127, 128
Cannula, 357, 392
Capillary blood gas analysis, 253
Carbohydrates
  on food labels, 371
  function of, 366, 368
Carcinoma in situ, 76
Cardinal signs. See Vital signs
Cardiology, 380
Cardiology procedures
  exercise tolerance stress tests as, 384–386
  Holter monitor application as, 382,
    384, 385
  12-lead electrocardiogram as, 380–384
Cardiopulmonary resuscitation (CPR)
  for adults, 182–183
  barrier devices to perform, 174
  for children, 184
  for infants, 184–185
  training in, 170
  when to use, 172

Cardiovascular disease, 297, 380
Casts
  application of, 138, 140
  classification of, 221
  explanation of, 138
  removal of, 140–141
Catalysts, 369
Catheterization
  explanation of, 83
  on females, 83–85
  kit for, 84
  on males, 86, 87
  for urine specimen collection, 212
Catheters
  central venous, 346
  over-the-needle, 349, 355–356
  peripheral, 346
Catheter sets, 349
Celsius/Fahrenheit temperature conversions,
    A-13
Centers for Disease Control (CDC), 9,
    344, 350
Centers for Medicare and Medicaid Services
    (CMS), 260–261
Central vascular devices (CVADs), 346
Centrifuge, 206
Cerebral spinal fluid (CSF), 72, 73
Cerumen, 93
Cervical biopsy
  assisting with, 82–83
  explanation of, 81
Cervical collars, 144
Chain of custody (COC), 202
Chair, transferring patient from wheelchair
    to, 135
Charting, SOAP, 47
Chemical disinfectants, 17
Chemical disposable thermometers, 21–22
Chemical name, of drugs, 310
Chemical pack, cold, 125–126
Chemical reagent strips, 219, 221–224
Chemistry analyzers, 208, 288
Chemistry tests. See Blood chemistry tests
Chest circumference, 105–107
Chest thrusts
  for conscious infants, 176–177
  for unconscious infants, 177–178
Chevron method, for intravenous
    therapy, 350
Chief complaint (CC)
  documentation of, 48–49
  explanation of, 43
Children. See also Infants
  abdominal thrusts for, 176, 178–179
  airways in, 172
  CPR for, 184
  growth and development of, 106,
    107–108
  head and chest circumference of, 104–107
  height and weight of, 102, 104
  hematocrit level in, 257–258

immunizations for, 107–113
medication administration to, 324
medication dosages for, 315
rescue breathing for, 180–181
skin puncture for, 239–240
urine collection procedure for, 112–114
vital signs for, 101–104
Chlamydia, 77–80
Chloride (Cl), 344
Choking
  abdominal thrusts for, 175–176, 178–179
  back blows and chest thrusts for, 176–178
  in children, 175, 178–179
  explanation of, 174
  in infants, 176–178
Cholangiography, 308
Cholecystogram, 305–306
Cholestech LDX Analyzer, 297–299
Cholesterol
  explanation of, 296–297
  on food labels, 371
Chorionic villi sampling (CVS), 80
Circulation, assessment of, 171–172
Clean-catch midstream specimen (CCMS)
  explanation of, 212, 233
  for female patients, 213–214
  for male patients, 212–213
Cleaning
  examination room, 43, 46–47
  minor wounds, 156–158
  skin prior to surgery, 155–156
CLIA Waived Tests (WTs), 199, 218, 224, 233, 258, 277–282, 288, 297
Clinical laboratories
  departments in, 199–200
  equipment in, 206–208
  proficiency testing in, 200
  quality control in, 200, 205–206
  safety in, 200
  types of, 198–199
Clinical Laboratory Improvement Amendments (CLIA) (1988), 199, 200
Clinical laboratory tests. See also Phlebotomy; Specimens
  chain of custody for, 202
  control values for, 205–206
  cycle for, 202, 203
  function of, 198
  monitoring and following up on, 202, 204
  patient preparation and specimen handling for, 202
  qualitative, 198
  quantitative, 198
  requisitions for, 200–201, 203–204
Clinitest Tablet Test, 221–222
Clot formation, 273, 274
Coagulation studies, 273, 274
Coagulation testing, 274

Cold Agglutinins tests, 282
Cold chemical pack, 125–126
Cold compress, 124
Cold emergencies, 193–194
Cold therapies
  application of, 124–126
  explanation of, 122–123
Colonoscopy, 67, 69
Colony
  explanation of, 228, 233
  isolation of, 232
Color vision acuity, 88–90
Colposcopy
  assisting with, 82–83
  explanation of, 81
Communication
  with culturally diverse patients, 58
  with elderly patients, 59
  importance of, 2
Compendium of Drug Therapy, 310
Complete blood count (CBC)
  explanation of, 257
  use of QBC STAR to perform, 264–267
Compliance, 375
Compound microscope, 206
Computed tomography (CT), 302
Consciousness, 173
Contact dermatitis, 62
Contact precautions, 11
Contraindicated drugs, 317
Contrast studies, 305–306
Controlled substances. See also Medications
  categories of, 310, 311
  monitoring of, 310–311, 316, 318, 320
  registration of, 310
Controlled Substances Act (1970), 310
Corpuscular, 271
Coulter Counters, 262
CPR. See Cardiopulmonary resuscitation (CPR)
C-Reactive protein (CRP), 282
Creams/ointments, for surgery, 147
Crutches
  explanation of, 128
  instructing patient in use of, 132–133
  measuring patient for, 131
  types of, 128–129
  walking gaits with, 129–130
Crutch walking gaits, 129–130
Cryosurgery, 168
Cryotherapy, 122–123
Crystals, urine, 221
Culturally diverse patients
  communicating with, 58
  expression of pain in, 38
  nutrition and, 375
Culture
  blood, 253–254
  explanation of, 227
  preparation of, 228–230, 233–234
Culture media, 230, 231
Cysts, sebaceous, 165

D

Daily value, on food labels, 371
Debridement, 162–163
Deltoid muscle, 339
Department of Agriculture (USDA), 370–372
Department of Health and Human Services (HHS), 2, 372
Dermal temperature, 27
Dermatology, 64–65
Dermis, 64
Desensitization injections, 64
Diabetes mellitus (DM)
  characteristics and treatment for, 290
  explanation of, 288
  testing for, 289
  types of, 289
Diagnostic imaging. See Radiologic procedures
Diagnostic imaging centers, 302
Diastolic blood pressure, 34, 36
Diazo tablets, 223–224
Dietary fats. See also Lipids
  equivalent services for, 372
  explanation of, 366, 369
  on food labels, 371, 372
Dietary fiber, 369, 376–377
Dietetics, 372
Diets. See also Nutrients; Nutrition
  guidelines for, 372–373
  modifications to, 373–374
  therapeutic, 374
Differential blood smears, 269–271
Digestive system
  examinations associated with, 66–71
  function of, 66
Digital sphygmomanometers, 34
Digital thermometers
  explanation of, 21–22
  to measure oral temperature, 25
  to measure rectal temperature, 26, 203
Dipstick tests, urine, 218, 219
Direct smear
  preparation of, 228
  staining of, 229–230
Discretion, 3
Disease prevention, 377–378
Disposable enema, 66–67
Disposable thermometers, 21, 27
Distance vision acuity (DVA), 86–88
Distribution, drug, 316
Diversity. See Culturally diverse patients
Documentation
  basic information related to, 3–4
  of medical emergencies, 170
Dorsal recumbent position, 51–52
Dorsogluteal muscle, 339
Dosimeter, 302
Drainage. See Exudate
Dressings. See Sterile dressings
Drip chambers, 347

Droplet precautions, 11
Drug administration. *See* Medication administration
Drug collection kits, 214
Drug Enforcement Agency (DEA), 310, 316
Drugs. *See* Medications
Drug screen, urine specimen for, 214–215
Dysplasia, 76
Dyspnea, 62

E

Ears
    instilling medication in, 93, 95–96
    irrigation of, 93–95
Earthquakes, 195
Eczema, 62
Elderly patients
    communicating with, 59
    medication issues for, 317, 318
Electrocardiograms (ECG or EKG)
    explanation of, 380–382
    procedures for, 383–384
Electrodes, 381–382
Electrolytes, 344–345
Electronic infusion devices (EIDs), 347–349, 357
Electronic medical records (EMRs), 47
Electronic thermometers
    explanation of, 21, 22
    glass nonmercury, 28
    to measure oral temperature, 25
    to measure rectal temperature, 26
Emergencies
    action plans for, 170
    anaphylactic, 188–189
    asthma attack, 187, 188
    automated external defibrillators for, 185–186
    bandages and splints for, 194, 195
    burn, 189–192
    choking, 174–176
    CPR for, 182–185
    equipment and supplies for, 171, 172, 186–187
    fainting, 187
    heat and cold, 193–194
    overview of, 170
    poisoning, 191, 193
    primary assessment for, 171–172
    recovery position for, 173–174
    rescue breathing techniques for, 180–182
    secondary assessment for, 172–173
    seizure, 190–193
    severe bleeding, 189, 190
Emergency calls, 7
Emergency crash carts
    explanation of, 171
    guidelines to maintain, 186–187
    supplies and equipment for, 171, 172

Emergency medical services (EMS), 170
Emergency preparedness, 195, 196
EMLA, 240, 349
Empathy, 3
Enemas, 66–67
Enterobius vermicularis, 235
Enzyme immunoassay test, 224, 225
Enzyme-linked immunosorbent assay (ELISA) tests, 276
Enzymes, 369
Epidermis, 64
Epidurals, 353
Epilepsy, 190
Epistaxis, 95, 97
Epithelial cells, in urine, 221
Epstein-Barr virus (EBV), 277
Equipment
    adaptive, 127–130, 132–133
    for blood drawing, 237–239, 241, 244–246
    for clinical laboratories, 206–208
    for emergencies, 170–171, 186, 187
    for intravenous therapy, 346–349
    for minor surgery, 146–148
    for parenteral medications, 329–330
    for physical examinations, 44
Erythrocytes, 257
Erythrocyte sedimentation rate (ESR), 271–273
Estimated date of delivery (EDD), 80
Evacuated tube collection method, 248–249
Examination table
    transferring patient from wheelchair to, 135
    transferring patient to bed or wheelchair from, 136–137
Excision, 65
Excretion, drug, 316
Exercise tolerance stress test, 384–386
Expectorate, 393
External controls, 276
Exudate
    explanation of, 157
    types of, 159
    wounds producing, 162, 163
Eye patch dressings, 92–93
Eyes. *See also* Ophthalmology
    instilling medication in, 89, 91
    irrigation of, 90–91
    pupil check of, 71–72

F

Face mask, 174
Face shield, 174
Facultative anaerobes, 230
Fainting, 187, 252
Falls, assisting patients with, 138
False-negative reactions, 276
False-positive reactions, 276
Family history (FH), 43

Fasting blood glucose (FBS or FBG) test, 289
Fat fold measurement, 39, 40
Fats. *See also* Lipids
    equivalent services for, 372
    explanation of, 366, 369
    on food labels, 371, 372
Female reproductive system. *See* Obstetrics and gynecology (OB/Gyn)
Females, urinary catheterization on, 83–85
Fetal heart rate, 80
Fetid, 216
Fiber, 369, 376–377
Figure-eight bandages, 143
Fires, 195–196
First aid, training in, 170
First responders, 170
First voided morning urine specimen, 210–211
Floods, 196
Flow rates, intravenous, 356–357
Fluid imbalances, 345
Fluids, electrolytes in, 344–345
Fluoroscopy, 302, 308
Fontanels, 100
Food and Drug Administration (FDA), 310
Food groups, 372
Food labels
    information on, 371–372
    teaching patients to read, 375–376
Food Pyramid, 370–373
Forced vital capacity (FVC), 387
Forceps, sterile transfer, 152–153
Forearm crutches, 128
Four-point gait, 129
Fowler's position, 50–51
Fractures, types of, 139
Freezers, in clinical laboratories, 208
Fruits, 372
Fundal height, 80
Fungi, 231

G

Gait belt, 127, 134
Gaits, crutch walking, 129–130
Gastroenterology
    explanation of, 66
    procedures related to, 66–71
Generic name, of drugs, 310
Genital herpes, 78
Genitalia, 113
Genital warts, 78
Germicidal wipes, 12
Gestational diabetes, 290
GI series, 305
Glass nonmercury thermometers
    cleaning and storing, 24
    explanation of, 21
    to measure axillary temperature, 28
    to measure oral temperature, 22–23
    to measure rectal temperature, 23–24

Gloves
    applying and removing nonsterile, 14
    applying and removing sterile, 149–150
Glucose, in urine, 221–222
Glucose tolerance test (GTT), 289
Glycemic index, 368
Glycosylated hemoglobin (hgbA1c), 290
Glycosylated hemoglobin test, 290, 294–296
Goniometer, 116
Gonorrhea
    amplified DNA probe test for, 77–80
    symptoms and diagnosis of, 78
Good Samaritan laws, 170
Grains, 372
Gram stain, 229
Gravida, 76
Growth charts, for infants and children, 107
Gynecology (Gyn). *See also* Obstetrics and
        gynecology (OB/Gyn)
    breast examinations and, 75–76
    colposcopies and cervical biopsies and,
        81–83
    explanation of, 75
    pelvic examinations and PAP tests and,
        76–77
    procedures related to, 75–83
    urinary catheterization and, 83–85

H

Hand sanitizing, waterless-based, 13
Hand washing
    aseptic, 12–13, 237
    surgical, 146, 148, 149
Headaches, following lumbar puncture, 73
Head circumference, 104–106
Health Care Financing Administration
        (HCFA), 199
Health Insurance Portability and
        Accountability Act (HIPAA)
    confidentiality requirements of, 202
    provisions of, 2–3
Heart attacks, 297
Heat emergencies, 193
Heat exhaustion, 193
Heating pads, 121, 123
Heat stroke, 193
Heelstick procedure
    explanation of, 240, 241
    for PKU screening, 242
Height measurement
    in adults, 21, 39
    in infants and children, 102, 104
Heimlich maneuver. *See* Abdominal thrusts
Helicobacter pylori test, 281–282
Hematocrit
    explanation of, 257–258
    HemataSTAT II to perform, 259–260
Hematology
    coagulation studies and, 273, 274
    coagulation testing and, 274

erythrocyte sedimentation rate and,
        271–273
    explanation of, 257
    hemoglobin and, 260–262
    microhematocrit and, 257–259
    peripheral blood smears and, 267–271
    QBC STAR, 264–267
    red blood cell indices and, 271
    Unopette System and, 262–264
    white and red blood cell counts and,
        260–262
Hematomas, 252
Hematopoiesis, 257
HemataSTAT II, 258–260
Hematuria, 218, 220
HemoCue system, 260–262
Hemogard closures, 244
Hemoglobin, 260
Hemoglobinometer, 260
Hemoglobin test, 261–262
Hemorrhage. *See* Severe bleeding
Hemorrhoid thrombectomy, 166–167
HemoSense INR, 274
Heparin lock, 359
HGB Meter, 260
High-density lipoproteins (HDLs), 297
HIPAA. *See* Health Insurance Portability
        and Accountability Act (HIPAA)
HIV/AIDS, 77. *See also* Acquired immune
        deficiency syndrome (AIDS)
H method, for intravenous therapy, 351
Holter monitor
    application of, 385
    explanation of, 382, 384
Home monitoring devices, 238
Homeostasis, 21
Horizontal recumbent position, 50
Hot compress, 121
Hot soaks, 120, 122
Hurricane preparedness, 196
Hyperglycemia, 288
Hyperinsulinemia, 368
Hypersensitivity, 61
Hyperthermia, 193
Hypertonic solutions, 345
Hypoglycemia, 288
Hypothermia, 193–194
Hypothyroidism, 240
Hypotonic solutions, 345
Hypovolemic shock, 189

I

Ice bags, 124–125
Ictotest, 223–224
Idiopathic conditions, 190
Idiosyncratic reactions, to drugs, 317
Immobilizing devices
    arm slings, 141–142
    cervical collars, 144
    explanation of, 141

    figure-eight bandages, 143
    spiral bandages, 142–143
Immune system, 276
Immunizations
    administration records of, 111–112
    administration route for, 335
    function of, 107
    recommended schedules for, 107–111
Immunohematology department, 276
Immunology department, 276
Impaired glucose tolerance (IGT), 290
Incision and drainage (I&D), 163
Incubator, 208
Indices, 271
Infants. *See also* Children
    abdominal thrusts for conscious, 176–177
    airways in, 172
    Apgar scoring for, 100
    back blows and chest thrusts for
        unconscious, 177–178
    CPR for, 184–185
    growth and development of, 106, 107–108
    head and chest circumference of, 104–107
    height and weight of, 102, 104, 105
    immunizations for, 109
    rescue breathing for, 181–182
    safety of, 100
    skin puncture for, 240–242
    vital signs for, 101–104
    wrapping procedure for, 100–102
Infection control procedures
    to apply and remove nonsterile gloves, 14
    for aseptic hand washing, 12–13
    to chemically sterilize instruments, 17
    explanation of, 11
    for infectious waste disposal, 12
    for isolation, 18–19
    overview of, 9
    to sanitize instruments, 15
    standard precautions for, 9–11
    to sterilize instruments in autoclave, 16–17
    transmission-based precautions for, 11, 18–19
    for waterless-based hand sanitizing, 13
    to wrap instruments for autoclaving, 15–16
Infections, nosocomial, 11
Infectious waste disposal, 12
Influenza, 235
Influenza tests, 235, 282
Ingredients, on food labels, 372
Inhalation, of medication, 325
Inhalation treatments
    explanation of, 389
    metered-dose, 389–391
    nebulized, 389, 391
    oxygen administration by nasal cannula or
        face mask as, 392
Injections
    intradermal, 335–337
    intramuscular, 337, 339–341
    subcutaneous, 335, 337–339
    Z-track, 339, 341–342

Inspection, 43
Instillation of medication
    in ears, 93, 95–96
    explanation of, 325
    in eyes, 89, 91
    in nose, 96
Institute for Healthcare Improvement
    (IHI), 155
Institute for Safe Medication Practices, 313,
    A-4–A-7
Instruments, 15–16. *See also* Equipment
Insufflator, 68
Insulin dependent diabetes mellitus (IDDM),
    288–289
Insulin levels, 288, 289, 368
Integrity, 3
Intermittent infusion lock, 359, 360
Internal controls, 276
International normalized ratio (INR), 274
Interstitial fluid, 237
Intradermal injections
    administration of, 336–337
    for allergy testing, 64, 335
    body sites for, 336
    explanation of, 335
Intramuscular injections
    administration of, 340–341
    body sites for, 339
    explanation of, 337, 339
Intravascular fluid, 344
Intravenous administration sets
    adding extension tubing to, 358
    explanation of, 347–349
Intravenous containers, 346–349
Intravenous pyelogram (IVP), 305
Intravenous therapy
    adding extension tubing for, 358
    adjusting flow rate for, 356–357
    changing solution for, 359
    containers and administration sets for,
        346–349
    converted to saline lock, 359, 360
    explanation of, 344
    for fluid and electrolyte balance, 344–345
    legal regulations for, 344
    medication administration methods for,
        360–363
    method to discontinue, 363–364
    monitoring, 358–359
    over-the-needle catheter for, 349, 355–356
    peripheral sites for, 347
    peripheral vascular access devices for, 346
    preparing infusion for, 351–353
    preparing venipuncture site for, 353–354
    procedures for, 345–346
    securing venus access device for, 350–351
    solutions for, 345
    uses for, 345
    vein puncture for, 349–350
    venus access devices for, 349
    winged needles for, 354–355

Intubate, 170
In utero, 283
In vitro tests, 276
In vivo tests, 276
Iodine, 367
Iontophoresis, 349–350
Ipecac, syrup of, 193
Iron, 367
Iron deficiency anemia, 260
Irrigation
    of ears, 93–95
    of eyes, 89, 90–91
    of wounds, 162, 163
Ishihara method, to test color deficits, 88
Isolation techniques
    Centers for Disease Control on, 9
    guidelines for, 18–19
Isotonic solutions, 345
I-STAT Point-of-Care analyzer, 260

J

Jaundice, 240
Joint Commission, 314, 344, A-3
Joint fluid, aspiration of, 165–166

K

Ketones, in urine, 222
Knee–chest position, 54–55
KOH slides, 79
Korotkoff sounds, 34
Kyphosis, 56

L

Laboratory requisition forms, 246
Laboratory tests. *See* Clinical laboratory tests;
        Specimens
Lancers, 238
Laser surgery, 167–168
Lateral position, 302, 303
Latex, sensitivity to, 11
Lavage, 89–91
Leads, 382
Legal issues
    related to intravenous therapy, 355, 361
    related to medication, 315–316, 335
Leukocytes, 257
Leukocytosis, 262
Leukopenia, 262
Level I Tests, 199
Level II Tests, 199–200
Lipemic serum, 276
Lipidemia, 290
Lipids, 296–297, 369. *See also* Fats
Lipid tests, 298–299
Lipoproteins, 297
Liquid medication dosages, 315
Lithotomy position, 52
Lochia, 80–81
Lofstrand crutches, 128

Logrolling, 172
Lordosis, 56
Low-density lipoproteins (LDLs), 297
Lower GI series, 305
Lumbar puncture
    assisting with, 74
    explanation of, 72–73

M

Magnesium (Mg), 344
Magnetic resonance imaging (MRI), 302
Male reproductive system
    explanation of, 83–84
    team approach to, 83
    testicular self-examination and, 84–86
Males, urinary catheterization on, 86, 87
Mammography, 308
Manipulation, 43
Mantoux test, 337
Measurement, metric units of, 198, 314, 315
Meats, 372
Medical assistants
    intravenous therapy protocols for, 344
    x-rays taken by, 302
Medical history, 43, 47–49
Medical history sheets, 49
Medical terminology
    analysis of, A-14–A-15
    to describe body direction, A-16–A-17
    to describe diseases and disease conditions,
        A-16
    to describe major body systems, A-16
    explanation of, A-14
    for planes of body, A-17, A-18
    prefixes for, A-19
    root words for, A-19–A-21
    singular and plural endings for,
        A-15–A-16
    suffixes for, A-15, A-21, A-22
Medication administration
    buccal, 324–325
    calculating dosages for, 315
    following exact guidelines for, 320–321
    intravenous, 345, 360–363 (*See also*
        Intravenous therapy)
    measurement and conversion system for,
        314–315
    oral, 321–324
    parenteral, 329–342 (*See also* Parenteral
        medication administration)
    for pediatric patients, 315, 324
    preparation for, 320
    routes of, 316–317
    safety aspects of, 318, 320
    sublingual, 324
    suppository, 325, 327–328
    topical, 325–326
    transdermal, 326–327
Medication administration record (MAR),
    318, 319

Medications
 actions on body, 316
 adverse reactions to, 317, 318
 buccal, 324–325
 classifications for, 310–313
 contraindicated, 317
 controlled substance, 310–311, 316, 318, 320
 for elderly individuals, 318
 inhalation of, 325
 installation of, 89, 91, 93, 95–96, 325
 legal implications related to, 315–316
 monitoring of, 310, 316
 names for, 310
 oral, 321–324
 over-the-counter, 95, 310
 parenteral, 329–342 (*See also* Parenteral medications)
 powdered, 329–331
 preparing physician orders for, 322–323
 prescriptions for, 311–314
 reference materials for, 310
 safety issues related to, 310, 316, 318
 sublingual, 324
 suppository, 325, 327–328
 teratogenic, 317
 topical, 325
Medline, 310
Menarche, 76
Menses, 75
Mensuration, 43
Mercury sphygmomanometers, 34, 35
Metabolic syndrome, 290, 368
Metabolism, drug, 316
Metered-dose inhaler (MDI), 389–391
Metric units of measurement, 198, 314, 315
Microbiology, 227
Microhematocrit
 explanation of, 257–258
 performing manual, 258–259
Microorganisms
 classes of, 231
 explanation of, 227
 growth of, 230
 procedure for naming, 227
Microscopes
 components of, 207
 explanation of, 206
 for urinalysis, 218
 use and cleaning of, 207
Microtainer unit, 243
Milk, 372
Minerals
 explanation of, 366–367, 369
 on food labels, 372
Minor surgery. *See* Surgical procedures
Mobility aids, 127
Mononucleosis tests
 BioStar Acceava, 278–279
 explanation of, 277–278
Mons pubis, 114

Morphology, 229
Mucus, in urine, 221
Multichannel electrocardiogram, 381, 383–384
Mycobacterium, 229
Myelography, 308

N

Naegele's rule, 80
Narcotics. *See* Controlled substances
Nasal irrigation, 95
Nasal sprays, over-the-counter, 95
National Childhood Vaccine Injury Act (NCVIA), 108, 111
Near vision acuity (NVA), 88, 89
Nebulizers, 389, 391
Needles
 for blood drawing, 244–246
 for surgery, 147
Nervous system
 explanation of, 71
 procedures related to, 71–74
Neurological examination, assisting with, 72–73
Neurology
 explanation of, 71–72
 procedures related to, 71–74
Newborns. *See also* Infants
 Apgar scoring for, 100
 vital signs for, 101–104
Niacin, 367
Nitroprusside reaction, 222
Nomogram, 315
Noncompliance, 375
Noninsulin dependent diabetes mellitus (NIDDM), 289
Nonpathogens, 227
Nonsterile gloves, 14
Nonverbal communication, 37
Normal blood values, A-8–A-12
Normal flora, 227
Nose, 95, 96
Nosebleed, 95, 97
Nosocomial infections, 11
Nuclear blasts, 196
Nuclear medicine, 308
Nutrients
 carbohydrates as, 368
 classes of, 366–368
 fats as, 369
 fiber as, 369, 376–377
 minerals as, 369
 proteins as, 369
 vitamins as, 369
 water as, 368, 369
Nutrition
 calories and, 370
 dietary guidelines for, 372–373
 explanation of, 366
 food labels with information on, 371–372

 Food Pyramid guidelines for, 370–371
 modifications for good, 373–374
 patient education on, 374–377
 role in wellness and prevention, 377–378
Nutritionists, 372
Nutrition Labeling and Education Act (1994), 372

O

Obesity, 297, 368
Oblique position, 302, 303
Obstetrics and gynecology (OB/Gyn)
 breast examinations and, 75–76
 colposcopies and cervical biopsies and, 81–83
 explanation of, 73, 75
 pelvic examinations and PAP tests and, 76–77
 postpartum examinations and, 80–82
 prenatal examinations and, 78, 80, 81
 procedures related to, 75, 78–82
 sexually transmitted diseases and, 77–80
 urinary catheterization and, 83–85
Obturator, 68
Occult blood
 explanation of, 66
 testing for, 70–71
Occupational Safety and Health Administration (OSHA), 9
Oliguria, 216
One Touch Ultra device, 291–292
Ophthalmology
 applying eye patch dressings and, 92
 assisting vision-impaired patients and, 89, 92
 color vision acuity testing and, 88–90
 distance vision acuity testing and, 86–88
 explanation of, 86–88
 instilling eye medication and, 89, 91
 irrigation of eye and, 89–91
 near vision acuity testing and, 88, 89
Oral medications. *See also* Medication administration; Medications
 administered to adults, 323–324
 administered to children, 324
 calculating dosages for, 315
 preparation of, 321–322
Oral thermometers, 22–23
Orifices, 227
Osmolarity, 345
Otorhinolaryngology
 assisting with audiometry, 93, 94
 assisting with treatment of epistaxis, 97
 examination of nose and throat, 95
 explanation of, 92–93
 instilling ear medication, 93, 95–96
 instilling nasal medication, 96
 irrigating the ear, 93–95
 obtaining throat culture, 98
Outside laboratories, 198–199

Ova, stool specimen for, 234
Over-the-counter (OTC) medications, 95, 310. *See also* Medications
Over-the-needle catheter, 349, 355–356
Oximeter, 38
Oxygen administration, 392
Oxygen saturation measurement, 38

P

Pain
  explanation of, 37
  location and level of, 173
  measurement of, 37–38
Palpation method, 43
Palpatory method, to measure systolic blood pressure, 35–36
Pap smear, 76, 81
Pap test, 76–77
Papules, 62
Para, 76
Paracentesis, abdominal, 168
Paramedics, 170
Parasites, 221, 234
Parenteral medication administration
  explanation of, 329–330, 335
  intradermal, 335–337
  intramuscular, 337, 339–341
  subcutaneous, 335, 337–339
  Z-track, 339, 341–342
Parenteral medications
  calculating dosages for, 315
  combined in one syringe using two different vials, 333
  equipment for, 329–330
  explanation of, 329
  in prefilled disposable cartridge syringe, 334–335
  reconstituting powdered, 329–331
  of two medications in two syringes and combined into one syringe, 334
  withdrawn from ampule, 332, 333
  withdrawn from vial, 331–332
Partial thromboplastin time (PTT), 273, 274
Passive range of motion (PROM)
  explanation of, 116
  lower body, 119–120
  upper body, 117–118
Past medical history (PH), 43
Patch tests, 63, 64
Patency, 357
Pathogens, 227
Patient-centered care, 2
Patient-controlled analgesia (PCA), 353
Patient database, 43
Patient examination positions
  dorsal recumbent, 51–52
  explanation of, 43
  Fowler's, 50–51
  illustrations of, 45–46
  knee–chest, 54–55

  lithotomy, 52
  prone, 53
  Sims', 53–54
  supine, 50
Patient interviews, 43, 47–49
Patient records, radiographic, 306–308
Patients
  assisting ambulating, 137
  assisting falling, 138
  culturally diverse, 38, 58, 375
  identification of, 246–247
  nutrition information for, 374–377
  recovery position for, 173–174
  wellness and disease prevention education for, 377–378
Patient's Bill of Rights (American Hospital Association), 3
Patient transfers
  from examination table or bed to wheelchair, 136–137
  guidelines for, 134
  from wheelchair to chair or examination table, 135
Peak flow measurement, 388–389
Pediatric cuff, 104
Pediatrics, 100. *See also* Children; Infants
Pelvic examination, 76–77
Percussion, 43
Periosteum, 139
Peripheral blood smears, 267–268, 271
Peripheral catheters, 346
Peripheral insertion of central catheter (PICC) line, 346
Peripheral parenteral nutrition (PPN), 345
Peripheral saline lock, 362–363
Peripheral vascular access devices, 346
Personal protective equipment (PPE)
  for emergencies, 171
  function of, 11
  use of, 9
Petri dish, 230, 231
Pharmacodynamics, 316
Pharmacokinetics, 316
Pharmacology. *See also* Medication administration; Medications
  abbreviations used in, 313, 314
  explanation of, 310
Phenylketonuria (PKU), 240, 242
Phlebotomists, 237
Phlebotomy. *See also* Clinical laboratory tests; Skin puncture
  equipment for, 237
  explanation of, 237
  needles, holders, and syringes for, 244–246
  order of draw for, 244
  patient identification and laboratory test orders for, 246–247
  problems and complications related to, 252–253
  procedural steps for, 237

  skin puncture for, 237–244
  special collection procedures for, 253–255
  venipuncture sites for, 247–252
Phosphorus (P), 344, 367
Physical examination
  assisting with, 49, 55–56
  cleaning examination room for, 43, 46–47
  documenting chief complaint and, 48–49
  of elderly and culturally diverse patients, 58–59
  equipment and supplies used for, 44
  function of, 43
  interviewing patient for, 43, 47–49
  positioning patient and methods of, 43, 45–46, 50–55
  for scoliosis, 56, 57
  of vomiting patient, 56, 57
Physical therapy, 116
Physicians' Desk Reference (PDR), 310
Physician's office laboratory (POL), 198, 206, 208
Piggyback bag, 361–362
Piggyback sets, 349
Pinworm specimens, 235
Plasma, 257
Platelets, 257, 270
Platform crutches, 129
Point of care testing (POCT) site, 206
Poisoning, 191, 193
Polycythemia, 257–258
Polyuria, 216
Portion sizes, 371, 373
Posteroanterior (PA) position, 302, 303
Postpartum examination, 80–82
Postprandial blood glucose test, 289
Potassium (K), 344
Potentiation, 317
PPE. *See* Personal protective equipment (PPE)
Prediabetes, 289
Pregnancy
  examinations during, 78, 80
  gestational diabetes during, 290
  postpartum visits following, 80–81
Pregnancy test kits, 224
Pregnancy tests, 224, 225
Prenatal examinations
  assisting with, 81
  explanation of, 78, 80
Prescription drugs. *See also* Medication administration; Medications
  authorization for, 311, 313–314
  explanation of, 310
Prescriptions
  elements of, 311, 313–314
  prepared for physician's signature, 322–323
Present illness (PI), 43
Privacy, requirements related to patient, 2–3
Privacy Rule (Department of Health and Human Services), 2
ProAct testing device, 297

Problem-oriented medical record (POMR), 47
Proctosigmoidoscopy, 66
Professionalism, 3
Proficiency testing (PT), 200
Prone position, 53
Protected Health Information (PHI), 2
Proteins
    on food labels, 372
    function of, 366, 369
    in urine, 223
Prothrombin time (PT), 273, 274
ProTime Microcoagulation time device, 274
Protozoa, 231
Provider-performed microscopic procedure
    (PPMP) certificate, 218
Puerperium, 73, 75
Pulmonary procedures
    collecting sputum specimen as, 393
    inhalation treatments as, 389–392
    peak flow measurement as, 388–389
    spirometry test as, 386–388
Pulmonology, 386
Pulse
    apical, 31–32, 104
    apical-radial, 32
    explanation of, 29
    in infants and children, 101–102
    radial, 30–31
    sites for measuring, 29, 30
Pulse deficit, 29
Pulse oximetry, 38
Pulse pressure, 34–35
Punch biopsy, 65
Pupil check, 71–72
Purified protein derivative (PPD), 335, 337
Purosanguineous exudate, 159
Purulent exudate, 159
Pyuria, 220

Q

QBC STAR Centrifugal Hematology System,
    261, 264–267
Qualitative tests, 198
Quality control (QC)
    for blood glucose testing, 293
    in clinical laboratories, 200, 205–206
    for serology tests, 276
Quantitative tests, 198
Quantity not sufficient (QNS), 202
Queckenstedt test, 73
QuickVue *Helicobacter pylori* Test (Quidel),
    281–282
QuickVue+ Mononucleosis Test (Quidel), 278

R

Radial pulse
    explanation of, 29
    measurement of, 30–31
Radiation therapy, 308
Radioallergosorbent (RAST) tests, 64

Radio frequency identification (RFID)
    tags, 247
Radiologic procedures
    contract studies as, 305–306
    explanation of, 302
    flat-plate, 306
    list of, 308
    maintaining records for, 306–308
    patient positions for, 302–303, 305
    scheduling multiple, 306, 307
    steps in general, 304
Radiology, 302
Random urine specimen, 210
Range-of-motion (ROM) exercises
    categories of, 116
    explanation of, 116
    passive, 117–120
    performing and instructing, 116
Rapid strep testing, 233
Recovery position, 173–174
Rectal suppositories, 327–328
Rectal temperature
    in infants and children, 103
    measurement of, 23–24
    when to measure, 23
Rectal thermometers
    care of, 22
    glass nonmercury, 23–24
Red blood cell indices, 271
Red blood cell (RBC) count,
    260–262
Red blood cells (RBCs)
    agglutination of, 282
    erythrocyte sedimentation rate and,
        271–272
    explanation of, 257
    hemoglobin in, 260
    in peripheral smear, 270
    in urine, 218, 220
Reference laboratories, 198, 199
Refractometer, 216, 217
Refrigerators, 208
Registered dietitians (RDs), 372
Rehabilitation, 116
Reproductive system
    female, 75–85
    male, 83–87
Rescue breathing
    for adults, 180
    barrier devices to perform, 174
    for children, 180–181
    for infants, 181–182
    when to use, 172
Respiration
    abnormal patterns of, 33
    explanation of, 32–33
    measurement of, 33–34
Restoration, 116
Retrograde pyelogram, 308
Review of systems (ROS), 47, 49
Rh antibodies, 282, 283

Rhinorrhea, 62
Rh typing, 285–286
Rickets, 366
Ringer's solution, 162
Romberg test, 73
Rule of nines, for burns, 189, 190

S

Safety issues
    in blood tube evacuation, 257
    in clinical laboratories, 200
    for infants and children, 110
    related to intravenous therapy, 364
    related to medication, 318, 320
    related to radiation, 302
Saline lock, 359, 360
Sanguineous exudate, 159
Saturated fats, 369
Scoliosis, 56, 57
Scoliosis examination, 56, 57
Scratch tests, 62–64
Scurvy, 366
Sebaceous cysts, 165
Secondary administration sets, 349
Sediment, in urine, 215
Seizures
    assisting patients during, 192–193
    explanation of, 190–191
Self-examinations
    breast, 75–76
    testicular, 84–86
Sensitivity, 276
Sensitivity test, 230–232
Septicemia, 253
Serology, 276
Serology tests
    CLIA waived, 277–282
    examples of frequently performed, 282
    explanation of, 276
    Helicobacter pylori, 281–282
    list of common, 277
    mononucleosis, 277–279
    quality control for, 276
    safety warning for, 277
    strep, 279–281
Serous exudate, 159
Serum, 257
Serum separator tube (SST), 288
Serving sizes, 371, 373
Severe bleeding
    evaluation for, 172
    explanation of, 189
    method to control, 190
Sexually transmitted diseases (STDs)
    list of, 78
    obtaining specimens to check for,
        77–80
Sick-child visits, 112
Sickle cell anemia, 260
Side effects, of drugs, 317, 318

Sigmoidoscopy
    assisting with, 67–68
    explanation of, 67
    function of, 66
Sims' position, 53–54
Sitz baths, 120
Skin
    conditions affecting, 65
    evaluation of, 173
    layers of, 64–65
    preparation for minor surgery, 155–156
    taking wound culture of, 65–66
Skin biopsy, 65
Skin puncture. *See also* Phlebotomy;
        Venipuncture
    for adults or children, 239–240
    equipment for, 237–239, 241,
        244–246
    explanation of, 237–238
    failure to obtain blood following, 252
    heelstick procedure for, 240–242
    on infants, 240–241
    sites for, 247–248
Snellen chart, 88
SOAP charting, 47
Social history (SH), 47
Sodium (Na), 344, 371
Solutes, 344
Solutions, for surgery, 147
Solvent, 344
Sonography, 302, 308
Specific gravity (SG), of urine, 216, 217
Specificity, 276
Specimens. *See also* Clinical laboratory tests
    blood, 237–255 (*See also* Phlebotomy)
    collection of, 227–228
    pinworm, 235
    preparation of, 228–230
    sensitivity testing for, 230–234
    sputum, 393
    stool, 234
    to test for influenza, 235
    urine, 210–215, 220–225, 233
Specula, 147
Spermatozoa, in urine, 221
Sphygmomanometers
    explanation of, 34
    use of, 35–36
Spiral bandages, 142–143
Spirometry tests
    explanation of, 386–387
    method to perform, 387–388
Splints, arm, 194
Sponges, for surgery, 147
Sputum specimen, 393
Squamous cell carcinoma, 65
Squamous epithelial cells, in urine, 221
Standard deviation, 200
Standard Precautions, 9–11
Staples, removal of, 159–161
Stat procedures, 73

Sterile adhesive skin closures, removal
        of, 162
Sterile dressings
    explanation of, 147
    method to change, 159–160
Sterile field, 152, 153
Sterile gloves, 149–150
Sterile items, 152–153
Sterile packets, 151
Sterile strips, for surgery, 147
Sterilization, 16–17
Stool specimens
    collection of, 69, 70
    for ova and parasite testing, 234
Strabismus, 92
Strep tests
    BioStar Acceava Strep A, 280–281
    explanation of, 279
Streptococci, 231–233
Streptococci pyogenes, 232
Streptococcus pyogenes, 97
Subcutaneous injections
    administration of, 338–339
    body sites for, 337–339
    explanation of, 335, 337
Subcutaneous layer, 64
Sublingual medications, 324, 325
Sulfosalicylic acid (SSA), 223
Supine position, 50
Supplies, minor surgery, 146–148
Suppositories
    explanation of, 325, 327
    rectal, 327–328
    vaginal, 328
SureStep Flexx Monitor, 293, 294
Surgical asepsis, 146–147
Surgical hand scrub/sterile scrub, 148–149
Surgical procedures
    applying and removing sterile adhesive
        skin closures, 162
    assisting with aspiration of joint fluid,
        165–166
    assisting with excision of sebaceous
        cyst, 165
    assisting with hemorrhoid thrombectomy,
        166–167
    assisting with minor, 154–155
    assisting with sutures, 157–159
    biopsy procedures, 164, 168
    changing dressings, 159–160
    cleaning minor wounds, 156–157
    cryosurgery, 168
    donning and removing sterile gloves,
        149–150
    dropping sterile item onto sterile field, 152
    laser, 167–168
    opening sterile packets, 151
    patient skin preparation, 155–156
    pouring from sterile container onto sterile
        field, 153–154
    procedures for minor, 146, 154

removing sutures and staples, 159–161
    supplies and instruments for minor, 147
    surgical hand scrub/sterile scrub, 148–149
    transferring sterile items with sterile
        transfer forceps, 152–153
    wound irrigation and packing, 162–164
Surgical staplers, 147
Surgicutt device, 255
Sutures
    assisting with, 157–159
    removal of, 160–161
    for surgery, 147
Swing gait, 130
Syncope, 252, 382
Synergism, 317
Syphilis, 78
Syringes
    combining medications in one, 333
    explanation of, 245, 246
    for parenteral medications, 329, 330
    preparing medications in two syringes and
        combining into one, 334
    setting up prefilled disposable medication
        cartridge, 334–335
    for venipuncture, 249–250
Syrup of ipecac, 193
Systolic blood pressure
    explanation of, 34
    measurement of, 35–36

T

Telephone procedures
    to answer and screen calls, 5–6
    to call pharmacy for prescriptions, 6
    for emergency calls, 7
    guidelines for, 4–6
Temperature, 21
Temperature conversions, A-13
Temperature measurement
    aural, 26–27
    axillary, 28
    dermal, 27
    in infants and children, 101, 103–104
    oral, 22–23, 25
    rectal, 21, 23–24, 26
    temporal artery, 21, 28–29
Temporal artery thermometers, 28–29,
        103–104
Teratogenic drugs, 317
Terrorist attacks, 196
Testicular self-examinations, 84–86
Theft, of medications, 316
Therapeutic diets, 374
Thermometers
    digital or electronic, 6, 21–22,
        25–26, 103
    disposable, 27
    glass nonmercury, 22–24, 28
    temporal artery, 28–29, 103–104
    tympanic membrane, 26–27, 103
    types of, 21–22

Thoracentesis, 164, 168
3-channel electrocardiogram, 381
Three-point gait, 129
Throat, examination of, 95
Throat culture, 97, 98
Thrombectomy
    explanation of, 146
    hemorrhoid, 166–167
Thrombocytes, 257
Timed urine specimen, 211–215
Tine test, 337
Tissue biopsy, 65
Topical medications, 325–326
Total cholesterol, 297
Total parenteral nutrition (TPN), 345
Tourniquets, 246, 349
Trade name, of drugs, 310
Transdermal medications
    application of, 326–327
    explanation of, 325
Trans fat, 369
Transmission-based precautions, 11, 18–19
Transparent membrane dressings
    (TMDs), 350
Transudates, 227
Trauma, evaluation for, 172
Treadmill stress tests, 385, 386
Trendelenburg position, 43, 45
Trichomonas vaginalis, 221
Trichomoniasis, 78
Trocars, 147
Tuberculin (TB) tests, 335, 337
Tubular gauze bandages, 194
Turbidity, 215
Turnaround time, in clinical
    laboratories, 198
12-lead electrocardiogram, 381, 383–384
24-hour urine specimen, 211–212
2-hour postprandial urine specimen, 212
Two-point gait, 130
Tympanic thermometers, 21, 22, 103

U

Ubiquitous, 227
Ultrasound, 308
Ultrasound therapy, 123, 126
U method, for intravenous therapy, 350
Universal Precautions, 9
Unopette System
    to count blood cells, 262–264
    preparing dilution of whole blood using
        WBC, 263–264
Unsaturated fats, 369
Upper GI series, 305
Urinalysis
    collecting specimen for, 210–215
    complete, 218, 220–221
    confirmation of chemical reagent stick
        testing and, 221–224
    explanation of, 210

pregnancy testing and, 224, 225
    routine, 215–219
Urinary catheterization. *See* Catheterization
Urinary tract infections (UTIs),
    221, 233
Urine
    bilirubin in, 223–224
    chemical characteristics of, 218
    glucose in, 221–222
    ketones in, 222
    physical characteristics of, 215–217
    protein in, 223
Urine analyzer, 208
Urine containers, 210
Urine crystals, 221
Urine pregnancy tests, 224, 225
Urine specimens
    clean-catch midstream, 212–214, 233
    for drug screen, 214–215
    first voided morning, 210–211
    guidelines for collecting, 210
    patient instructions for, 211–214
    pediatric, 112–114
    random, 210
    timed, 211–215
    24-hour, 211–212
    2-hour postprandial, 212
Urticaria, 62
*U.S. Pharmacopeia and National Formulary
    (USPNF),* 310

V

Vaccine Administration Record for Children
    and Teens, 111
Vaccine information statements (VIS),
    109, 111
Vacuum tubes
    explanation of, 241, 244
    type of, 288
    use designations for, 244, 245
Vaginal suppositories, 328
Vaginitis, 79
Vascular access port (VAP), 346
Vastus lateralis muscle, 339
Vegans, 375
Vegetables, 372
Vegetarians, 375
Venipuncture. *See also* Phlebotomy;
        Skin puncture
    butterfly/winged infusion method for,
        251–252
    evacuated tube collection method for,
        248–249
    explanation of, 241
    failure to obtain blood following, 252
    method for, 349–350, 353–354
    sites for, 247–248
    syringe method for, 249–250
Venous access device
    explanation of, 349

method to secure, 350–351
Ventrogluteal muscle, 339
Vertex, 104
Very-low-density lipoproteins (VLDLs), 297
Vesicants, 346
Vesicles, 62
Vials
    combining medications in one syringe
        using two different, 333
    explanation of, 329
    withdrawing medication from, 331–332
Viruses, 231
Vision-impaired patients, 89, 92
Visual acuity. *See also* Ophthalmology
    color vision, 88–90
    distance vision, 86–88
    near vision, 88, 89
    Snellen eye chart to screen for, 86–88
Vital signs
    blood pressure as, 34–37
    evaluation of, 173
    explanation of, 21
    pain as, 37–38
    pediatric, 101–104
    pulse as, 29–32, 104
    respiration as, 32–34
    temperature as, 21–29
    variations in, 21
Vitamin A, 367, 369
Vitamin B_1, 367
Vitamin B_2, 367
Vitamin B_{12}, 368
Vitamin B complex, 367
Vitamin C, 368, 369
Vitamin D, 368, 369
Vitamin E, 369
Vitamin K, 369
Vitamins, 369, 372
Volume-control sets, 349
Vomiting
    caring for patients who are, 56, 57
    method to induce, 193
Vomitus, 56

W

Walkers, 133
Water, as nutrient, 368, 369
Waterless-based hand sanitizing, 13
WebMD, 310
Web sites
    for drug information, 310
    for nutrition information, 371, 375
Weight
    in infants and children, 102, 104, 105
    measurement of, 39
    variations in, 21
Wellness, 377–378
Westergren method, to perform erythrocyte
        sedimentation rate, 273
Wet mount preparations, 79

Wheelchair
  transferring patient from examination table or bed to, 136–137
  transferring patient to chair or examination table from, 135
White blood cells (WBCs)
  in differential smear, 271
  explanation of, 257
  Unopette dilution, 263–264
  in urine, 220
White blood cell (WBC) count, 260–262

Wicks, 147
Winged infusion sets, 246, 251–252, 349
Winged needles, 354–355
Wood's light, 65
Wound culture, 65–66
Wounds
  cleaning minor, 156–158
  irrigation and packing of, 162–164
  packing, 162–164
Wright-Giemsa stain, 267, 270
Wright's stain, 267, 270

X

X-rays, 302. *See also* Radiologic procedures

Y

Yeast, in urine, 221

Z

Z-track injections, 339, 341–342